河南省癌症中心、河南省肿瘤医院
Henan Cancer Center，Henan Cancer Hospital
河南省肿瘤防治研究办公室
Office for Cancer Control and Research, Henan

2017
河南省肿瘤登记年报
Henan Cancer Registry Annual Report

主编　张建功　刘曙正

河南科学技术出版社
· 郑州 ·

图书在版编目（CIP）数据

2017河南省肿瘤登记年报 / 张建功，刘曙正主编. —郑州：河南科学技术出版社，2018.4
ISBN 978-7-5349-8948-3

Ⅰ. ①2… Ⅱ. ①张… ②刘… Ⅲ. ①肿瘤—卫生统计—河南—2017—年报 Ⅳ. ①R73-54

中国版本图书馆CIP数据核字（2018）第048028号

出版发行：河南科学技术出版社
地址：郑州市经五路66号 邮编：450002
电话：（0371）65788673 65788613
网址：www.hnstp.cn
策划编辑：李 林
责任编辑：李 林
责任校对：金兰苹
封面设计：张 伟
责任印制：朱 飞
印 刷：河南安泰彩印有限公司
经 销：全国新华书店
幅面尺寸：210 mm × 285 mm 印张：15.5 字数：423 千字
版 次：2018 年 4 月第 1 版 2018 年 4 月第 1 次印刷
定 价：160.00 元

编委会
Editorial Board

序

肿瘤随访登记是一项收集、分析、评价肿瘤发病、死亡和生存资料的统计制度。通过肿瘤随访登记可以全面、准确和及时地掌握居民恶性肿瘤发生与死亡等相关信息，它是恶性肿瘤预防和控制的基础，并为制定卫生事业发展规划、肿瘤防治及其防治效果评价提供科学依据。

在国家卫生和计划生育委员会和河南省卫生和计划生育委员会的全力支持下，河南省癌症中心、河南省肿瘤防治研究办公室于1988年在林县（现林州市）建立了全人群肿瘤登记系统。2015年2月5日国家卫生和计划生育委员会联合国家中医药管理局印发了《肿瘤登记管理办法》，河南省卫生和计划生育委员会和河南省中医管理局结合我省实际情况，组织制定了《河南省肿瘤登记实施方案》（豫卫疾控〔2015〕10号）。河南省肿瘤防治研究办公室按照《河南省肿瘤登记实施方案》的要求，制定了具体的实施方案和各项规章制度，建立了河南省肿瘤随访登记网络直报系统，要求全省各地市和省直管县成立肿瘤登记处，开展肿瘤随访登记工作，通过河南省肿瘤随访网络直报系统上报当地的肿瘤发病、死亡和随访数据。

目前在河南省已建立了32个国家级和省级肿瘤登记处，开展以人群为基础的肿瘤登记工作，初步形成了反映河南省城乡居民恶性肿瘤发病与死亡基本信息的肿瘤随访登记系统。

《2017河南省肿瘤登记年报》系统地报告了2014年河南省肿瘤登记地区人群恶性肿瘤发病与死亡的流行情况，为恶性肿瘤的控制与研究提供了基础数据。

河南省卫生和计划生育委员会疾病预防控制处

2017年11月

Preface

Cancer registration is a statistical system to collect, analyze and evaluate related information including cancer incidence, mortality and survival, through which cancer occurrence and death in the population could be obtained completely, accurately and timely. It is the basis for cancer prevention and control, and it also provides scientific evidence for health development planning, cancer prevention and control and the effect evaluation.

Supported by National Health and Family Planning Commission (Health and Family Planning Commission, HFPC) and Henan Provincial HFPC, Henan Cancer Center and Office for Cancer Control and Research established the first population based Cancer Registry in Linzhou city (the former Lin county) in 1988.

The National HFPC and National Administration of Traditional Chinese Medicine (ATCM) issued "Approaches for Cancer Registration Management" on February 5th, 2015. Henan Province HFPC and ATCM made the implementation plan according to the Approaches. Office for Cancer Control and Research in Henan made the regulations and relevant specific procedures, and established the Provincial Electronic Cancer Registration System (ECRS) .All the city and provincial county in Henan are required to set up cancer registries, and to carry out cancer registration project and report new cancer cases through ECRS.

Now 32 population based cancer registries have been established in Henan Province, and the data basically reflected the cancer incidence and mortality in Henan.

Henan Cancer Registry Annual Report, 2017 reported the cancer incidence and mortality in Henan cancer registration areas in 2014 completely and systematically, and provided basic data for cancer control and research.

Department of Disease Control and Prevention,

Henan Province Health and Family Planning Commission

November, 2017

前　言

肿瘤随访登记报告是恶性肿瘤预防控制工作的基础工程，完整、有效的肿瘤登记数据可以系统地反映登记地区居民肿瘤发病、死亡和生存状况，了解人群癌症流行规律和时间变化趋势，探索病因，为政府制定癌症控制措施和防治效果评价提供科学依据。

为进一步加强全国肿瘤登记工作规范化管理，获得及时、统一、准确的肿瘤发病、死亡和生存信息，2015 年 2 月 5 日国家卫生和计划生育委员会联合国家中医药管理局印发的《肿瘤登记管理办法》，要求各级卫生计生行政部门和中医药管理部门负责全国肿瘤登记体系建设、组织协调和监督管理全国肿瘤登记工作。各省（区、市）指定相关部门成立省级肿瘤登记中心，实施全省肿瘤登记工作。省会城市、地级市为城市肿瘤登记地区，指定相关部门设立肿瘤登记处，开展市辖区的肿瘤登记报告工作。县级市和县为农村肿瘤登记地区，指定相关部门设立肿瘤登记处，开展辖区内的肿瘤登记报告工作。登记处所在的疾病预防控制中心负责提供死因数据。肿瘤登记处辖区内所有医疗机构需定期向肿瘤登记处报告所有恶性肿瘤（包括中枢神经系统良性肿瘤）病例的发病和死亡信息。

2017 年河南省 32 个登记处上报了 2014 年的肿瘤随访登记资料，其中 29 个登记处的资料由市县疾病预防控制中心上报，3 个由肿瘤防治专业机构上报。登记处分布在 17 个市，其中地级以上城市 8 个，县及县级市 24 个。符合登记质量要求的登记处有 27 个，覆盖人口 21 044 835 人，约占河南省 2014 年人口总数的 19.73%。

《2017 河南省肿瘤登记年报》（以下简称《年报》）共分六个部分：第一章为概述，简要介绍了河南省肿瘤登记系统及居民全死因登记系统的发展情况；第二章介绍资料的来源及资料的收集方法；第三章介绍数据质量控制指标及评价方法和常用统计学指标的计算方法；第四章描述河南省主要肿瘤的发病和死亡水平；第五章对各部位肿瘤的发病和死亡进行描述；第六章为年报附录，包含河南省各个登记处发病和死亡的主要统计结果。

《2017 河南省肿瘤登记年报》的顺利出版，凝聚着全省各登记处工作人员的辛勤劳动，在此谨表示衷心的感谢！

张建功

2017 年 11 月

Foreword

Cancer registration is foundamental for cancer prevention and control. Complete and effective cancer registration data can reflect cancer incidence, mortality and survival, and the epidemic characteristics and temporal trend were also acquired. Therefore, it could provide evidence to inform strategies for cancer prevention and control.

In order to standardize cancer registration work, acquire accurate and consistant cancer incidence, mortality and survival data timely,national HFPC (Health and Family Planning Commission, HFPC) and national ATCM (Administration of Traditional Chinese Medicine, ATCM) issued "Approaches for Cancer Registration Management" on February 5th, 2015. According to the "Approaches", administrative departments of HFPC and ATCM are responsible for building cancer registration system, organizing, coordinating and supervising cancer registration implementation and management. Provincial cancer registry was first established, responsible for cancer registration in whole province. Urban cancer registries were established in provincial capital and prefecture-level cities, and the rural cancer rigistries in the counties or county-level cities, responsible for cancer registration within their municipal districts, respectively. Centers for Disease Control and Prevention (CDCP) in the registration areas take the responsibilities of providing vital statistics data.All medical institutions within municipal district need to report all malignant tumors (including central nervous system benign cancers) to the cancer registry center regularly.

Since the National Health and Family Planning Commission (the former Ministry of Health) initiated national cancer registration project in 2009, the number of cancer follow-up registries in Henan Province has been gradually developed from 6 to 27 and the population coverage from 6 million to 26 million or so.

In 2017, there were 32 cancer registries reported cancer registration data of 2014 in Henan province, among which 29 cancer registries belong to the CDCPs and 3 belong to cancer control offices. All the cancer registries covered 17 cities in Henan, including 8 cities and 24 counties or county-level cities.There were 27registries satisfied registration quality requirements with a population coverage of 21 044 835, accounting for 19.73%

of the total population in the end of 2014 in Henan (Statistical Communique on national economic and social development of Henan Province in 2014: 106 million 620 thousand).

Henan Cancer Registry Annual Report, 2017 includes six chapters:

Chapter 1 is an overview of the development of cancer registration system and the vital statistics system in Henan Province; Chapter 2 introduces data source and collecting methods; Chapter 3 introduces the index system of data quality, methods for evaluating data quality and the statistical methods; Chapter 4 describes the incidence and mortality of main cancer 5 in Henan Province; Chapter 5 describes incidence and mortality of cancers in each anatomic site, and chapter 6 is appendix, which describes the incidence and mortality of each cancer registry in Henan Province.

In order to understand the cancer burden of cancer registration area in Henan Province comprehensively, the report describes the main causes of death and their level and distribution in 2014 among the registration population, including the mortality and the constituent ratio of the top five major causes, which reflects hazard rating of each type of main causes of death.

The work presented in this report derived from data collected by all registries in Henan Province. We are grateful to all the staffs who had contributed to and supported the work of Henan cancer registry and looking forward to close cooperation in the future.

Jiangong Zhang

November, 2017

鸣　谢
Acknowledgement

河南省肿瘤登记年报编委会对各肿瘤登记处的相关工作人员在本次年报出版过程中给予的大力协助，尤其是在数据收集、整理、补充、审核登记资料，以及建档、建库等方面所做出的贡献表示感谢！衷心感谢编写组成员在本次年报撰写工作中付出的辛苦努力！

The editorial committee of Henan cancer report express their gratitude to all the staff working in cancer registries, Henan province, who made great contribution on data collecting, sorting, completing, crediting and filing. Sincere thanks to all compilation group members for their hard working.

肿瘤登记处名单

地区	肿瘤登记处	登记处所在单位	成员
洛阳市	洛阳市	洛阳市 CDC	李爱红　闫云燕　常　颖　程先景　杨　浩　温　丹　陈亚揃　韩迎霞　陈　均　何桂婷　邢建乐
	偃师市	偃师市 CDC	段凤玲　秦艳锦　周艳艳
	嵩县	嵩县 CDC	乔幸石　梦　瑶　安转霞
	栾川县	栾川县 CDC	刘爱坡　黄建生　田　森
	宜阳县	宜阳县 CDC	楚玉梅　陈　培
	孟津县	孟津县 CDC	许瑞瑞　张琰琰
	汝阳县	汝阳县 CDC	李白鸟　郭晓娅
	吉利区	吉利区 CDC	席永娟　张菲菲
	新安县	新安县 CDC	翟亚楠
济源市	济源市	济源市 CDC	陈正文　郑莹如　黄艳芳
驻马店	西平县	西平县 CDC	邵天堂　赵春玲　毛小辉　王中梅　夏耀华　康文昊
新乡市	辉县市	辉县市 CDC	孙花荣　赵小聪　顾伟嘉
三门峡市	三门峡市	三门峡市 CDC	刘存棣　陈士艳　吴彦领　陈　震　武恕星　郭振平　刘润娣　何建磊　罗　丹　姚晓云
漯河市	漯河市	漯河市 CDC	代　莹　孙路平　胡　昕　孟　蕾　杨俊蝶　张起行
	源汇区	源汇区 CDC	刘伟飞　李　冬　王春玲　李　彤　牛艳丽　李凯歌
	召陵区	召陵区 CDC	任东洋　杨红宇　程　果　党丽媛

续表

地区	肿瘤登记处	登记处所在单位	成员
	郾城区	郾城区 CDC	姬建国 庞 静 宋哲奥 常帅奇
周口市	郸城县	郸城县 CDC	郭德银 陈 静 张 建 顾雅靖 张吉志
	沈丘县	沈丘县 CDC	程 麟 薛玉堂 胡晓岚 马 平 王振远
安阳市	林州市	林州市肿瘤医院	程兰萍 李变云 未建荣 于晓东 侯 凯 王 丽
	安阳市	安阳市肿瘤医院	王建坡 王 强 潘鹏飞 付 维 任晓光 阎焕勤
信阳市	固始县	固始县 CDC	李程鹏 张 柯 沈 玉
	罗山县	罗山县 CDC	曹世明 李晓航
许昌市	禹州市	禹州市 CDC	杨安锋 赵江珍 杨宗慧 李晓蕊
南阳市	内乡县	内乡县 CDC	李亚波 张永庆 张 骏
	方城县	方城县 CDC	李 谱 田向阳 倪林静
	卧龙区	卧龙区 CDC	刘 凯 周 静 张飞虎
商丘市	虞城县	虞城县 CDC	张亚威 冯金洪 王立新 王士刚 毕兴华 马 宁 刘 威 江 培
	睢县	睢县 CDC	郇树青 蔡 蕾 祝海松 周 康
开封市	祥符区	祥符区 CDC	马 师 李慎榜 田艳玲 代 蒙 王晓倩
濮阳市	濮阳市	濮阳市 CDC	岳 磊 梁 森 张玉华
	华龙区	华龙区 CDC	王培贤 王新杰 毛丽娟
鹤壁市	鹤壁市	鹤壁市人民医院	钞利娜 王冰冰 董雪萍 武亚鑫 胡凤琴 裴树英
平顶山	鲁山县	鲁山县 CDC	郭启民 李果果 田大广 侯永春 马亚飞

目　录
Contents

第一章 概述

Chapter 1 Summary

一、河南省肿瘤登记系统介绍

肿瘤登记报告是按照统一的技术与方法在目标人群中开展经常性的收集、储存、整理、统计分析和评价肿瘤发病、死亡及生存资料的统计制度。肿瘤登记是国际公认的关于人群肿瘤发病信息收集的标准方法，在慢性非传染病中，只有肿瘤疾病采用该方法。其目的是了解人群中恶性肿瘤的发病、死亡和生存状况，为肿瘤病因研究提供依据，为制订卫生工作规划和肿瘤防治计划、评价和考核肿瘤防治效果提供服务。

20 世纪 50 年代末，由河南医学院、河南中医学院、河南省人民医院等单位的科研人员组成的河南省食管癌防治研究协作组，参加了由中国医学科学院组织的华北四省市食管癌普查大协作，深入林县山区，开展了食管癌流行病学的调查和防治研究工作，组织实施了林县食管癌单病种发病及死亡登记工作。1959—1962 年林县人群食管癌发病、死亡病例的收集主要依靠回顾性调查。随着县、乡、村三级肿瘤防治网的建立，1963—1966 年食管癌 / 贲门癌的发病、死亡登记报告工作基本稳定。1967—1969 年，由于“文化大革命”的原因，使登记工作受到了严重影响，发病、死亡登记资料漏报严重，经后期回顾调查补报得以完善。1977 年根据全国的统一部署，河南省卫生厅领导组织了覆盖河南省 6 000 多万人口的 3 年（1974—1976 年）全死因回顾调查。

在 3 年全死因回顾调查的基础上，河南省

1. Introduction to Henan cancer registration system

Cancer registry report is a statistical system for constant collection, storage, sorting, statistical analysis to evaluate cancer incidence, mortality and survival data in the target population according to the unified technology and method. Cancer registration is generally acknowleged as a standardized method for collecting information on cancer incidence all around the world. It aims to know cancer incidence, mortality, and survival in the population, and to provide scientific basis for cancer etiology study, health policy development on cancer prevention and control, and for the relevant practice effect evaluation and assessment on cancer prevention and control.

In the late 1950s, a cooperative esophageal cancer screening in Northern China was organized by Chinese Academy of Medical Sciences. The Henan research representives were mainly from Henan Medical College, Henan College of Traditional Chinese Medicine, and Henan Provincial People’ s Hospital. They penetrated into Linxian County mountainous areas and carried out esophageal cancer epidemiological investigation to explore cancer prevention and control strategies. From then on esophageal cancer incidence and mortality registration was initiated in Linxian County. During 1959 to 1962, the information was mainly collected depending on retrospective survey. During 1963 to 1966, cancer registration and reporting system had basically spread in the three administrative levels of county, township and village. During 1967 to 1969, cancer registration system was severely affected by the “Cultural Revolution” and many cases had been reported under surveillance. Anyhow, the missed cases had been supplemented later through retrospective investigation. In 1977, Henan Provincial Health Bureau organized a retrospective survey on all causes of death from 1974 to 1976 with a coverage of 60 000 000 population according to the national unified deployment.

Whereafter, in order to know all the deaths caused by

肿瘤医院/研究院于1983年在全省抽样选取了林县、济源市、禹州市、洛阳市、偃师市、罗山县、鲁山县、内乡县等15个县市，约占河南省人口1/10的地区开展了居民全死因登记工作，建立起了河南省以肿瘤为主的全死因登记报告系统。目的是掌握人群死亡原因及恶性肿瘤死亡的基础数据。

1988年，林县在全死因登记系统的基础上，参照国际癌症中心（IARC）/国际癌症登记协会（IACR）推荐的肿瘤随访登记方法与原则，建立起了以人群为基础的肿瘤发病登记报告系统，按照国际疾病分类方法对恶性肿瘤及中枢神经系统良性肿瘤进行登记报告和编码。2004年4月1日，河南省癌症及生命统计中心成立，并在15个市县建立了癌症及生命统计登记处。2004年10月7日，河南省卫生厅印发《河南省癌症及生命统计登记工作规范》的通知，下发到市、县卫生局及各登记处并落实执行。

2008年，河南省肿瘤医院/研究院在偃师市、禹州市、内乡县、开封市、鲁山县开始实施人群肿瘤登记报告工作。2009年国家卫生部在全国范围内启动了中央财政转移支付地方的肿瘤随访登记项目工作，中央财政对登记市县给予经费支持。河南省林州市、洛阳市、偃师市、禹州市、西平县和沈丘县纳入国家肿瘤随访登记项目市县。在2009年的基础上，2010年将济源市、鲁山县、漯河市、内乡县、郸城县、罗山县、三门峡市、虞城县列入河南省肿瘤登记系统。2012—2013年又有开封县、鹤壁市区、睢县及郑州市四个市县进入全省的肿瘤登记系统。

为进一步加强全国肿瘤登记工作规范化管理，获得及时、统一、准确的肿瘤发病、死亡和生存信息，2015年2月5日国家卫生和计划生育委员会联合国家中医药管理局印发了《肿瘤登记管理办法》，河南省卫生和计划生育委员会和河南省中医管理局结合我省实际情况，组织制定了《河南省肿瘤登记实施方案》（豫卫疾控〔2015〕10号）。河南省肿瘤防治研究

cancers and other causes, Henan Cancer Hospital / Henan Cancer Institute established cancer-centering vital statistics in 1983. It covered one tenth of Henan provincial population, comprised 15 selected counties / cities, Linxian County, Jiyuan City, Yuzhou City, Luoyang City, Yanshi City, Luoshan County, Lushan County and Neixiang County.

In 1988, the first population based cancer registration system was established based on the vital statistics system in Linxian County. Under this system, all cancer registration and follow-up principles were refered to International Agency for Research on Cancer (IARC) / International Association of Cancer Registries (IACR), and all cancers (including central nervous system benign cancers) were classified and reported by the codes in accordance with the International Classification of Disease. On April 1, 2004, Henan Provincial Cancer and Vital Statistics Center was set up. Meanwhile, 15 city / county Cancer and Vital Statistics Registries were opened. On October 7, 2004, Henan Provincial Health Bureau issued the "Methods for Cancer and Vital Statistics Registration, Henan", which was sent out to each registry as work specification.

In 2008, Henan Cancer Hospital / Institute built the population based cancer registration and reporting system in Yanshi City, Yuzhou City, Neixiang County and Lushan County. In 2009, the registries could be supported by the central government finance, as Ministry of Health launched the transfer payments on cancer follow-up registration program to local governments. In Henan province, the funded registries located in Linzhou City, Luoyang City, Yanshi City, Yuzhou City, Xiping County and Shenqiu County. The funded registries were added up gradually. In 2010, Jiyuan City, Lushan County, Luohe City, Neixiang County, Dancheng County, Luoshan County, Sanmenxia City and Yucheng County were added, and Hebi City, Kaifeng County, Suixian County and Zhengzhou City were contained during 2012 to 2013.

In order to strengthen cancer registration specification to obtain accurate, prompt and unified cancer incidences, mortalities and survival data, the National Health and Family Planning Commission and National Administration of Traditional Chinese Medicine issued "Cancer Registration Management and Methods" on February 5, 2015. Henan Province Health and Family Planning Administrative Departments and Henan Province Administrative Departments for Traditional Chinese Medicine schemed out "Cancer Registration Management and Specifications" applicable to Henan Province. Correspondingly, Office for Cancer Control and Research, Henan trained all the staffs

办公室按照《河南省肿瘤登记实施方案》的要求对全省各级医疗机构相关人员进行了业务培训，要求各地市和省直管县成立肿瘤登记处，开展肿瘤随访登记工作，并通过河南省网络直报系统（http://218.28.13.204:35556）上报当地的肿瘤发病、死亡和随访数据。

2017 年河南省 32 个登记处上报了 2014 年的肿瘤随访登记资料，其中 29 个登记处的资料由市县疾病预防控制中心上报，3 个为肿瘤防治专业机构上报。登记处分布在 17 个市，其中地级以上城市 8 个，县及县级市 24 个。符合登记质量要求的登记处有 27 个，有效覆盖人口 21 044 835 人，约占河南省 2014 年人口总数的 19.73%（2014 年河南省国民经济和社会发展统计公报：10 662 万）。

各级肿瘤登记处要履行肿瘤登记报告职责，建立健全肿瘤登记报告工作管理制度，明确本单位肿瘤登记报告管理科室及管理人，明确诊疗机构科室责任。

从早期林县食管癌 / 贲门癌的单癌种登记系统，发展到目前的全部位的肿瘤随访登记系统，是为了满足肿瘤预防控制工作的实际需求。肿瘤随访登记工作以政府为主导，河南省卫生和计划生育委员会作为项目主管单位全面负责肿瘤登记报告工作，制定相关政策和规划，组织开展考核和评估。

河南省肿瘤医院，肿瘤防治研究办公室作为技术指导单位，负责全省肿瘤登记系统的建立和工作的实施；制订及修订肿瘤登记报告实施方案和年度工作计划；负责开展全省肿瘤登记工作业务培训、技术指导等工作。

河南省各市、县（区）卫生行政部门负责辖区内肿瘤登记报告系统的建立及项目工作的管理和实施；对肿瘤登记报告工作进行督导检查和考核评估；协调相关机构和部门，为肿瘤登记报告工作的正常运行提供保障。

市、县（区）肿瘤登记处负责制订本辖区肿瘤登记报告工作计划和实施方案；指导辖区内各级医疗机构开展肿瘤登记报告工作；确定

who worked in cancer Registries or the relevant medical institutions regarding to the cancer follow-up and reporting management specifications and Henan Cancer Reporting System (http://218.28.13.204:35556) , which was the dedicated network for the registries to report all the cancer incidences, deaths and survival.

There were 32 cancer registration reported the cancer follow-up data, among which 29 cancer registries data were reported by the city or county disease prevention and control centers and 3 were reported by cancer control office. The registries distribute in 17 cities, including 8 cities and 24 counties or county level cities. According to the quality requirement, 27 cancer registries satisfied the criteria. The qualified data covered the population of 21 044 835, accounting for 19.73 percent of total population of Henan province in 2014, which was 106 million 620 thousand according to Statistical Communique on national economic and social development of Henan Province in 2014.

All the registries took responsibilities of cancer reporting, such as drawing cancer reporting management specifications, assigning the person-in-charge and specifying the work in medical institutions, and so on.

Whether it was in the early stage for single cancer type of esophageal cancer in Linxian County, or the present status for all cancer types, the cancer reporting system is designed to meet the actual needs of cancer prevention and control. The work of cancer follow-up registration is led by the government. The Henan Provincial Health and Family Planning Commission is in charge of the entire project, responsible for formulating relevant regulations and plans, and for organizing the work appraisal.

Office for Cancer Control and Research, Henan Cancer Hospital, is in charge of the technical support and guidance, which takes responsibilities of developing cancer reporting and registration system and its application, making implementation schedule and annual work plan, and carrying out relevant professional and technological training.

The city or county administrative agencies are responsible for establishing the local cancer registration reporting system and the registration practice and management, for supervising, inspecting and appraising the work, and for coordinating the agencies for the normal operation of cancer registration.

The city or county cancer registries have the responsibility for cancer registration management and technical guidance under the jurisdiction. They formulate the specifications and work plan, supervise the medical institutions to carry out cancer registration, and designate

辖区内肿瘤登记报告单位、报告人、联系方式、并登记建档；负责肿瘤登记的业务管理和技术指导等工作。

各级医疗机构为登记病例的上报单位，要求各级医疗机构在当地肿瘤登记处的指导下，利用河南省肿瘤随访登记网络直报系统开展肿瘤登记报告工作，按照项目内容要求，提供及时、准确、完整的肿瘤登记信息。建立、健全机构内的登记报告管理组织制度和技术规范，将资料登记及死亡报告工作纳入本单位内部考核管理内容，并制定相关的奖励管理措施。

二、河南省居民死因登记系统简介

居民病伤死因登记是系统性、经常性收集居民病伤死亡信息的统计制度，目的是了解城乡居民各种疾病的死亡原因、分布状况和流行动态。完整、准确的人群死亡信息对于制定人口和卫生政策、合理配置资源具有非常重要的意义。

河南省在 1975—1977 年第一次死因回顾调查的基础上，于 1983 年在 15 个县市建立了居民病伤死亡登记报告制度，在当地政府和卫生行政部门配合下，经过 30 年不断的努力已经形成了县、乡、村三级死因登记上报体系，建立、完善了各项登记报告制度。死因统计资料基本可以反映河南省人群各种死亡原因的死亡水平。

肿瘤随访登记是在具备完善、规范的居民全死因登记的基础上建立的，肿瘤随访登记中肿瘤死亡数据来源于人群全死因登记系统，死因登记系统也是肿瘤随访登记补充、完善发病资料的途径之一，健全、完整的死因登记系统是全面评价肿瘤随访登记资料质量的主要基础数据系统。

本次年报按照要求应该上报资料的市县为洛阳市、孟津县、新安县、栾川县、嵩县、汝阳县、宜阳县、吉利区（洛阳市）、偃师市、鲁山县、林州市、鹤壁市、辉县市、禹州市、漯河市、漯河市郾城区、三门峡市、南阳市、方城县、内乡县、睢县、虞城县、罗山县、沈丘县、郸

cancer reporting institutions and reporting personnel to put on records.

The medical institutions are responsible for cancer case reporting. They report cancer registration data under supervision of Cancer Registries through cancer registration and reporting system timely and precisely. They establish and improve the mechanism of the registration management system and technical specifications, and they incorporate cancer registration and death report into the internal examination and management to formulate relevant reward management measures.

2. Introduction to the vital statistics system in Henan

Vital statistics is a systematic and statistical system to collect the residents' death information caused by diseases or injuries on a recurring basis, which aims at monitoring death causes, distribution and disease epidemic dynamics in urban and rural areas. The integracy and accuracy of the vital information is of great significance for population health policies and resources allocation.

Vital statistics in Henan province had been developed in 15 cities and counties till 1983, since the first retrospective deaths survey was conducted during 1975~1977. With the thirty years' continuous efforts, in coordination with the support from local government and the health administration, vital statistics system has formed the county-township-village registration and reporting network and perfect management regulations, which now basically delineates all death causes among Henan residents.

Cancer registry bases on the standard and perfect vital statistics system, because cancer registration contains cancer death cases on the one hand, on the other hand, vital statistics system is an important route to supplement cancer incidences and passive follow-up. So a perfect vital statistics system is the vital basis for cancer registration when assess its data quality.

The annual report 2017 include the cancer data reported from 32 cancer registries, they are Luoyang City, Mengjin County, Xin'an County, Luanchuan County, Songxian County, Ruyang County, Yiyang County, Jili District (Luoyang City), Yanshi County, Lushan County, Linzhou City, Hebi City, Huixian City, Yuzhou City, Luohe City, Yancheng District (Luohe City), Sanmenxia City, Nanyang City, Fangcheng County, Neixiang County, Suixian County, Yucheng County, Luoshan County, Shenqiu County, Dancheng County, Xiping County, Jiyuan City, Xiangfu District (Kaifeng City), Anyang City Proper, Hualong District (Puyang City), Gushi County and Zhengzhou City Proper.

城县、西平县、济源市、开封市祥符区、安阳市城区、濮阳市华龙区、固始县、郑州市城区。

死因统计按照国际疾病分类（international Classification of diseases,ICD–10）方法进行分类编码，将死因分类为 18 大类，101 种疾病进行统计。

Death cause statistics were classified into 18 categories and 101 diseases in accordance with international classification of diseases, ICD–10.

第二章　肿瘤登记的方法和统计学指标

Chapter 2　Data collection methods and statistical indicators

肿瘤登记是系统性、经常性收集有关肿瘤及肿瘤患者信息的统计制度。目的是了解我省城乡居民癌症发病、死亡情况和生存状态，掌握癌症的疾病负担与变化趋势，以及在不同地区和人群中的分布特征，为政府和卫生行政部门制订癌症防治策略、规划与计划，为癌症基础研究及临床研究提供基本信息，为监测和评价癌症控制措施的效果提供基本依据。

Cancer registration is a kind of statistical system regarding how to collect information of cancer and cancer cases systematically and constantly. It aims to master the data about cancer incidence, mortality and survival in the urban and rural areas in Henan province, to analyze cancer burden, dynamic trends and distribution characteristics in different regions and populations, hence to provide evidence to inform strategies for cancer prevention and control for government and the health administrative departments, provide basic information for fundamental and clinical cancer research, and cancer surveillance effective appraisal.

一、建立肿瘤登记处

1. Establishment of a cancer registry

肿瘤登记处是连续性收集、储存、整理、统计分析、评价、阐述及报告肿瘤发病、死亡和生存信息资料的部门。

肿瘤登记地区应具备完善的县、乡、村三级死因登记系统，同时能够获取准确的人口学资料。肿瘤登记地区覆盖管辖范围内全部户籍人口。

当地政府或卫生行政部门应制定和颁布实行肿瘤登记报告制度的法律法规或规范性文件，设立肿瘤登记处，并配备相应的工作人员、经费及设备，同时制定肿瘤登记报告实施细则。

A cancer Registry is an organization that bear the responsibility to collect, store, sort, analyze, appraise, elaborate and report dynamical cancer incidences, mortalities and survival information constantly.

A cancer registry should possess a perfect three-level of county-township-village death surveillance system, bear the capability of obtaining the demographic data accurately. A cancer registry should cover all the registered population in the whole administrative region either in urban area or rural area cancer registries.

The local governments or health administrative departments should make and issue the specification and regulations on cancer registration and report system, set up the cancer registries, allocate necessary personnel, funds and equipment, and draw up the relevant implementing measures.

二、登记资料收集方法

2. Methods of cancer registration data collection

河南省肿瘤登记地区资料收集采用被动和主动收集相结合的方法。由各医疗机构定期报送肿瘤发病登记卡片到肿瘤登记处，或由登记处工作人员主动到各医疗单位查阅肿瘤新发病例的诊疗病史，摘录肿瘤发病信息。同时，登记处还定期通过保险机构（新农合医疗保险、城镇居民医疗保险、职工医疗保险及商业医疗

Cancer registration data are mainly collected through a combination of passive and active collection method. On the one hand, medical institutions report cancer incidence registration cards to the cancer registry periodically, or the staff in the cancer registry go for cancer information through abstracting the newly diagnosed cancer cases file in medical institutions. On the other hand, cancer registries supplement

保险）及居民死因报告系统获取相关因肿瘤疾病报销及死亡医学证书中提及肿瘤发病信息的个体补充新发病例登记，保证肿瘤登记的完整性。

（一）建立信息收集渠道

肿瘤登记处从相关部门收集辖区内肿瘤新发病例、死亡病例、生存信息和相关人口资料。病例资料的收集渠道包括登记地区各级医疗机构、医疗保险数据库、死因监测数据库、新型农村合作医疗及城镇居民 / 职工医疗保险数据库等。人口资料的来源包括人口普查资料、公安及统计部门有关资料等。

（二）开展病例核实工作

肿瘤登记处负责肿瘤病例的建卡和分类编码、剔除重复记录病例。应用死因监测数据库进行死亡补发病流程。

（三）开展随访工作

通过电话、书信、电子邮件，以及社区居委会、基层医疗卫生机构开展随访工作，获取病例的生存情况。

肿瘤登记工作流程见图 2-1。

三、登记资料收集内容

肿瘤登记主要收集的是登记覆盖范围内全部恶性肿瘤（ICD-10：C00-C96）和中枢神经系统良性肿瘤及中枢神经系统动态未定或未知的肿瘤（ICD-10：D32-D33.9；D42.0-D43.9）的发病、死亡和生存信息，以及登记覆盖人群的相关人口资料。

（一）新发病例资料

个人信息包括姓名、性别、出生日期、年龄、身份证号码、住址、出生地、民族、婚姻状况、职业等；肿瘤信息包括发病日期、解剖学部位（亚部位）、组织学类型、诊断依据、临床分期等；报告单位信息包括报告日期、诊断单位、报告单位、报告医生等；随访信息包括随访患者的死亡日期及生命状态等。

and complete cancer incidence information through the related death certification in the death surveillance system or the related reimbursement credentials in medical assurance agencies, including new rural cooperative medical insurance, urban residents medical insurance, basic medical insurance for urban workers and commercial medical insurance.

2.1 Data collection channels

Cancer registries collect cancer incidence, mortality, survival and related demographic data from certain departments.Cancer information collection channels include medical institutions at different levels, medical insurance database, death surveillance database, rural cooperative medical system or urban residents or employee medical insurance database. The demographic datasources include census data, public security or bureaus of statistics.

2.2 Cancer cases ascertainment

Cancer registries establish and classify registration cards. The cases are ascertained, with identified card number as identification code, through which the duplicated are deleted. And the cases are verified by the death surveillance database, through which the missed are supplemented.

2.3 Cancer case follow-up

Home visiting, phone calls, letter or Email correspondence can all be follow-up methods for survival information collection by the community committee or primary health care institutions.

Cancer registration process was shown in figure 2-1.

3. Collection contents of cancer registration

Cancer registration mainly collect sincidence, mortality, and survival of all cancer cases(ICD-10: C00-C96) and neoplasms and uncertain behaviors of the central nervous systems (ICD-10：D32-D33.9；D42.0-D43.9) in the registration areas, and the related demographic information of the covering population as well.

3.1 The incidence data

The incidence data are as follows: the individual information includes name, gender, date of birth, age, identified card number, address, place of birth, race, marital status, professional career, etc; cancer information includes date of onset, anatomical site and sub-site, histological type, diagnosing evidences, clinical stages, etc; reporting unit information includes reporting date, diagnosing department, reporting institution,reporting physician, etc; follow-up information include survival status, date of death, etc.

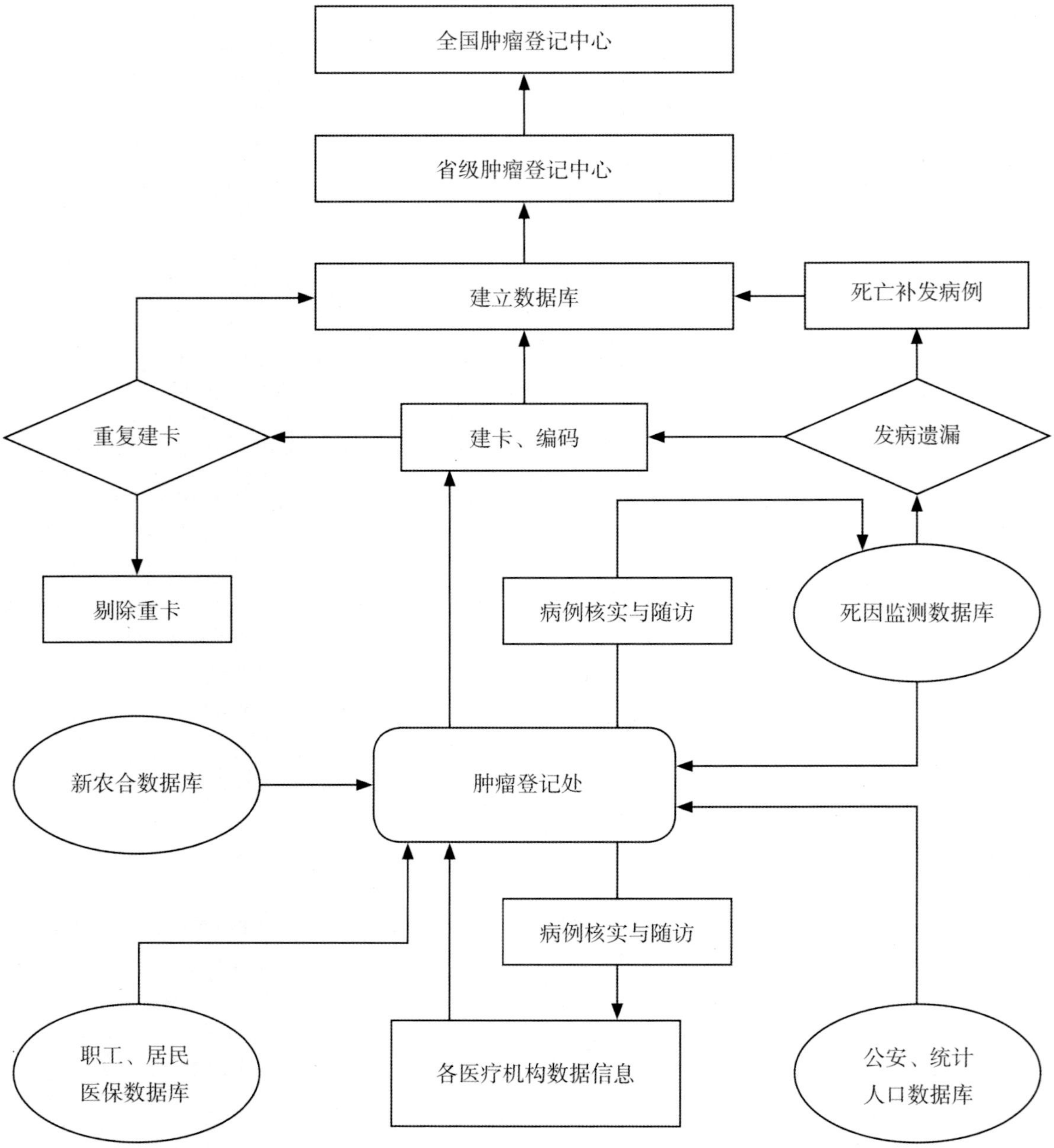

图 2-1　肿瘤登记工作流程

（二）死亡资料

肿瘤死亡资料来源于全人口死因登记报告，包括根本死因为非肿瘤原因的肿瘤病例的死亡资料。除发病信息外，还应包括死亡日期、实足年龄、死亡原因、主要诊断、诊断级别和依据、

3.2 The mortality data

Cancer mortality data are mainly from vital statistical system, including the cancer cases who died of causes other than cancers. Besides incidence information, the motality data includes date, age of death, cause of death, place of death, major diagnoses, diagnostic level, diagnostic evidences, etc.

死亡地点等。

（三）人口资料

人口资料指辖区覆盖的户籍人口。资料来源于我国人口普查资料和公安、统计部门逐年提供的人口资料。人口资料应包括居民人口总数及其性别、年龄。年龄组按 0~、1~4、5~9、10~14、…、75~79、80~84、85+ 分组。

四、登记数据的质量控制

质量控制贯穿肿瘤登记工作的全过程。肿瘤登记地区应在各个环节制定工作规范和质量控制程序，并严格执行。质量控制从登记资料的可比性、完整性、有效性和时效性等四个方面进行系统评估。

（一）登记资料的质量控制

1. 可比性

数据结果真实可比的基本先决条件是采用通用的标准或定义。通常而言，可比性是指不同地区或不同时间人群发病率的差异不是因登记数据质量、采用的编码标准及运用规则不同所产生。可比性涉及以下几个指标：对“发病”的定义，对原发、复发和转移的诊断标准、分类与编码、死亡证明等。

2. 完整性

完整性是指在登记地区资料库中目标人群内所有新发病例被记录的完整程度。常用的评价指标有死亡 / 发病比（M：I）、只有死亡证明比例（DCO%）、组织学诊断确认比例（HV%）、病例的来源数与报告单数、不同时间发病率的稳定性、不同人群发病率的比较、年龄别发病率曲线、儿童癌症发病率评价等。

3. 有效性

有效性是指登记病例中具有给定特征（如肿瘤部位、年龄）真正属性的病例所占的比例。常用的评价指标有组织学诊断确认比例（HV%）、只有死亡证明比例（DCO%）、部位不明的百分比 (UK%)、年龄不明的百分比等。

3.3 The population information

The population refers to household registered people covered in the registration area. The data originate from census data, public security or bureaus of statistics. The population information includes overall population coverage, gender and age composition. The population are divided into groups by age as: 0~, 1~4, 5~9, 10~14, ···, 75~79, 80~84 and 85+ age group.

4. Quality control of cancer registration

Quality control goes through all along cancer registration. Each step of cancer registration observes specified regulations and procedure for quality control. Quality control on registration data are systematically assessed from four aspects of comparability, completeness,validity and timeliness.

4.1 Quality control of registration data

4.1.1 Comparability

The basic prerequisite for the true comparability of data results is the use of universal standards or definitions. Generally speaking, comarability refers to the difference in the difference of population in different regions or at different times, not because of the quality of registration data, the different coding standards or the rules of use. Comparability involves the following indicators: the definition of “onset”, diagnostic criteria about primary, recurrent and metastatic, classification and coding, death certification, etc.

4.1.2 Completeness

The completeness refers that to what extent all of the incident cancers are included and recorded in the whole objective covering population in the registration areas. The common evaluating indicators include mortality / incidence ratios (M：I), the proportion of death certification only (DCO%), histological verified diagnoses (HV%), the number of sources and notifications per case, the stability of incidence rates over time, a comparison of incidence rates in different populations, age-specific incidence curves, and incidence rate of childhood cancers evaluation.

4.1.3 Validity

Validity is defined as the proportion of cases in a dataset with a given characteristic that truly have the attribute. The common evaluation indicators include ratio of histological verified diagnoses (HV%), proportion of the death certification only (DCO%), proportion of unspecific site diagnoses(UK%), unspecific age proportion, etc. Cancer registries must evaluate validity of data for information consistency, for example, age/date of birth, gender/anatomic site, anatomic site/histologic diagnosis, anatomic site/histologic diagnosis/age, and the

对各登记处的数据进行内部一致审核，检查数据库中无效编码或组合及可疑的编码组合，如年龄 / 出生日期、性别 / 部位、部位 / 组织学，以及部位 / 组织学 / 年龄等。

4. 时效性

时效性一般指发病日期（诊断日期）到数据被利用时（年报、研究报告、论文）的间隔。登记地区及时获取并报告癌症信息，会提高肿瘤登记工作的效率，但是新发病例登记流程自身存在滞后性，时效性考虑的就是在效率与完整性间取得平衡。目前对时效性无统一的国际标准。为平衡完整性和准确性的关系，全国肿瘤登记中心要求各登记地区于诊断年份后的 30 个月内提交数据。

（二）登记资料的审核流程

河南省肿瘤登记中心收到各登记地区的上报资料后，首先检查资料的完整性。在确认资料完整后，使用 IARC/IACR 工具软件中的 Check 程序逐一检查所有记录的变量是否完整和有效，同时对不同变量之间是否合乎逻辑的一致性进行检查。然后使用数据分析软件及数据库软件生成统一表格，对登记数据的完整性和可靠性做出评估。各登记地区根据评估结果，对登记资料进行核实、补充与修改，将修改后的资料再次上报省级肿瘤登记中心，河南省肿瘤登记中心将全省各登记地区数据进行汇总分析，并撰写年度报告（图 2-2）。

（三）统计分类

1. 肿瘤分类

参照 ICD-10 国际统计分类的肿瘤学类目的内容，根据 ICD-10 前三位“C”类编码，将包括男、女性肿瘤细分类为 59 部位及 25 个大类，其中脑和神经系统包括良性及良恶性未定肿瘤（表 2-1、表 2-2）。

completeness of all basic variables.

4.1.4 Timeliness

Timeliness refers to time interval between the date of onset / diagnosis and data utilization (annual report, research report or papers). Timely access to and reporting cancer information can improve the efficiency of cancer registration work, but the new case registration process has its own lag, and the timeliness consideration is to balance the efficiency and integrity. There are no international guidelines yet for the timeliness of cancer registration data. Now, NCCR (National Central Cancer Registry) requires a reporting interval within 30 months after diagnosing under consideration of the data integrity.

4.2 Audit process of registration data

After receiving cancer registration data, HNCCR checks the data' s completeness firstly. IARC/IACR check software are used to determine whether all the variables are complete and valid. The internal logical consistency of the dataset is also checked. HNCCR further generates a unified form to assess integrity and reliability of the registration data with the using data analysis software and database software. Then, the local registries revise the cancer datasets following the assessment form till it is satisfied with the requirements. Qualified cancer datasets are pooled together for Henan provincial annual cancer report analysis (Figure 2-2).

4.3 Data classification and coding

4.3.1 Cancer classification and coding

According to the first three “C” class codes of ICD-10, male and female tumors were subdivided into 59 parts and 25 major categories, including neoplasms, uncertain whether benign or malignant, of brain and nervous system(Table 2-1, Table2-2).

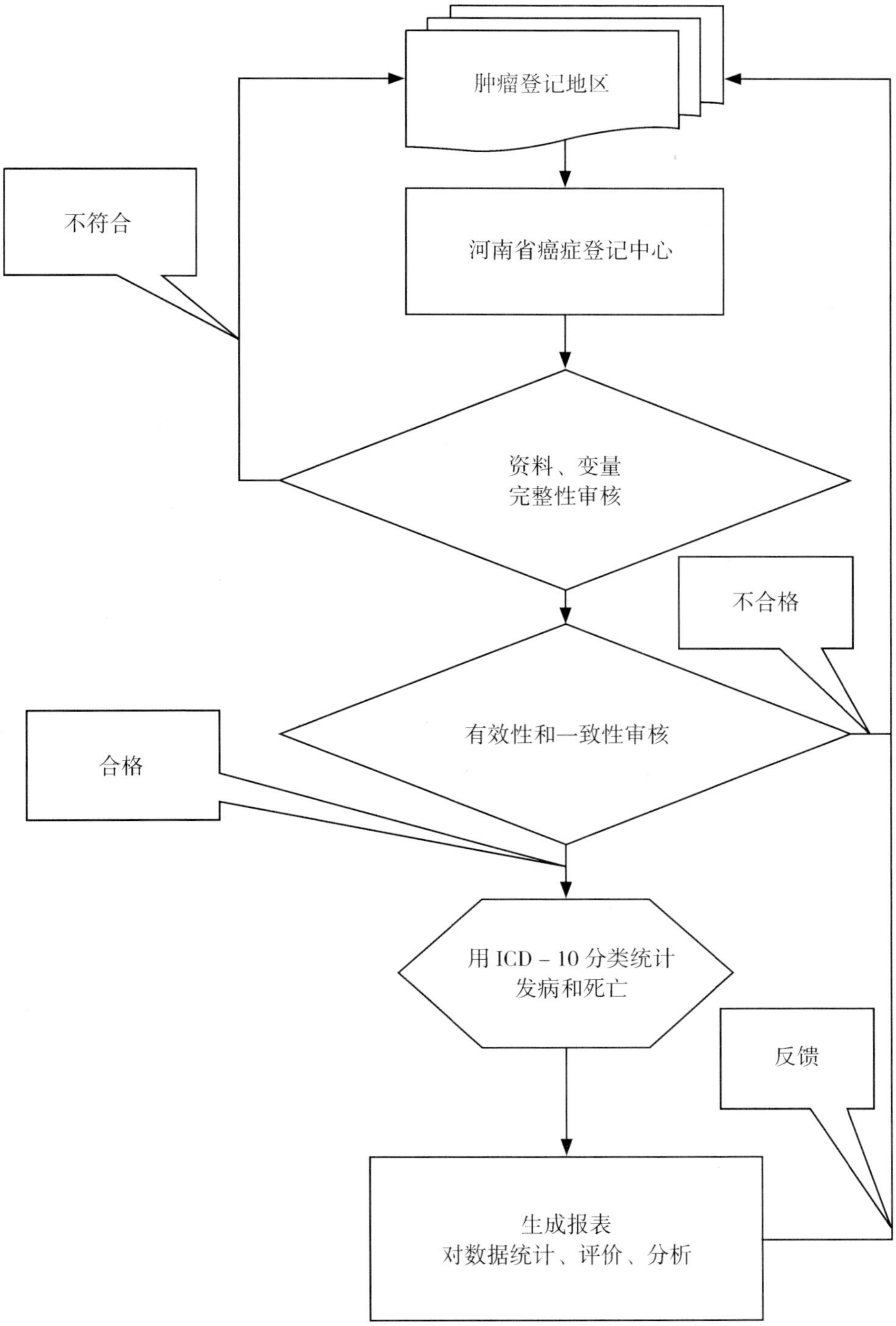

图 2-2　登记资料的审核流程

表 2-1 常用癌症分类统计表（细分类）

部位	编码范围（ICD-10）	部位	编码范围（ICD-10）
唇	C00	间皮瘤	C45
舌	C01-C02	卡波西肉瘤	C46
口	C03-C06	周围神经、其他结缔组织、软组织	C47，C49
唾液腺	C07-C08	乳房	C50
扁桃体	C09	外阴	C51
其他的口咽	C10	阴道	C52
鼻咽	C11	子宫颈	C53
喉咽	C12-C13	子宫体	C54
咽，部位不明	C14	子宫，部位不明	C55
食管	C15	卵巢	C56
胃	C16	其他的女性生殖器	C57
小肠	C17	胎盘	C58
结肠	C18	阴茎	C60
直肠	C19-C20	前列腺	C61
肛门	C21	睾丸	C62
肝脏	C22	其他的男性生殖器	C63
胆囊及其他	C23-C24	肾	C64
胰腺	C25	肾盂	C65
鼻、鼻窦及其他	C30-C31	输尿管	C66
喉	C32	膀胱	C67
气管、支气管、肺	C33-C34	其他的泌尿器官	C68
其他的胸腔器官	C37-C38	眼	C69
骨	C40-C41	脑、神经系统	C70-C72
皮肤的黑色素瘤	C43	甲状腺	C73
其他的皮肤	C44	肾上腺	C74
其他的内分泌腺	C75	髓样白血病	C92-C94
霍奇金病	C81	白血病，未特指	C95
非霍奇金淋巴瘤	C82-C85，C96	其他的或未指明部位的	O&U
免疫增生性疾病	C88	骨髓增殖性疾病	MPD
多发性骨髓瘤	C90	骨髓增生异常综合征	MDS
淋巴样白血病	C91		
合计	ALL	所有部位除外 C44	ALL but C44

表 2–2　常用癌症分类统计表（大类）

部位	编码范围（ICD–10）
口腔和咽(除外鼻咽癌和喉癌)	C00–10，C12–14（除外 C10.1）
鼻咽癌	C11
食管	C15
胃	C16
结直肠肛门	C18–21
肝脏	C22
胆囊及其他	C23–C24
胰腺	C25
喉	C32，C10.1
气管、支气管、肺	C33–C34
骨	C40–C41
乳房	C50
子宫颈	C53
子宫体及子宫部位不明	C54–55
卵巢	C56
前列腺	C61
睾丸	C62
肾及泌尿系统不明	C64–66，68
膀胱	C67
脑,神经系统	C70–C72
甲状腺	C73
淋巴瘤	C81–85，88，90，96
白血病	C91–C95
其他	Other（除外以上）
所有部位合计	ALL

2. 登记地区分类

城市与农村的分类标准：根据国家标准 GB 2260—2009，将地级以上城市归于城市地区，县及县级市归于农村地区。按照此项标准我们把洛阳市、三门峡市、鹤壁市、漯河市（召陵区和源汇区）、郑州市、安阳市、濮阳市华龙区、南阳市归类为城市地区；林州市、开封市（祥符区）、内乡县等地区归类为农村地区。

4.3.2 Cancer registration area classification

The urban area and rural area difinition standards: according to national standard GB 2260–2009, prefecture-level cities are classified into the urban areas, whereas counties and county-level cities are classified into the rural areas. Accordingly, the urban areas include Luoyang city, Sanmenxia City, Hebi City and Luohe City (Shaoling District and Yuanhui District), and the rural areas include Linzhou City, Kaifeng City (Xiangfu District), Neixiang County, etc.

（四）常用统计指标

1. 年平均人口数

年均人口数是计算发病（死亡）率指标的分母，常用年初和年末人口数的算术平均数作为年平均人口数的近似值。

$$年均人口数=\frac{年初（上年末）人口数+年末人口数}{2}$$

如果人口数变化均匀，年中人口数（7 月 1 日零时人口数）等于年平均人口数，可以用年中人口数代替年平均人口数。

2. 性别、年龄别人口数

性别、年龄别人口数是指按男、女性别和不同年龄分组的人口数。性别年龄的分组，除 0 岁组、1~4 岁组及 85 岁及以上年龄组外，常用 5 岁一个年龄组分组。常用的 19 个年龄分组分别为：不满 1 岁、1~4 岁、5~9 岁、10~14 岁……75~79 岁、80~84 岁、85 岁及以上。

3. 发病（死亡）率

发病（死亡）率又称粗发病（死亡）率，是人口发病（死亡）情况的基本指标，反映了人群的疾病发病（死亡）水平。发病（死亡）率是一定期间内，某人群发生某疾病新病例（死亡）的频率，通常以十万分率表示，整数后保留小数点两位，计算公式为

$$恶性肿瘤发病（死亡）率=\frac{某年某地恶性肿瘤新病例（死亡）数}{某年某地平均人口数}\times 100\,000(1/10^5)$$

4. 性别年龄别发病（死亡）率

人口的性别年龄结构是影响癌症发病（死亡）水平的重要因素，性别年龄别发病（死亡）率是统计研究的重要指标，计算公式如下：

$$某年龄组发病（死亡）率=\frac{某年龄组发病（死亡）人数}{同年龄组人口数}\times 100\,000(1/10^5)$$

5. 年龄调整率（标准化率）

由于年龄因素影响癌症的发病率与死亡率，因此在分析比较不同地区的发病（死亡）率或

4.4 Common statistical indicators

4.4.1 Average annual population

Average annual population is the denominator of the incidence (mortality) rates. We often use the arithmetic mean of the population at the beginning of the year and the end of the year as the approximate value of the annual average population.The formula is:

$$\text{Average annual population}=\frac{\text{Population at the beginning of the year}+\text{Population at the end of the year}}{2}$$

If the population changes evenly, the mid-year population, population at 00:00, July 1, can substitute for average annual population.

4.4.2 Sex- and age-specific population

Sex- and age-specific population is the population categorized by sex and different age groups and it can be calculated by interpolation. Age specific population is grouped by age groups of 5 years as follows: 0~1 years old, 1~4 years old, 5~9 years old, 10~14 years old…75~79 years old, 80~84 years old and 85+ years old.

4.4.3 Incidence (mortality) rate

Incidence (mortality) rate,also known as crude incidence (mortality) rate, is a measure of the frequency of an event, such as a new case of cancer (cancer death) occurring in a population over a period of time. The incidence is usually expressed as one hundred thousand points, and two decimal digits are retained after integer. The formula is:

$$\text{The incidence/mortality rate per 100 000}=\frac{\text{New cases(cancer deaths)occuring during a given time period}}{\text{Population at risk during the same time period}}\times 100\,000$$

4.4.4 Sex- and age-specific incidence (mortality) rates

Sex and age are important factors influencing cancer incidence and mortality. Sex-and age-specific rates are important indicators in cancer statistics. The formula is:

$$\text{Age-specific incidence/mortality rate per 100 000}=\frac{\text{Cases in a specific age group}}{\text{Population in the age group}}\times 100\,000$$

4.4.5 Age-standardized rate or age-adjusted rate (ASR)

Standardization is necessary when comparing several populations with different age structures because age has such a powerful influence on cancer incidence and mortality. ASR is a summary measure of the rate that a population

同一地区人群不同时期的发病（死亡）水平时，为消除人口年龄结构对发病（死亡）水平的影响，需要计算年龄标准化发病（死亡）率，即指按照某一标准人口的年龄结构所计算的发病（死亡）率。本年报使用的中国标准人口是 2000 年全国第五次人口普查的人口年龄构成，世界标准人口采用 Segi's 标准人口构成。表 2–3 为中国人口和世界人口年龄构成，可供计算年龄标化率时选用。

would have if it had a standard age structure. In this report, the population standards we used are Segi's population and the fifth Chinese national census of 2000 for the world and China, respectively (Table 2–3).

表 2–3　标准人口构成

年龄组（岁）	中国人口构成（2000 年）	世界人口构成 (Segi's)
0~	13 793 799	2 400
1~	55 184 575	9 600
5~	90 152 587	10 000
10~	125 396 633	9 000
15~	103 031 165	9 000
20~	94 573 174	8 000
25~	117 602 265	8 000
30~	127 314 298	6 000
35~	109 147 295	6 000
40~	81 242 945	6 000
45~	85 521 045	6 000
50~	63 304 200	5 000
55~	46 370 375	4 000
60~	41 703 848	4 000
65~	34 780 460	3 000
70~	25 574 149	2 000
75~	15 928 330	1 000
80~	7 989 158	500
85+	4 001 925	500
合计	1 242 612 226	100 000

年龄标化发病(死亡)率的计算(直接法):

(1)计算年龄组发病(死亡)率。

(2)以各年龄组发病(死亡)率乘相应的标准人口年龄构成百分比,得到相应的理论发病(死亡)率。

(3)将各年龄组的理论发病(死亡)率相加之和,即是年龄标化发病(死亡)率。

$$\text{标准化发病(死亡)率} = \frac{\sum \text{标准人口年龄构成} \times \text{年龄别发病(死亡)率}}{\sum \text{标准人口年龄构成}}$$

6. 分类构成

各类癌症发病(死亡)构成百分比可以反映各类癌症对居民健康危害的情况。癌症发病(死亡)分类构成百分比的计算公式如下:

$$\text{某癌症构成} = \frac{\text{某癌症发病(死亡)人数}}{\text{总发病(死亡)人数}} \times 100\%$$

7. 累积发病(死亡)率

累积发病(死亡)率是指某病在某一年龄阶段内按年龄(岁)的发病(死亡)率进行累积的总指标。累积发病(死亡)率消除了年龄构成不同的影响,故不需要标准化便可以与不同地区直接进行比较。癌症一般是计算 0 ~74 岁的累积发病(死亡)率。

$$\text{累积发病(死亡)率} = \sum \text{年龄组发病(死亡)率} \times \text{年龄组距} \times 100\%$$

8. 截缩发病(死亡)率

通常对癌症是截取 35 ~64 岁这一易发年龄段计算,其标准人口常用世界人口年龄构成。

$$\text{截缩发病(死亡)率} = \frac{\sum \text{截缩段各年龄组发病(死亡)率} \times \text{各段标准年龄构成}}{\sum \text{各段标准年龄构成}} \times 100\%$$

因为癌症在 35 岁以前发生频率较低,而在 65 岁以后其他疾病较多,干扰较大,所以采用 35 ~64 岁这一阶段的截缩发病(死亡)率比较稳定(截缩率是标化率),便于率的比较。

Calculating ASR incidence (mortality) (direct method):

(Ⅰ)Calculating the incidence (mortality) rates in each specific age groups.

(Ⅱ) Multiplying incidence (mortality) rate of each age group by the corresponding age group composition of standard population is the theoretical incidence (mortality) rate.

(Ⅲ) Adding up the theoretical incidence (mortality) rate in each age group is the age-standardized incidence (mortality) rate.

$$\text{Age-standarized rate} = \frac{\sum \text{Standard population in the correspon ding age group} \times \text{Age-specific rate}}{\sum \text{Standard population}}$$

4.4.6 Proportions

Proportional distribution indicates the site-specific percentage level of incident cases (deaths) compared with total cases (deaths) recorded, reflecting the hazards of various cancer types to people health. The formula is:

$$\text{Proportion of a certain type of cancer} = \frac{\text{Cases of a particular cancer}}{\text{Cases of all cancers}} \times 100\%$$

4.6.7 Cumulative rate

A cumulative incidence or death rate indicates the probability of onset of cancer between birth and a specifc age. The rate can be compared without age standardization because it is not affected by age structures. Cancer generally calculates cumulative rates at 0~74 years of age.

$$\text{Cumulative rate} = \sum (\text{Age-specific rate} \times \text{Width of the age group}) \times 100\%$$

4.4.8 Truncated incidence/mortality rate

Truncated rate is the calculation of rates over the truncated age of 35~64 years old, generally for cancer, using WHO world standard population. The data are presented as truncated rates mainly because the accuracy of age-specific rates in the elderly may be much less certain and the rates in the younger age groups may be rare.

$$\text{Truncated incidence/mortality rate} = \frac{\sum \text{Truncated in a specific age group} \times \text{Standard proportion of the age group}}{\sum \text{Standard proportion}} \times 100\%$$

第三章　数据质量评价

Chapter 3　Data quality evaluation

一、数据来源

2017 年河南省有 32 个市县登记处上报了 2014 年肿瘤登记资料，分别是洛阳市、孟津县、新安县、栾川县、嵩县、汝阳县、宜阳县、洛阳市吉利区、偃师市、鲁山县、林州市、鹤壁市、辉县市、禹州市、漯河市、漯河市郾城区、三门峡市、南阳市、方城县、内乡县、睢县、虞城县、罗山县、沈丘县、郸城县、西平县、济源市、开封市祥符区、安阳市城区、濮阳市华龙区、固始县、郑州市城区（表 3-1）。

1. Data sources

A total of 32 cancer registries submited cancer registration data of 2014 to HNCCR in 2017. They are Luoyang City, Mengjin County, Xin' an County, Luanchuan County, Songxian County, Ruyang County, Yiyang County, Jili District, Yanshi City, Lushan County, Linzhou City, Hebi City, Huixian City, Yuzhou City, Luohe City, Yancheng District, Sanmenxia City, Nanyang City, Fangcheng County, Neixiang County, Suixian County, Yucheng County, Luoshan County, Shenqiu County, Dancheng County, Xiping County, Jiyuan City, Xiangfu district of Kaifeng City, Urban district of Anyang City, Hualong district of Puyang City, Gushi County and Urban district of Zhengzhou City (Table 3-1).

表 3-1　2014 年河南省提交肿瘤登记资料的地区

地区	登记地区	登记机构名单
洛阳市	洛阳市	洛阳市疾控中心
	偃师市	偃师市疾控中心
	孟津县	孟津县疾控中心
	新安县	新安县疾控中心
	栾川县	栾川县疾控中心
	嵩县	嵩县疾控中心
	汝阳县	汝阳县疾控中心
	宜阳县	宜阳县疾控中心
	吉利区	吉利区疾控中心
济源市	济源市	济源市疾控中心
驻马店市	西平县	西平县疾控中心
新乡市	辉县市	辉县市疾控中心

续表

地区	登记地区	登记机构名单
漯河市	漯河市	漯河市疾控中心
	郾城区	郾城区疾控中心
周口市	郸城县	郸城县疾控中心
	沈丘县	沈丘县疾控中心
安阳市	安阳市	安阳市肿瘤医院
	林州市	林州市肿瘤医院
信阳市	罗山县	罗山县疾控中心
	固始县	固始县疾控中心
许昌市	禹州市	禹州市疾控中心
南阳市	内乡县	内乡县疾控中心
	卧龙区	卧龙区疾控中心
	方城县	方城县疾控中心
商丘市	虞城县	虞城县疾控中心
	睢县	睢县疾控中心
开封市	开封县	开封县疾控中心
鹤壁市	鹤壁市	鹤壁市人民医院
郑州市	郑州市	郑州市疾控中心
濮阳市	华龙区	华龙区疾控中心
三门峡市	三门峡市	三门峡市疾控中心
平顶山市	鲁山县	鲁山县疾控中心

二、《年报》数据质量分级

全国肿瘤登记中心肿瘤登记专家组和《中国肿瘤登记年报》编委会，根据《卫生部肿瘤随访登记技术方案》（卫生部疾病预防控制局2009）中的要求，参照《中国肿瘤登记工作指导手册》，以及国际癌症研究中心（IARC）/ 国际癌症登记协会（IACR）的《五大洲癌症发病率》数据入选标准，结合我国肿瘤登记实际情况，修改了新的《年报》数据入选标准，并根据标准对登记地区进行质量分级标注（表 3–2）。

2. Classification of data quality

The detailed data inclusion criteria were based on "Technical Protocols of Cancer Registration and Follow up" by Ministry of Health 2009, "Guideline for Chinese Cancer Registration" and "Cancer Incidence in Five Continents Volume IX" by The International Agency for Research on Cancer (IARC)/ the International agency for Cancer Registry (IACR). Accordingly, the data were classified into three categories (Table 3–2).

表 3-2　《年报》数据质量分级

A 级	B 级	D 级
覆盖全部人口	覆盖全部人口或特定人口	覆盖人口不明确
有可靠的人口数据来源，已建立完善、规范的全死因监测系统	死因监测系统不够完善，数据质量较差	无死因监测系统
诊断依据不明比例 <10%	诊断依据不明比例 <20%	诊断依据不明比例≥ 20%
0<DCO<10%	DCO<20%	DCO ≥ 20%
部位不明比例 <10%	部位不明比例 <20%	部位不明比例≥ 20%
0.60<M/I<0.80，主要癌症 M/I 合理	0.55<M/I<0.85，主要癌症 M/I 比较合理	M/I ≤ 0.55,M/I ≥ 0.85，主要癌症 M/I 不合理
66%<MV%<85%	55%<MV<95%	MV% ≤ 55%，MV% ≥ 95%
癌症变化趋势稳定，水平合理	癌症变化趋势相对稳定，水平比较合理	癌症变化趋势不稳定，水平不合理
死亡率不低于 $120/10^5$	死亡率不低于 $100/10^5$	

注：M/I 为死亡 / 发病比。

三、2014 年肿瘤登记资料评价

（一）《年报》收录登记地区的选取

河南省肿瘤登记中心有 32 个登记处提交了 2014 年登记资料。

参照全国登记资料《年报》数据入选标准，根据数据的病理学诊断比例（MV%）、只有死亡医学证明书比例（DCO%）、死亡 / 发病比（M/I）、人口数、发病率和死亡率水平、逐年变化趋势，以及我们平时对各个登记点制度建设与落实、经费保障、机构建设、岗位职责、人员配备及稳定性等指标进行综合评价，分为 A 级、B 级和 D 级，其中 A 级、B 级纳入年报，D 级拒绝，其中南阳市、禹州市、漯河市郾城区、鹤壁市、辉县市、罗山县、偃师市、虞城县、济源市、洛阳市、林州市、西平县、沈丘县、嵩县、郸城县、新安县被评为 A 级；方城县、鲁山县、开封市祥符区、栾川县、漯河市、睢县、三门峡市、汝阳县、宜阳县、孟津县、内乡县被评为 B 级。郑州市、安阳市、固始县、濮阳市华龙区上报数据资料，经过统计，恶性肿瘤发病率、死亡率低，漏报较多，很多指标不符合逻辑，资料没有正确反映当地居民恶性肿瘤的危害程度，被评为 D 级，资料没有收录《年报》。

3. Quality evaluation of cancer registration data of 2014

3.1 Selection of cancer registries for Annual Report

A total of 32 cancer registries submitted registration data to HNCCR. The data quality evaluation indicators include MV%, DCO%, M/I, population, incidence rate, mortality rates and stability, etc., and a comprehensive evaluation of system construction and implementation, funds guarantee, organization construction, job responsibilities, staffing and personnel stabilization as well. 16 registries were classified as level “A”, they were Nanyang City, Yuzhou City, Yancheng District, Hebi City, Huixian City, Luoshan County, Yanshi City, Yucheng County, Jiyuan City, Luoyang City, Linzhou City, Xiping County, Shenqiu County, Songxian County, Dancheng and Xin’an County. 11 cancer registries were classified as class B, which were Fangcheng County, Lushan county, Xiangfu District, Luanchuan County, Luohe City, Suixian County, Sanmenxia City, Ruyang County, Yiyang County, Mengjin County and Neixiang County. 4 cancer registries were classified as level “D”, they are Zhengzhou City, Anyang City, Gushi County, and Hualong District, where

需要指出的是，漯河市包括源汇区和召陵区，由于源汇区数据不符合质量要求，所以本年报中所提及漯河市的数据均以召陵区的数据代表。

按照全国登记资料《年报》的选取标准，河南省有 32 个登记处上报资料，其中 27 个符合《年报》报告要求，因此我们选取这 27 个登记处的资料作为河南省肿瘤登记样本数据，以分析河南省癌症的发病与死亡水平。

（二）有效覆盖人口、发病数和死亡数

2014 年，纳入年报分析的登记地区人口为 21 044 835 人（其中，男性 10 851 503 人，女性 10 193 332 人），约占河南省 2014 年人口总数的 19.73%（2014 年河南省国民经济和社会发展统计公报：10 662 万）。其中城市地区为 3 435 270 人，占登记人口的 16.32%，农村地区为 17 609 565 人，占 83.68%。

2014 年报告癌症新发病例数合计 53 200 例，其中城市地区 8 969 例，占 16.86%，农村地区报告癌症新发病 44 231 例，农村地区占 83.14%。上报癌症死亡病例合计 32 952 例，其中城市地区上报 5 452 例，城市地区占 16.55%，农村地区上报 27 500 例，农村地区占 83.45%。详见表 3–3。

the data failed to reflect local cancer epidemiological status because of low incidence rates or mortality rates, omissions, out of logical consistency, etc.

Annual report included registration data from the 27 registries classified as level "A" and level "B". The data were pooled for cancer incidence and mortality analysis.

3.2 Population coverage, new cancer cases and cancer deaths

Population coverage of Cancer Registries in Henan Province was 21 044 835 (10 851 503 males and 10 193 332 females), accounting for 19.73% of the provincial population in 2014, with 3 435 270 (16.32%) in urban areas and 17 609 596 (83.68%) in rural areas.

A total of 53 200 new cancer cases were reported in 2014, among which 8 969 (16.86%) were from urban areas, and 44 231 (83.14%) were from rural areas. There were 32 952 new cancer deaths in 2014, with 5 452 (16.55%) in urban areas and 27 500 (83.45%) in rural areas (Table 3–3).

表 3–3　2014 年各肿瘤登记地区覆盖人口、发病数和死亡数

单位：（人）

序号	登记市县	肿瘤登记机构	人口数	发病数	死亡数
1	开封市	祥符区疾控中心	703 906	1 632	792
2	洛阳市	洛阳市疾控中心	1 119 126	2 880	1 887
3	孟津县	孟津县疾控中心	459 600	1 121	662
4	新安县	新安县疾控中心	534 291	1 200	921
5	栾川县	栾川县疾控中心	346 991	823	404
6	嵩县	嵩县疾控中心	598 981	1 330	1 003
7	汝阳县	汝阳县疾控中心	509 917	1 278	733
8	宜阳县	宜阳县疾控中心	695 512	2 015	1 176
9	偃师市	偃师市疾控中心	620 440	1 416	908

续表

序号	登记市县	肿瘤登记机构	人口数	发病数	死亡数
10	鲁山县	鲁山县疾控中心	897 305	2 254	1 070
11	林州市	林州市肿瘤医院	1 093 727	3 224	2 178
12	鹤壁市	鹤壁市人民医院	634 834	1 646	1 042
13	辉县市	辉县市疾控中心	856 425	2 271	1 426
14	禹州市	禹州市疾控中心	1 134 293	2 840	1 721
15	漯河市	漯河市疾控中心	476 579	1 155	597
16	漯河市郾城区	郾城区疾控中心	476 339	1 202	740
17	三门峡市	三门峡市疾控中心	292 686	818	441
18	南阳市	卧龙区疾控中心	912 045	2 470	1 485
19	方城县	方城县疾控中心	1 135 497	2 965	1 246
20	内乡县	内乡县疾控中心	718 859	1 902	1 130
21	睢县	睢县疾控中心	849 995	2 176	1 155
22	虞城县	虞城县疾控中心	1 105 661	2 604	1 660
23	罗山县	罗山县疾控中心	745 553	1 777	1 121
24	沈丘县	沈丘县疾控中心	1 177 710	3 197	2 366
25	郸城县	郸城县疾控中心	1 373 054	3 416	2 629
26	西平县	西平县疾控中心	874 824	1 971	1 402
27	济源市	济源市疾控中心	700 685	1 617	1 057
	合计		20 144 835	53 200	32 952

（三）各登记地区数据质量评价

病理诊断比例（MV%）是指病理组织学诊断的病例占全部病例的百分比，是评价登记资料完整性和有效性的重要指标，全国肿瘤登记中心主要质控指标要求在 66%~85%。

仅有死亡医学证明书比例（DCO%）是指仅有死亡医学证明书的发病病例数占全部新发病例的比例。它也是评价登记资料完整性和有效性的重要指标，此项指标要求大于 0 且小于 10%。

死亡 / 发病比（M/I）是指同期登记的恶性肿瘤死亡数与新病例数之比。死亡 / 发病比既是评价完整性的指标，也是评价可靠性的重要

3.3 Data quality evaluation in each cancer registry

Morphologically verified case proportion (MV%) refers to the proportion of cases verified by histological, cytological and haematological evidence accounting for all cancer cases. MV% is an important indicator to evaluate data integrity and effectiveness. The index requirement of MV% of National Central Cancer Registry (NCCR) is between 66% and 85%.

Percentage of death certificate only (DCO%) refers to the proportion of cancer cases completed by death certificate only among all newly diagnosed cases. It is also an important index to evaluate the integrity and effectiveness of registration data, which is required less than 10%.

Mortality to incidence ratio (M/I) refers to the ratio of cancer deaths to new cancer cases in a certain period. It is an important index to evaluate data inteterity and reliability. It is

指标。一般此项指标在 0.60~0.80。

在有完善、规范的死因监测系统条件下，河南省肿瘤登记中心要求 M/I 在 0.60~0.80；MV% 在 66%~85%，DCO% 大于 0 且小于 10% 为 A 级；病理诊断比例（MV%）在 55%~95%，DCO% 小于 20%，M/I 在 0.55~0.85 为 B 级，数据达到入《年报》登记质量要求。无死因资料或死因资料不完整，MV% 小于等于 55% 或大于等于 95%，DCO% 大于等于 20%，M/I 小于等于 0.55 或大于等于 0.85 为 D 级，数据不被接受。详见表 3–4。

required between 0.60 and 0.80.

HNCCR classified the data into three categories. Category A or B were qualified and deemed acceptable, whereas category D was rejected. Briefly, category "A" requires M/I between 0.60~0.80, MV% between 66%~85%, DCO% less than 10% and with a complete and solid death surveillance system. Category "B" requires M/I between 0.55~0.85, MV% between 55%~95%, DCO% less than 20%. Category "D" means MV% less than 55% or no less than 95%, DCO% no less than 20%, M/I no more than 0.55 or no less than 0.85 and with no death surveillance system or incomplete death surveillance data (Table 3–4).

表 3–4　2014 年肿瘤登记地区资料主要质控指标

序号	登记地区	登记机构	人口数	MV%	DCO%	M/I	级别
1	开封市祥符区	祥符区疾控中心	703 906	66.24	1.1	0.49	B
2	洛阳市	洛阳市疾控中心	1 119 126	74.38	3.89	0.66	A
3	孟津县	孟津县疾控中心	459 600	58.61	5.44	0.59	B
4	新安县	新安县疾控中心	534 291	33.92	0.25	0.77	B
5	栾川县	栾川县疾控中心	346 991	62.33	11.3	0.49	B
6	嵩县	嵩县疾控中心	598 981	69.02	1.35	0.75	A
7	汝阳县	汝阳县疾控中心	509 917	70.42	2.97	0.57	B
8	宜阳县	宜阳县疾控中心	695 512	65.91	1.29	0.58	B
9	偃师市	偃师市疾控中心	620 440	59.18	4.73	0.64	A
10	鲁山县	鲁山县疾控中心	897 305	75.29	1.29	0.47	B
11	林州市	林州市肿瘤医院	1 093 727	74.66	1.15	0.68	A
12	鹤壁市	鹤壁市人民医院	634 834	66.52	3.83	0.63	A
13	辉县市	辉县市疾控中心	856 425	69.48	0.31	0.63	A
14	禹州市	禹州市疾控中心	1 134 293	69.26	3.35	0.61	A
15	漯河市	漯河市疾控中心	476 579	64.33	0	0.52	B
16	漯河市郾城区	郾城区疾控中心	476 339	68.89	2.66	0.62	A
17	三门峡市	三门峡疾控中心	292 686	81.78	0	0.54	B
18	南阳市	南阳市疾控中心	912 045	64.49	1.78	0.60	A
19	方城县	方城县疾控中心	1 135 497	59.33	0.03	0.42	B
20	内乡县	内乡县疾控中心	718 859	76.92	0.47	0.59	B

续表

序号	登记地区	登记机构	人口数	MV%	DCO%	M/I	级别
21	睢县	睢县疾控中心	849 995	85.29	0.05	0.53	B
22	虞城县	虞城县疾控中心	1 105 661	60.37	1.00	0.64	A
23	罗山县	罗山县疾控中心	745 553	69.27	2.59	0.63	A
24	沈丘县	沈丘县疾控中心	1 177 710	69.38	4.16	0.74	A
25	郸城县	郸城县疾控中心	1 373 054	68.12	1.79	0.77	A
26	西平县	西平县疾控中心	874 824	71.03	2.18	0.71	A
27	济源市	济源市疾控中心	700 685	65.99	6	0.65	A

注：根据其上报发病率、死亡率等数据，按照数据质量评价标准，表中所列地区数据分别评为 A 级、B 级。郑州市、安阳市、濮阳市华龙区和固始县发病率、死亡率较低，漏报较多，其数据被评为 D 级。

（四）肿瘤登记地区2009—2014年癌症发病率与死亡率稳定性评价

2009 年卫生部在全国范围内启动了中央财政转移支付地方的肿瘤随访登记项目，我省的洛阳市、偃师市、禹州市、济源市、鲁山县、内乡县等地区先后被纳入国家肿瘤随访登记项目点。除了林州市开展肿瘤登记工作较早以外，河南省其他地区的登记处于 2008 年以后开始实施人群肿瘤登记。

2009 年登记地区覆盖人口只有 600 万，占全省人口的 6% 左右，由于覆盖人口较少，各项统计指标的代表性不能全面反映我省各种肿瘤的发病率、死亡率和生存状态。2010 年新增加 10 个登记点，上报点数为 16 个，登记地区覆盖人口达到 1 300 多万，占当年全省人口的 15% 左右。

2011 年没有新增登记点，肿瘤登记工作重点是加强了肿瘤登记基础工作建设，包括制度建设与落实，机构建设，人员培训，岗位职责，人员配备及稳定性等。目的是建立起完善的、及时的、系统的肿瘤登记报告系统，能准确、及时反映我省城乡居民肿瘤发病、死亡、生存状态，并提供满足我省肿瘤防治需求的基本信息。2012—2013 年增加鹤壁市、开封县、睢县及郑州市为肿瘤登记点，上报单位为 20 个。

2013 年，登记地区覆盖人口达到 16 225 815 人（其中，男性 8 370 772 人，女性 7 855 043 人）约占河南省 2013 年年底总人口的 15.31%。

2014 年，登记地区人口为 21 044 835 人（其

3.4 Stability of incidences and mortalities in cancer registries, 2009—2014

When central financing supported local cancer registries establishment by Ministry of Health in 2009, Luoyang City, Yanshi City, Yuzhou City, Jiyuan City, Lushan County and Neixiang County were subsumed into national cancer follow-up registration project. Other cancer registries in Henan Province carried out population-based cancer registration in 2008 except Linzhou City, which started earlier.

In 2009, the registries covered 6% of the population (6 000 000). Due to the less population coverage, the statistical indicators had less power to reflect the overall cancer incidences, mortalities and survival conditions in Henan Province. In 2010, ten more cancer registries were established and cancer registries increased to sixteen, when the population coverage was 13 million, accounting for about 15 percent of the population in Henan, 2010.

In 2011, there were no new cancer registries established. Cancer registration focused on foundamental construction of system implementation, institution, personnel training, job responsibility, staff stabilization, etc, aiming at constructing a complete, timely and systematic cancer registration and reporting system with the capabilility of reflecting cancer incidence, mortality and survival of Henan residents to provide basic information for cancer control and research. In 2012 and 2013, new cancer registries of Hebi City, Kaifeng County, Sui County and Zhengzhou City developed, and the number of cancer registries increased to 20 in Henan Province.

In 2013, the population coverage was 16 225 815 (Male:

中，男性 10 851 503 人；女性 10 193 332 人），约占河南省 2014 年人口总数的 19.73%。

2009—2014 年河南省肿瘤发病率分别是 199.47/10^5、239.00/10^5、246.12/10^5、247.51/10^5、250.34/10^5、252.79/10^5；死亡率分别是 132.64/10^5、153.65/10^5、159.62/10、158.83/10^5、161.00/10^5、156.58/10^5，发病率与死亡率基本处于稳定状态。各个登记处随着登记系统和登记制度的不断完善，登记质量明显提高，漏报减少。表 3-5、表 3-6、图 3-1~ 图 3-20 显示各个登记点开展肿瘤随访登记工作以来每年肿瘤发病率及死亡率的变动情况，从上报数据分析各个登记处发病率及死亡率没有明显的波动，数据都呈现小幅上升，发病率与死亡率的水平基本稳定，显示各个地方的登记质量在不断地提高，漏报逐渐减少。肿瘤登记资料的可比性、完整性与有效性得到了基本保证。

8 370 772; Female: 7 855 043), accounting for 15.31% of the population in the end of 2013.

In 2014, the population coverage was 21 044 835 (Male: 10 851 503; Female: 10 193 332), accounting for 19.73% of the population in 2014.

During 2009—2014, cancer incidences in Henan Province were 199.47/10^5, 239.00/10^5, 246.12/10^5, 247.51/10^5, 250.34/10^5 and 252.79/10^5, respectively, and mortalities were 132.64/10^5, 153.65/10^5, 159.62/10^5, 158.83/10^5, 161.00/10^5 and 156.58/10^5,which were relatively stable. With the construction of registration system and regularities, data quality improved greatly, missing cases shortened. Table 3-5, table 3-6 and figures 3-1 to 3-20 showed the changes of cancer incidence and mortality each year since cancer registration had been carried out. From the statistical data, the incidence and mortality rates kept stable relatively and the cases increased slightly, which reflected an increasing trend of data quality and a decreasing trend of case omissions. The comparability, completeness and validity of cancer registration data are basically guaranteed.

表 3-5 登记地区的 2009 — 2014 年恶性肿瘤发病率（1/10^5）

序号	登记地区	2014 年	2013 年	2012 年	2011 年	2010 年	2009 年
1	林州市	294.77	301.52	324.93	288.69	264.66	248.18
2	洛阳市	257.34	240.57	262.30	232.42	243.84	240.93
3	偃师市	228.23	234.48	228.73	224.89	219.24	185.47
4	禹州市	250.38	255.59	235.96	240.84	229.94	166.36
5	沈丘县	271.46	288.47	263.69	278.52	246.77	162.00
6	西平县	225.30	219.16	218.37	217.39	220.38	189.39
7	鲁山县	251.20	239.64	245.88	246.89	248.64	
8	辉县市	265.17	252.23	242.62	252.47	247.23	
9	济源市	230.77	225.26	234.27	241.12	236.75	
10	漯河市	242.35	222.73	226.16	239.96	225.90	
11	漯河市郾城区	252.34	234.05	237.72	223.25	225.82	
12	三门峡市	279.48	269.16	231.14	247.63	232.36	
13	虞城县	235.52	239.06	241.40	244.22	239.48	
14	郸城县	248.79	251.33	247.68	242.11	243.15	
15	内乡县	264.59	258.22	242.74	237.14	226.45	
16	罗山县	238.35	255.95	251.22	250.66	233.64	

续表

序号	登记地区	2014 年	2013 年	2012 年	2011 年	2010 年	2009 年
17	开封县	231.85	226.02	227.34			
18	鹤壁市	259.28	257.82	259.77			
19	睢县	256.00	255.09	239.89			
20	孟津县	243.91					
21	新安县	224.60					
22	栾川县	237.18					
23	嵩县	222.04					
24	汝阳县	250.63					
25	宜阳县	289.71					
26	南阳市	270.82					
27	方城县	261.12					
	合计	252.79	250.34	247.51	246.12	239.00	199.47

表 3-6　登记地区的 2009—2014 年恶性肿瘤死亡率（$1/10^5$）

	登记地区	2014年	2013年	2012年	2011年	2010年	2009年
1	林州市	199.14	183.31	203.85	184.9	179.14	165.1
2	洛阳市	168.61	157.17	172.77	142.02	151.33	96.94
3	偃师市	146.35	157.88	143.38	142.74	141.19	122.87
4	禹州市	151.72	160.31	158.95	181.98	152.16	86.08
5	沈丘县	200.90	206.31	168.00	184.78	149.44	148.39
6	西平县	160.26	128.95	136.94	141.45	113.40	157.11
7	鲁山县	119.25	149.37	159.92	162.02	164.03	
8	辉县市	166.51	155.77	149.05	150.91	153.26	
9	济源市	150.85	149.16	145.58	146.22	146.06	
10	漯河市	125.27	131.28	139.34	143.05	143.55	
11	漯河市郾城区	155.35	154.63	153.08	148.34	145.17	
12	三门峡市	150.67	161.16	150.70	148.77	151.77	
13	虞城县	150.14	148.23	157.12	156.13	158.62	
14	郸城县	191.47	193.42	177.43	163.81	157.70	

续表

	登记地区	2014年	2013年	2012年	2011年	2010年	2009年
15	内乡县	157.19	155.75	155.09	155.56	157.30	
16	罗山县	150.36	164.01	156.84	157.11	152.92	
17	开封县	112.52	149.31	138.56			
18	鹤壁市	164.14	165.96	152.89			
19	睢县	135.88	142.26	149.57			
20	孟津县	144.04					
21	新安县	172.38					
22	栾川县	116.43					
23	嵩县	167.45					
24	汝阳县	143.75					
25	宜阳县	169.08					
26	南阳市	162.82					
27	方城县	109.73					
	合计	156.58	161.00	158.83	159.62	153.65	132.64

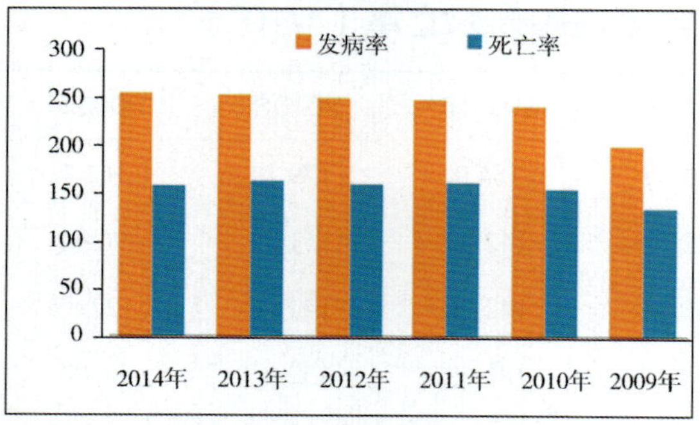

图 3-1 河南省 2009—2014 年恶性肿瘤的发病（死亡）率（$1/10^5$）

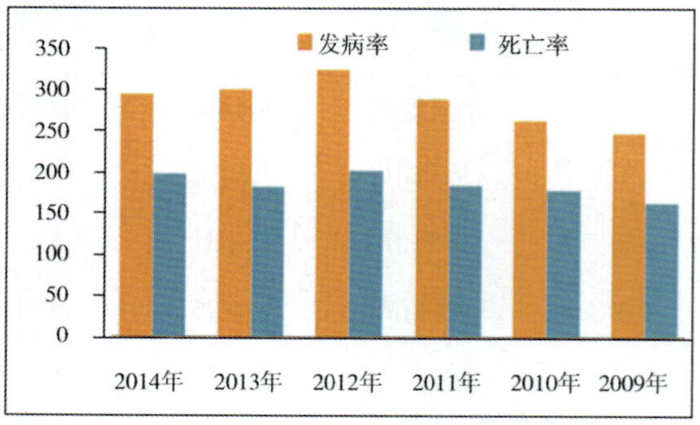

图 3-2 林州市 2009—2014 年恶性肿瘤的发病（死亡）率（$1/10^5$）

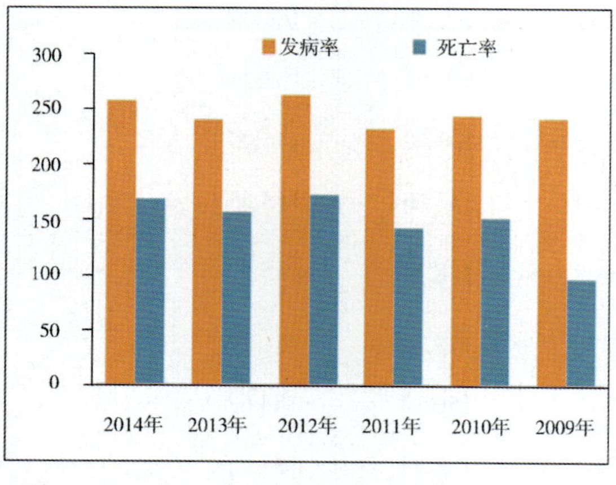

图 3-3 洛阳市 2009—2014 年恶性肿瘤的发病（死亡）率（$1/10^5$）

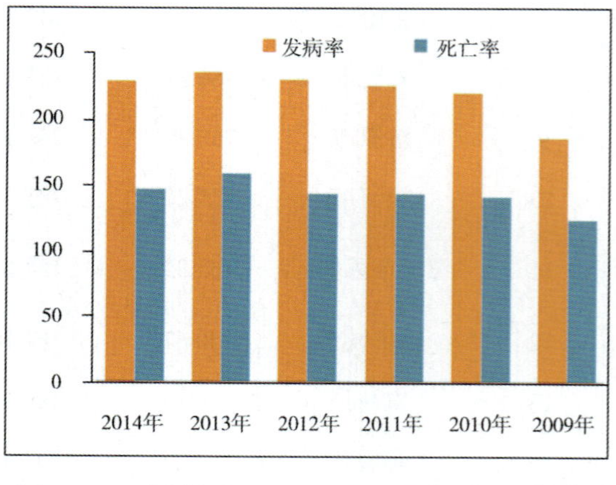

图 3-4 偃师市 2009—2014 年恶性肿瘤的发病（死亡）率（$1/10^5$）

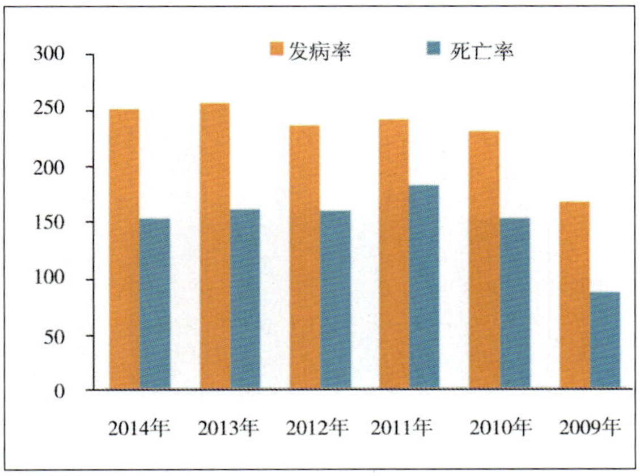

图 3-5　禹州市 2009—2014 年恶性肿瘤的发病（死亡）率（$1/10^5$）

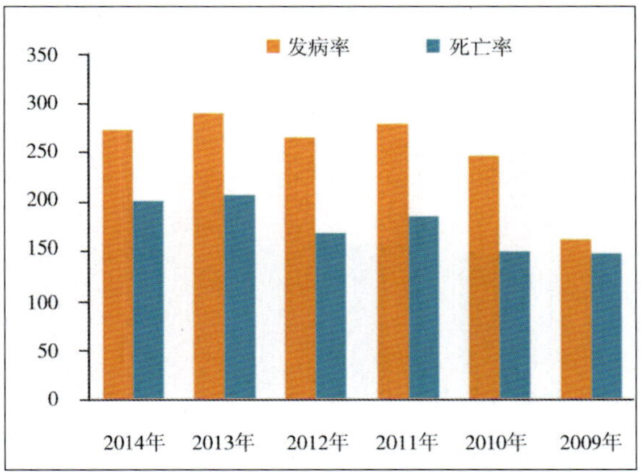

图 3-6　沈丘县 2009—2014 年恶性肿瘤的发病（死亡）率（$1/10^5$）

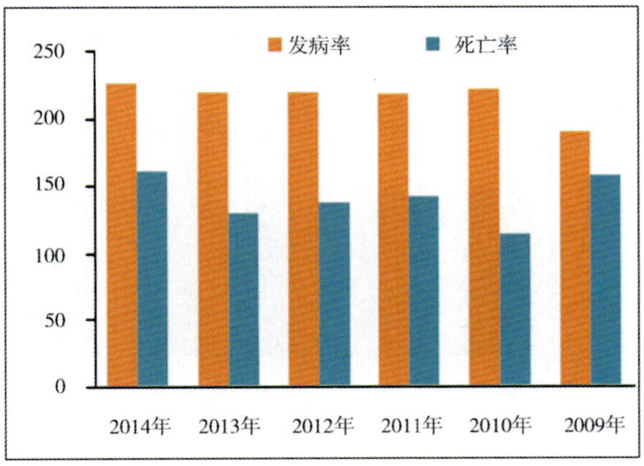

图 3-7　西平县 2009—2014 年恶性肿瘤的发病（死亡）率（$1/10^5$）

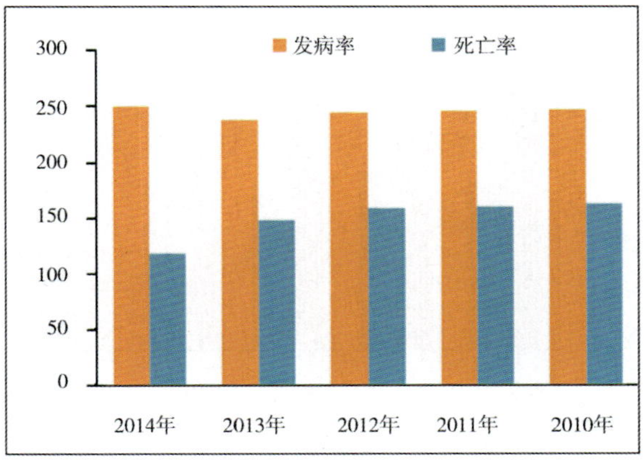

图 3-8　鲁山县 2010—2014 年恶性肿瘤的发病（死亡）率（$1/10^5$）

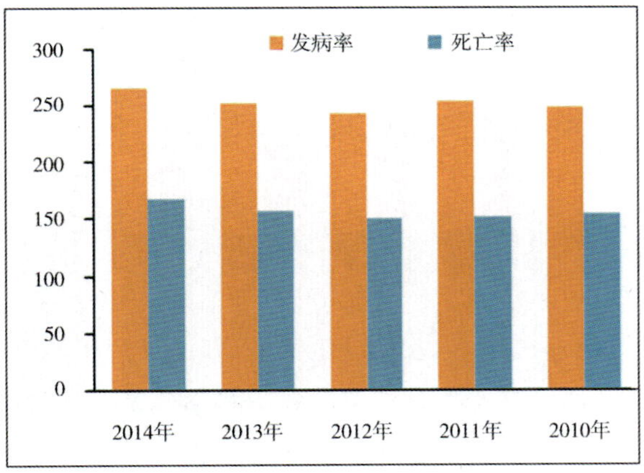

图3-9　辉县市2010—2014年恶性肿瘤的发病（死亡）率（$1/10^5$）

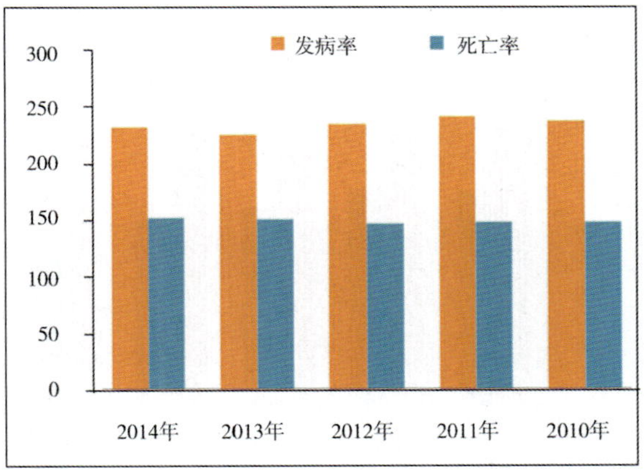

图 3-10　济源市 2010—2014 年恶性肿瘤的发病（死亡）率（$1/10^5$）

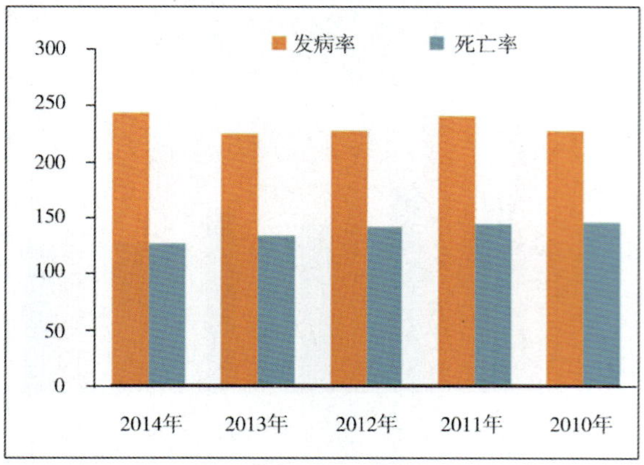

图 3-11 漯河市 2010—2014 年恶性肿瘤的发病（死亡）率（$1/10^5$）

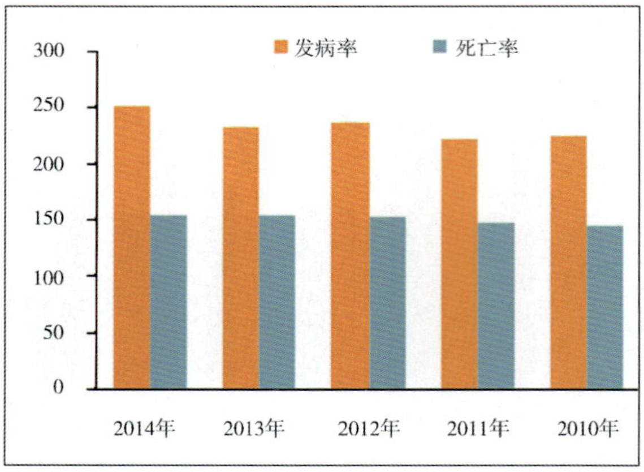

图 3-12 漯河市郾城区 2010—2014 年恶性肿瘤的发病（死亡）率（$1/10^5$）

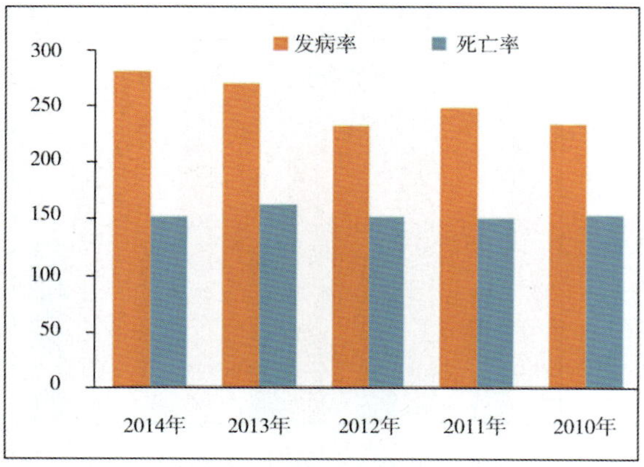

图 3-13 三门峡市 2010—2014 年恶性肿瘤的发病（死亡）率（$1/10^5$）

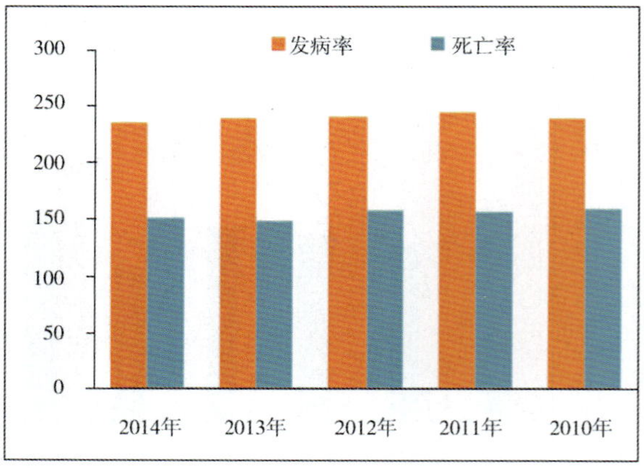

图 3-14 虞城县 2010—2014 年恶性肿瘤的发病（死亡）率（$1/10^5$）

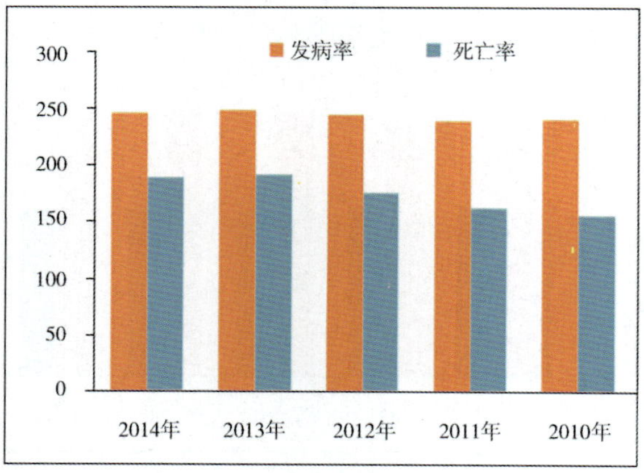

图 3-15 郸城县 2010—2014 年恶性肿瘤的发病（死亡）率（$1/10^5$）

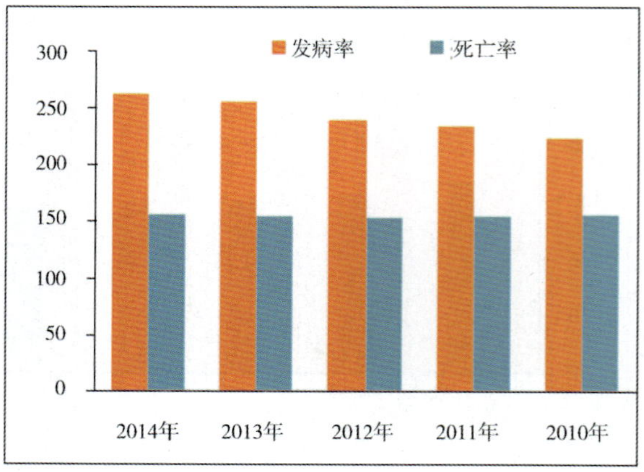

图 3-16 内乡县 2010—2014 年恶性肿瘤的发病（死亡）率（$1/10^5$）

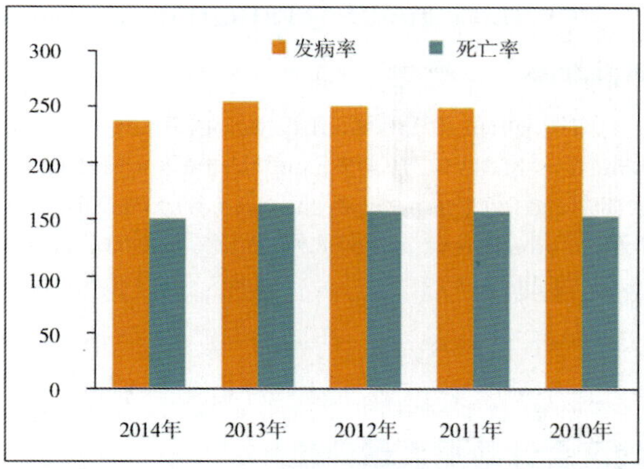

图 3-17 罗山县 2010—2014 年恶性肿瘤的发病(死亡)率($1/10^5$)

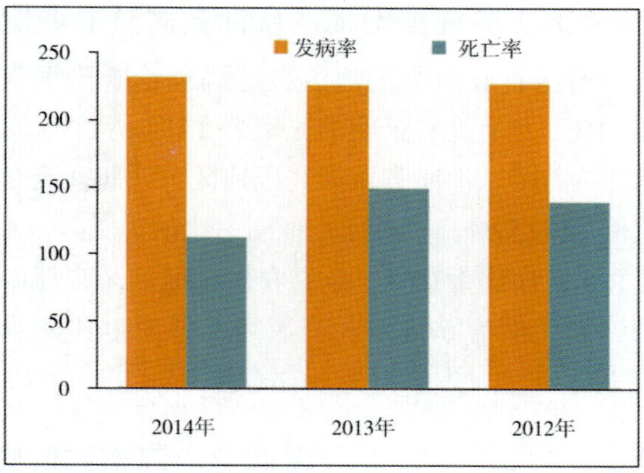

图 3-18 开封县 2012—2014 年恶性肿瘤的发病(死亡)率($1/10^5$)

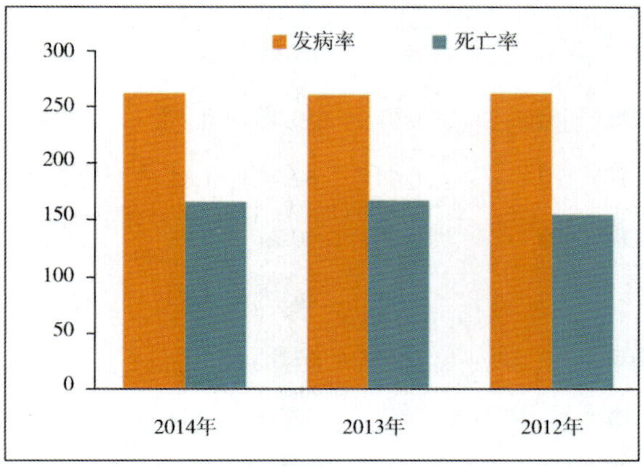

图 3-19 鹤壁市 2012—2014 年恶性肿瘤的发病(死亡)率($1/10^5$)

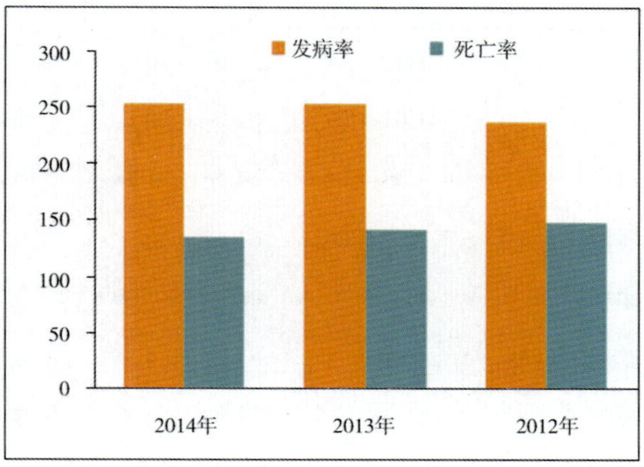

图 3-20 睢县 2012—2014 年恶性肿瘤的发病(死亡)率($1/10^5$)

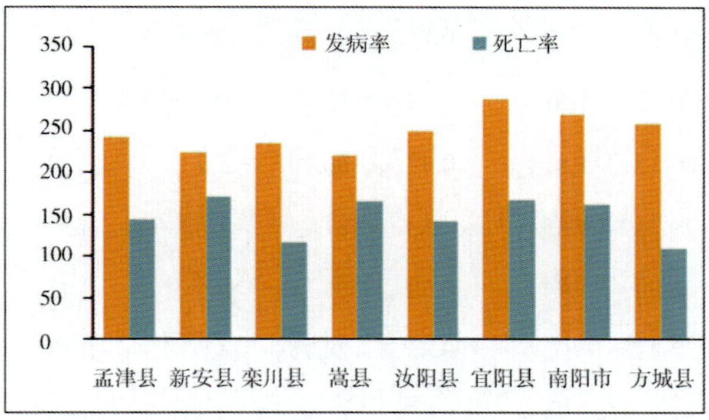

图 3-21 2014 年新增肿瘤登记地区恶性肿瘤的发病(死亡)率($1/10^5$)

（五）肿瘤登记地区合计数据质量评价

河南省肿瘤登记地区合计病理诊断比例为 68.11%，只有死亡证明书比例为 2.18%，死亡 / 发病比为 0.62。河南省城市登记地区合计病理诊断比例为 69.57%，只有死亡证明书比例为 2.44%，死亡 / 发病比为 0.61；全省农村登记地区合计病理诊断比例为 67.82%，只有死亡证明书比例为 2.13%，死亡 / 发病比为 0.62（表 3-7）。

3.5 Data quality evaluation of Henan registries

The general data quality was evaluated and the indicators of MV%, DCO%, and M/I ratio were 68.11%, 2.18% and 0.62, respectively,they were 69.57%,2.44% and 0.61 in urban areas, and 67.82%, 2.13% and 0.62 in rural areas（Table 3-7）.

表 3-7 河南省肿瘤登记地区合计数据质量评价

部位	ICD-10	全省合计			城市			农村		
	编码范围	MV%	DCO%	M/I	MV%	DCO%	M/I	MV%	DCO%	M/I
唇	C00	66.67	0	0.37	100	0	0	65.52	0	0.38
舌	C01–C02	64.04	0	0.46	86.96	0	0.61	56.06	0	0.41
口	C03–C06	64.14	1.38	0.46	70.27	0	0.49	62.04	1.85	0.44
唾液腺	C07–C08	61.47	0	0.24	65.38	0	0.19	60.24	0	0.25
扁桃体	C09	46.15	7.69	0.77	0	0	—	46.15	7.69	0.77
其他的口咽	C10	67.39	4.35	0.59	66.67	0	0.83	67.5	5	0.55
鼻咽	C11	72.53	3.3	0.46	71.43	4.76	0.5	72.73	3.03	0.45
喉咽	C12–C13	60.98	0	0.56	50	0	0.3	64.52	0	0.65
咽，部位不明	C14	47.62	2.38	0.86	87.5	0	1	38.24	2.94	0.82
食管	C15	79.64	1.45	0.69	75.11	3.93	0.65	80.37	1.05	0.69
胃	C16	81.8	1.49	0.72	77.78	2.56	0.65	82.44	1.32	0.73
小肠	C17	70.22	1.57	0.42	75.61	0	0.59	69.42	1.8	0.4
结肠	C18	80.13	1.81	0.47	80.19	2.2	0.59	80.12	1.7	0.44
直肠	C19–C20	79.76	1.65	0.53	81.94	1.62	0.57	79.2	1.66	0.52
肛门	C21	66.99	1.94	0.52	64.29	0	0.43	67.42	2.25	0.54
肝脏	C22	32.23	4.02	0.84	28.75	4.03	0.78	32.9	4.02	0.85
胆囊及其他	C23–C24	54.1	2.94	0.67	51.92	4.81	0.63	54.51	2.58	0.67
胰腺	C25	50.75	4.08	0.75	62.42	1.34	0.88	47.78	4.78	0.72
鼻、鼻窦及其他	C30–C31	57.33	1.33	0.43	72.73	9.09	0.18	54.69	0	0.47
喉	C32	60.26	2.93	0.52	65.63	6.25	0.75	59.64	2.55	0.49
气管、支气管、肺	C33–C34	60.98	2.88	0.75	72.27	2.36	0.74	58.38	3	0.75

续表

部位	ICD-10 编码范围	全省合计			城市			农村		
		MV%	DCO%	M/I	MV%	DCO%	M/I	MV%	DCO%	M/I
其他的胸腔器官	C37–C38	47.22	2.08	0.51	59.46	2.7	0.54	42.99	1.87	0.5
骨	C40–C41	43.74	2.24	0.5	38.67	4	0.65	44.57	1.96	0.48
皮肤的黑色素瘤	C43	100	0	0.44	100	0	0.71	100	0	0.4
其他的皮肤	C44	75.51	2.04	0.47	75	2.27	0.48	75.62	1.99	0.47
间皮瘤	C45	100	0	0.78	100	0	1	100	0	0.67
卡波西肉瘤	C46	100	0	0	0	0	—	100	0	0
周围神经，其他结缔组织软组织	C47;C49	62.92	0	0.29	66.67	0	0.24	61.76	0	0.31
乳房	C50	86.47	0.59	0.29	81.95	0.85	0.33	87.53	0.53	0.28
外阴	C51	64	0	0.32	100	0	1.5	60.87	0	0.22
阴道	C52	38.1	4.76	0.57	50	0	0.5	36.84	5.26	0.58
子宫颈	C53	84.37	0.92	0.3	82.77	0.37	0.34	84.66	1.02	0.29
子宫体	C54	81.13	0.45	0.25	82.41	0	0.36	80.88	0.53	0.22
子宫，部位不明	C55	53.8	3.51	0.5	81.48	0	0.37	48.61	4.17	0.52
卵巢	C56	72.96	1.42	0.43	72.32	0	0.46	73.09	1.72	0.42
其他的女性生殖器	C57	37.04	11.11	0.41	80	0	0.4	27.27	13.64	0.41
胎盘	C58	77.78	0	0.22	0	0	—	77.78	0	0.22
阴茎	C60	68.42	0	0.26	85.71	0	0.57	66	0	0.22
前列腺	C61	55.88	2.65	0.56	68.27	0.96	0.44	50.42	3.39	0.62
睾丸	C62	55.81	0	0.47	70	0	0.7	51.52	0	0.39
其他的男性生殖器	C63	55.56	0	0.56	100	0	0	50	0	0.63
肾	C64	57.32	1.49	0.43	73.33	0	0.5	51.68	2.01	0.4
肾盂	C65	57.14	1.79	0.5	50	0	0.36	59.52	2.38	0.55
输尿管	C66	58.14	0	0.67	87.5	0	0.69	40.74	0	0.67
膀胱	C67	62.41	2.27	0.45	69.7	4.55	0.42	60.23	1.59	0.45
其他的泌尿器官	C68	45.83	4.17	0.42	61.54	7.69	0.38	27.27	0	0.45
眼	C69	47.37	0	0.24	75	0	0.13	40	0	0.27
脑、神经系统	C70–C72	28.2	3.69	0.59	41.01	1.38	0.51	25.86	4.11	0.6
甲状腺	C73	79.15	0.62	0.16	80	0	0.21	78.93	0.79	0.15

续表

部位	ICD-10	全省合计			城市			农村		
	编码范围	MV%	DCO%	M/I	MV%	DCO%	M/I	MV%	DCO%	M/I
肾上腺	C74	50	6.52	0.5	44.44	0	0.33	51.35	8.11	0.54
其他的内分泌腺	C75	45.76	1.69	0.25	36.36	0	0.18	47.92	2.08	0.27
霍奇金病	C81	100	0	0.51	100	0	0.67	100	0	0.44
非霍奇金淋巴瘤	C82–C85;C96	98.8	0.72	0.59	97.22	1.39	0.56	99.13	0.58	0.6
免疫增生性疾病	C88	100	0	1	100	0	0	100	0	2
多发性骨髓瘤	C90	99.13	0.87	0.55	100	0	0.32	98.96	1.04	0.59
淋巴样白血病	C91	100	0	0.68	100	0	0.55	100	0	0.73
髓样白血病	C92–C94	100	0	0.54	100	0	0.36	100	0	0.59
白血病，未特指	C95	95.7	1.38	0.57	95.05	3.96	0.7	95.82	0.91	0.54
其他的或未指明部位	O&U	46.25	6.9	0.37	20	8.57	0.59	49.81	6.67	0.34
骨髓增殖性疾病骨髓	MPD	100	0	0.21	100	0	0.2	100	0	0.21
骨髓增生异常综合征	MDS	100	0	1.42	100	0	1	100	0	1.71
合计	ALL	68.15	2.18	0.62	69.6	2.44	0.61	67.85	2.13	0.62
所有部位除外C44	ALL but C44	68.11	2.18	0.62	69.57	2.44	0.61	67.82	2.13	0.62

第四章　河南省登记地区恶性肿瘤发病与死亡

Chapter 4　Incidences and Mortalities in Henan registries

2014 年河南省共有 32 个市县肿瘤登记处提交了肿瘤登记发病和死亡数据，27 个登记处数据质量控制指标符合中国肿瘤登记年报的质量标准要求。全省各登记处数据合并得到的河南省肿瘤发病与死亡的统计指标基本反映了我省人群恶性肿瘤的流行情况。

一、河南省肿瘤登记地区覆盖人口

2014 年，登记地区人口为 21 044 835 人（其中，男性 10 851 503 人，女性 10 193 332 人），约占河南省 2014 年人口总数的 19.73%（2014 年河南省国民经济和社会发展统计公报：10 662 万）。其中城市地区为 3 435 270 人，占登记人口的 16.32%；农村地区为 17 609 565 人，占 83.68%（表 4-1，图 4-1a ~ 图 4-1c）。

A total of 32 cancer registries submitted cancer registration data to HNCCR in 2014 and 27 satisfied data quallity requirements by national cancer registration annual report. The data can basically reflect cancer prevalence in Henan Province.

1. Population coverage in Henan cancer registries

The population in Henan Province cancer registration areas in 2014 was 21 044 835 (10 851 503 males and 10 193 332 females), accounting for 19.73% of the provincial population, 2014, with 3 435 270 (16.32 %) in urban areas and 17 609 565 (83.68%) in rural areas (Table 4-1, Figure 4-1a~Figure 4-1c).

表 4-1　河南省肿瘤登记地区覆盖人口（2014 年）

年龄组	全省			城市			农村		
	合计	男性	女性	合计	男性	女性	合计	男性	女性
合计	21 044 835	10 851 503	10 193 332	3 435 270	1 757 181	1 678 089	17 609 565	9 094 322	8 515 243
0-	256 123	136 121	120 002	40 018	21 073	18 945	216 105	115 048	101 057
1-	1 198 165	653 382	544 783	179 824	96 425	83 399	1 018 341	556 957	461 384
5-	1 418 466	763 129	655 337	217 728	117 000	100 728	1 200 738	646 129	554 609
10-	1 324 354	717 250	607 104	193 974	105 058	88 916	1 130 380	612 192	518 188
15-	1 470 297	764 838	705 459	232 818	117 677	115 141	1 237 479	647 161	590 318
20-	1 843 918	950 578	893 340	318 724	162 268	156 456	1 525 194	788 310	736 884

续表

年龄组	全省			城市			农村		
	合计	男性	女性	合计	男性	女性	合计	男性	女性
25–	1 824 500	934 377	890 123	295 456	150 899	144 557	1 529 044	783 478	745 566
30–	1 534 735	788 972	745 763	242 284	121 375	120 909	1 292 451	667 597	624 854
35–	1 603 915	837 123	766 792	283 574	147 255	136 319	1 320 341	689 868	630 473
40–	1 708 216	883 772	824 444	310 606	159 722	150 884	1 397 610	724 050	673 560
45–	1 668 618	845 012	823 606	287 400	146 129	141 271	1 381 218	698 883	682 335
50–	1 284 794	653 224	631 570	217 120	110 561	106 559	1067 674	542 663	525 011
55–	1 152 518	586 964	565 554	200 107	99 684	100 423	952 411	487 280	465 131
60–	934 282	473634	460 648	144 759	72 999	71 760	789 523	400 635	388 888
65–	652 060	326 155	325 905	99 777	49 404	50 373	552 283	276 751	275 532
70–	481 643	237 935	243 708	75 807	36 892	38 915	405 836	201 043	204 793
75–	363 158	169 448	193 710	56 476	26 514	29 962	306 682	142 934	163 748
80–	206 329	88 493	117 836	26 517	11 642	14 875	179 812	76 851	102 961
85+	118 744	41 096	77 648	12 301	4 604	7 697	106 443	36492	69 951

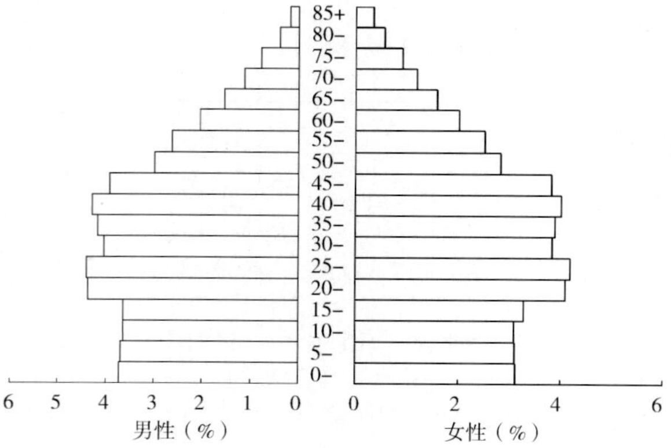

图 4–1a　河南省肿瘤登记地区人口金字塔

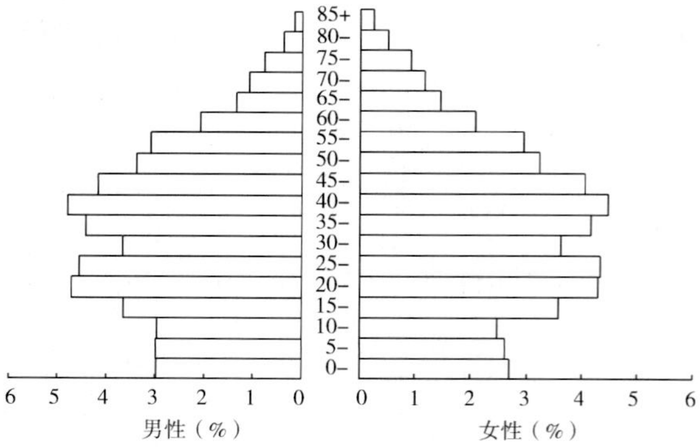

图 4–1b　河南省城市肿瘤登记地区人口金字塔

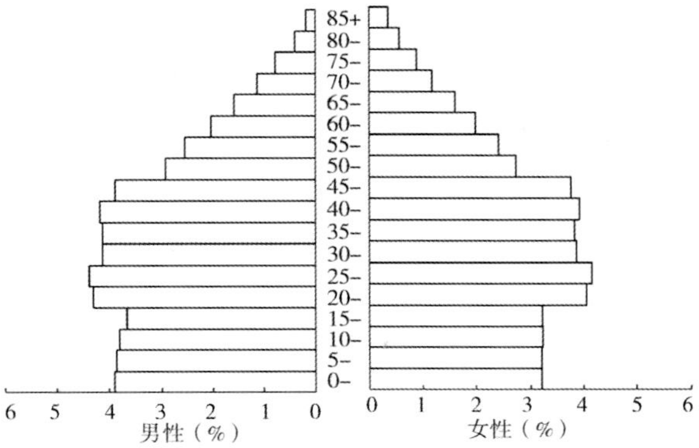

图 4-1c 河南省农村肿瘤登记地区人口金字塔

二、恶性肿瘤发病（ICD-10：C00-C96）

（一）全部恶性肿瘤（ICD-10：C00-C96）发病情况

河南省肿瘤登记地区 2014 年报告癌症新发病例数合计 53 200 例，其中男性 29 684 例，女性 23 516 例。城市地区上报 8 969 例，占 16.86%；农村地区报告癌症新发病 44 231 例，农村地区占 83.14%。

河南省肿瘤登记地区恶性肿瘤发病率为 252.79 /10^5（男性 273.55/10^5，女性 230.70 /10^5），中标率为 205.27/10^5，世标率为 203.78 /10^5，累积率（0~74 岁）为 24.17%。

城市地区发病率为 261.09 /10^5（男性 290.47/10^5，女性 230.32/10^5），中标率为 219.31/10^5，世标率为 216.64/10^5，累积率（0 ~ 74 岁）为 24.52%。

农村地区发病率为 251.18/10^5（男性 270.28/10^5，女性 230.77/10^5），中标率为 203.35/10^5，世标率为 202.16/10^5，累积率（0~74 岁）为 24.12%。

城市与农村相比，城市男性及男女合计发病率、中标率、世标率、累积率均高于农村地区，城市女性中标率、世标率高于农村女性，发病率及累积率略低于农村女性（表 4-2）。

2. Cancer incidences (ICD-10: C00-C96)

2.1 Incidences of all cancers (ICD-10: C00-C96)

In 2014, there were a total of 53 200 (Male: 29 684, Female: 23 516) new cancer cases in Henan cancer registration areas, among which 8 969 (16.86%) were from urban areas and 44 231 (83.14%) from rural areas.

The incidence rate of all cancer sites was 252.79/10^5(273.55/10^5 for males and 230.70/10^5 for females). The ASR China was 205.27/10^5 and ASR World was 203.78/10^5. The cumulative rate (0~74 years old) for both sexes was 24.17%.

The incidence rate of all cancers in urban areas was 261.09/10^5 (290.47/10^5 for males and 230.32/10^5 for females). The ASR China was 219.31/10^5 and ASR World was 216.64/10^5. The cumulative rate (0~74 years old) for both sexes was 24.52%.

The incidence rate of all cancer sites in rural areas was 251.18/10^5 (270.28/10^5 for males and 230.77/10^5 for females). The ASR China was 203.35/10^5 and ASR World was 202.16/10^5. The cumulative rate (0~74 years old) for both sexes was 24.12%.

In urban areas, the crude incidence rates, ASR China, ASR World and cumulative rate for males and both genders of all cancer sites were higher than those in the rural areas. For females, the ASR China, ASR World in the urban areaswere higher than those in the rural areas, whilethe crude incidence and cumulative rate in the urban areas were slightly lower than those in the rural areas (Table4-2).

表 4-2 河南省肿瘤登记地区全部恶性肿瘤（ICD-10: C00-C96）发病主要指标

地区	性别	发病数（人）	发病率 (1/10^5)	中标率 (1/10^5)	世标率 (1/10^5)	累积率 0-74 (%)
全省	合计	53 200	252.79	205.27	203.78	24.17
	男性	29 684	273.55	231.62	232.51	28.02
	女性	23 516	230.70	181.91	178.08	20.37
城市	合计	8 969	261.09	219.31	216.64	24.52
	男性	5 104	290.47	257.81	257.44	28.90
	女性	3 865	230.32	186.38	181.75	20.30
农村	合计	44 231	251.18	203.35	202.16	24.12
	男性	24 580	270.28	227.65	228.89	27.87
	女性	19 651	230.77	181.55	177.93	20.39

（二）全部恶性肿瘤（ICD-10：C00-C96）年龄别发病率

河南省肿瘤登记地区恶性肿瘤年龄别发病率在 34 岁以下年龄组低于 $45/10^5$，35 岁以上年龄组发病率快速升高，在 80 岁年龄组时达到最高峰，为 1 698.74 $/10^5$，85 岁及以上年龄组发病率有所下降。男、女性年龄别发病率的年龄变化趋势基本相同，二者均在 35 岁年龄组时呈现快速上升，在 80 岁年龄组时达到最高峰，其中男性发病率为 2 265.72/10^5，女性发病率为 1 272.96/10^5，85 岁及以上年龄组显现下降趋势。

河南省城市登记地区年龄别发病率在 35 岁以下较低，35 岁以后呈现明显升高，男性在 85 岁年龄组达到最高，发病率为 4 126.85/10^5。女性在 85 岁年龄组时达到最高，发病率为 1 808.40/10^5。

河南省农村登记地区的年龄别发病率变化模式与城市大体一致。发病率最高年龄组为 80 岁，发病率为 1 542.17 /10^5，85 岁之后发病率开始下降。农村男性和女性的年龄别发病率高峰都是 80 岁，发病率分别为 2 006.48/10^5 和 1 195.60/10 万。

2.2 Age-specific incidences of all cancer sites (ICD-10：C00-C96)

The age-specific incidence rate of all cancer sites in Henan cancer registration areas was lower than $45/10^5$ at 0~34 age group. It increased dramatically after 35 years old, reaching the peak at the age group of 80-, with a rate of 1 698.74/10^5, and then decreased slightly after 85+ years old. The age-specific incidence rate for males is similar to that for females, increasing dramatically after 35 years old and reached the peak at the age group of 80-, with a peak rate of 2 265.72/10^5 for males and 1 272.96/10^5 for females, and then decreased slightly after 85+ years old.

The age-specific incidence rate in urban areas was relatively low before 34, it increased dramatically after 35 years old. The peak incidence rates were at the age group of 85-. with the peak rates were of 4 126.85/10^5 formales and 1808.40/10^5 for females.

The trend of age-specific incidence in rural areas was similar to that in urban areas. It reached the peak at the age group of 80- and decreased after 85 years old for both males and females. The peak rates were 1 542.17/10^5 for both genders,2 006.48/10^5 for males and 1 195.60 /10^5 for females.

When compare the age-specific incidence rates between males and females, they were slightly lower for males than those for females at the age groups of 20- to 54-, while obviously higher for males than those for females after 55 years old.

性别间的年龄别发病率比较显示在20~54岁年龄组时，女性的发病率轻微高于男性，55岁以后则发生逆转，男性的发病率明显高于女性，城市和农村登记地区男、女性的年龄别发病率的分布特征均基本一致。

城乡间的年龄别发病率比较显示：69岁以下大部分年龄组城市地区略微低于农村地区，70岁组及以上各年龄组城市地区的发病率明显高于农村地区；男性和女性的年龄别发病率的分布特征基本一致（表4–3，图4–2a~图4–2d）。

This characteristic was seen in both urban areas and rural areas.

When compare the age-specific incidence rates between the urban areas and the rural areas, the age-specific rates in urban areas were slightly lower than those in rural areas before 69 years old and reversely, they were obviously higher in urban areas than those in rural areas after 70 years old. There were similar characteristics in both males and females (Table 4–3, Figures 4–2a~Figure4–2d).

表4–3　河南省肿瘤登记地区恶性肿瘤年龄别发病率（$1/10^5$）

年龄组	全省			城市			农村		
	合计	男性	女性	合计	男性	女性	合计	男性	女性
合计	252.79	273.55	230.70	261.09	290.47	230.32	251.18	270.28	230.77
0–	7.03	7.35	6.67	10.00	14.24	5.28	6.48	6.08	6.93
1–	10.10	10.25	9.91	5.00	3.11	7.19	11.00	11.49	10.40
5–	9.24	11.79	6.26	6.43	7.69	4.96	9.74	12.54	6.49
10–	9.14	10.04	8.07	6.70	4.76	9.00	9.55	10.94	7.91
15–	9.39	9.41	9.36	5.15	5.95	4.34	10.18	10.04	10.33
20–	15.56	11.68	19.70	8.79	7.40	10.23	16.98	12.56	21.71
25–	25.43	18.84	32.36	24.37	17.89	31.13	25.64	19.02	32.59
30–	44.11	30.17	58.87	44.16	32.13	56.24	44.10	29.81	59.37
35–	74.63	55.43	95.59	72.64	47.54	99.77	75.06	57.11	94.69
40–	144.71	112.25	179.51	128.14	100.17	157.74	148.40	114.91	184.39
45–	234.09	206.39	262.50	204.94	173.13	237.84	240.15	213.34	267.61
50–	353.75	348.43	359.26	363.39	358.17	368.81	351.79	346.44	357.33
55–	572.49	637.01	505.52	520.22	595.88	445.12	583.47	645.42	518.56
60–	918.46	1 067.28	765.44	875.94	1 024.67	724.64	926.26	1 075.04	772.97
65–	1 146.37	1 441.65	850.86	1 142.55	1 477.61	813.93	1 147.06	1 435.23	857.61
70–	1 267.95	1 633.64	910.93	1 494.58	1 921.83	1 089.55	1 225.62	1 580.76	876.98
75–	1 422.80	1 846.58	1 052.09	1 921.17	2 587.31	1 331.69	1 331.02	1 709.18	1 000.93
80–	1 698.74	2 265.72	1 272.96	2 760.49	3 976.98	1 808.40	1 542.17	2 006.48	1 195.60
85–	1 423.23	2 080.49	1 075.37	2 674.58	4 126.85	1 805.90	1 278.62	1 822.32	994.98

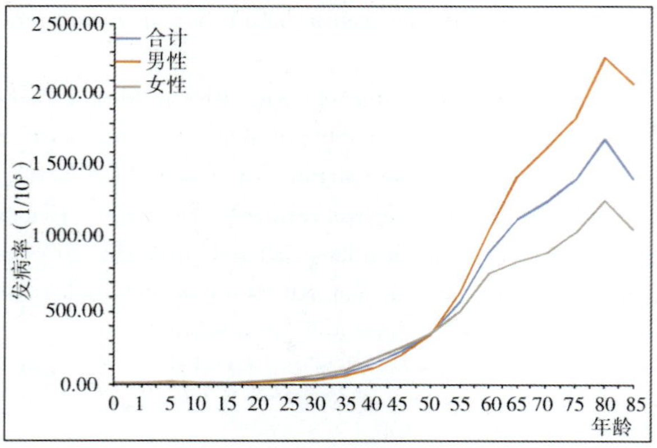

图 4–2a　河南省肿瘤登记地区恶性肿瘤年龄别发病率

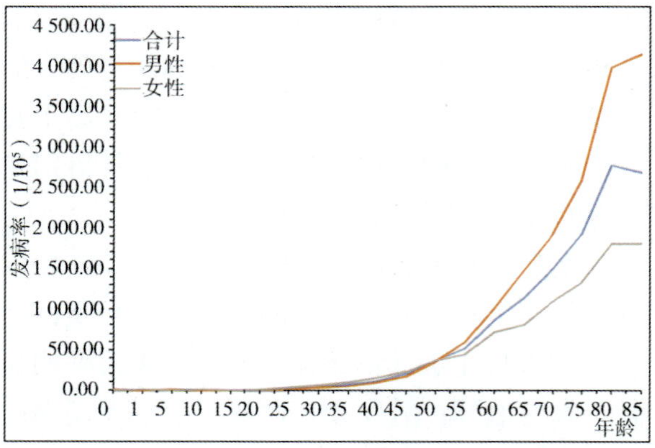

图 4–2b　城市肿瘤登记地区恶性肿瘤年龄别发病率

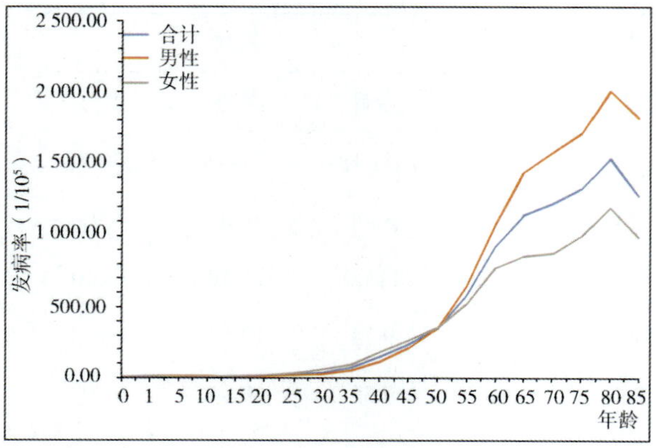

图 4–2c　农村肿瘤登记地区恶性肿瘤年龄别发病率

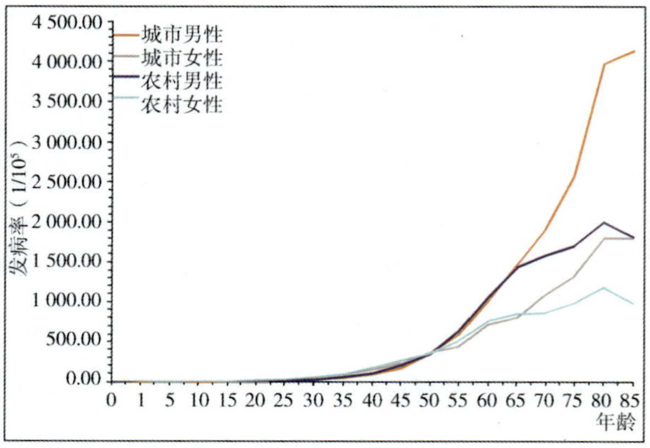

图 4–2d　河南省城市和农村肿瘤登记地区恶性肿瘤年龄别发病率

（三）河南省前 10 位恶性肿瘤发病情况

2014年河南省地区恶性肿瘤发病第1位的是肺癌，其次为胃癌、食管癌、肝癌和乳腺癌，前10位恶性肿瘤占全部恶性肿瘤的82.93%。男性恶性肿瘤发病第1位的是肺癌，其次为胃癌、食管癌、肝癌和结直肠肛门癌，男性前10位恶性肿瘤占全部恶性肿瘤的87.82 %；女性恶性肿瘤发病第1位的是乳腺癌，其次为肺癌、食管癌、胃癌和子宫颈癌，女性前10位恶性肿瘤占全部恶性肿瘤的82.01 %（表4–4，图4–3a~图4–3f）。

2.3 Incidence of the 10 most common cancers

In Henan cancer registration areas in 2014, lung cancer was the most common cancer followed by cancers of stomach, esophagus, liver and breast. The 10 most common cancers accounted for 82.93% of all cancers. For males, lung cancer was the most common cancer followed by cancers of stomach, esophagus, liver and colorectum. The 10 most common cancers accounted for 87.82% of all cancers in males. For females, breast cancer was the most common cancer followed by cancers of lung, esophagus, stomach and cervix. The 10 most common cancers accounted for 82.01% of all cancers (Table 4–4, Figure 4–3a ~ Figure4–3f) .

表 4-4　河南省肿瘤登记地区前 10 位恶性肿瘤发病主要指标

顺位	合计 部位	合计 发病率 (1/10^5)	合计 构成 (%)	合计 中标率 (1/10^5)	男性 部位	男性 发病率 (1/10^5)	男性 构成 (%)	男性 中标率 (1/10^5)	女性 部位	女性 发病率 (1/10^5)	女性 构成 (%)	女性 中标率 (1/10^5)
1	气管、支气管、肺 (C33–C34)	48.28	19.10	38.41	气管、支气管、肺 (C33–C34)	64.88	23.72	54.57	乳房 (C50)	36.39	15.77	30.29
2	胃 (C16)	39.32	15.55	31.30	胃 (C16)	54.54	19.94	45.70	气管、支气管、肺 (C33–C34)	30.61	13.27	23.00
3	食管 (C15)	38.06	15.06	30.03	食管 (C15)	45.78	16.74	38.28	食管 (C15)	29.84	12.94	22.20
4	肝脏 (C22)	26.23	10.38	21.08	肝脏 (C22)	34.98	12.79	29.49	胃 (C16)	23.11	10.02	17.40
5	乳房 (C50)	36.39	6.97	30.29	结直肠肛门 (C18–C21)	16.85	6.16	14.27	子宫颈 (C53)	17.07	7.40	14.37
6	结直肠肛门 (C18–C21)	16.21	6.41	13.04	脑及中枢神经系统 (C70–C72)	6.50	2.38	5.75	肝脏 (C22)	16.91	7.33	12.68
7	子宫颈 (C53)	17.07	3.27	14.37	白血病 (C91–C95)	5.63	2.06	5.27	结直肠肛门 (C18–C21)	15.53	6.73	11.88
8	脑及中枢神经系统 (C70–C72)	6.69	2.65	5.71	膀胱 (C67)	3.97	1.45	3.36	脑及中枢神经系统 (C70–C72)	6.90	2.99	5.68
9	白血病 (C91–C95)	5.12	2.03	4.70	胰腺 (C25)	3.91	1.43	3.31	子宫体 (C54)	6.60	2.86	5.31
10	甲状腺 (C73)	3.81	1.51	3.38	前列腺 (C61)	3.13	1.15	2.66	卵巢 (C56)	6.24	2.70	5.17
	前 10 位	209.60	82.93		前 10 位	240.16	87.82	202.67	前 10 位	189.20	82.01	147.97

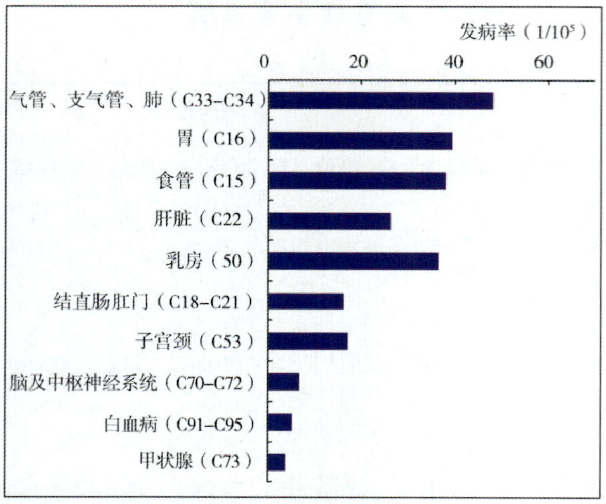

图 4–3a　河南省肿瘤登记地区前 10 位恶性肿瘤发病率

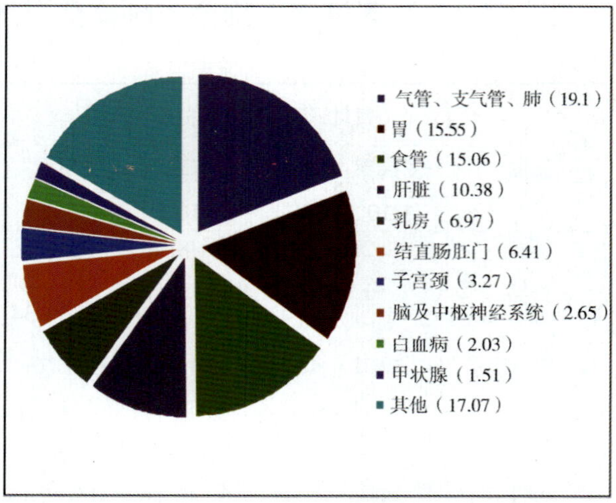

图 4–3d　河南省肿瘤登记地区恶性肿瘤发病构成 (%)

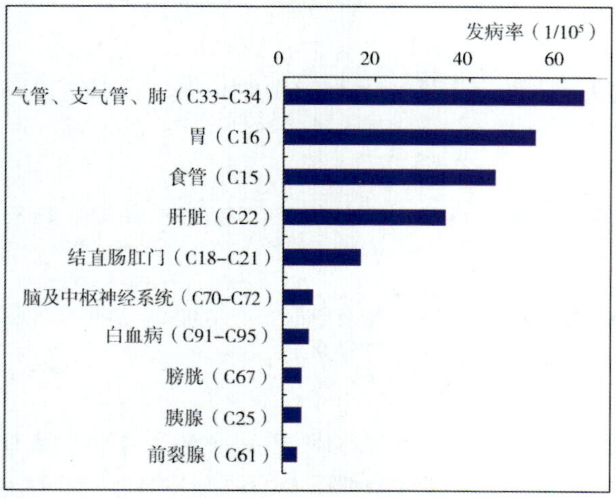

图 4–3b　河南省肿瘤登记地区男性前 10 位恶性肿瘤发病率

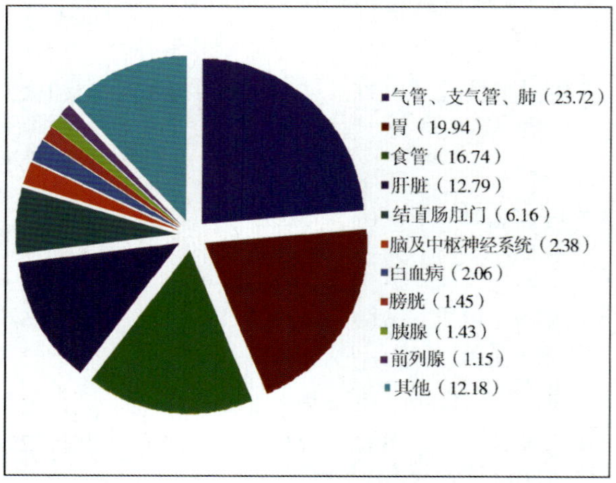

图 4–3e　河南省肿瘤登记地区男性恶性肿瘤发病构成 (%)

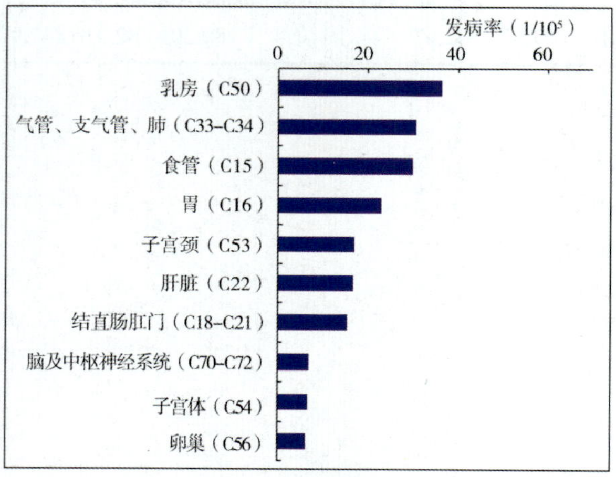

图 4–3c　河南省肿瘤登记地区女性前 10 位恶性肿瘤发病率

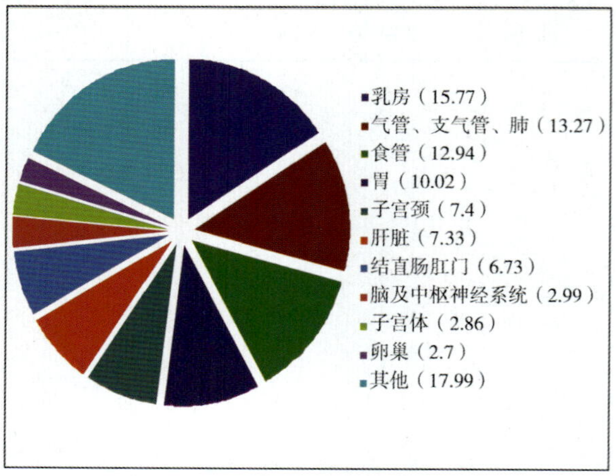

图 4–3f　河南省肿瘤登记地区女性恶性肿瘤发病构成 (%)

（四）城市地区前 10 位恶性肿瘤发病情况

2014 年河南省城市地区恶性肿瘤发病第 1 位的是肺癌，其次为胃癌、食管癌、肝癌和乳腺癌，前 10 位恶性肿瘤占全部恶性肿瘤的 81.67%。男性恶性肿瘤发病第 1 位的是肺癌，其次为胃癌、食管癌、肝癌和结直肠肛门癌，男性前 10 位恶性肿瘤占全部恶性肿瘤的 87.85 %；女性恶性肿瘤发病第 1 位的是乳腺癌，其次为肺癌、食管癌、胃癌和结直肠肛门癌，女性前 10 位恶性肿瘤占全部恶性肿瘤的 80.95 %（表 4-5，图 4-4a~ 图 4-4f）。

2.4 Incidence of the 10 most common cancers in urban areas

In Henan urban cancer registration areas in 2014, lung cancer was the most common cancer followed by cancers of stomach, esophagus, liver and breast. The 10 most common cancers accounted for 81.67 % of all cancers. For males, lung cancer was the most common cancer followed by cancers of stomach, esophagus, liver and colorectum. The 10 most common cancers accounted for 87.85 % of all cancers in males. For females, breast cancer was the most common cancer followed by cancers of lung, esophagus, stomach and colorectum. The 10 most common cancers accounted for 80.95 % of all cancers (Table 4-5, Figure 4-4a ~ Figure4-4f) .

表4-5　河南省城市肿瘤登记地区前10位恶性肿瘤发病主要指标

顺位	合计				男性				女性			
	部位	发病率 $(1/10^5)$	构成 (%)	中标率 $(1/10^5)$	部位	发病率 $(1/10^5)$	构成 (%)	中标率 $(1/10^5)$	部位	发病率 $(1/10^5)$	构成 (%)	中标率 $(1/10^5)$
1	气管、支气管、肺 (C33–C34)	55.43	21.23	46.34	气管、支气管、肺 (C33–C34)	77.62	26.72	68.94	乳房 (C50)	42.25	18.34	34.50
2	胃 (C16)	33.01	12.64	27.63	胃 (C16)	46.32	15.95	41.10	气管、支气管、肺 (C33–C34)	32.18	13.97	25.50
3	食管 (C15)	32.63	12.50	27.35	食管 (C15)	41.66	14.34	36.92	食管 (C15)	23.18	10.06	18.25
4	肝脏 (C22)	26.02	9.97	21.58	肝脏 (C22)	36.65	12.62	32.00	胃 (C16)	19.07	8.28	15.11
5	乳房 (C50)	42.25	7.91	34.50	结直肠肛门 (C18–C21)	22.19	7.64	19.58	结直肠肛门 (C18–C21)	18.65	8.10	14.84
6	结直肠肛门 (C18–C21)	20.46	7.84	17.03	白血病 (C91–C95)	7.23	2.49	6.56	子宫颈 (C53)	15.91	6.91	13.33
7	子宫颈 (C53)	15.91	2.98	13.33	脑及中枢神经系统 (C70–C72)	6.54	2.25	5.82	肝脏 (C22)	14.90	6.47	11.63
8	脑及中枢神经系统 (C70–C72)	6.32	2.42	5.40	前列腺 (C61)	5.92	2.04	5.63	甲状腺 (C73)	7.21	3.13	6.44
9	白血病 (C91–C95)	6.11	2.34	5.51	肾及泌尿系统不明 (C64–C66,C68)	5.63	1.94	4.88	卵巢 (C56)	6.67	2.90	5.57
10	甲状腺 (C73)	4.80	1.84	4.27	膀胱 (C67)	5.41	1.86	4.82	子宫体 (C54)	6.44	2.79	5.11
	前 10 位	213.20	81.67		前 10 位	255.18	87.85	226.25	前 10 位	186.46	80.95	150.27

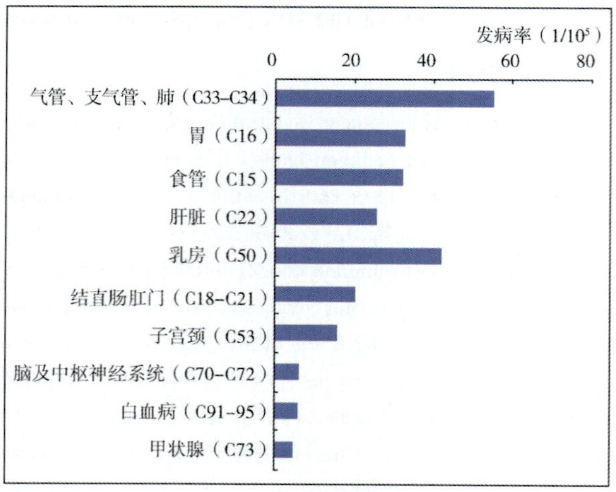

图 4–4a 河南省城市肿瘤登记地区前 10 位恶性肿瘤发病率

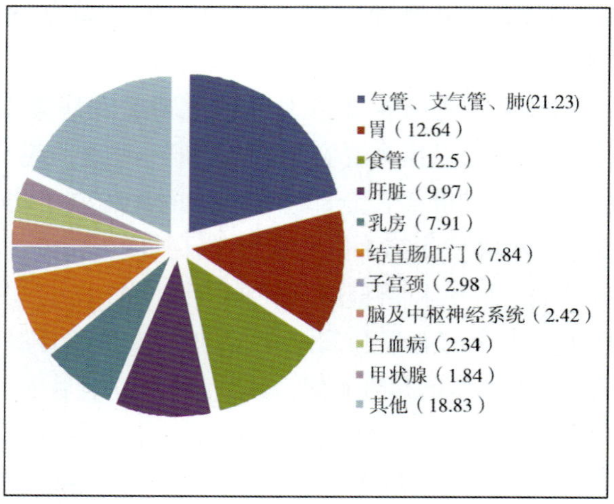

图 4–4d 河南省城市肿瘤登记地区恶性肿瘤发病构成 (%)

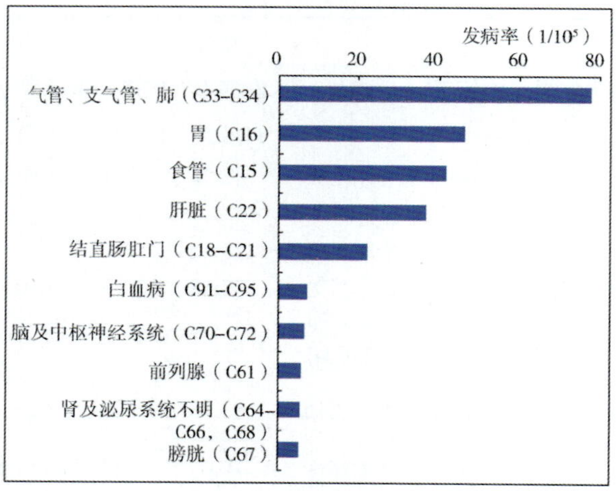

图 4–4b 河南省城市肿瘤登记地区男性前 10 位恶性肿瘤发病率

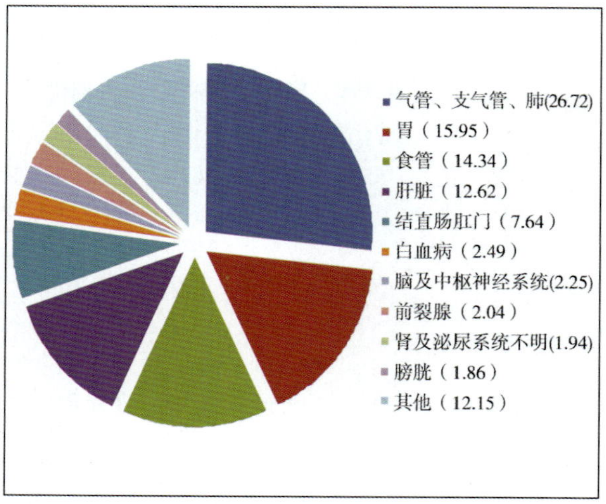

图 4–4e 河南省城市肿瘤登记地区男性恶性肿瘤发病构成 (%)

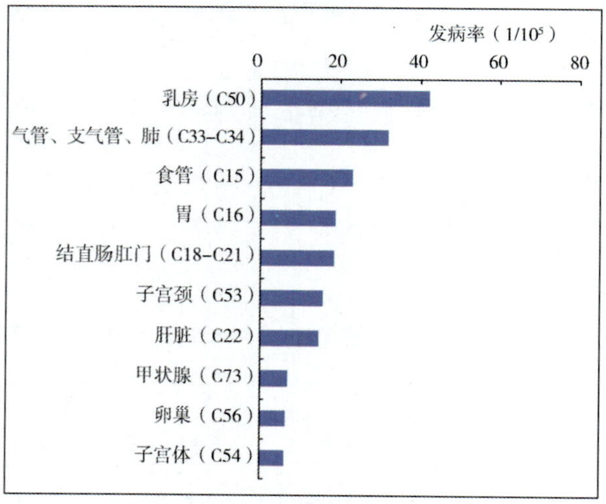

图 4–4c 河南省城市肿瘤登记地区女性前 10 位恶性肿瘤发病率

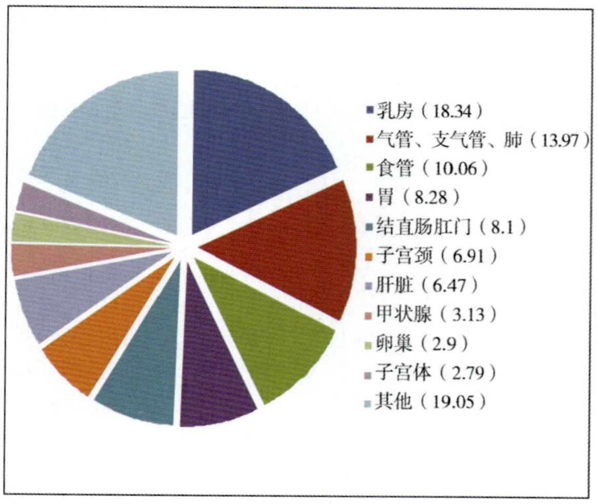

图 4–4f 河南省城市肿瘤登记地区女性恶性肿瘤发病构成 (%)

（五）农村地区前10位恶性肿瘤发病情况

2014 年河南省农村地区恶性肿瘤发病第 1 位的是肺癌，其次为胃癌、食管癌、肝癌和乳腺癌，前 10 位恶性肿瘤占全部恶性肿瘤的 83.17%。男性恶性肿瘤发病第 1 位的是肺癌，其次为胃癌、食管癌、肝癌和结直肠肛门癌，男性前 10 位恶性肿瘤占全部恶性肿瘤的 87.94 %；女性恶性肿瘤发病第 1 位的是乳腺癌，其次为食管癌、肺癌、胃癌和肝癌，女性前 10 位恶性肿瘤占全部恶性肿瘤的 82.33 %（表 4–6，图 4–5a~ 图 4–5f）。

2.5 Incidence of the 10 most common cancers in rural areas

In Henan rural cancer registration areas in 2014, lung cancer was the most common cancer followed by cancers of stomach, esophagus, liver and breast. The 10 most common cancers accounted for 83.17% of all cancers. For males, lung cancer was the most common cancer followed by cancers of stomach, esophagus, liver and colorectum. The top 10 most common cancers accounted for 87.94% of all cancers in males. For females, breast cancer was the most common cancer followed by cancers of esophagus,lung, stomach and liver. The 10 most common cancers accounted for 82.33% of all cancers (Table 4–6, Figure 4–5a~Figure 4–5f) .

表 4–6 河南省农村肿瘤登记地区前 10 位恶性肿瘤发病主要指标

顺位	合计				男性				女性			
	部位	发病率 (1/10^5)	构成 (%)	中标率 (1/10^5)	部位	发病率 (1/10^5)	构成 (%)	中标率 (1/10^5)	部位	发病率 (1/10^5)	构成 (%)	中标率 (1/10^5)
1	气管、支气管、肺 (C33–C34)	46.88	18.67	37.08	气管、支气管、肺 (C33–C34)	62.41	23.09	52.13	乳房 (C50)	35.23	15.27	29.48
2	胃 (C16)	40.55	16.14	32.09	胃 (C16)	56.12	20.76	46.70	食管 (C15)	31.16	13.50	23.06
3	食管 (C15)	39.12	15.58	30.63	食管 (C15)	46.58	17.23	38.62	气管、支气管、肺 (C33–C34)	30.30	13.13	22.61
4	肝脏 (C22)	26.27	10.46	21.06	肝脏 (C22)	34.66	12.82	29.14	胃 (C16)	23.91	10.36	17.88
5	乳房 (C50)	35.23	6.78	29.48	结直肠肛门 (C18–C21)	15.81	5.85	13.41	肝脏 (C22)	17.31	7.50	12.91
6	结直肠肛门 (C18–C21)	15.38	6.12	12.39	脑及中枢神经系统 (C70–C72)	6.49	2.40	5.75	子宫颈 (C53)	17.30	7.50	14.60
7	子宫颈 (C53)	17.30	3.33	14.60	白血病 (C91–C95)	5.32	1.97	5.02	结直肠肛门 (C18–C21)	14.91	6.46	11.38
8	脑及中枢神经系统 (C70–C72)	6.76	2.69	5.78	胰腺 (C25)	3.69	1.37	3.12	脑及中枢神经系统 (C70–C72)	7.06	3.06	5.81
9	白血病 (C91–C95)	4.93	1.96	4.56	膀胱 (C67)	3.69	1.37	3.10	子宫体 (C54)	6.64	2.88	5.36
10	甲状腺 (C73)	3.61	1.44	3.20	骨 (C40–C41)	2.91	1.08	2.63	卵巢 (C56)	6.15	2.67	5.09
	前 10 位	208.90	83.17		前 10 位	237.70	87.94	199.62	前 10 位	189.97	82.33	148.17

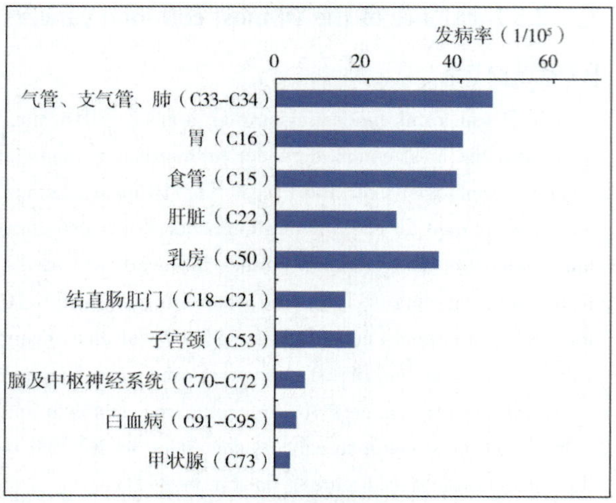

图 4-5a　河南省农村肿瘤登记地区前 10 位恶性肿瘤发病率

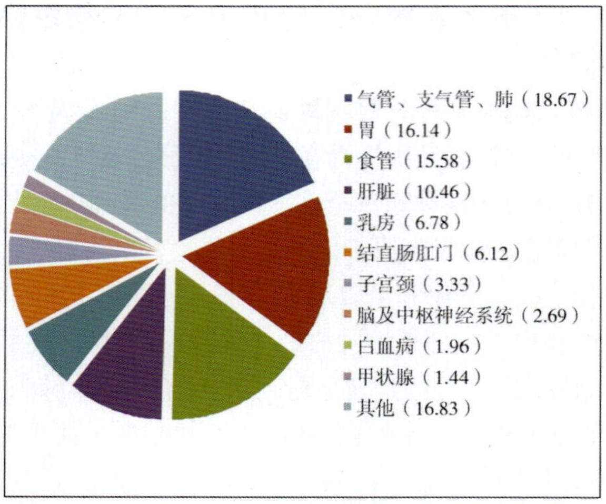

图 4-5d　河南省农村肿瘤登记地区恶性肿瘤发病构成 (%)

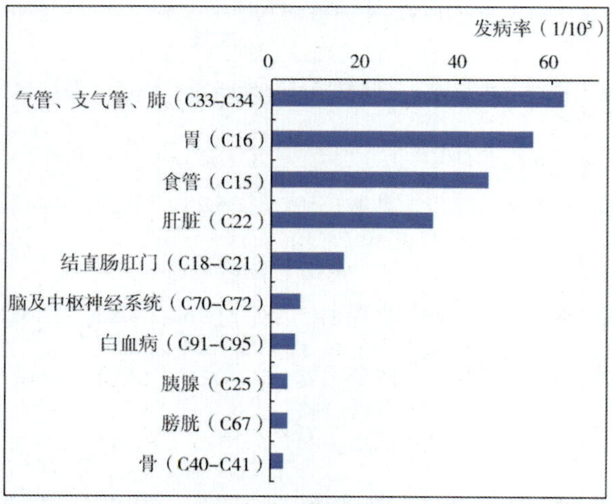

图 4-5b　河南省农村肿瘤登记地区男性前 10 位恶性肿瘤发病率

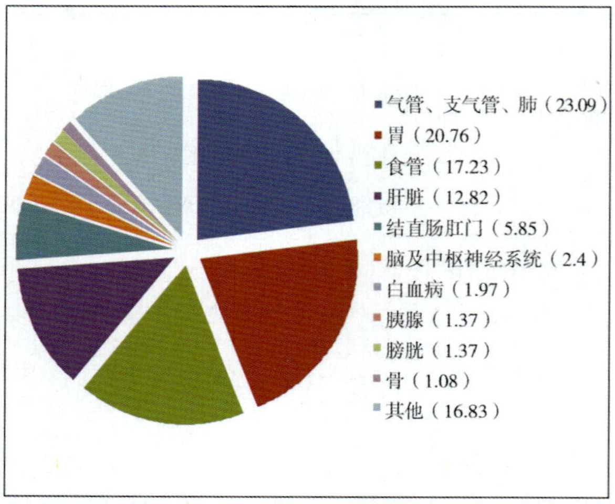

图 4-5e　河南省农村肿瘤登记地区男性恶性肿瘤发病构成 (%)

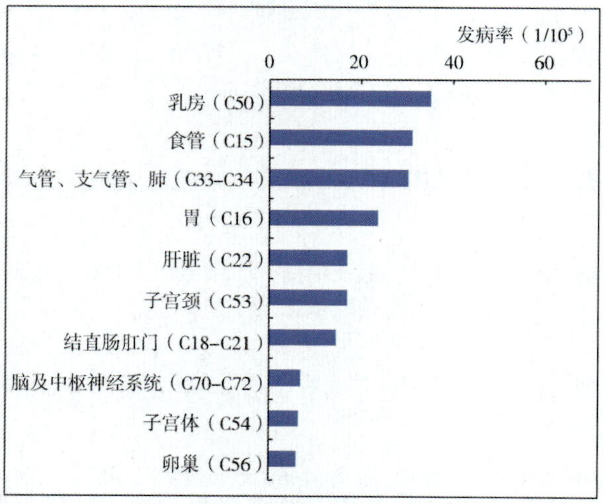

图 4-5c　河南省农村肿瘤登记地区女性前 10 位恶性肿瘤发病率

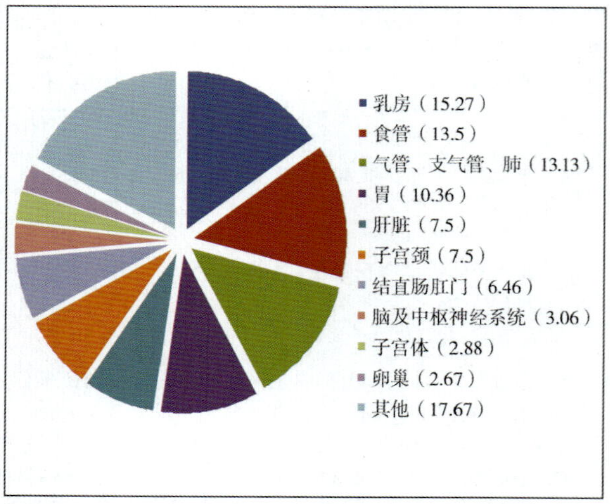

图 4-5f　河南省农村肿瘤登记地区女性恶性肿瘤发病构成 (%)

三、恶性肿瘤死亡(ICD-10：C00-C96)

(一)登记地区恶性肿瘤死亡(ICD-10：C00-C96)

河南省肿瘤登记地区 2014 年报告恶性肿瘤死亡病例 32 952(男性 20 412 例，女性 12 540 例)，其中城市地区 5 452 例，占登记地区全部恶性肿瘤死亡的 16.42%；农村地区 27 500 例，占登记地区全部恶性肿瘤死亡的 83.58%。

2014 年河南省肿瘤登记地区恶性肿瘤死亡率为 $156.58/10^5$(男性 $188.10/10^5$，女性 $123.02/10^5$)，中标率为 $123.94/10^5$，世标率为 $123.80/10^5$，累积率(0~74 岁)为 14.30%。

城市地区恶性肿瘤死亡率为 $158.71/10^5$(男性 $194.69/10^5$，女性 $121.03/10^5$)，中标率为 $133.56/10^5$，世标率为 $133.12/10^5$，累积率(0~74 岁)为 13.90%。

农村地区恶性肿瘤死亡率为 $156.17/10^5$(男性 $186.83/10^5$，女性 $123.41/10^5$)，中标率为 $122.67/10^5$，世标率为 $122.68/10^5$，累积率(0~74 岁)为 14.38%。

城市与农村相比，城市地区的男性和女性恶性肿瘤死亡粗率、中标率、世标率和累积率均高于农村地区恶性肿瘤死亡率水平(表 4-7)。

3. Cancer mortality (ICD-10：C00-C96)

3.1 Mortality of all cancer sites (ICD-10：C00-C96)

In 2014, there were a total of 32 952 death cases (20 412 males and 12 540 females) of all cancer sites in Henan cancer registration areas, among which 5 452 (16.42%) were from the urban areas and 27 500 (83.58%) from rural areas.

The mortality rate of all cancer sites was $156.58/10^5$ ($188.10/10^5$ for males and $123.02/10^5$ for females). The ASR China was $123.94/10^5$ and ASR World was $123.80/10^5$. The cumulative rate (0~74 years old) was 14.30%.

The mortality rate of all cancer sites in urban areas was $158.71/10^5$ ($194.69/10^5$ for males and $121.03/10^5$ for females). The ASR China was $133.56/10^5$ and ASR World was $133.12/10^5$. The cumulative rate (0~74 years old) was 13.90%.

The mortality rate of all cancer sites in rural areas was $156.17/10^5$ ($186.83/10^5$ for males and $123.41/10^5$ for females). The ASR China was $122.67/10^5$ and ASR World was $122.68/10^5$. The cumulative rate (0~74 years old) for both sexes was14.38%.

The crude mortality rate, ASR China, ASR World and cumulative rate for both males and females in urban areas were higher than those in rural areas, except that the crude mortality rate and cumulative rate for females in urban areas were slightly lower than those in rural areas (Table 4-7).

表 4-7 河南省肿瘤登记地区恶性肿瘤(ICD-10：C00-C96)死亡主要指标

地区	性别	死亡数	死亡率 ($1/10^5$)	中标率 ($1/10^5$)	世标率 ($1/10^5$)	累积率(0~74 岁) (%)
全省	合计	32 952	156.58	123.94	123.80	14.30
	男性	20 412	188.10	159.10	159.47	18.24
	女性	12 540	123.02	91.52	91.13	10.36
城市	合计	5 452	158.71	133.56	133.12	13.90
	男性	3 421	194.69	176.09	176.57	17.83
	女性	2 031	121.03	96.39	95.60	10.06
农村	合计	27 500	156.17	122.67	122.68	14.38
	男性	16 991	186.83	156.76	157.24	18.32
	女性	10 509	123.41	90.83	90.60	10.42

（二）恶性肿瘤（ICD-10：C00-C96）年龄别死亡率

河南省肿瘤登记地区恶性肿瘤男女年龄别死亡率随着年龄增长而增加。在 30- 岁年龄组死亡率为 14.70/10^5，此后快速上升，50- 年龄组死亡率为 199.32/10^5，到 85+ 年龄组死亡率达到最高值，死亡率为 2 467.39/10^5。

恶性肿瘤年龄别死亡率城乡比较，35 岁以前死亡率处于较低水平，城乡差别较小。男性在 40~69 岁年龄段城市死亡率低于农村，75 岁以后城市男性高于农村；女性在 40~64 岁组的各年龄组城市的死亡率均低于农村，65 岁以上的各年龄组城市女性的恶性肿瘤死亡率高于农村地区死亡水平（表 4-8，图 4-6a~ 图 4-6d）。

3.2 Age-specific mortality rate of all cancer sites（ICD-10: C00-C96）

The age-specific mortality rate of all cancer sites in Henan increased with age. It was 14.70/10^5 at age group of 30- and 199.32/10^5 at 50-, it reached the peak of 2 467.39/10^5 when at age group of 85+.

When assessing the mortality in urban and rural areas, the age-specific mortality rate was relatively low before 35 years old with less differences between the urban and rural areas. For males, the mortality rates in urban areas was lower than those in urban areas at the age group of 40~69 years old and they were higher after 75 years old. For females, the mortality rates in urban areas were lower than those in rural areas between 40~64 years old and they were higher after 65 years old in urban areas than those in rural areas (Table 4-8, Figure 4-6a~Figure4-6d).

表 4-8 河南省肿瘤登记地区恶性肿瘤年龄别死亡率（1/10^5）

年龄组	全省			城市			农村		
	合计	男性	女性	合计	男性	女性	合计	男性	女性
合计	156.58	188.10	123.02	158.71	194.69	121.03	156.17	186.83	123.41
0-	1.95	2.94	0.83	2.50	4.75	0.00	1.85	2.61	0.99
1-	3.17	2.91	3.49	3.34	2.07	4.80	3.14	3.05	3.25
5-	3.81	4.32	3.20	4.13	4.27	3.97	3.75	4.33	3.07
10-	3.85	4.60	2.96	3.09	0.95	5.62	3.98	5.23	2.51
15-	2.86	3.27	2.41	0.86	0.85	0.87	3.23	3.71	2.71
20-	4.88	4.84	4.93	4.39	7.40	1.28	4.98	4.31	5.70
25-	8.00	8.24	7.75	10.15	10.60	9.68	7.59	7.79	7.38
30-	13.88	14.70	13.01	14.03	12.36	15.71	13.85	15.13	12.48
35-	23.69	24.25	23.08	25.04	21.73	28.61	23.40	24.79	21.89
40-	51.40	57.37	45.00	49.90	49.46	50.37	51.73	59.11	43.80
45-	96.31	108.87	83.41	90.47	95.81	84.94	97.52	111.61	83.10
50-	168.28	199.32	136.17	162.12	184.51	138.89	169.53	202.34	135.62
55-	275.74	343.63	205.29	254.36	324.02	185.22	280.24	347.64	209.62
60-	523.40	661.06	381.85	479.42	604.12	352.56	531.46	671.43	387.26
65-	753.00	998.30	507.51	699.56	955.39	448.65	762.65	10 05.96	518.27
70-	928.90	1 211.68	652.83	978.80	1 292.96	680.97	919.58	1 196.76	647.48
75-	1 186.81	1 595.77	829.07	1 473.19	1 965.00	1 037.98	1 134.07	1 527.28	790.85
80-	1 725.88	2 397.93	1 221.19	2 571.93	4 028.52	1 431.93	1 601.12	2 150.92	1 190.74
85-	1 653.14	2 467.39	1 222.18	2 885.94	4 561.25	1 883.85	1 510.67	2 203.22	1 149.38

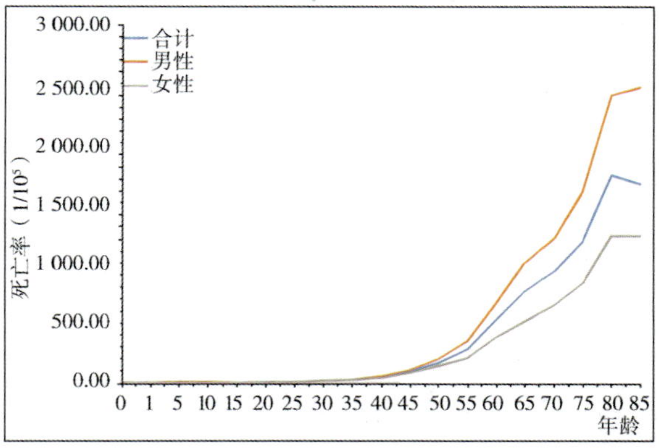

图 4-6a 河南省肿瘤登记地区恶性肿瘤年龄别死亡率

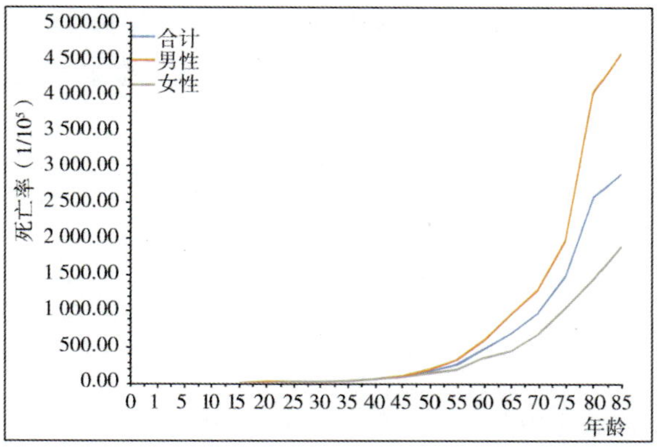

图 4-6b 河南省城市肿瘤登记地区恶性肿瘤年龄别死亡率

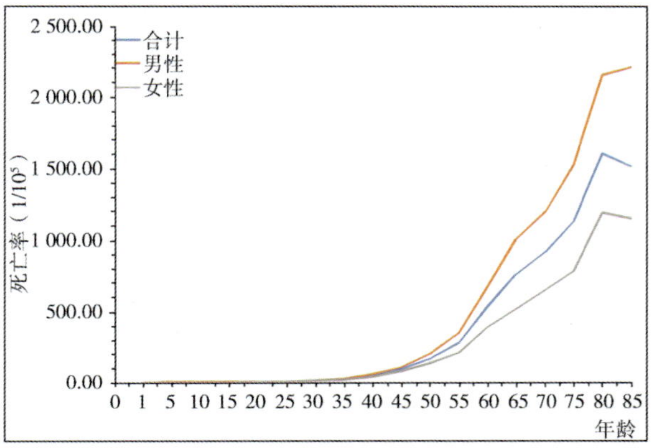

图 4-6c 河南省农村肿瘤登记地区恶性肿瘤年龄别死亡率

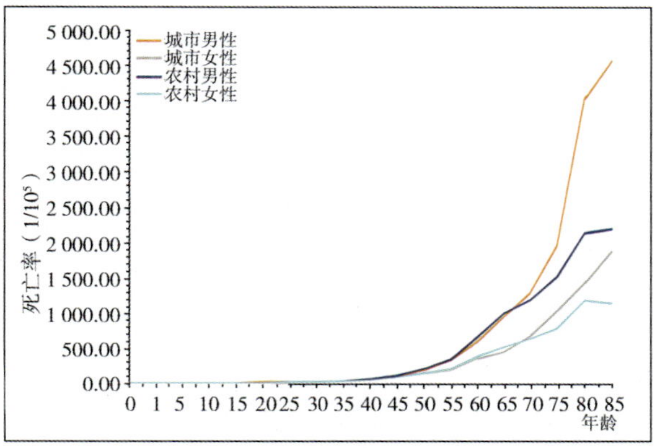

图 4-6d 河南省城市和农村肿瘤登记地区恶性肿瘤年龄别死亡率

（三）河南省前10位恶性肿瘤死亡情况

2014 年河南省恶性肿瘤死亡第 1 位的是肺癌，其次为胃癌、食管癌、肝癌和结直肠肛门癌，前 10 位恶性肿瘤占全部恶性肿瘤的 88.09%。男性恶性肿瘤死亡第 1 位的是肺癌，其次为胃癌、食管癌、肝癌和结直肠肛门癌，男性前 10 位恶性肿瘤占全部恶性肿瘤的 91.70 %；女性恶性肿瘤死亡第 1 位的是肺癌，其次为食管癌、胃癌、肝癌和乳腺癌，女性前 10 位恶性肿瘤占全部恶性肿瘤的 85.56 %（表 4-9，图 4-7a~ 图 4-7f）。

3.3 Mortality of the top 10 leading causes of cancer death

In Henan cancer registration areas in 2014, lung cancer was the leading cause of cancer deaths followed by cancers of stomach, esophagus, liver and colorectum. The top 10 leading causes of cancer accounted for 88.09% of all cancer deaths. For males, lung cancer was the leading cause of cancer death followed by cancers of stomach, esophagus,liver and colorectum, and the top 10 leading causes of cancer deaths accounted for 91.70% of all cancer deaths. For females, lung cancer was the leading cause of cancer death followed by cancers of esophagus, stomach, liver and breast. The top 10 leading causes of cancer deaths accounted for 85.56% of all cancer deaths (Table 4-9, Figure 4-7a~Figure4-7f).

表4-9　河南省肿瘤登记地区前10位恶性肿瘤死亡主要指标

顺位	合计				男性				女性			
	部位	死亡率 (1/10^5)	构成 (%)	中标率 (1/10^5)	部位	死亡率 (1/10^5)	构成 (%)	中标率 (1/10^5)	部位	死亡率 (1/10^5)	构成 (%)	中标率 (1/10^5)
1	气管、支气管、肺 (C33–C34)	36.30	23.19	28.46	气管、支气管、肺 (C33–C34)	49.61	26.37	41.90	气管、支气管、肺 (C33–C34)	22.14	18.00	15.98
2	胃 (C16)	28.25	18.04	22.09	胃 (C16)	38.73	20.59	32.53	食管 (C15)	20.16	16.39	14.46
3	食管 (C15)	26.14	16.70	20.36	食管 (C15)	31.77	16.89	26.70	胃 (C16)	17.10	13.90	12.37
4	肝脏 (C22)	21.96	14.03	17.51	肝脏 (C22)	29.50	15.68	24.79	肝脏 (C22)	13.94	11.33	10.34
5	结直肠肛门 (C18–C21)	8.16	5.21	6.42	结直肠肛门 (C18–C21)	9.05	4.81	7.66	乳房 (C50)	10.46	8.50	8.28
6	乳房 (C50)	10.46	3.24	8.28	脑及中枢神经系统 (C70–C72)	4.20	2.23	3.73	结直肠肛门 (C18–C21)	7.21	5.86	5.29
7	脑及中枢神经系统 (C70–C72)	3.93	2.51	3.30	白血病 (C91–C95)	3.16	1.68	2.97	子宫颈 (C53)	5.15	4.19	4.04
8	白血病 (C91–C95)	2.97	1.90	2.65	胰腺 (C25)	2.89	1.54	2.48	脑及中枢神经系统 (C70–C72)	3.64	2.96	2.89
9	胰腺 (C25)	2.63	1.68	2.11	恶性淋巴瘤 (C81–C85, C88,C90, C96)	1.83	0.97	1.55	白血病 (C91–C95)	2.77	2.25	2.31
10	子宫颈 (C53)	5.15	1.59	4.04	前列腺 (C61)	1.77	0.94	1.49	卵巢 (C56)	2.68	2.18	2.10
	前 10 位	137.92	88.09		前 10 位	172.51	91.70	145.80	前 10 位	105.25	85.56	78.07

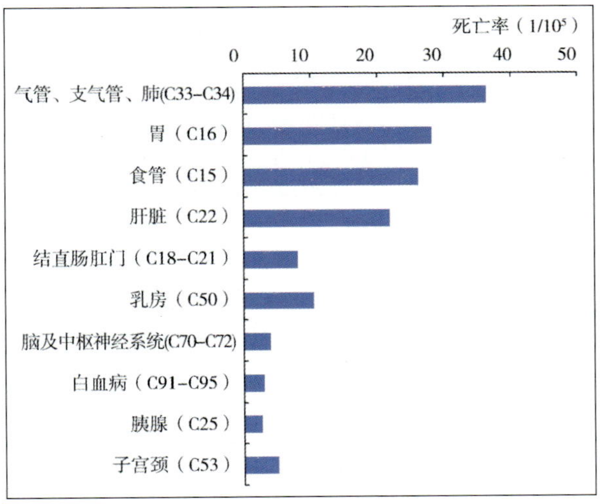

图 4-7a 河南省肿瘤登记地区前 10 位恶性肿瘤死亡率

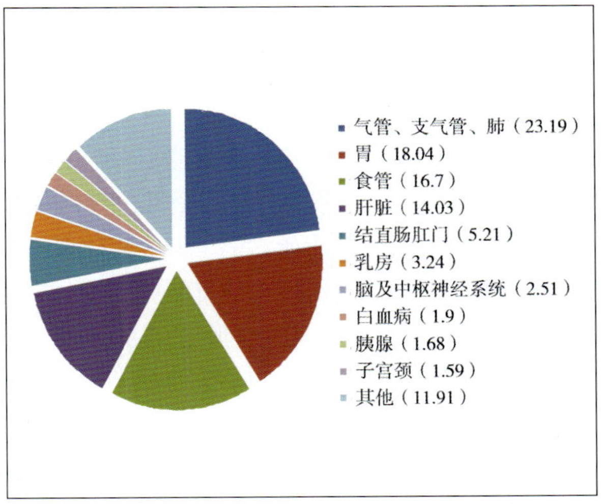

图 4-7d 河南省肿瘤登记地区恶性肿瘤死亡构成 (%)

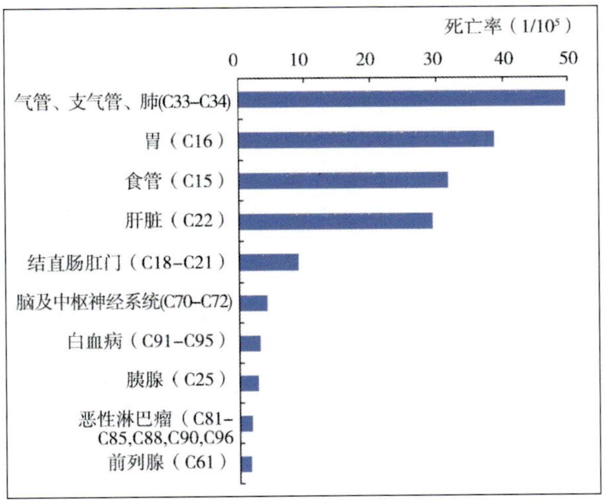

图 4-7b 河南省肿瘤登记地区男性前 10 位恶性肿瘤死亡率

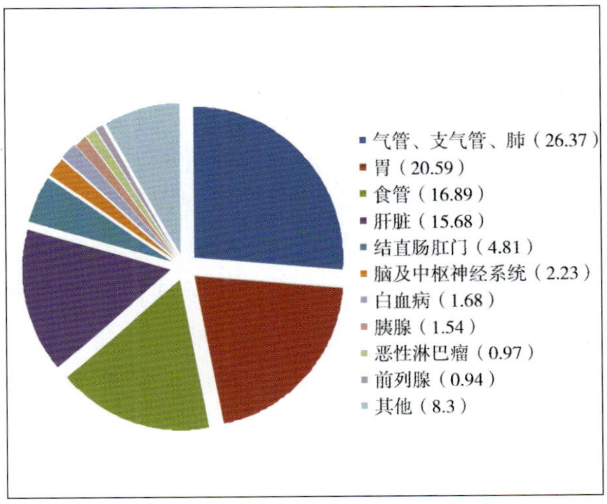

图 4-7e 河南省肿瘤登记地区男性恶性肿瘤死亡构成 (%)

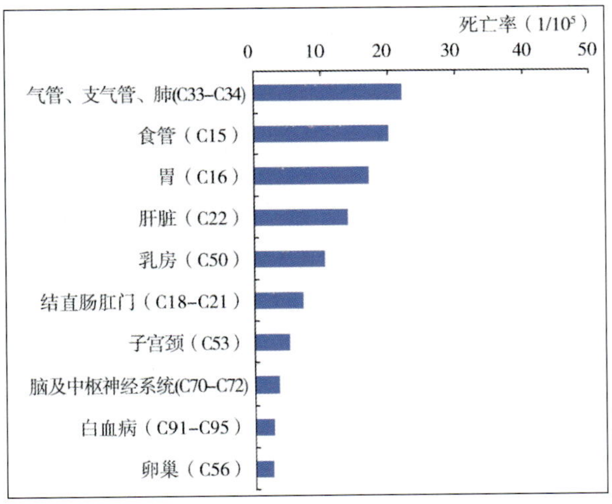

图 4-7c 河南省肿瘤登记地区女性前 10 位恶性肿瘤死亡率

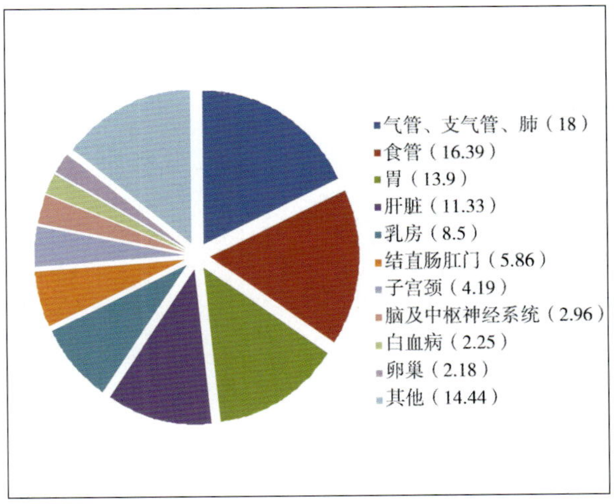

图 4-7f 河南省肿瘤登记地区女性恶性肿瘤死亡构成 (%)

（四）城市地区前 10 位恶性肿瘤死亡情况

2014 年河南省城市地区恶性肿瘤死亡第 1 位的是肺癌，其次为胃癌、食管癌、肝癌和结直肠肛门癌，前 10 位恶性肿瘤占全部恶性肿瘤的 85.66%。男性恶性肿瘤死亡第 1 位的是肺癌，其次为胃癌、肝癌、食管癌和结直肠肛门癌，男性前 10 位恶性肿瘤占全部恶性肿瘤的 90.47%；女性恶性肿瘤死亡第 1 位的是肺癌，其次为食管癌、乳腺癌、胃癌和肝癌，女性前 10 位恶性肿瘤占全部恶性肿瘤的 82.62%（表 4–10，图 4–8a~ 图 4–8f）。

（五）农村地区前 10 位恶性肿瘤死亡情况

2014 年河南省农村地区恶性肿瘤死亡第 1 位的是肺癌，其次为胃癌、食管癌、肝癌和结直肠肛门癌，前 10 位恶性肿瘤占全部恶性肿瘤的 88.56%。男性恶性肿瘤死亡第 1 位的是肺癌，其次为胃癌、食管癌、肝癌和结直肠肛门癌，男性前 10 位恶性肿瘤占全部恶性肿瘤的 92.10%；女性恶性肿瘤死亡第 1 位的是肺癌，其次为食管癌、胃癌、肝癌和乳腺癌，女性前 10 位恶性肿瘤占全部恶性肿瘤的 86.20%（表 4–11，图 4–9a~ 图 4–9f）。

3.4 Mortality of the top 10 leading causes of cancer death in urban areas

In the urban areas of Henan cancer registries in 2014, lung cancer was the leading cause of cancer deaths followed by cancers of stomach, esophagus, liver and colorectum. The top 10 leading causes of cancer accounted for 85.66% of all cancer deaths. For males, lung cancer was the leading cause of cancer death followed by cancers of stomach, liver, esophagus and colorectum, and the top 10 leading causes of cancer deaths accounted for 90.47% of all cancer deaths. For females, lung cancer was the leading cause of cancer death followed by cancers of esophagus, breast,stomach and liver. The top 10 leading causes of cancer deaths accounted for 82.62% of all cancer deaths (Table 4–10, Figure 4–8a~Figure4–8f).

3.5 Mortality of the top 10 leading causes of cancer death in rural areas

In Henan rural cancer registration areas in 2014, lung cancer was the leading cause of cancer deaths followed by cancers of stomach, esophagus, liver and colorectum. The top 10 leading causes of cancer deaths accounted for 88.56% of all cancer deaths. For males, lung cancer was the leading cause of cancer death followed by cancers of stomach, esophagus, liver, and colorectum, and the top 10 leading causes of cancer deaths accounted for 92.10% of all cancer deaths. For females, lung cancer was the leading cause of cancer death followed by cancers of esophagus, stomach, liver and breast, and the top 10 leading causes of cancer deaths accounted for 86.20% of all cancer deaths (Table 4–11, Figure 4–9a~Figure 4–9f).

表 4–10　河南省城市肿瘤登记地区前 10 位恶性肿瘤死亡主要指标

顺位	合计 部位	死亡率 (1/10⁵)	构成 (%)	中标率 (1/10⁵)	男性 部位	死亡率 (1/10⁵)	构成 (%)	中标率 (1/10⁵)	女性 部位	死亡率 (1/10⁵)	构成 (%)	中标率 (1/10⁵)
1	气管、支气管、肺 (C33–C34)	41.10	25.90	34.45	气管、支气管、肺 (C33–C34)	58.56	30.08	52.79	气管、支气管、肺 (C33–C34)	22.82	18.86	17.99
2	胃 (C16)	21.60	13.61	18.21	胃 (C16)	30.50	15.67	27.71	食管 (C15)	14.78	12.21	11.63
3	食管 (C15)	21.13	13.32	17.82	肝脏 (C22)	28.91	14.85	25.38	乳房 (C50)	13.88	11.47	11.05
4	肝脏 (C22)	20.29	12.78	16.85	食管 (C15)	27.20	13.97	24.59	胃 (C16)	12.28	10.14	9.63
5	结直肠肛门 (C18–C21)	11.85	7.47	9.95	结直肠肛门 (C18–C21)	13.54	6.96	12.36	肝脏 (C22)	11.26	9.31	8.81
6	乳房 (C50)	13.88	4.27	11.05	胰腺 (C25)	4.44	2.28	4.14	结直肠肛门 (C18–C21)	10.07	8.32	7.90
7	胰腺 (C25)	3.81	2.40	3.25	脑及中枢神经系统 (C70–C72)	3.76	1.93	3.39	子宫颈 (C53)	5.48	4.53	4.45
8	白血病 (C91–C95)	3.49	2.20	3.09	白血病 (C91–C95)	3.76	1.93	3.45	白血病 (C91–C95)	3.22	2.66	2.73
9	脑及中枢神经系统 (C70–C72)	3.20	2.02	2.76	肾及泌尿系统不明 (C64–C66,C68)	2.85	1.46	2.54	胰腺 (C25)	3.16	2.61	2.50
10	子宫颈 (C53)	5.48	1.69	4.45	前列腺 (C61)	2.62	1.34	2.57	卵巢 (C56)	3.04	2.51	2.54
	前 10 位	135.94	85.66		前 10 位	176.13	90.47	158.90	前 10 位	99.99	82.62	79.24

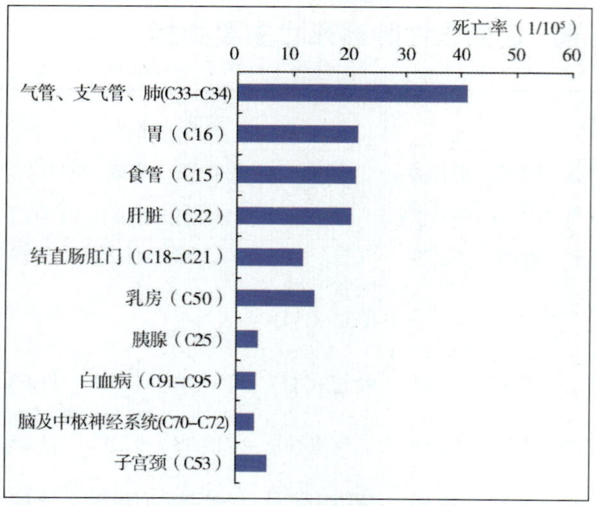

图 4–8a　河南省城市肿瘤登记地区前 10 位恶性肿瘤死亡率

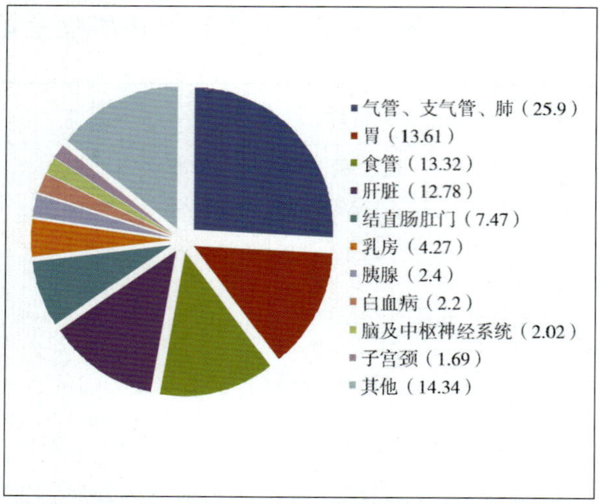

图 4–8d　河南省城市肿瘤登记地区恶性肿瘤死亡构成 (%)

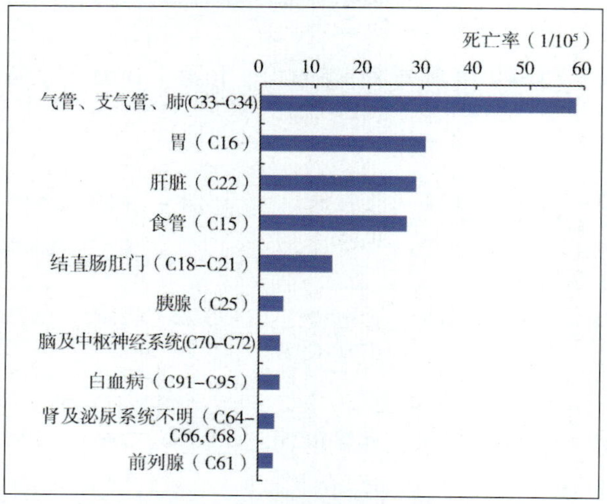

图 4–8b　河南省城市肿瘤登记地区男性前 10 位恶性肿瘤死亡率

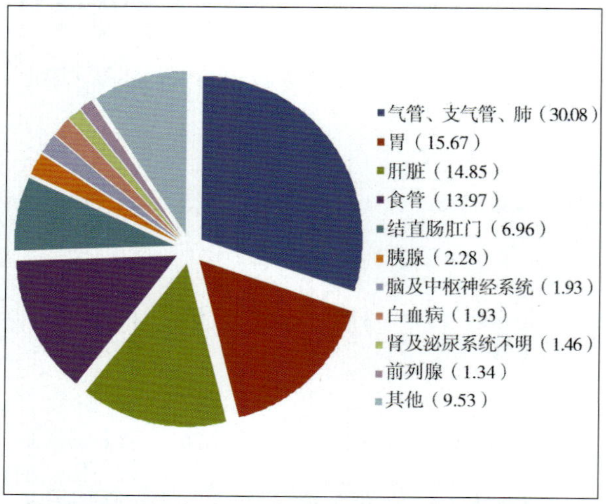

图 4–8e　河南省城市肿瘤登记地区男性恶性肿瘤死亡构成 (%)

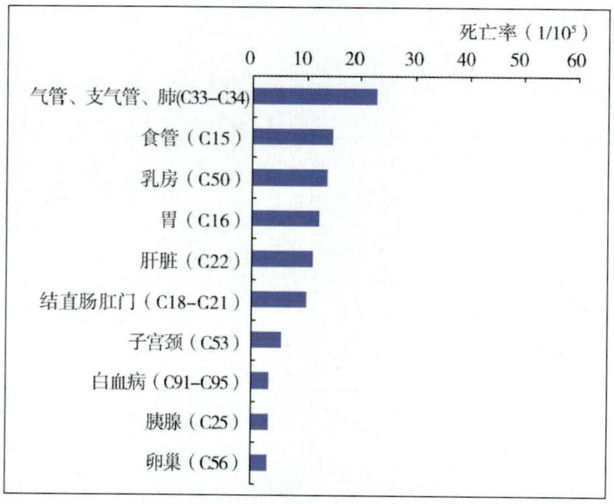

图 4–8c　河南省城市肿瘤登记地区女性前 10 位恶性肿瘤死亡率

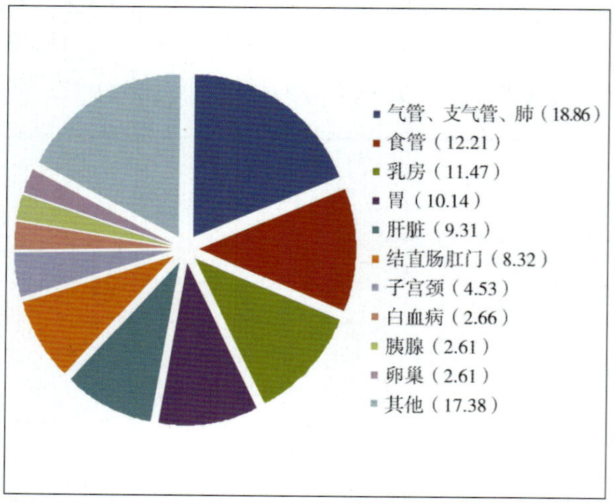

图 4–8f　河南省城市肿瘤登记地区女性恶性肿瘤死亡构成 (%)

表 4-11　河南省农村肿瘤登记地区前 10 位恶性肿瘤死亡主要指标

顺位	合计 部位	死亡率 (1/10^5)	构成 (%)	中标率 (1/10^5)	男性 部位	死亡率 (1/10^5)	构成 (%)	中标率 (1/10^5)	女性 部位	死亡率 (1/10^5)	构成 (%)	中标率 (1/10^5)
1	气管、支气管、肺 (C33–C34)	35.37	22.65	27.47	气管、支气管、肺 (C33–C34)	47.88	25.63	40.08	气管、支气管、肺 (C33–C34)	22.01	17.83	15.63
2	胃 (C16)	29.55	18.92	22.88	胃 (C16)	40.32	21.58	33.51	食管 (C15)	21.22	17.19	15.04
3	食管 (C15)	27.12	17.37	20.89	食管 (C15)	32.65	17.47	27.16	胃 (C16)	18.05	14.63	12.92
4	肝脏 (C22)	22.29	14.27	17.69	肝脏 (C22)	29.61	15.85	24.79	肝脏 (C22)	14.47	11.72	10.65
5	结直肠肛门 (C18–C21)	7.44	4.76	5.84	结直肠肛门 (C18–C21)	8.18	4.38	6.89	乳房 (C50)	9.78	7.93	7.77
6	乳房 (C50)	9.78	3.03	7.77	脑及中枢神经系统 (C70–C72)	4.29	2.30	3.81	结直肠肛门 (C18–C21)	6.65	5.39	4.85
7	脑及中枢神经系统 (C70–C72)	4.07	2.61	3.42	白血病 (C91–C95)	3.05	1.63	2.90	子宫颈 (C53)	5.08	4.12	3.94
8	白血病 (C91–C95)	2.87	1.84	2.59	胰腺 (C25)	2.60	1.39	2.20	脑及中枢神经系统 (C70–C72)	3.84	3.11	3.04
9	子宫颈 (C53)	5.08	1.57	3.94	恶性淋巴瘤 (C81–C85, C88,C90, C96)	1.86	0.99	1.56	白血病 (C91–C95)	2.68	2.17	2.25
10	胰腺 (C25)	2.40	1.54	1.91	膀胱 (C67)	1.65	0.88	1.39	卵巢 (C56)	2.61	2.11	2.01
	前 10 位	138.30	88.56		前 10 位	172.07	92.10	144.29	前 10 位	106.39	86.20	78.11

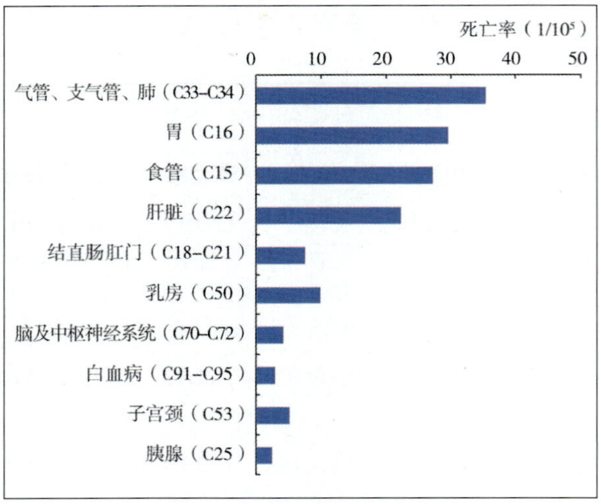

图 4–9a 河南省农村肿瘤登记地区前 10 位恶性肿瘤死亡率

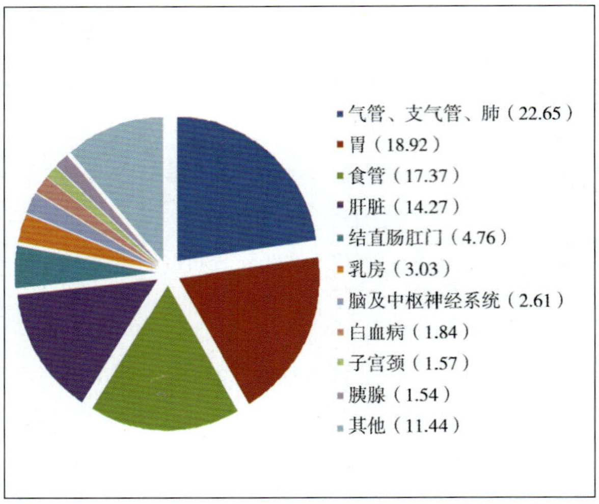

图 4–9d 河南省农村肿瘤登记地区恶性肿瘤死亡构成 (%)

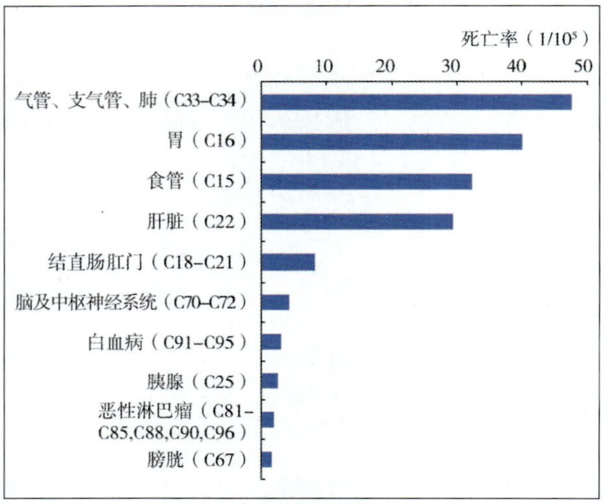

图 4–9b 河南省农村肿瘤登记地区男性前 10 位恶性肿瘤死亡率

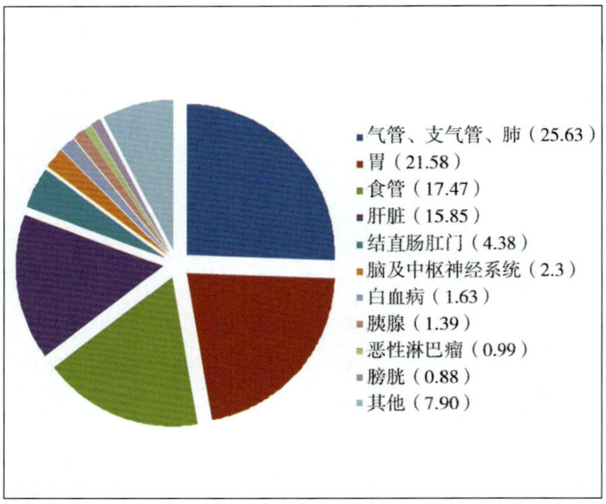

图 4–9e 河南省农村肿瘤登记地区男性恶性肿瘤死亡构成 (%)

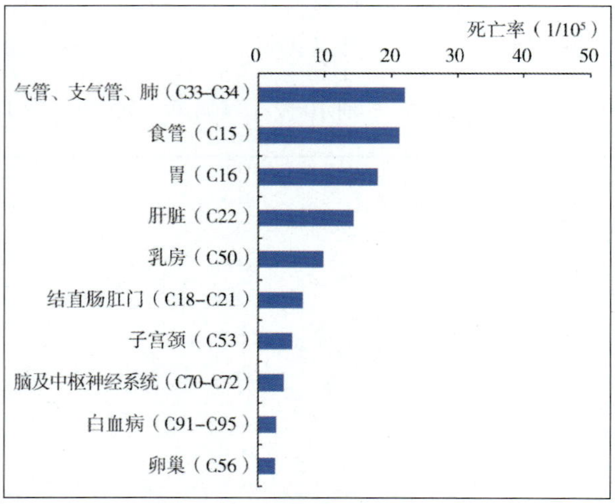

图 4–9c 河南省农村肿瘤登记地区女性前 10 位恶性肿瘤死亡率

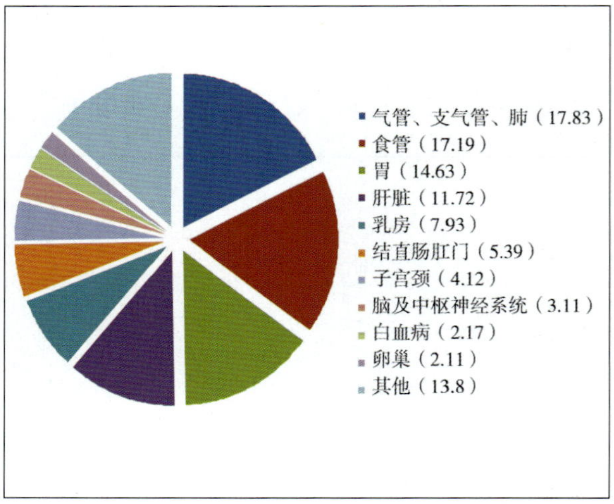

图 4–9f 河南省农村肿瘤登记地区女性恶性肿瘤死亡构成 (%)

第五章　各部位恶性肿瘤发病与死亡

Chapter 5　Incidence and mortality of each kind of cancers

一、口腔和咽（除外鼻咽）（C00–C10；C12–C14）

2014 年，河南省肿瘤登记地区口腔和咽（除外鼻咽）恶性肿瘤的发病率为 2.43/10^5，中标率为 2.02/10^5，世标率为 1.97/10^5，占全部恶性肿瘤发病的 0.96%。其中男性发病率为 2.71/10^5，女性为 2.14/10^5。男性中标率为女性的 1.35 倍，城市为农村的 1.47 倍。同期口腔和咽（除外鼻咽）恶性肿瘤的死亡率为 1.13/10^5，中标率为 0.89/10^5，世标率为 0.88/10^5。其中男性死亡率为 1.27/10^5，女性为 0.98/10^5。口腔和咽（除外鼻咽）恶性肿瘤发病和死亡的 0~74 岁累积率分别为 0.21% 和 0.09%（表 5–1）。

1. Oral Cavity & Pharynx but Nasopharynx (C00–C10; C12–C14)

In 2014, oral cavity and pharyngeal cancer cases accounted for 0.96% of all cancer cases in Henan cancer registration areas with the crude incidence 2.43/10^5, the ASR China 2.02/10^5 and ASR for World 1.97/10^5. The incidence in males was 2.71/10^5, and 2.14/10^5 in females. It was 1.35 times in males as high as that in females and it was 1.47 times in urban areas as that in rural areas. The crude mortality of oral cavity and pharyngeal cancers in 2014 was 1.13/10^5, The ASR China was 0.89/10^5 and ASR for World was 0.88/10^5. The mortality in males was 1.27/10^5, and 0.98/10^5 in females. The cumulative rates of incidence and mortality from 0 to 74 years old were 0.21% and 0.09%, respectively (Table 5–1).

表 5–1　河南省肿瘤登记地区口腔和咽（除外鼻咽）恶性肿瘤发病与死亡

地区	性别	病例数	粗率（1/10^5）	构成（%）	中标率（1/10^5）	世标率（1/10^5）	累积率 0~74（%）
发病							
全省	合计	512	2.43	0.96	2.02	1.97	0.21
	男性	294	2.71	0.99	2.33	2.30	0.25
	女性	218	2.14	0.93	1.73	1.64	0.17
城市	合计	111	3.23	1.24	2.78	2.68	0.25
	男性	60	3.41	1.18	3.05	3.06	0.29
	女性	51	3.04	1.32	2.52	2.32	0.21
农村	合计	401	2.28	0.91	1.89	1.85	0.20
	男性	234	2.57	0.95	2.20	2.17	0.25
	女性	167	1.96	0.85	1.59	1.53	0.16

续表

地区	性别	病例数	粗率（$1/10^5$）	构成（%）	中标率（$1/10^5$）	世标率（$1/10^5$）	累积率 0~74（%）
死亡							
全省	**合计**	**238**	**1.13**	**0.72**	**0.89**	**0.88**	**0.09**
	男性	138	1.27	0.68	1.07	1.07	0.11
	女性	100	0.98	0.80	0.73	0.72	0.08
城市	**合计**	**53**	**1.54**	**0.97**	**1.30**	**1.30**	**0.11**
	男性	29	1.65	0.85	1.54	1.60	0.11
	女性	24	1.43	1.18	1.14	1.12	0.11
农村	**合计**	**185**	**1.05**	**0.67**	**0.82**	**0.81**	**0.09**
	男性	109	1.20	0.64	1.00	0.99	0.11
	女性	76	0.89	0.72	0.66	0.65	0.07

口腔和咽（除外鼻咽）恶性肿瘤年龄别发病率和死亡率在 0~44 岁年龄段处于较低水平，45 岁以后快速上升，在 80- 岁或 85+ 岁组达到高峰，男性高于女性。城乡和不同地区年龄别率的水平虽然有一定的差异，但总体趋势类同（图 5-1a~ 图 5-1f）。

The age-specific incidence and mortality rates of oral cavity and pharyngeal cancers were relatively low before 45 years old and increased dramatically since 45 years old, reaching the peak at the age group of 80 and 85, respectively. Incidence and mortality rates in male were generally higher than those in female, and higher in the urban areas than in the rural areas. The age-specific incidence and mortality rates varied in urban and rural areas with similar curves (Figure 5-1a ~ Figure5-1f).

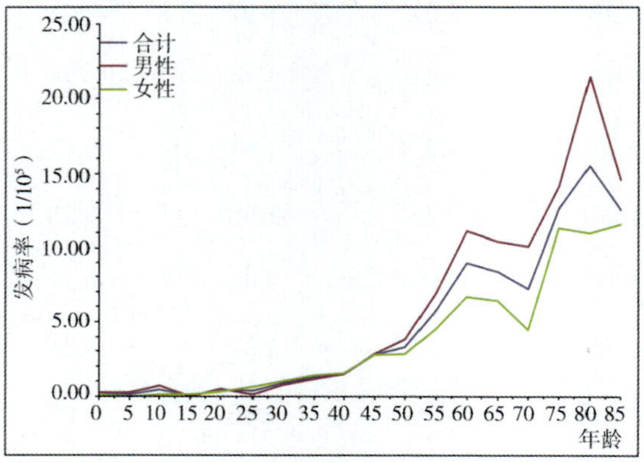

图 5-1a 河南省肿瘤登记地区口腔和咽（除外鼻咽）恶性肿瘤年龄别发病率，2014

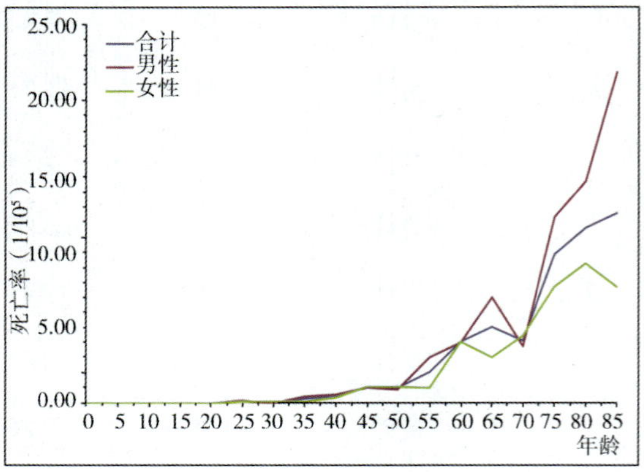

图 5-1d 河南省肿瘤登记地区口腔和咽（除外鼻咽）恶性肿瘤年龄别死亡率，2014

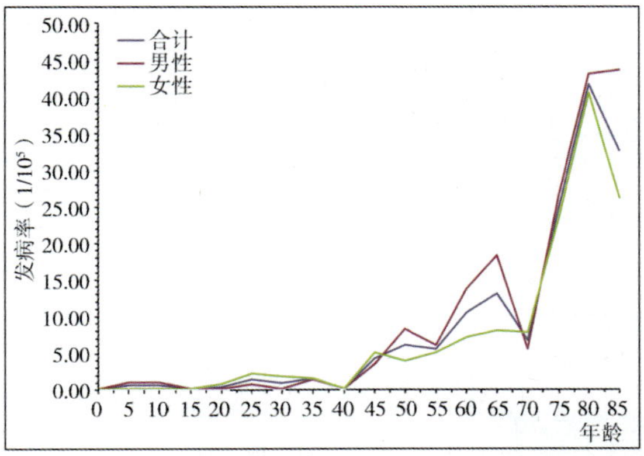

图 5-1b 城市肿瘤登记地区口腔和咽（除外鼻咽）恶性肿瘤年龄别发病率，2014

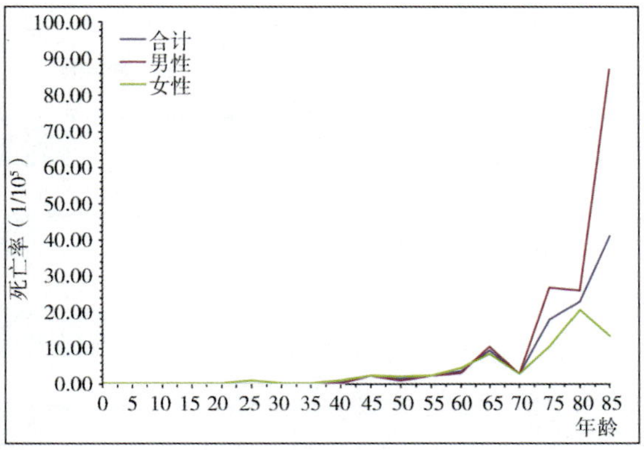

图 5-1e 城市肿瘤登记地区口腔和咽（除外鼻咽）恶性肿瘤年龄别死亡率，2014

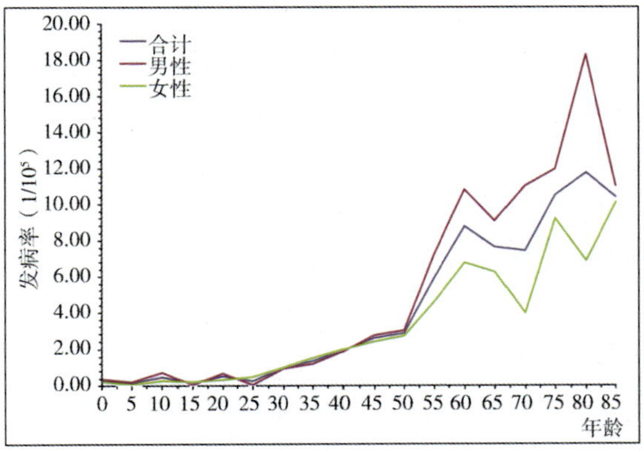

图 5-1c 农村肿瘤登记地区口腔和咽（除外鼻咽）恶性肿瘤年龄别发病率，2014

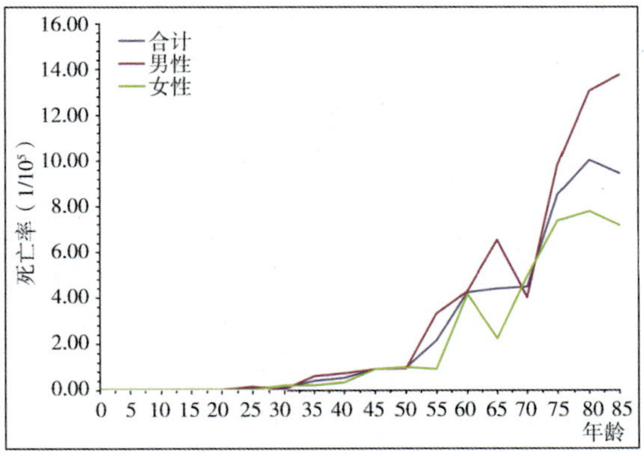

图 5-1f 农村肿瘤登记地区口腔和咽（除外鼻咽）恶性肿瘤年龄别死亡率，2014

在 5 个城市肿瘤登记地区中，男性口腔和咽（除外鼻咽）恶性肿瘤标化发病率最高的是鹤壁市（$4.40/10^5$），其次是三门峡市；女性发病率最高的是漯河市（$4.55/10^5$），其次是鹤壁市和南阳市。男性标化死亡率最高的是洛阳市（$2.44/10^5$），女性死亡率最高的是南阳市（$1.88/10^5$）（图 5-1g）。

在 22 个农村肿瘤登记地区中，男性口腔和咽（除外鼻咽）恶性肿瘤标化发病率最高的是郸城县（$4.54/10^5$），其次是虞城县和开封市祥符区；女性发病率最高的是郸城县（$4.88/10^5$），其次是开封市祥符区和汝阳县。男性和女性标化死亡率最高的均是郸城县，分别为 $2.91/10^5$ 和 $3.13/10^5$（图 5-1h）。

Among the 5 urban cancer registration areas, the ASR China incidence rate of oral cavity and pharyngeal cancers was the highest in Hebi City ($4.40/10^5$), followed by Sanmenxia City. In females, it was the highest in Luohe City ($4.55/10^5$), followed by Hebi City and Nanyang City. The ASR China mortality was the highest in Luoyang City for both males ($2.44/10^5$) and females ($1.88/10^5$) (Figure 5-1g).

Among the 22 rural cancer registration areas, the ASR China incidence rate of oral cavity and pharyngeal cancers was the highest in Dancheng County ($4.54/10^5$), followed by Yucheng County and Xiangfu District. For females, it was the highest in Dancheng County ($4.88/10^5$), followed by Xiangfu District and Ruyang County. The ASR China mortality was the highest in Dancheng County for both males ($2.91/10^5$) and females ($3.13/10^5$) (Figure 5-1h).

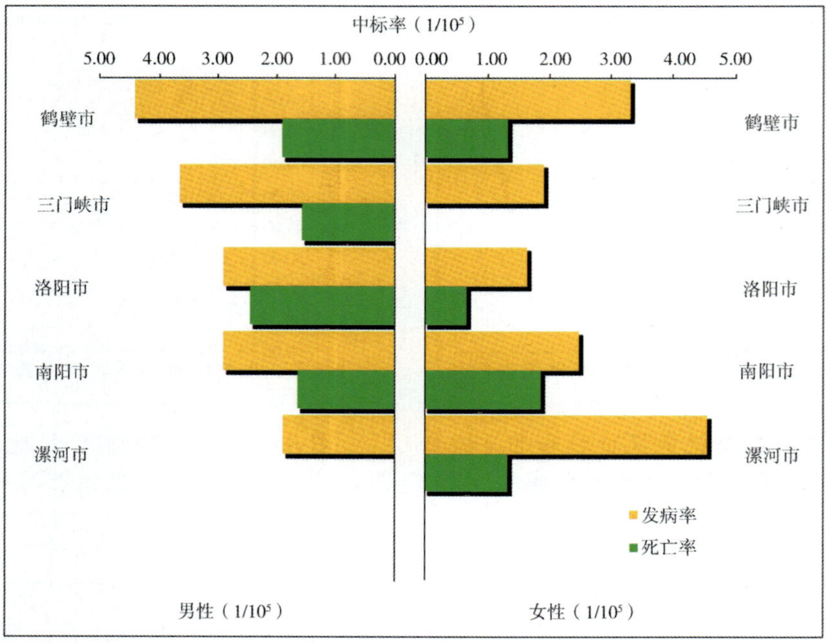

图 5-1g 城市肿瘤登记地区口腔和咽（除外鼻咽）恶性肿瘤发病率与死亡率

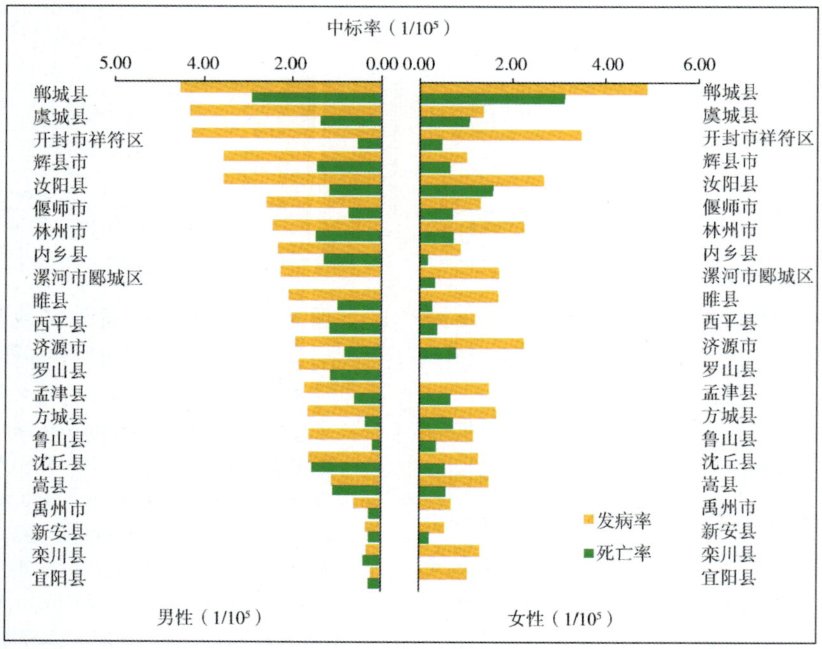

图 5-1h 农村肿瘤登记地区口腔和咽（除外鼻咽）恶性肿瘤发病率与死亡率

二、鼻咽（C11）

2014 年，河南省肿瘤登记地区鼻咽恶性肿瘤的发病率为 1.30/10^5，中标率为 1.12/10^5，世标率为 1.05/10^5，占全部恶性肿瘤发病的 0.51%。其中男性发病率为 1.62/10^5，女性为 0.95/10^5。男性中标率为女性的 1.82 倍，城市为农村的 0.94

2. Nasopharynx (C11)

In 2014, nasopharyngeal cancer cases accounted for 0.51% of all cancer cases in Henan cancer registration areas with the crude incidence of 1.30/10^5, ASR for China 1.12/10^5 and ASR for World 1.05/10^5. The crude incidence in males was 1.62/10^5, and 0.95/10^5 in females. It was 1.82 times in males as high as that in females and it was 0.94 times in urban areas as that in rural areas. The crude mortality

倍。同期鼻咽恶性肿瘤的死亡率为 $0.6/10^5$，中标率为 $0.49/10^5$，世标率为 $0.49/10^5$。其中男性死亡率为 $0.67/10^5$，女性为 $0.52/10^5$。鼻咽恶性肿瘤发病和死亡的 0~74 岁累积率分别为 0.11% 和 0.06%（表 5–2）。

of nasopharyngeal cancer in 2014 was $0.60/10^5$, ASR for China was $0.49/10^5$ and ASR for World was $0.49/10^5$.The mortality in males was $0.67/10^5$, and $0.52/10^5$ in females. The cumulative rates of incidence and mortality from 0 to 74 years old were 0.11% and 0.06%, respectively (Table 5–2).

表 5–2　河南省肿瘤登记地区鼻咽恶性肿瘤发病与死亡

地区	性别	病例数	粗率 ($1/10^5$)	构成 (%)	中标率 ($1/10^5$)	世标率 ($1/10^5$)	累积率 0~74 (%)
发病							
全省	合计	273	1.30	0.51	1.12	1.05	0.11
	男性	176	1.62	0.59	1.44	1.35	0.14
	女性	97	0.95	0.41	0.79	0.75	0.08
城市	合计	42	1.22	0.47	1.06	1.00	0.12
	男性	28	1.59	0.55	1.42	1.36	0.16
	女性	14	0.83	0.36	0.70	0.67	0.08
农村	合计	231	1.31	0.52	1.13	1.06	0.11
	男性	148	1.63	0.60	1.45	1.36	0.14
	女性	83	0.97	0.42	0.81	0.76	0.08
死亡							
全省	合计	126	0.60	0.38	0.49	0.49	0.06
	男性	73	0.67	0.36	0.58	0.58	0.07
	女性	53	0.52	0.42	0.42	0.41	0.05
城市	合计	21	0.61	0.39	0.55	0.53	0.06
	男性	14	0.80	0.41	0.80	0.78	0.08
	女性	7	0.42	0.34	0.32	0.31	0.04
农村	合计	105	0.60	0.38	0.49	0.48	0.06
	男性	59	0.65	0.35	0.55	0.55	0.07
	女性	46	0.54	0.44	0.43	0.43	0.05

鼻咽恶性肿瘤年龄别发病率和死亡率在 0~35 岁年龄段处于较低水平，35 岁以后逐渐上

The age-specific incidence and mortality rates of nasopharyngeal cancer were relatively low before 35 years old and increased gradualy since 35 years old with obvious fluctuation,

升，在 75- 岁及 85+ 岁组分别达到高峰，除 80 岁以上男性发病率低于女性以外，男性发病率及死亡率均高于女性。城乡和不同地区年龄别率的水平虽然有一定的差异，但总体呈现波动趋势（图 5-2a ~ 图 5-2f）。

reached the peak at the age group of 75 and 85+ , respectively. The incidence rate and mortality rate in males generally were higher than that in females except for the incidence in age group of 80 and above. The age-specific incidence and mortality rates in rural areas and urban areas both refluctuated with different values (Figure 5-2a~Figure5-2f).

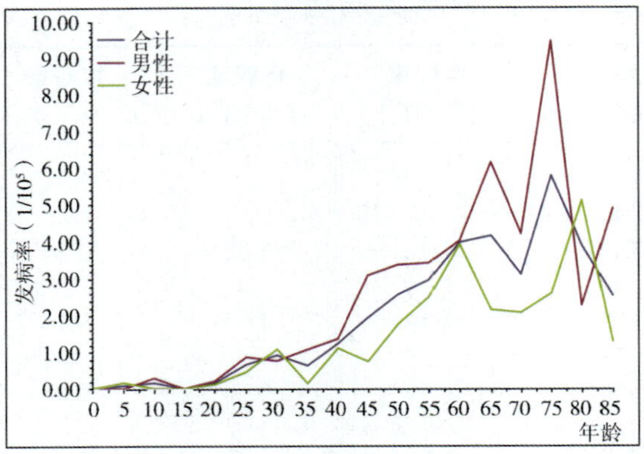

图 5-2a 河南省肿瘤登记地区鼻咽恶性肿瘤年龄别发病率，2014

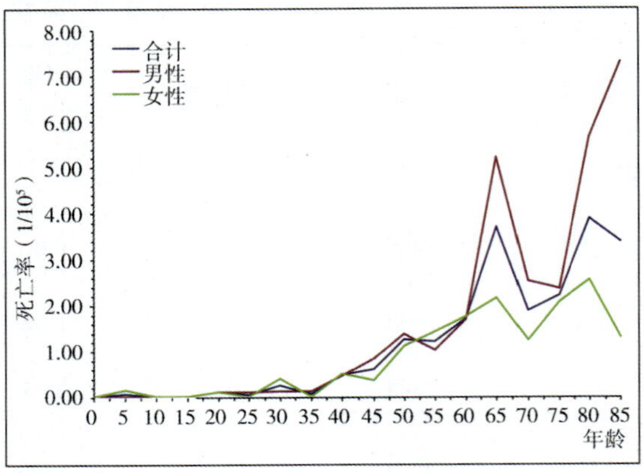

图 5-2d 河南省肿瘤登记地区鼻咽恶性肿瘤年龄别死亡率，2014

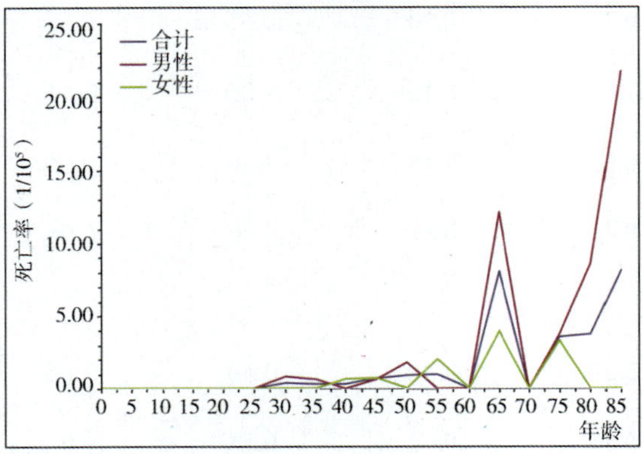

图 5-2b 城市肿瘤登记地区鼻咽恶性肿瘤年龄别发病率，2014

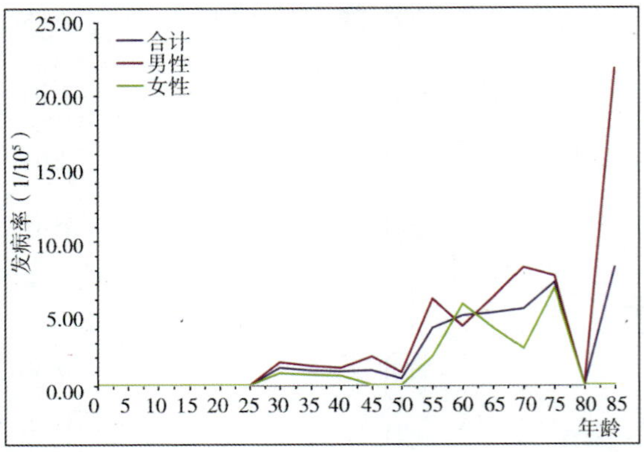

图 5-2e 城市肿瘤登记地区鼻咽恶性肿瘤年龄别死亡率，2014

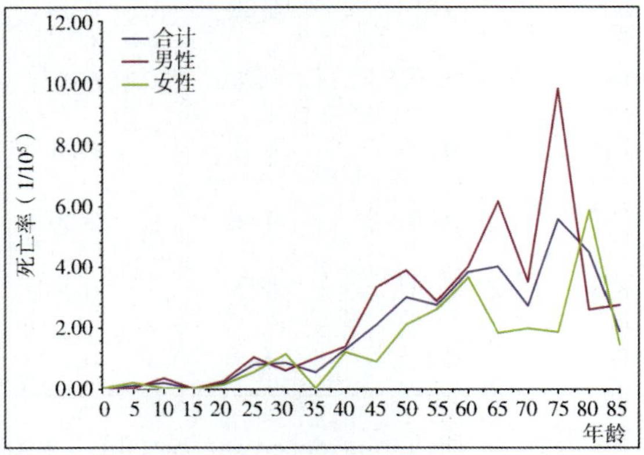

图 5-2c 农村肿瘤登记地区鼻咽恶性肿瘤年龄别发病率，2014

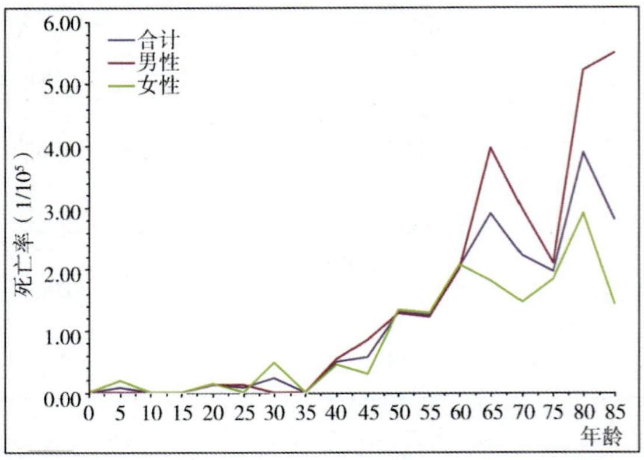

图 5-2f 农村肿瘤登记地区鼻咽恶性肿瘤年龄别死亡率，2014

在 5 个城市肿瘤登记地区中，男性鼻咽恶性肿瘤标化发病率最高的是漯河市（$2.00/10^5$），其次是洛阳市和三门峡市；女性发病率最高的是漯河市（$0.96/10^5$），其次是洛阳市和南阳市。男性标化死亡率最高的是洛阳市（$1.61/10^5$），女性死亡率最高的是南阳市（$0.76/10^5$）（图 5–2g）。

Among the 5 urban cancer registration areas, the ASR China incidence rate of nasopharyngeal cancer in males was the highest in Luohe City ($2.00/10^5$), followed by Luo yang City and Sanmenxia City. In females, it was the highest in Luohe City ($0.96/10^5$), followed by Luoyang City and Nan yang City. The highest ASR China mortality in males was in Luoyang City ($1.61/10^5$) and in females it was in Nanyang City ($0.76/10^5$) (Figure 5–2g).

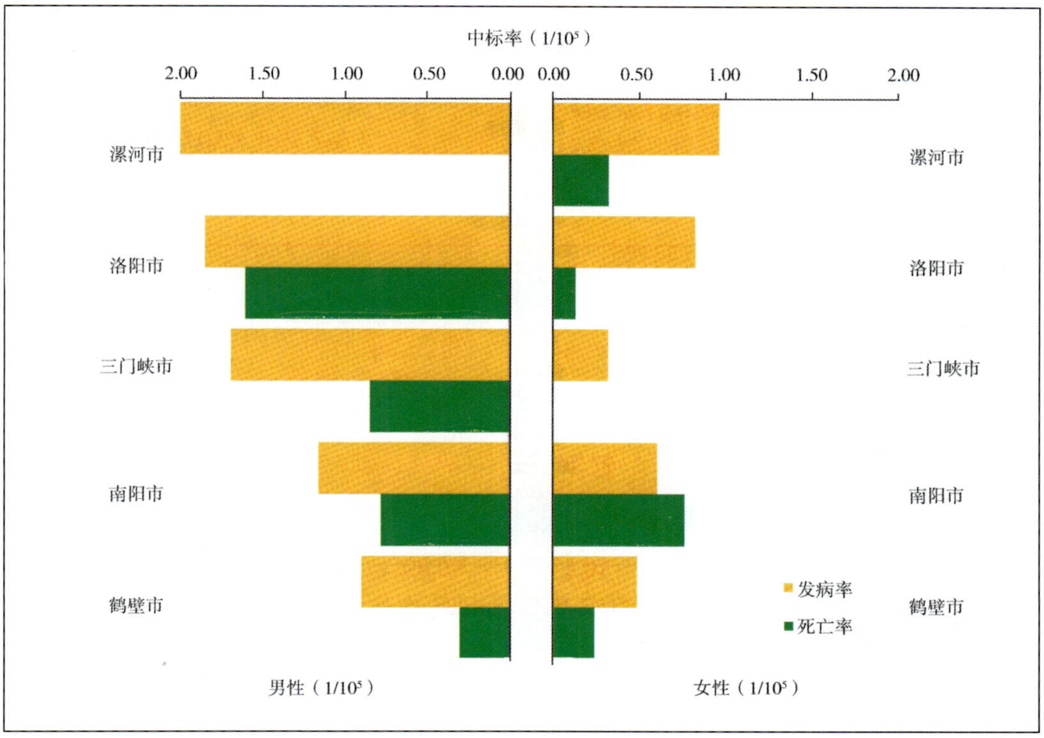

图 5–2g　城市肿瘤登记地区鼻咽恶性肿瘤发病率与死亡率

在 22 个农村肿瘤登记地区中，男性鼻咽恶性肿瘤标化发病率最高的是罗山县（$7.80/10^5$），其次是开封市祥符区和睢县；女性发病率最高的是虞城县（$2.53/10^5$），其次是罗山县和禹州市。男性标化死亡率最高的是罗山县（$1.98/10^5$），女性死亡率最高的是虞城县（$1.46/10^5$）（图 5–2h）。

Among the 22 rural cancer registration areas, the ASR China incidence rate of nasopharyngeal cancer in males was the highest in Luoshan County ($7.80/10^5$), followed by Xiangfu District, Kaifeng County and Suixian County. For females, it was the highest in Yucheng County ($2.53/10^5$), followed by Luoshan County and Yuzhou County. The ASR China mortality was the highest in Luoshan County for males ($1.98/10^5$) and Yucheng County for females ($1.46/10^5$) (Figure 5–2h).

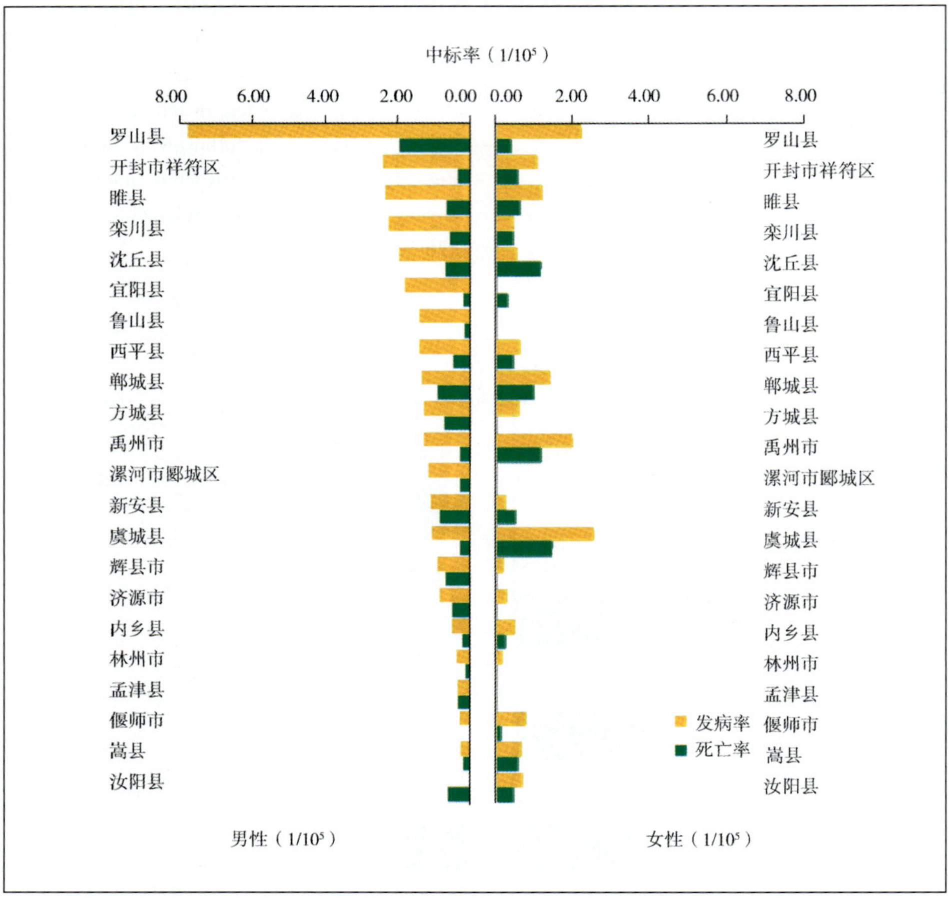

图 5-2h　农村肿瘤登记地区鼻咽恶性肿瘤发病率与死亡率

三、食管（C15）

2014 年，河南省肿瘤登记地区食管恶性肿瘤的发病率为 38.06/10^5，中标率为 30.03/10^5，世标率为 30.56/10^5，占全部恶性肿瘤发病的 15.06%。其中男性发病率为 45.78/10^5，女性为 29.84/10^5。男性中标率为女性的 1.72 倍，城市为农村的 0.89 倍。同期食管恶性肿瘤的死亡率为 26.14/10^5，中标率为 20.36/10^5，世标率为 20.53/10^5。其中男性死亡率为 31.77/10^5，女性为 20.16/10^5。食管恶性肿瘤发病和死亡的 0~74 岁累积率分别为 3.89% 和 2.44%（表 5-3）。

3. Esophagus (C15)

In 2014, esophageal cancer cases accounted for 15.06% of all cancer cases in Henan cancer registration areas with the crude incidence of 38.06/10^5, ASR for China 30.03/10^5 and ASR for World 30.56/10^5. The incidence in males was 45.78/10^5, and 29.84/10^5 in females. It was 1.72 times in males as high as that in females and it was 0.89 times in urban areas as that in rural areas. The crude mortality of esophageal cancer in 2014 was 26.14/10^5, ASR for China was 20.36/10^5 and ASR for World was 20.53/10^5. The mortality in males was 31.77/10^5, and 20.16/10^5 in females. The cumulative rates of incidence and mortality from 0 to 74 years old were 3.89% and 2.44%, respectively (Table 5-3).

表 5-3 河南省肿瘤登记地区食管恶性肿瘤发病与死亡

地区	性别	病例数	粗率（1/10^5）	构成（%）	中标率（1/10^5）	世标率（1/10^5）	累积率 0~74（%）
发病							
全省	合计	8 010	38.06	15.06	30.03	30.56	3.89
	男性	4 968	45.78	16.74	38.28	39.05	4.91
	女性	3 042	29.84	12.94	22.20	22.54	2.85
城市	合计	1 121	32.63	12.50	27.35	27.92	3.39
	男性	732	41.66	14.34	36.92	37.25	4.53
	女性	389	23.18	10.06	18.25	18.97	2.26
农村	合计	6 889	39.12	15.58	30.63	31.17	3.98
	男性	4 236	46.58	17.23	38.62	39.46	4.99
	女性	2 653	31.16	13.50	23.06	23.35	2.97
死亡							
全省	合计	5 502	26.14	16.70	20.36	20.53	2.44
	男性	3 447	31.77	16.89	26.70	27.01	3.18
	女性	2 055	20.16	16.39	14.46	14.53	1.70
城市	合计	726	21.13	13.32	17.82	17.99	1.90
	男性	478	27.20	13.97	24.59	24.44	2.57
	女性	248	14.78	12.21	11.63	12.03	1.25
农村	合计	4 776	27.12	17.37	20.89	21.08	2.54
	男性	2 969	32.65	17.47	27.16	27.54	3.29
	女性	1 807	21.22	17.19	15.04	15.08	1.79

食管恶性肿瘤年龄别发病率和死亡率在0~40岁年龄段处于较低水平，50岁以后快速上升，在80-岁组达到高峰，男性高于女性。城乡和不同地区年龄别率的水平虽然有一定的差异，但总体趋势类同（图5-3a ~图5-3f）。

The age-specific incidence and mortality rates of esophageal cancer were relatively low before 40 years old and increased dramatically since 50 years old, reaching the peak at the age group of 80. Incidence and mortality rates in males were generally higher than those in females. The age-specific incidence and mortality rates varied in urban and rural areas with similar curves (Figure 5-3a ~ Figure5-3f).

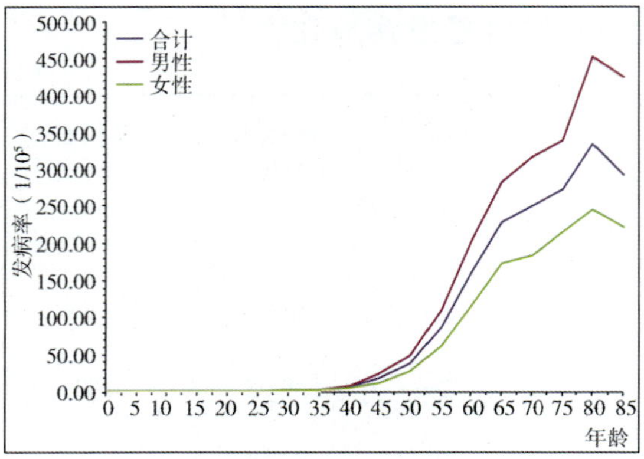

图 5-3a 河南省肿瘤登记地区食管恶性肿瘤年龄别发病率，2014

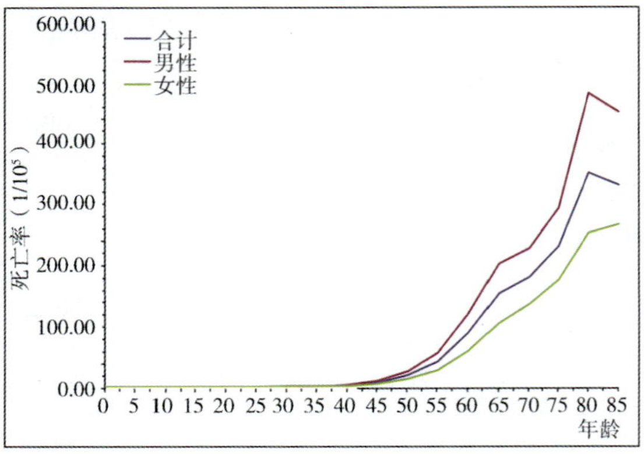

图 5-3d 河南省肿瘤登记地区食管恶性肿瘤年龄别死亡率，2014

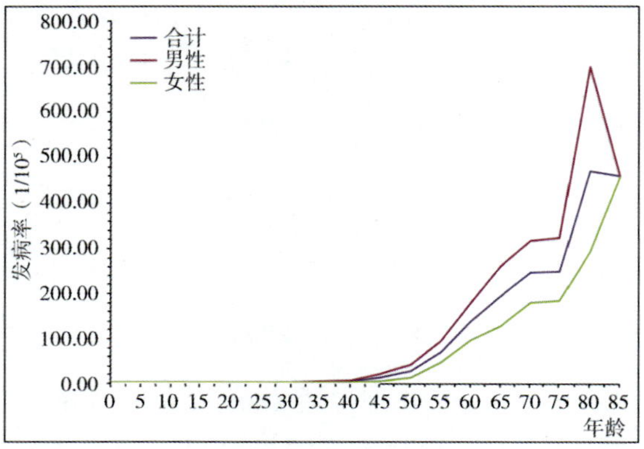

图 5-3b 城市肿瘤登记地区食管恶性肿瘤年龄别发病率，2014

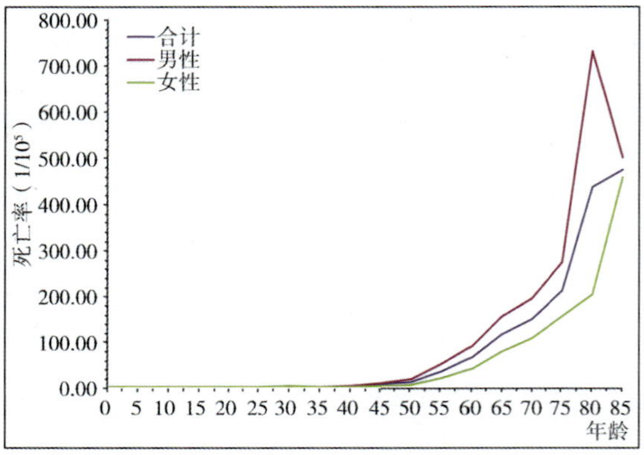

图 5-3e 城市肿瘤登记地区食管恶性肿瘤年龄别死亡率，2014

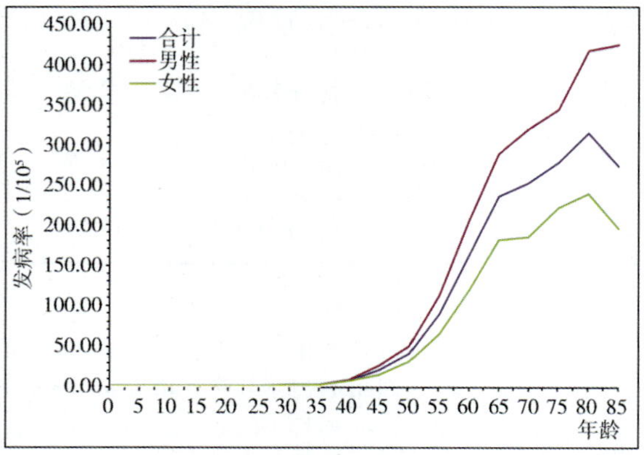

图 5-3c 农村肿瘤登记地区食管恶性肿瘤年龄别发病率，2014

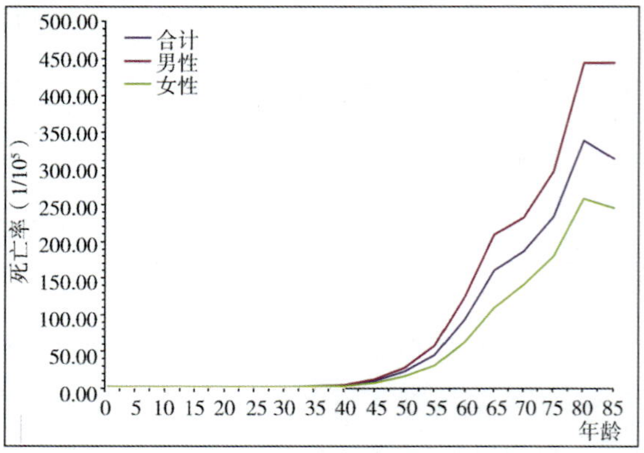

图 5-3f 农村肿瘤登记地区食管恶性肿瘤年龄别死亡率，2014

在5个城市肿瘤登记地区中，男性食管恶性肿瘤标化发病率最高的是鹤壁市（60.10/10⁵），其次是南阳市和洛阳市；女性发病率最高的是鹤壁市（35.31/10⁵），其次是南阳市和洛阳市。男性和女性标化死亡率最高的均是鹤壁市，分别为42.08/10⁵、23.92/10⁵（图5-3g）。

Among the 5 urban cancer registration areas, the ASR China incidence rate of esophageal cancer in both males ($60.10/10^5$) and females ($35.31/10^5$) was the highest in Hebi City, followed by Nanyang City and Luoyang City. The ASR China mortality was the highest in Hebi City for both males ($42.08/10^5$) and females ($23.92/10^5$) (Figure 5-3g).

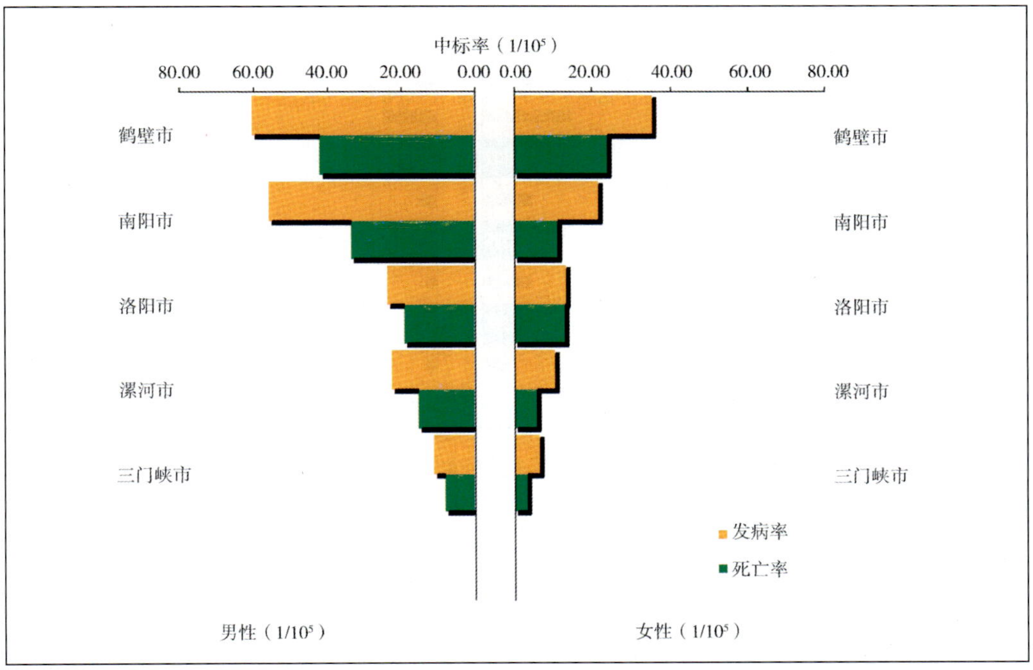

图5-3g 城市肿瘤登记地区食管恶性肿瘤发病率与死亡率

在22个农村肿瘤登记地区中，男性食管恶性肿瘤标化发病率最高的是宜阳县（87.56/10⁵），其次是内乡县和辉县市；女性发病率最高的是宜阳县（47.76/10⁵），其次是嵩县和林州市。男性标化死亡率最高的是宜阳县（61.44/10⁵），女性死亡率最高的是林州市（30.60/10⁵）（图5-3h）。

Among the 22 rural cancer registration areas, the ASR China incidence rate of esophageal cancer in males was the highest in Yiyang County ($87.56/10^5$), followed by Neixiang County and Huixian City . For females, it was the highest in Yiyang County ($47.76/10^5$), followed by Songxian County City and Linzhou City. The ASR China mortality was the highest in Yiyang County for males ($61.44/10^5$) and Linzhou City for females ($30.60/10^5$) (Figure 5-3h).

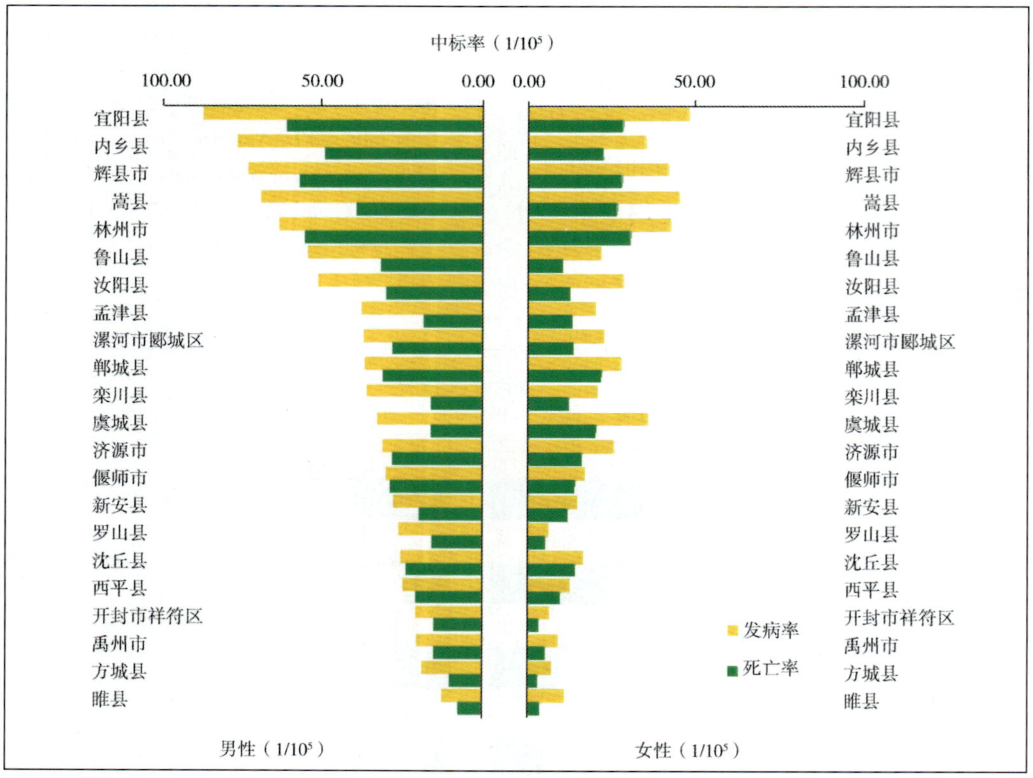

图 5-3h　农村肿瘤登记地区食管恶性肿瘤发病率与死亡率

2014 年肿瘤登记地区食管癌发病病例中有确切解剖学亚部位（C15.0–C15.5，C15.8）信息的占 62.3%，亚部位未特指（C15.9）的占 37.7%。在有亚部位的食管癌病例中，颈部食管癌（C15.0）占 5.9%，胸部食管癌（C15.1）占 3.9%，腹部食管癌（C15.2）占 7.2%，食管上三分之一（C15.3）的占 22.6%，食管中三分之一（C15.4）的占 37.1%，食管下三分之一（C15.5）的占 19.9%，食管交搭跨越（C15.8）的占 3.4%（图 5–3i）。

Among all the reported esophageal cancer cases in 2014, 62.3% had specific anatomic site information (C15.0~C15.5, C15.8) and the rest 37.7% didn't have. The specific anatomic sites of esophageal cancer included neck (C15.0) (5.9%), chest (C15.1) (3.9%), stomach (C15.2) (7.2%), upper esophagus (C15.3) (22.6%), middle esophagus (C15.4) (37.1%), lower esophagus (C15.5) (19.9%) and the overlapping part (C15.8) (3.4%) (Figure 5–3i).

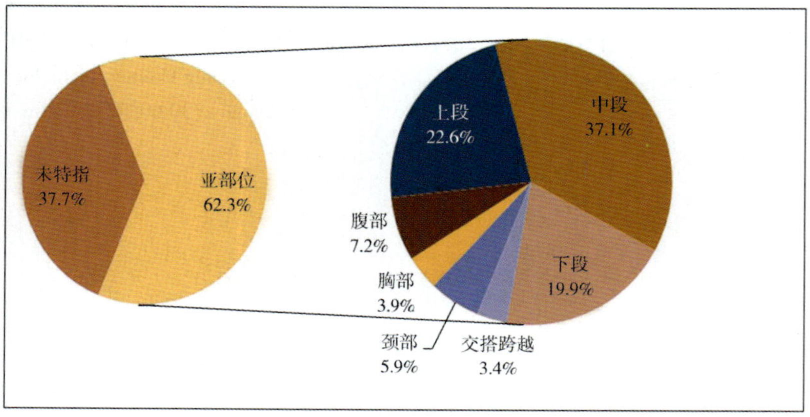

图 5-3i　河南省肿瘤登记地区食管癌发病亚部位构成 (%)

2014 年肿瘤登记地区食管癌发病病例中有明确组织病理学分型的占 77.3%，组织学类型未特指的占 22.7%。在有组织病理学分型的食管癌病例中，鳞状细胞癌占 87.4%，腺癌占 11.2%，腺鳞癌占 0.3%，其他类型的食管癌占 1.1%（图 5–3j）。

Among all cases, 77.3% had specific pathological diagnostic information and the rest 22.7% didn' t have. Squamous cell carcinoma accounted for 87.4% of the cases with specific pathological diagnostic information, adenocarcinoma accounted for 11.2%, adenosquamous carcinoma 0.3% and other pathological type 1.1% (Figure 5–3j).

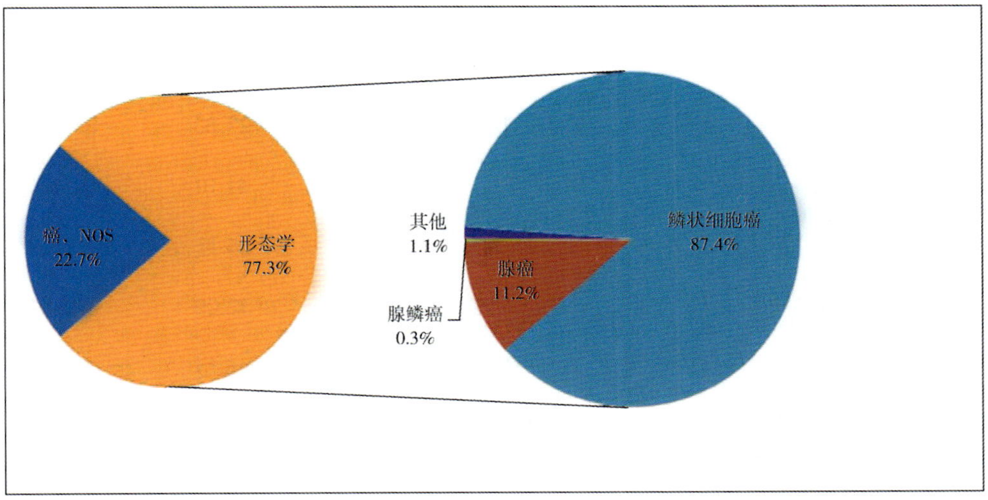

图 5–3j 河南省食管癌发病形态学构成 (%)

四、胃（C16）

2014 年，河南省肿瘤登记地区胃恶性肿瘤的发病率为 39.32/10^5，中标率为 31.30/10^5，世标率为 31.53/10^5，占全部恶性肿瘤发病的 15.55%。其中男性发病率为 54.54/10^5，女性为 23.11/10^5。男性中标率为女性的 2.63 倍，城市为农村的 0.86 倍。同期胃恶性肿瘤的死亡率为 28.25/10^5，中标率为 22.09/10^5，世标率为 22.06/10^5。其中男性死亡率为 38.73/10^5，女性为 17.1/10^5。胃恶性肿瘤发病和死亡的 0~74 岁累积率分别为 3.95% 和 2.57%（表 5–4）。

4. Stomach (C16)

In 2014, stomach cancer cases accounted for 15.55% of all cancer cases in Henan cancer registration areas with the crude incidence of 39.32/10^5, ASR for China 31.3/$10^5$and ASR for World 31.53/10^5. The incidence in males was 54.54/10^5, and 23.11/10^5 in females. It was 2.63 times in males as high as that in females and it was 0.86 times in urban areas as that in rural areas. The crude mortality rate of stomach cancer in 2014 was 28.25/10^5, ASR for China was 22.09/10^5 and ASR for World 22.06/10^5. The mortality in males was 38.73/10^5, and 17.1/10^5 in females. The cumulative rates of incidence and mortality from 0 to 74 years old were 3.95% and 2.57%, respectively (Table 5–4).

表 5-4 河南省肿瘤登记地区胃恶性肿瘤发病与死亡

地区	性别	病例数	粗率（1/10^5）	构成（%）	中标率（1/10^5）	世标率（1/10^5）	累积率 0~74（%）
发病							
全省	**合计**	**8 274**	**39.32**	**15.55**	**31.30**	**31.53**	**3.95**
	男性	5 918	54.54	19.94	45.70	46.23	5.83
	女性	2 356	23.11	10.02	17.40	17.34	2.06
城市	**合计**	**1 134**	**33.01**	**12.64**	**27.63**	**27.84**	**3.30**
	男性	814	46.32	15.95	41.10	41.60	4.86
	女性	320	19.07	8.28	15.11	15.13	1.76
农村	**合计**	**7 140**	**40.55**	**16.14**	**32.09**	**32.34**	**4.08**
	男性	5 104	56.12	20.76	46.70	47.26	6.01
	女性	2 036	23.91	10.36	17.88	17.81	2.12
死亡							
全省	**合计**	**5 946**	**28.25**	**18.04**	**22.09**	**22.06**	**2.57**
	男性	4 203	38.73	20.59	32.53	32.55	3.77
	女性	1 743	17.10	13.90	12.37	12.31	1.38
城市	**合计**	**742**	**21.60**	**13.61**	**18.21**	**18.14**	**1.88**
	男性	536	30.50	15.67	27.71	27.66	2.88
	女性	206	12.28	10.14	9.63	9.60	0.91
农村	**合计**	**5 204**	**29.55**	**18.92**	**22.88**	**22.85**	**2.70**
	男性	3 667	40.32	21.58	33.51	33.54	3.93
	女性	1 537	18.05	14.63	12.92	12.85	1.47

胃恶性肿瘤年龄别发病率和死亡率在 0~44 岁年龄段处于较低水平，45 岁以后快速上升，在 80- 岁组达到高峰，男性高于女性。城乡和不同地区年龄别率的水平虽然有一定的差异，但总体趋势类同（图 5-4a ~ 图 5-4f）。

The age-specific incidence and mortality rates of stomach cancer were relatively low before 44 years old and increased dramatically since 45 years old, reaching the peak at the age group of 80. Incidence and mortality rates in males were generally higher than those in females. The age-specific incidence and mortality rates varied in urban and rural areas with similar curves (Figure 5-4a~Figure5-4f).

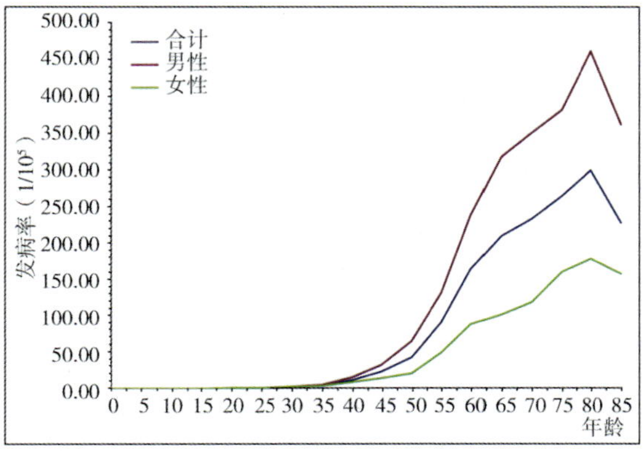

图 5-4a　河南省肿瘤登记地区胃恶性肿瘤年龄别发病率，2014

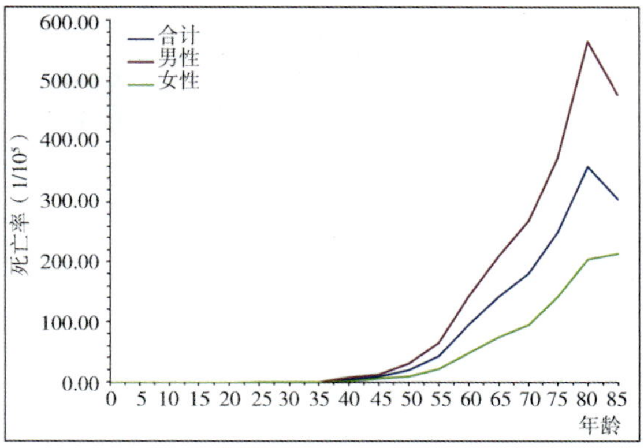

图 5-4d　河南省肿瘤登记地区胃恶性肿瘤年龄别死亡率，2014

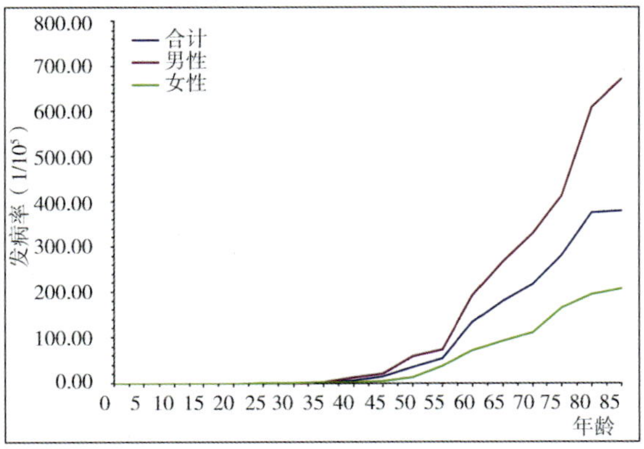

图 5-4b　城市肿瘤登记地区胃恶性肿瘤年龄别发病率，2014

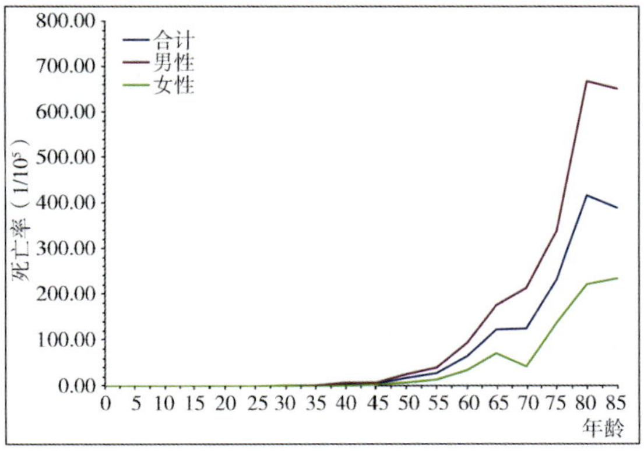

图 5-4e　城市肿瘤登记地区胃恶性肿瘤年龄别死亡率，2014

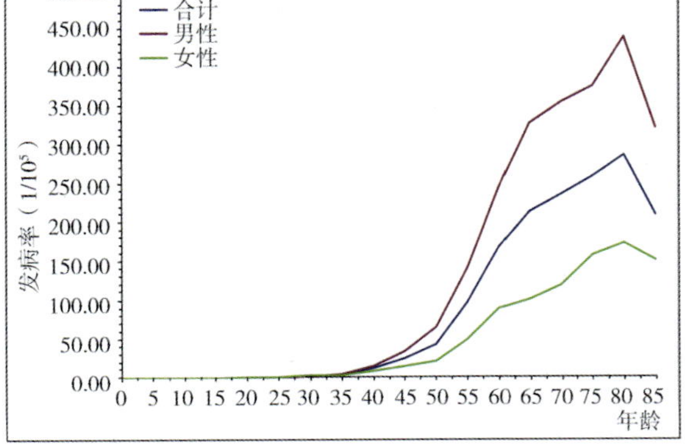

图 5-4c　农村肿瘤登记地区胃恶性肿瘤年龄别发病率，2014

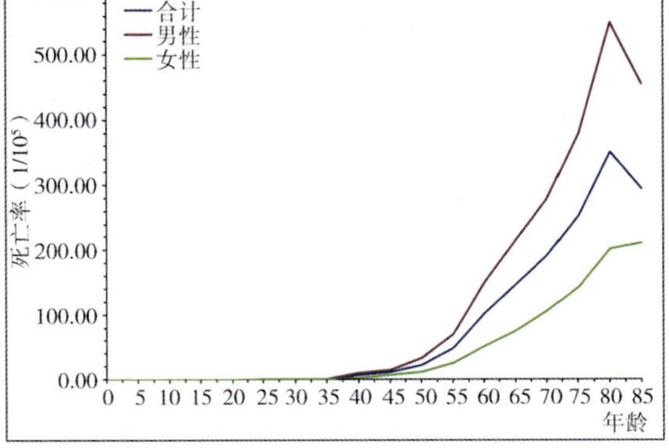

图 5-4f　农村肿瘤登记地区胃恶性肿瘤年龄别死亡率，2014

在 5 个城市肿瘤登记地区中，男性胃恶性肿瘤标化发病率最高的是南阳市（62.25/10^5），其次是鹤壁市和洛阳市；女性发病率最高的是南阳市（22.33/10^5），其次是鹤壁市和洛阳市。男性和女性标化死亡率最高的均是南阳市，分别为 39.83/10^5、13.91/10^5（图 5-4g）。

Among the 5 urban cancer registration areas, the ASR China incidence rate of stomach cancer in both males (62.25/10^5) and females (22.33/10^5) was the highest in Nanyang City, followed by Hebi City and Luoyang City. The highest ASR China mortalites were in Nanyang City for both males(39.83/10^5) and females (13.91/10^5) (Figure 5-4g).

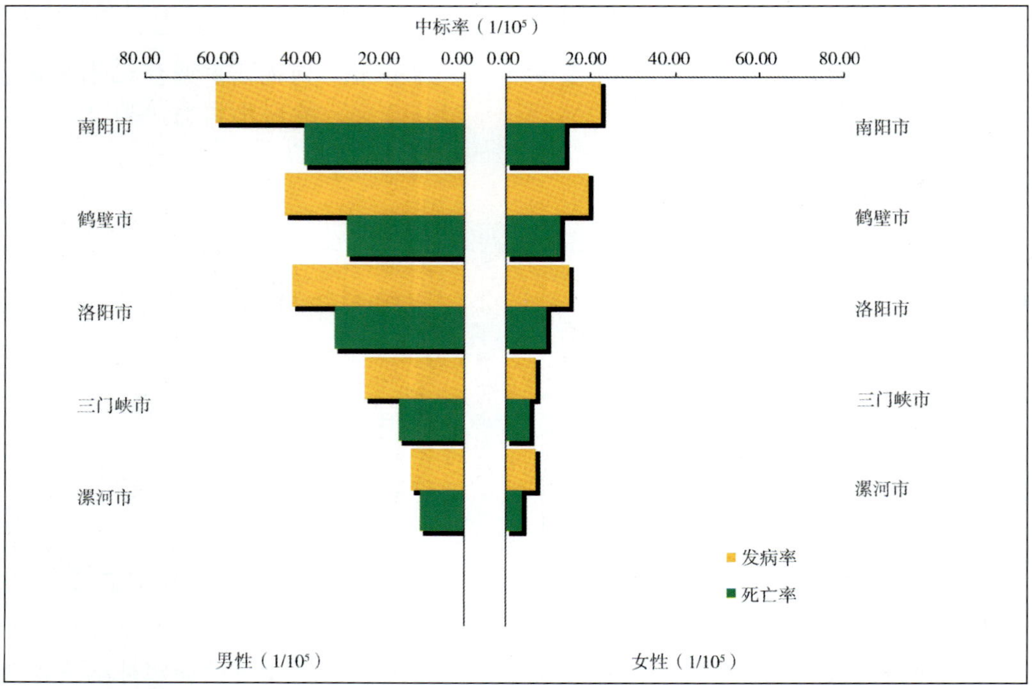

图 5-4g 城市肿瘤登记地区胃恶性肿瘤发病率与死亡率

在 22 个农村肿瘤登记地区中，男性胃恶性肿瘤标化发病率最高的是林州市（91.51/10^5），其次是济源市和内乡县；女性发病率最高的是林州市（34.27/10^5），其次是济源市和郸城县。男性和女性标化死亡率最高的均是林州市，分别为 68.57/10^5、24.83/10^5（图 5-4h）。

Among the 22 rural cancer registration areas, the ASR China incidence rate of stomach cancer in males was the highest in Linzhou City (91.51/10^5), followed by Jiyuan City and Neixiang County. For females, it was the highest in Linzhou City (34.27/10^5), followed by Jiyuan City and Dancheng County. TheASR China mortality was the highest in Linzhou City for males (68.57/10^5) and Linzhou City for females (24.83/10^5) (Figure 5-4h).

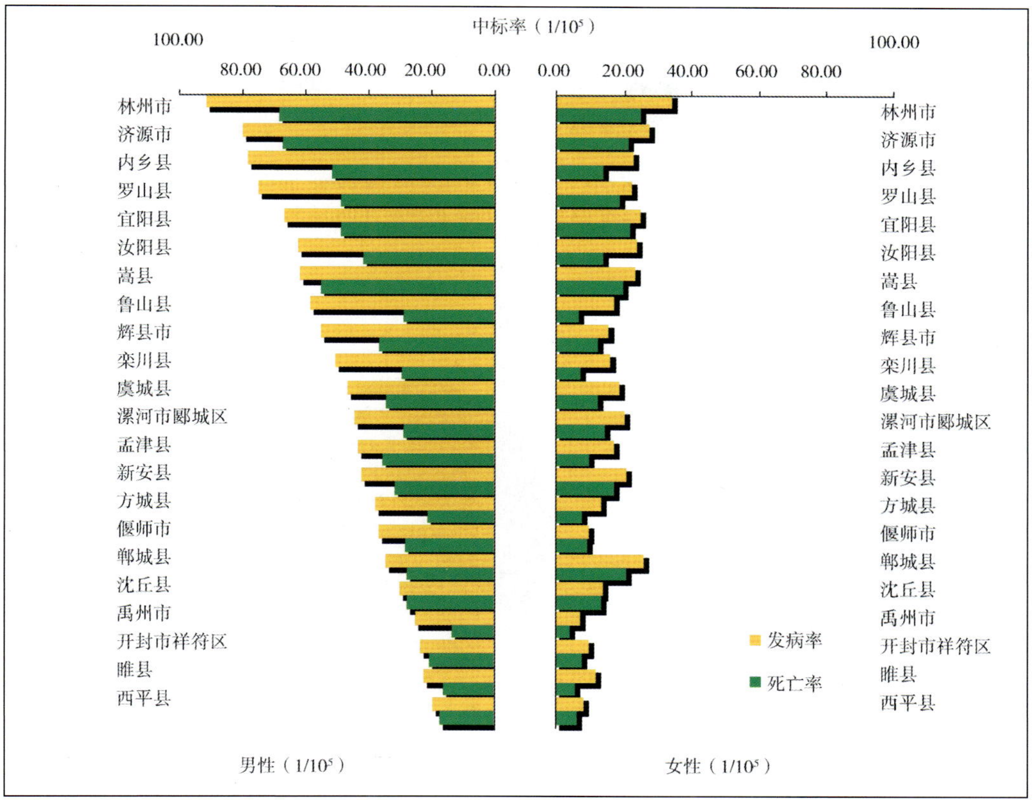

图 5-4h　农村肿瘤登记地区胃恶性肿瘤发病率与死亡率

2014 年肿瘤登记地区胃癌发病病例中有确切解剖学亚部位（C16.0~C16.6，C16.8）信息的占 68.4%，亚部位未特指（C16.9）的占 31.6%。在有亚部位的胃癌病例中，发生在胃贲门（C16.0）的占 55.9%，胃底（C16.1）占 8.2%，胃体（C16.2）占 16.4%，胃窦（C16.3）占 8.4%，胃幽门（C16.4）占 2.8%，胃小弯（C16.5）占 3.9%，胃大弯（C16.6）占 2.2%，胃交搭跨越（C16.8）的占 2.2%（图 5-4i）。

Among all the reported stomach cancer cases in 2014, 68.4% had specified subcategories (C16.0~C16.6, C16.8) and the rest 31.6% didn' t have. The specified subcategories of stomach cancer included cardia (C16.0) (55.9%), fundus (C16.1) (8.2%), body(C16.2) (16.4%), pylorus antrum (C16.3) (8.4%), pylorus (C16.4) (2.8%), lesser curvature (C16.5) (3.9%), greater curvature (C16.6) (2.2%), and overlapping part (C16.8) (2.2%) (Figure 5-4i).

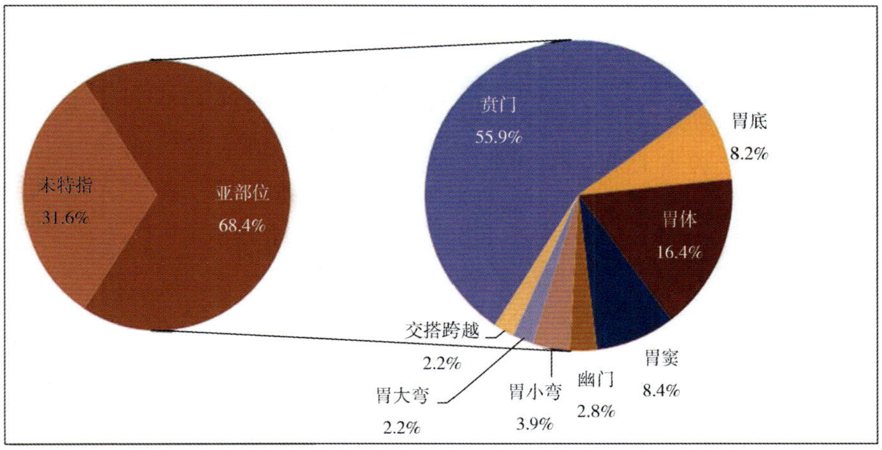

图 5-4i　河南省胃癌发病亚部位构成 (%)

2014 年肿瘤登记地区胃癌发病病例中有明确组织病理学分型的占 78.6%，组织学类型未特指的占 21.4%。在有组织病理学分型的胃癌病例中，腺癌占 92.1%，鳞状细胞癌占 6.5%，腺鳞癌占 0.2%，类癌占 0.2%，其他类型的胃癌占 0.9%（图 5-4j）。

Among all cases, 78.6% had specified pathological diagnostic information and the rest 21.4% didn' t have. The specified stomach pathological type include adenocarcinoma (92.1%), squamous cell carcinoma (6.5%), adenosquamous carcinoma (0.2%), carcinoid (0.2%) and other pathological type (0.9%) (Figure 5-4j).

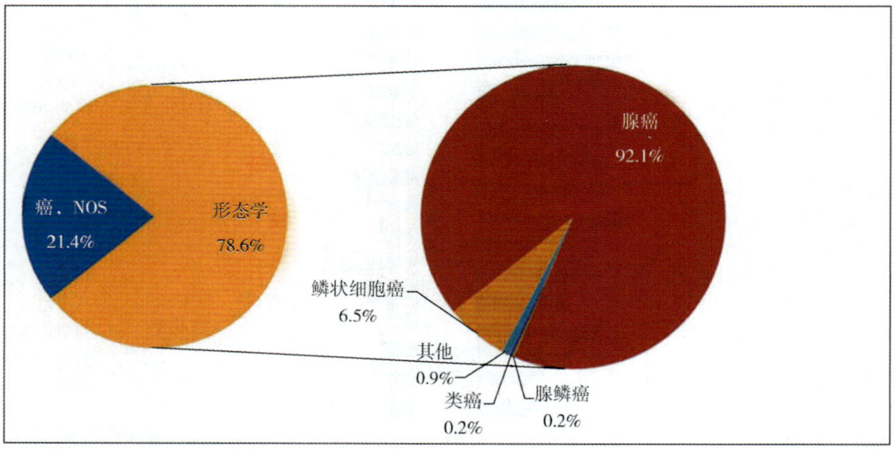

图 5-4j　河南省胃癌发病形态学构成 (%)

五、结直肠肛门（C18-C21）

2014 年，河南省肿瘤登记地区结直肠肛门恶性肿瘤的发病率为 16.21/10^5，中标率为 13.04/10^5，世标率为 12.88/10^5，占全部恶性肿瘤发病的 6.41%。其中男性发病率为 16.85/10^5，女性为 15.53/10^5。男性中标率为女性的 1.2 倍，城市为农村的 1.37 倍。同期结直肠肛门恶性肿瘤的死亡率为 8.16/10^5，中标率为 6.42/10^5，世标率为 6.36/10^5。其中男性死亡率为 9.05/10^5，女性为 7.21/10^5。结直肠肛门恶性肿瘤发病和死亡的 0~74 岁累积率分别为 1.53% 和 0.71%（表 5-5）。

5. Colon, Rectum & Anus (C18-C21)

In 2014, colorectal cancer cases accounted for 6.41% of all cancer cases in Henan cancer registration areas with the crude incidence of 16.21/10^5, ASR for China 13.04/10^5 and ASR for World 12.88/10^5. The incidence in males was 16.85/10^5, and 15.53/10^5 in females. It was 1.2 times in males as high as that in females and it was 1.37 times in urban areas as that in rural areas. The crude mortality of stomach cancer in 2014 was 8.16/10^5, ASR for China was 6.42/10^5 and ASR for World 6.36/10^5. The mortality in males was 9.05/10^5, and 7.21/10^5 in females. The cumulative rates of incidence and mortality from 0 to 74 years old were 1.53% and 0.71%, respectively (Table 5-5).

表 5-5 河南省肿瘤登记地区结直肠肛门恶性肿瘤发病与死亡

地区	性别	病例数	粗率（1/10⁵）	构成（%）	中标率（1/10⁵）	世标率（1/10⁵）	累积率 0~74（%）
发病							
全省	合计	3 411	16.21	6.41	13.04	12.88	1.53
	男性	1 828	16.85	6.16	14.27	14.08	1.68
	女性	1 583	15.53	6.73	11.88	11.74	1.39
城市	合计	703	20.46	7.84	17.03	16.78	1.81
	男性	390	22.19	7.64	19.58	19.55	2.07
	女性	313	18.65	8.10	14.84	14.40	1.56
农村	合计	2 708	15.38	6.12	12.39	12.25	1.48
	男性	1 438	15.81	5.85	13.41	13.20	1.61
	女性	1270	14.91	6.46	11.38	11.32	1.35
死亡							
全省	合计	1 717	8.16	5.21	6.42	6.36	0.71
	男性	982	9.05	4.81	7.66	7.58	0.84
	女性	735	7.21	5.86	5.29	5.25	0.58
城市	合计	407	11.85	7.47	9.95	9.95	0.96
	男性	238	13.54	6.96	12.36	12.35	1.09
	女性	169	10.07	8.32	7.90	7.93	0.82
农村	合计	1 310	7.44	4.76	5.84	5.78	0.67
	男性	744	8.18	4.38	6.89	6.82	0.79
	女性	566	6.65	5.39	4.85	4.81	0.54

结直肠肛门恶性肿瘤年龄别发病率和死亡率在 0~39 岁年龄段处于较低水平，40 岁以后快速上升，在 80- 岁组达到高峰，55 岁以上人群男性高于女性。城乡和不同地区年龄别率的水平虽然有一定的差异，但总体趋势类同，城市地区死亡率在 85+ 岁组达到高峰（图 5-5a ~ 图 5-5f）。

The age-specific incidence rate of colorectal cancer were relatively low before 39 years old and increased dramatically since 40 years old, reaching the peak at the age group of 80. Incidence and mortality rates in males were generally higher than those in females after 55 years old.The age-specific incidence and mortality rates varies between the urban and rural areas, but they have the similar trends except that it reached the peak at the age group of 85+ in the urban areas (Figure 5-5a~Figure5-5f).

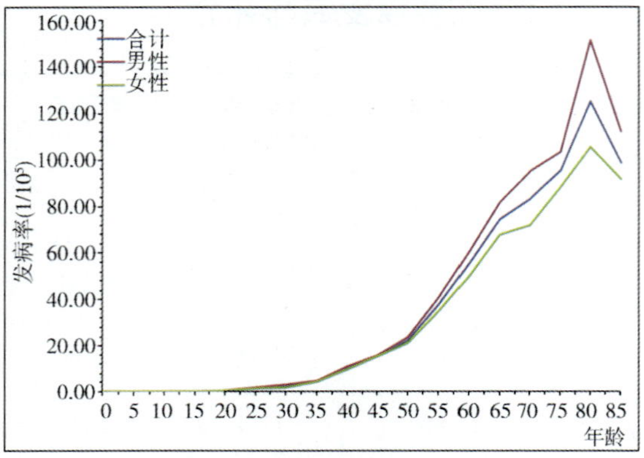

图 5-5a 河南省肿瘤登记地区结直肠肛门恶性肿瘤年龄别发病率，2014

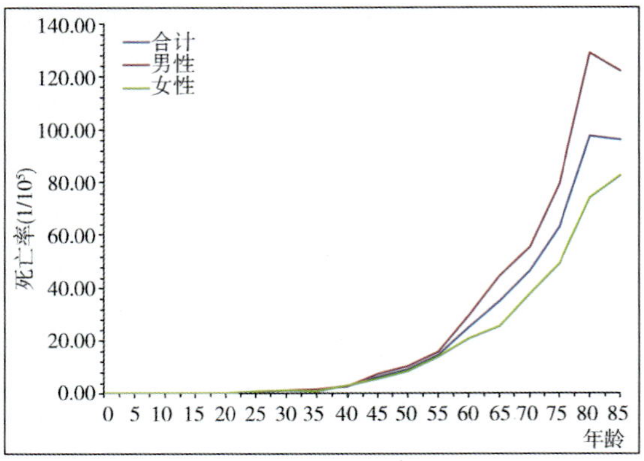

图 5-5d 河南省肿瘤登记地区结直肠肛门恶性肿瘤年龄别死亡率，2014

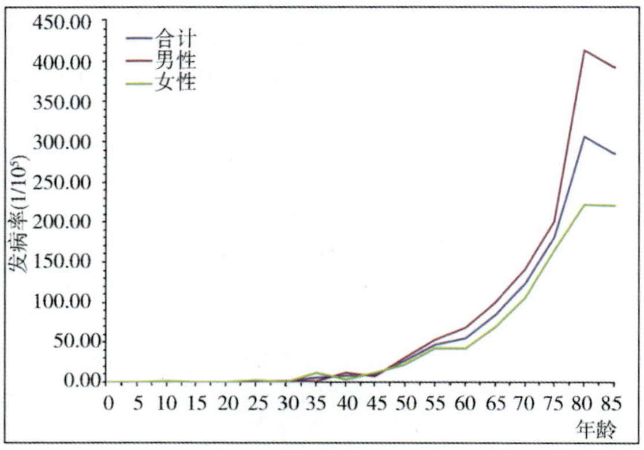

图 5-5b 城市肿瘤登记地区结直肠肛门恶性肿瘤年龄别发病率，2014

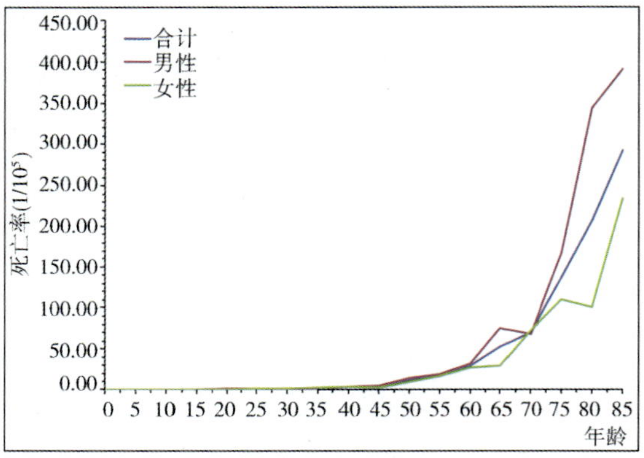

图 5-5e 城市肿瘤登记地区结直肠肛门恶性肿瘤年龄别死亡率，2014

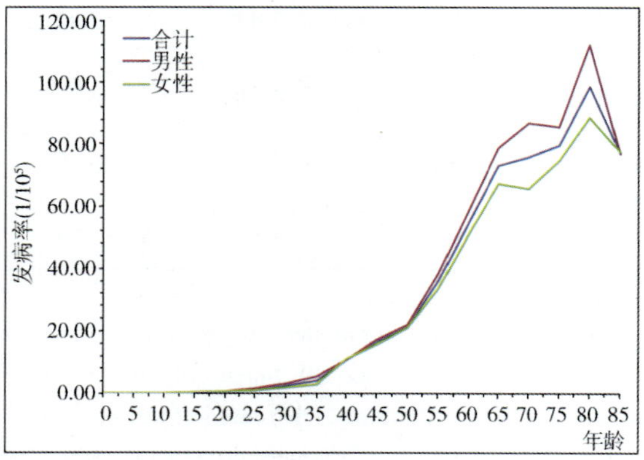

图 5-5c 农村肿瘤登记地区结直肠肛门恶性肿瘤年龄别发病率，2014

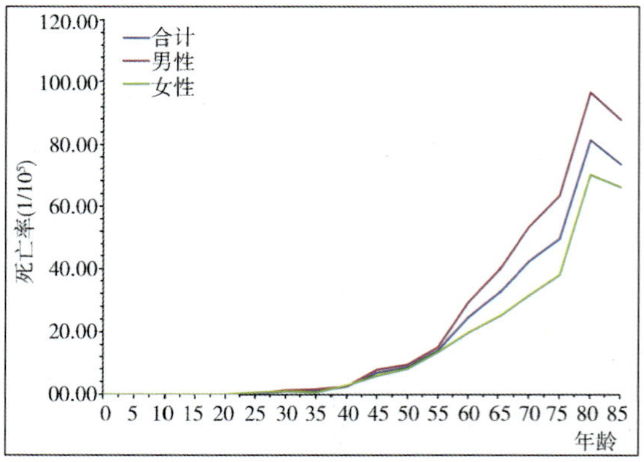

图 5-5f 农村肿瘤登记地区结直肠肛门恶性肿瘤年龄别死亡率，2014

在5个城市肿瘤登记地区中，男性结直肠肛门恶性肿瘤标化发病率最高的是洛阳市（28.43/10^5），其次是三门峡市和漯河市；女性发病率最高的是洛阳市（22.12/10^5），其次是漯河市和鹤壁市。男性和女性标化死亡率最高的均是洛阳市，分别为18.40/10^5、12.43/10^5（图5–5g）。

Among the 5 urban cancer registration areas, the age-specific incidence rate of colorectal cancer in males was the highest in Luoyang City (28.43/10^5), followed by Sanmenxia City and Luohe City. In females, it was the highest in Luoyang City (22.12/10^5), followed by Luohe City and Hebi City. The highest age-specific mortality in males was in Luoyang City (18.40/10^5) and in females it was in Luoyang City (12.43/10^5) (Figure 5–5g).

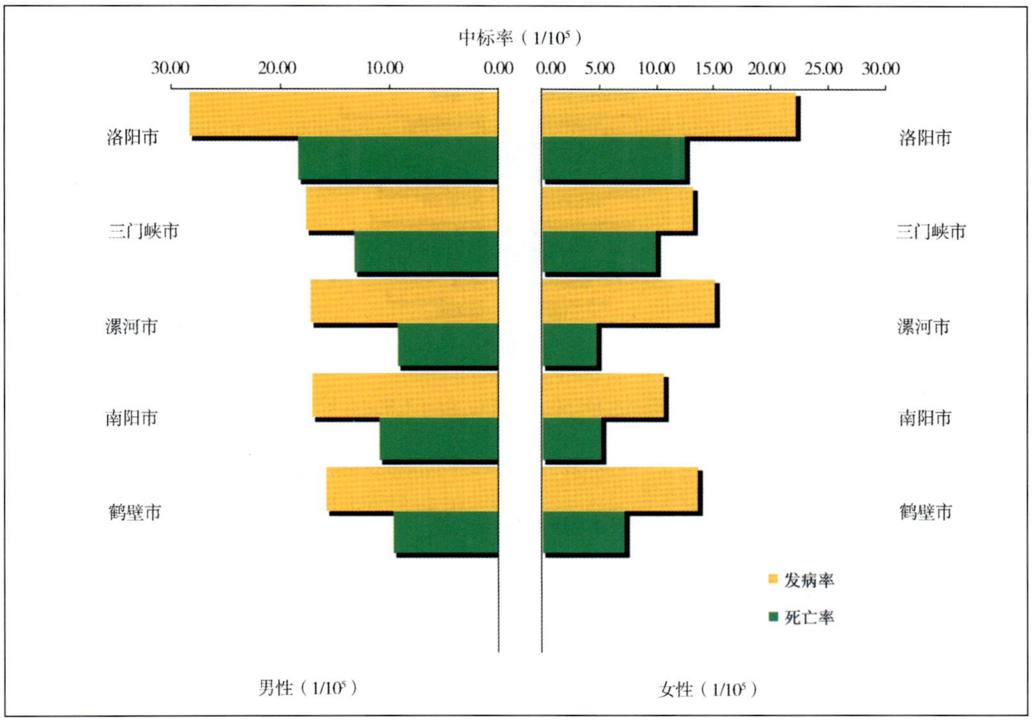

图5–5g　城市肿瘤登记地区结直肠肛门恶性肿瘤发病率与死亡率

在22个农村肿瘤登记地区中，男性结直肠肛门恶性肿瘤标化发病率最高的是罗山县（26.62/10^5），其次是开封市祥符区和虞城县；女性发病率最高的是罗山县（20.36/10^5），其次是郸城县和沈丘县。男性和女性标化死亡率最高的均是罗山县，分别为13.32/10^5、11.59/10^5（图5–5h）。

Among the 22 rural cancer registration areas, the ASR China incidence rate of colorectal cancer in males was the highest in Luoshan County (26.62/10^5), followed by Xiangfu District, Kaifeng and Yucheng County. For females, it was the highest in Luoshan County (20.36/10^5), followed by Dancheng County and Shenqiu County. The ASR China mortality was the highest in Luoshan County for both males (13.32/10^5) and females (11.59/10^5) (Figure 5–5h).

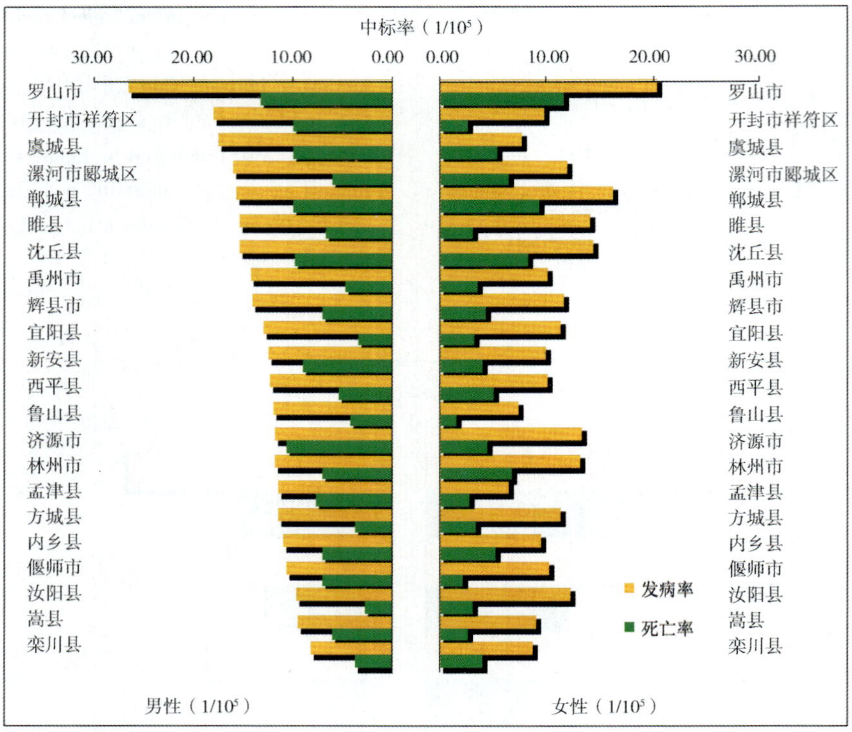

图 5-5h　农村肿瘤登记地区结直肠肛门恶性肿瘤发病率与死亡率

2014 年肿瘤登记地区结直肠癌发病病例中有确切解剖学亚部位（C18.0~C18.8，C19.9）信息的占 55.6%，亚部位未特指（C18.9，C20.9）的占 44.4%。在有亚部位的结直肠癌病例中，发生在盲肠（C18.0）的占 14.0%，阑尾（C18.1）的占 4.7%，升结肠（C18.2）的占 20.7%，结肠肝曲（C18.3）的占 3.9%，横结肠（C18.4）的占 6.7%，降结肠（C18.5）的占 7.1%，结肠脾曲（C18.6）的占 2.6%，乙状结肠（C18.7）的占 26.8%，结直肠交搭跨越（C18.8，C19.9）的占 13.5%（图 5-5i）。

Among all the reported colorectal cancer cases in 2014, 55.6% had specified subcategories (C18.0~C18.8, C19.9) and the rest 44.4% had unspecified anatomic sites (C18.9，C20.9). The specified subcategories of colorectal cancer included caecum (C18.0) (14.0%), appendix (C18.1) (4.7%), ascending colon (C18.2) (20.7%), hepatic flexure (C18.3) (3.9%), transverse colon (C18.4) (6.7%), descending colon(C18.5) (7.1%), splenic flexure (C18.6) (2.6%), sigmoid colon (C18.7) (26.8%), and overlapping part(C18.8,C19.9) (13.5%) (Figure 5-5i).

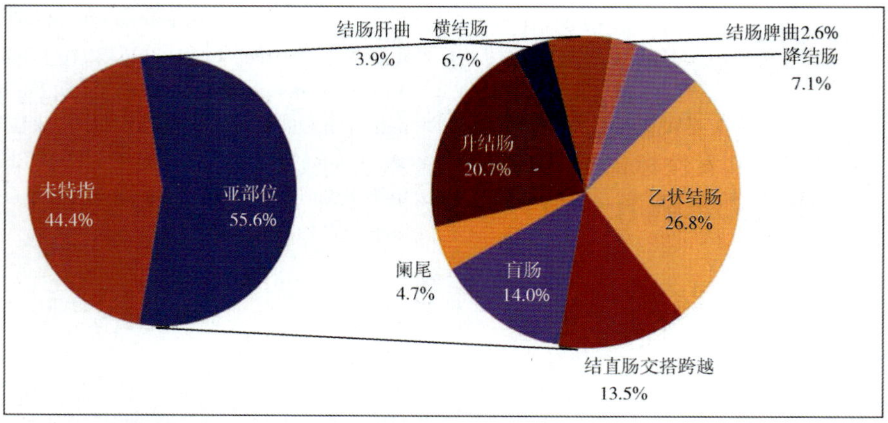

图 5-5i　河南省结直肠癌发病亚部位构成 (%)

六、肝脏（C22）

2014 年，河南省肿瘤登记地区肝脏恶性肿瘤的发病率为 26.23/10^5，中标率为 21.08/10^5，世标率为 21.03/10^5，占全部恶性肿瘤发病的 10.38%。其中男性发病率为 34.98/10^5，女性为 16.91/10^5。男性中标率为女性的 2.33 倍，城市为农村的 1.02 倍。同期肝脏恶性肿瘤的死亡率为 21.96/10^5，中标率为 17.51/10^5，世标率为 17.51/10^5。其中男性死亡率为 29.5/10^5，女性为 13.94/10^5。肝脏恶性肿瘤发病和死亡的 0~74 岁累积率分别为 2.53% 和 2.07%（表 5–6）。

6. Liver (C22)

In 2014, liver cancer cases accounted for 10.38% of all cancer cases in Henan cancer registration areas with the crude incidence of 26.23/10^5, ASR for China 21.08/10^5 and ASR for World 21.03/10^5. The incidence in males was 34.98/10^5, and 16.91/10^5 in females. It was 2.33 times in males as high as that in females and it was 1.02 times in urban areas as that in rural areas. The crude mortality of stomach cancer in 2014 was 21.96/10^5, ASR for China was 17.51/10^5 and ASR for World 17.51/10^5. The mortality in males was 29.5/10^5, and 13.94/10^5 in females. The cumulative rates of incidence and mortality from 0 to 74 years old were 2.53% and 2.07%, respectively (Table 5–6).

表 5–6　河南省肿瘤登记地区肝脏恶性肿瘤发病与死亡

地区	性别	病例数	粗率（1/10^5）	构成（%）	中标率（1/10^5）	世标率（1/10^5）	累积率 0~74（%）
发病							
全省	合计	5 520	26.23	10.38	21.08	21.03	2.53
	男性	3 796	34.98	12.79	29.49	29.37	3.50
	女性	1 724	16.91	7.33	12.68	12.71	1.54
城市	合计	894	26.02	9.97	21.58	21.61	2.50
	男性	644	36.65	12.62	32.00	32.10	3.62
	女性	250	14.90	6.47	11.63	11.72	1.39
农村	合计	4 626	26.27	10.46	21.06	20.99	2.54
	男性	3 152	34.66	12.82	29.14	29.00	3.48
	女性	1 474	17.31	7.50	12.91	12.92	1.57
死亡							
全省	合计	4 622	21.96	14.03	17.51	17.51	2.07
	男性	3 201	29.50	15.68	24.79	24.83	2.90
	女性	1 421	13.94	11.33	10.34	10.36	1.22
城市	合计	697	20.29	12.78	16.85	16.95	1.91
	男性	508	28.91	14.85	25.38	25.79	2.84
	女性	189	11.26	9.31	8.81	8.74	0.98
农村	合计	3 925	22.29	14.27	17.69	17.69	2.10
	男性	2 693	29.61	15.85	24.79	24.78	2.91
	女性	1 232	14.47	11.72	10.65	10.69	1.27

肝脏恶性肿瘤年龄别发病率和死亡率在0~34岁年龄段处于较低水平，35岁以后快速上升，在80-岁或85+岁组达到高峰，男性高于女性。城乡和不同地区年龄别率的水平虽然有一定的差异，但总体趋势类同（图5-6a ~图5-6f）。

The age-specific incidence and mortality rates of liver cancer were relatively low before 34 years old and increased dramatically since 35 years old, reaching the peak at the age group of 80 or 85. Incidence and mortality rates in male were generally higher than those in female. Although the age-specific incidence and mortality rates varied in urban and rural areas, they showed similar curves (Figure 5-6a ~ Figure5-6f).

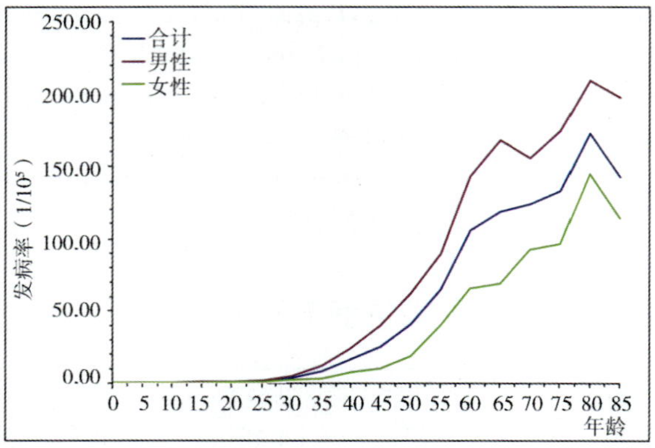

图5-6a 河南省肝脏恶性肿瘤年龄别发病率，2014

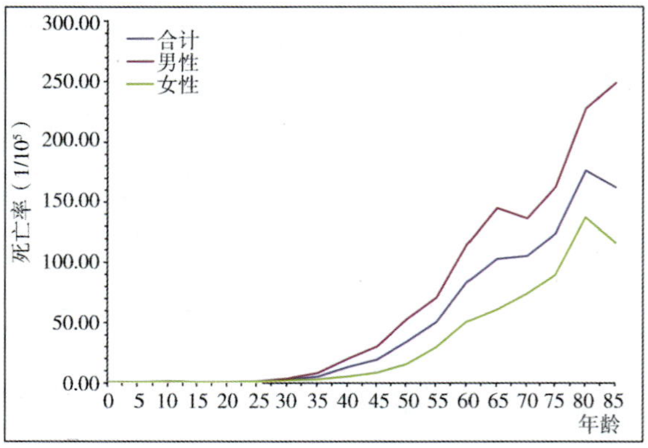

图5-6d 河南省肝脏恶性肿瘤年龄别死亡率，2014

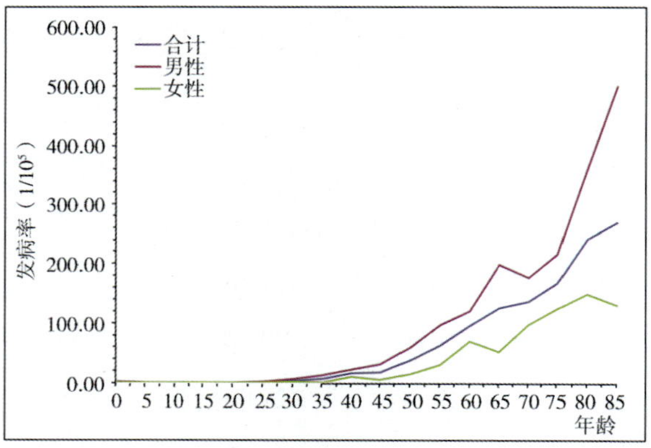

图5-6b 城市肿瘤登记地区肝脏恶性肿瘤年龄别发病率，2014

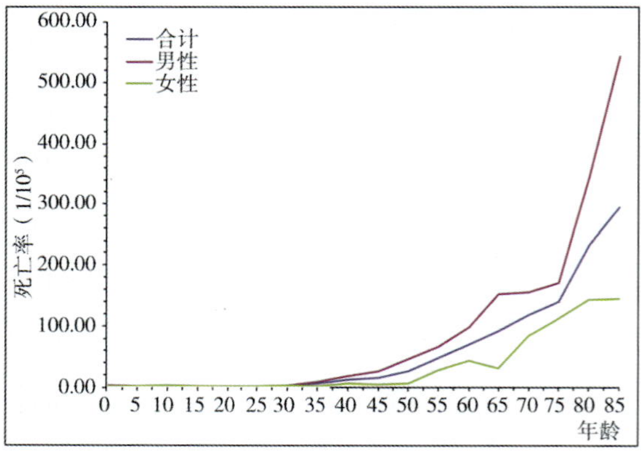

图5-6e 城市肿瘤登记地区肝脏恶性肿瘤年龄别死亡率，2014

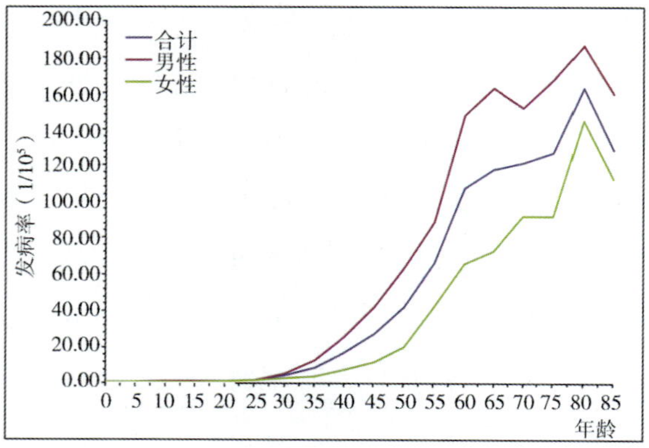

图5-6c 农村肿瘤登记地区肝脏恶性肿瘤年龄别发病率，2014

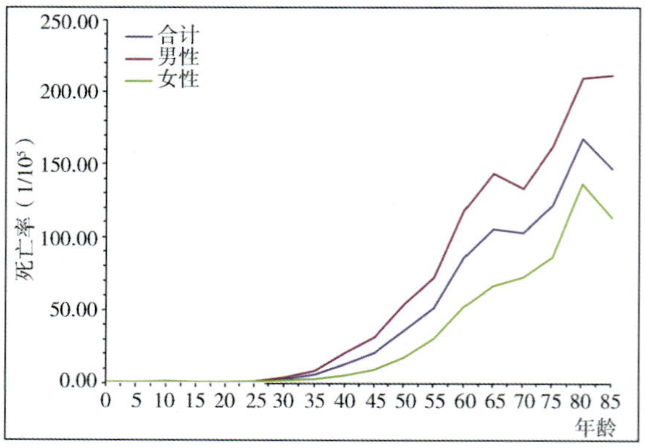

图5-6f 农村肿瘤登记地区肝脏恶性肿瘤年龄别死亡率，2014

在 5 个城市肿瘤登记地区中，男性肝脏恶性肿瘤标化发病率最高的是漯河市（$37.89/10^5$），其次是洛阳市和南阳市；女性发病率最高的是洛阳市（$15.57/10^5$），其次是三门峡市和南阳市。男性标化死亡率最高的是漯河市（$30.92/10^5$），女性死亡率最高的是洛阳市（$13.69/10^5$）（图 5–6g）。

Among the 5 urban cancer registration areas, the ASR China incidence rate of liver cancer in males was the highest in Luohe City ($37.89/10^5$), followed by Luoyang City and Nanyang City. In females, it was the highest in Luoyang City ($15.57/10^5$), followed by Sanmenxia City and Nanyang City. The highest ASR China mortality in males was in Luohe City ($30.92/10^5$) and in females it was in Luoyang City ($13.69/10^5$) (Figure 5–6g).

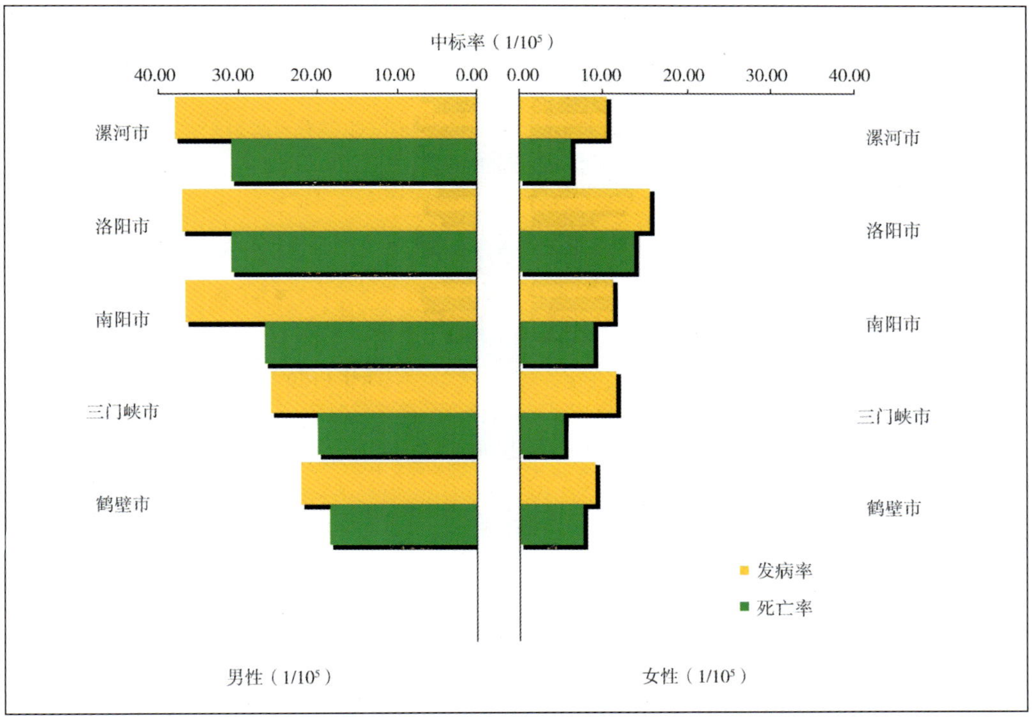

图 5–6g　城市肿瘤登记地区肝脏恶性肿瘤发病率与死亡率

在 22 个农村肿瘤登记地区中，男性肝脏恶性肿瘤标化发病率最高的是睢县（$52.80/10^5$），其次是沈丘县和罗山县；女性发病率最高的是郸城县（$22.94/10^5$），其次是虞城县和新安县。男性标化死亡率最高的是沈丘县（$49.94/10^5$），女性死亡率最高的是郸城县（$20.95/10^5$）（图 5–6h）。

Among the 22 rural cancer registration areas, the ASR China incidence rate of liver cancer in males was the highest in Suixian County ($52.80/10^5$), followed by Shenqiu County and Luoshan County. For females, it was the highest in Dancheng County ($22.94/10^5$), followed by Yucheng County and Xin'an County. The ASR China mortality was the highest in Shenqiu County for males ($49.94/10^5$) and Dancheng County for females ($20.95/10^5$) (Figure 5–6h).

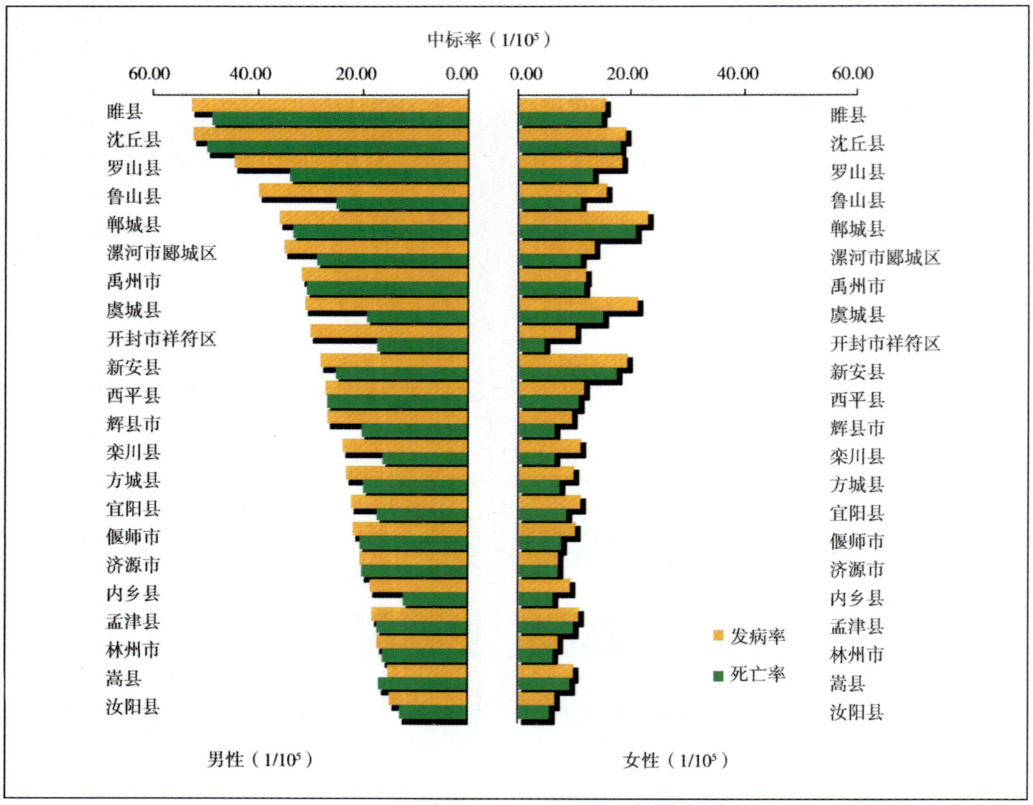

图 5-6h　农村肿瘤登记地区肝脏恶性肿瘤发病率与死亡率

七、胆囊及其他（C23–C24）

2014 年，河南省肿瘤登记地区胆囊及其他恶性肿瘤的发病率为 3.07/10^5，中标率为 2.40/10^5，世标率为 2.41/10^5，占全部恶性肿瘤发病的 1.22%。其中男性发病率为 2.51/10^5，女性为 3.68/10^5。男性中标率为女性的 0.79 倍，城市为农村的 1.05 倍。同期胆囊及其他恶性肿瘤的死亡率为 2.05/10^5，中标率为 1.58/10^5，世标率为 1.59/10^5。其中男性死亡率为 1.63/10^5，女性为 2.49/10^5。胆囊及其他恶性肿瘤发病和死亡的 0~74 岁累积率分别为 0.28% 和 0.18%（表 5–7）。

7. Gallbladder & Extrahepatic Bile Ducts (C23–C24)

In 2014, cancer cases of gallbladder and extrahepatic ducts (the following named as gallbladder cancer) accounted for 1.22% of all cancer cases in Henan cancer registration areas with the crude incidence of 3.07/10^5, ASR for China 2.4/10^5 and ASR for World 2.41/10^5. The incidence in males was 2.51/10^5, and 3.68/10^5 in females. It was 0.79 times in males as high as that in females and it was 1.05 times in urban areas as that in rural areas. The crude mortality of gallbladder cancer in 2014 was 2.05/10^5, ASR for China was 1.58/10^5 and ASR for World 1.59/10^5. The mortality in males was1.63/10^5, and 2.49/10^5 in females. The cumulative rates of incidence and mortality from 0 to 74 years old were 0.28% and 0.18%, respectively (Table 5–7).

表 5-7　河南省肿瘤登记地区胆囊及其他恶性肿瘤发病与死亡

地区	性别	病例数	粗率（1/10^5）	构成（%）	中标率（1/10^5）	世标率（1/10^5）	累积率 0~74（%）
发病							
全省	**合计**	**647**	**3.07**	**1.22**	**2.40**	**2.41**	**0.28**
	男性	272	2.51	0.92	2.11	2.13	0.26
	女性	375	3.68	1.59	2.68	2.69	0.30
城市	**合计**	**104**	**3.03**	**1.16**	**2.51**	**2.52**	**0.24**
	男性	44	2.50	0.86	2.20	2.26	0.20
	女性	60	3.58	1.55	2.79	2.76	0.26
农村	**合计**	**543**	**3.08**	**1.23**	**2.39**	**2.41**	**0.28**
	男性	228	2.51	0.93	2.10	2.11	0.27
	女性	315	3.70	1.60	2.68	2.70	0.30
死亡							
全省	**合计**	**431**	**2.05**	**1.31**	**1.58**	**1.59**	**0.18**
	男性	177	1.63	0.87	1.37	1.41	0.15
	女性	254	2.49	2.03	1.79	1.78	0.20
城市	**合计**	**65**	**1.89**	**1.19**	**1.58**	**1.59**	**0.18**
	男性	29	1.65	0.85	1.51	1.53	0.14
	女性	36	2.15	1.77	1.68	1.70	0.22
农村	**合计**	**366**	**2.08**	**1.33**	**1.58**	**1.59**	**0.18**
	男性	148	1.63	0.87	1.36	1.39	0.16
	女性	218	2.56	2.07	1.80	1.79	0.20

胆囊及其他恶性肿瘤年龄别发病率和死亡率在 0~49 岁年龄段处于较低水平，50 岁以后快速上升，在 80- 岁或 85+ 岁组达到高峰，男性低于女性。城乡和不同地区年龄别率的水平虽然有一定的差异，但总体趋势类同（图 5-7a ~ 图 5-7f）。

The age-specific incidence and mortality rates of gallbladder cancer were relatively low before 49 years old and increased dramatically since 50 years old, reaching the peak at the age group of 85. Incidence and mortality rates in males were lower than those in females. Although the age-specific incidence and mortality rates varied in urban and rural areas, they showed similar curves (Figure 5-7a~Figure5-7f).

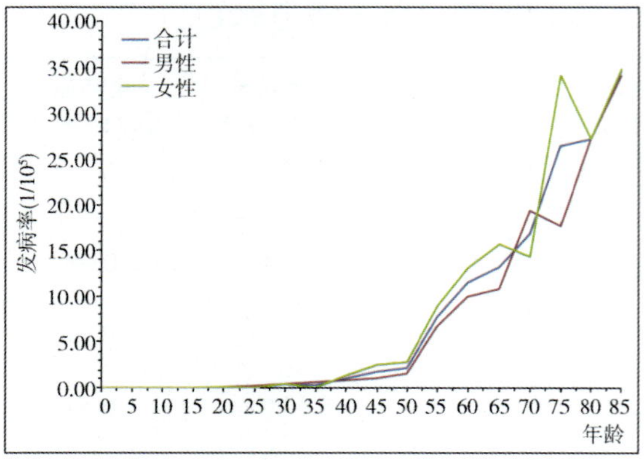

图 5-7a　河南省胆囊及其他恶性肿瘤年龄别发病率，2014

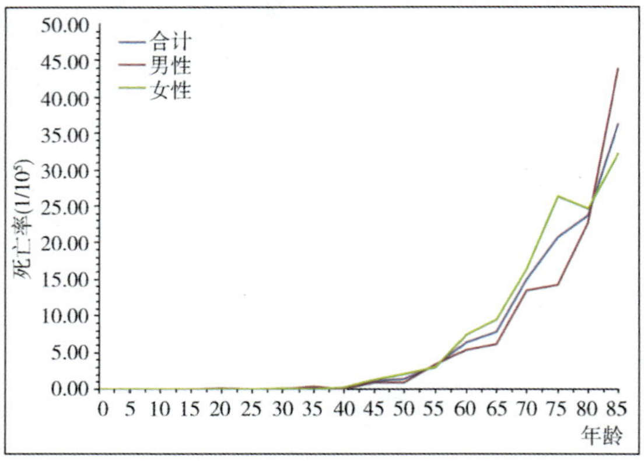

图 5-7d　河南省胆囊及其他恶性肿瘤年龄别死亡率，2014

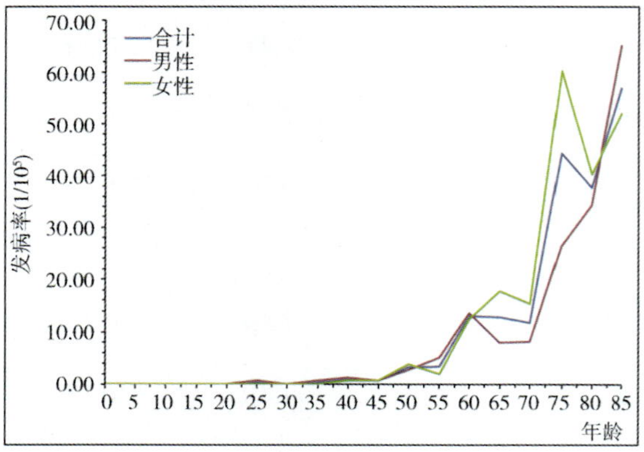

图 5-7b　城市肿瘤登记地区胆囊及其他恶性肿瘤年龄别发病率，2014

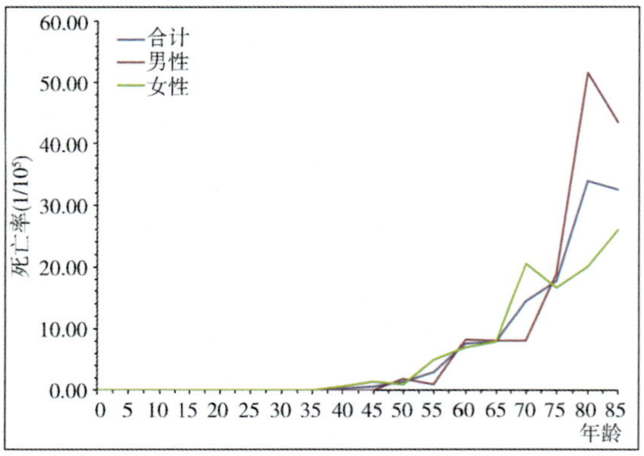

图 5-7e　城市肿瘤登记地区胆囊及其他恶性肿瘤年龄别死亡率，2014

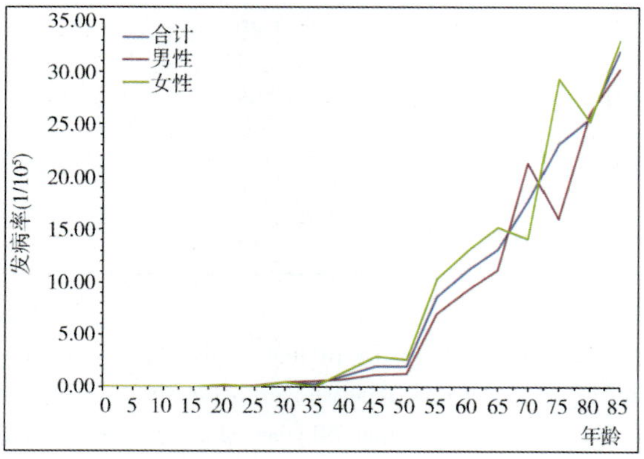

图 5-7c　农村肿瘤登记地区胆囊及其他恶性肿瘤年龄别发病率，2014

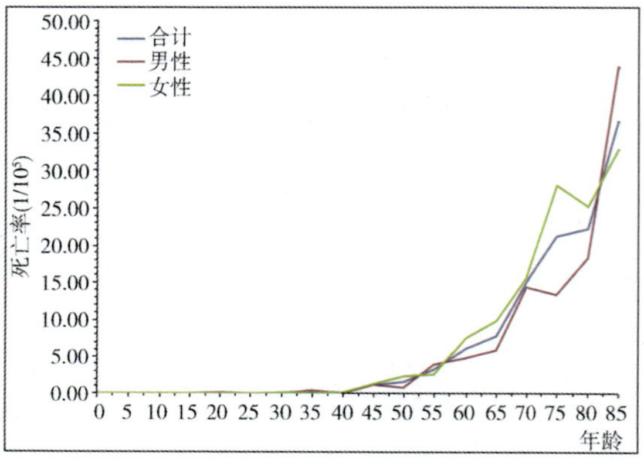

图 5-7f　农村肿瘤登记地区胆囊及其他恶性肿瘤年龄别死亡率，2014

在5个城市肿瘤登记地区中，男性胆囊及其他恶性肿瘤标化发病率最高的是洛阳市（4.68/10^5），其次是漯河市和鹤壁市；女性发病率最高的是洛阳市（6.22/10^5），其次是鹤壁市和三门峡市。男性和女性标化死亡率最高的均是洛阳市，分别为3.59/10^5、4.03/10^5（图5-7g）。

Among the 5 urban cancer registration areas, the ASR China incidence rate of gallbladder cancer in males was the highest in Luoyang City (4.68/10^5), followed by Luohe City and Hebi City. In females, it was the highest in Luoyang City (6.22/10^5), followed by Hebi City and Sanmenxia City. The highest ASR China mortality rates in both males (3.59/10^5) and females (4.03/10^5) were in Luoyang City (Figure 5-7g).

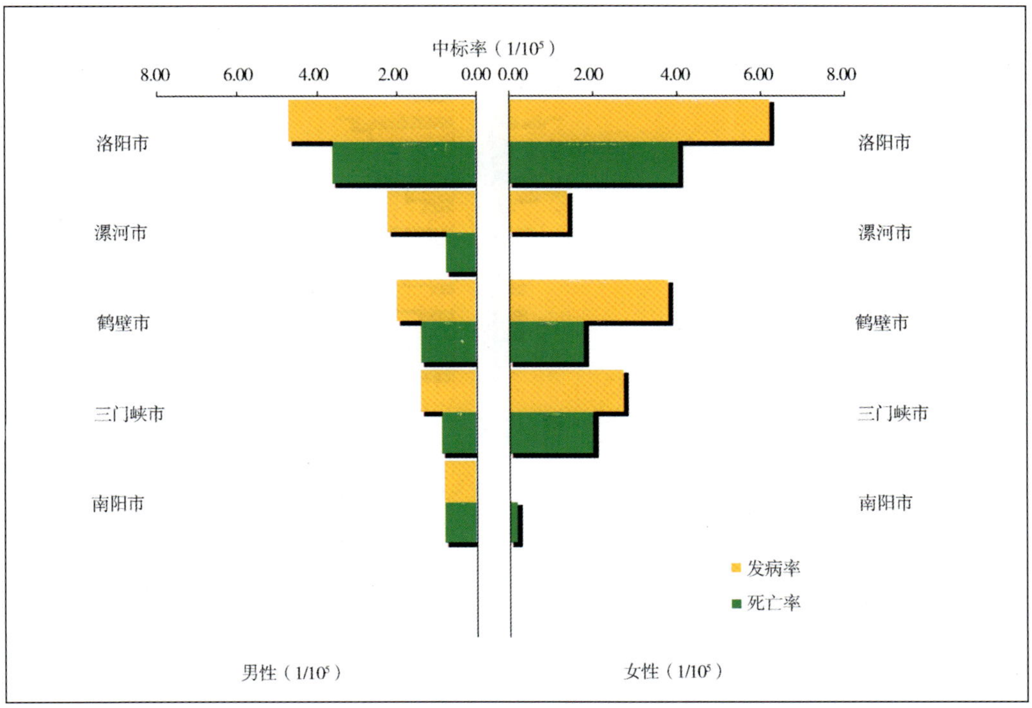

图5-7g　城市肿瘤登记地区胆囊及其他恶性肿瘤发病率与死亡率

在22个农村肿瘤登记地区中，男性胆囊及其他恶性肿瘤标化发病率最高的是孟津县（5.34/10^5），其次是睢县和开封市祥符区；女性发病率最高的是睢县（5.92/10^5），其次是西平县和新安县。男性标化死亡率最高的是孟津县（4.42/10^5），女性死亡率最高的是睢县（4.56/10^5）（图5-7h）。

Among the 22 rural cancer registration areas, the ASR China incidence rate of gallbladder cancer in males was the highest in Mengjin County (5.34/10^5), followed by Suixian County and Xiangfu District, Kaifeng. For females, it was the highest in Suixian County (5.92/10^5), followed by Xiping County and Xin'an County. The ASR China mortality was the highest in Mengjin County for males (4.42/10^5) and Suixian County for females (4.56/10^5) (Figure 5-7h).

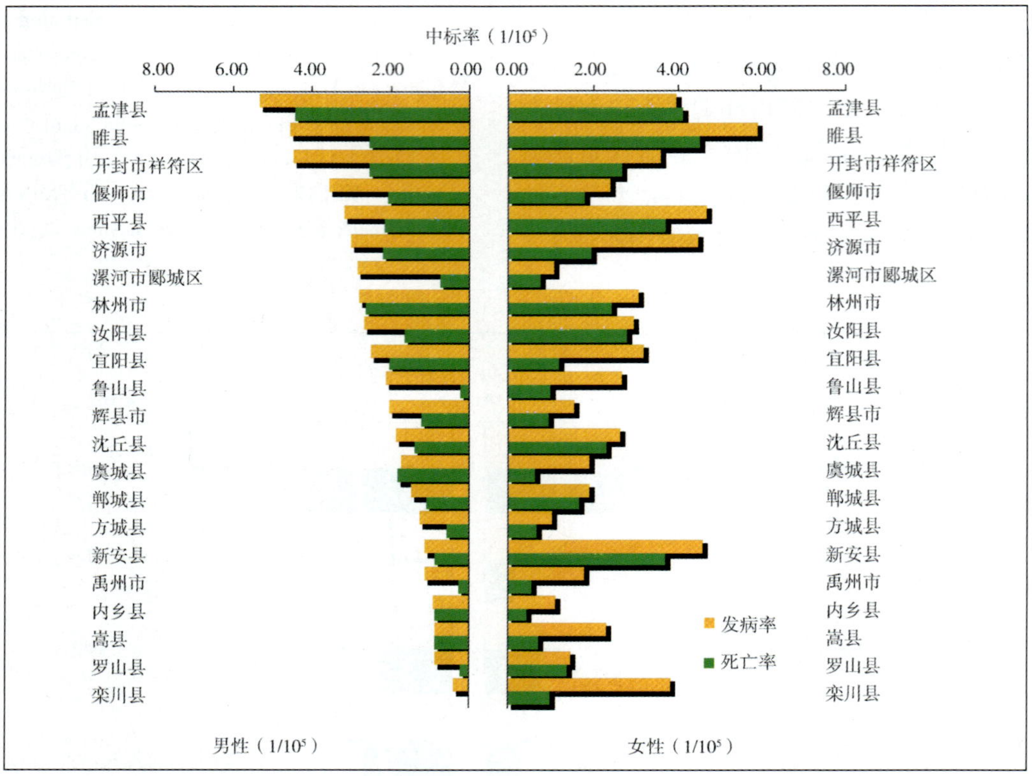

图 5-7h　农村肿瘤登记地区胆囊及其他恶性肿瘤发病率与死亡率

八、胰腺（C25）

2014 年，河南省肿瘤登记地区胰腺恶性肿瘤的发病率为 $3.49/10^5$，中标率为 $2.81/10^5$，世标率为 $2.81/10^5$，占全部恶性肿瘤发病的 1.38%。其中男性发病率为 $3.91/10^5$，女性为 $3.05/10^5$。男性中标率为女性的 1.42 倍，城市为农村的 1.38 倍。同期胰腺恶性肿瘤的死亡率为 $2.63/10^5$，中标率为 $2.11/10^5$，世标率为 $2.11/10^5$。其中男性死亡率为 $2.89/10^5$，女性为 $2.35/10^5$。胰腺恶性肿瘤发病和死亡的 0~74 岁累积率分别为 0.35% 和 0.26%（表 5-8）。

8. Pancreas (C25)

In 2014, pancreas cancer cases accounted for 1.38% of all cancer cases in Henan cancer registration areas with the crude incidence of $3.49/10^5$, ASR for China $2.81/10^5$ and ASR for World $2.81/10^5$. The incidence in males was $3.91/10^5$, and $3.05/10^5$ in females. It was 1.42 times in males as high as that in females and it was 1.38 times in urban areas as that in rural areas. The crude mortality of pancreas cancer in 2014 was $2.63/10^5$, ASR for China was $2.11/10^5$ and ASR for World $2.11/10^5$. The mortality in males was $2.89/10^5$, and $2.35/10^5$ in females. The cumulative rates of incidence and mortality from 0 to 74 years old were 0.35% and 0.26%, respectively (Table 5-8).

表 5-8　河南省肿瘤登记地区胰腺恶性肿瘤发病与死亡

地区	性别	病例数	粗率 (1/10^5)	构成 (%)	中标率 (1/10^5)	世标率 (1/10^5)	累积率 0~74 (%)
发病							
全省	合计	735	3.49	1.38	2.81	2.81	0.35
	男性	424	3.91	1.43	3.31	3.33	0.41
	女性	311	3.05	1.32	2.33	2.32	0.29
城市	合计	149	4.34	1.66	3.68	3.69	0.46
	男性	88	5.01	1.72	4.48	4.52	0.53
	女性	61	3.64	1.58	2.94	2.93	0.38
农村	合计	586	3.33	1.32	2.66	2.67	0.33
	男性	336	3.69	1.37	3.12	3.13	0.39
	女性	250	2.94	1.27	2.22	2.22	0.27
死亡							
全省	合计	554	2.63	1.68	2.11	2.11	0.26
	男性	314	2.89	1.54	2.48	2.51	0.30
	女性	240	2.35	1.91	1.76	1.75	0.22
城市	合计	131	3.81	2.40	3.25	3.29	0.36
	男性	78	4.44	2.28	4.14	4.30	0.43
	女性	53	3.16	2.61	2.50	2.45	0.28
农村	合计	423	2.40	1.54	1.91	1.92	0.24
	男性	236	2.60	1.39	2.20	2.22	0.28
	女性	187	2.20	1.78	1.62	1.63	0.20

胰腺恶性肿瘤年龄别发病率和死亡率在0~44岁年龄段处于较低水平，45岁以后快速上升，在85+岁组达到高峰，男性高于女性。城乡和不同地区年龄别率的水平虽然有一定的差异，但总体趋势类同（图5-8a ~ 图5-8f）。

The age-specific incidence and mortality rates of pancreas cancer were relatively low before 44 years old and increased dramatically since 45 years old, reaching the peak at the age group of 85 respectively. Incidence and mortality rates in males were generally higher than those in females. Although the age-specific incidence and mortality rates varied in urban and rural areas, they showed similar curves (Figure 5-8a~Figure 5-8f).

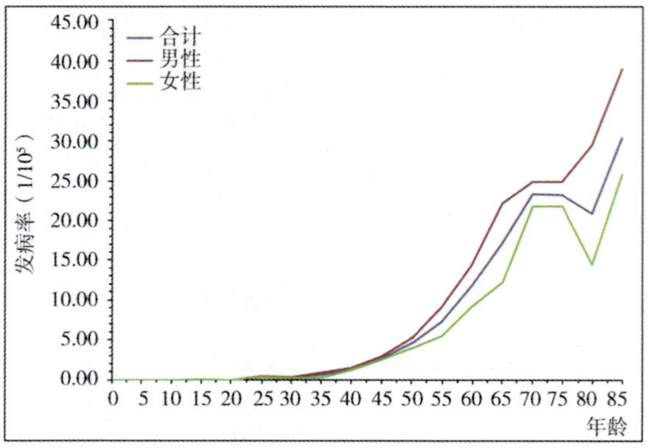

图 5-8a　河南省胰腺恶性肿瘤年龄别发病率，2014

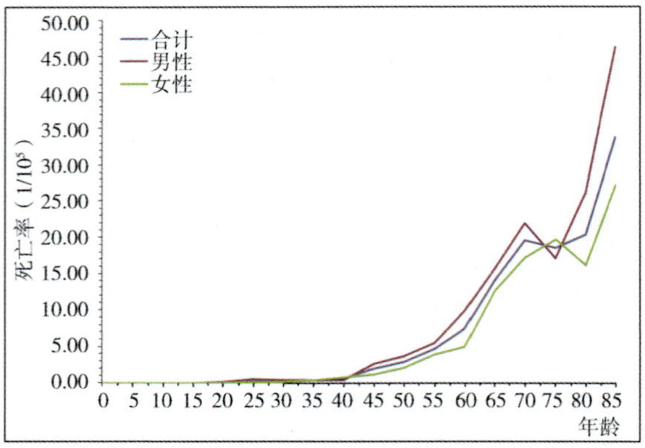

图 5-8d　河南省胰腺恶性肿瘤年龄别死亡率，2014

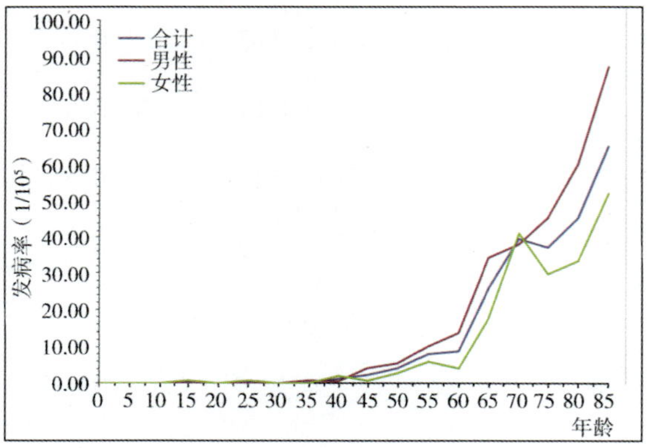

图 5-8b　城市肿瘤登记地区胰腺恶性肿瘤年龄别发病率，2014

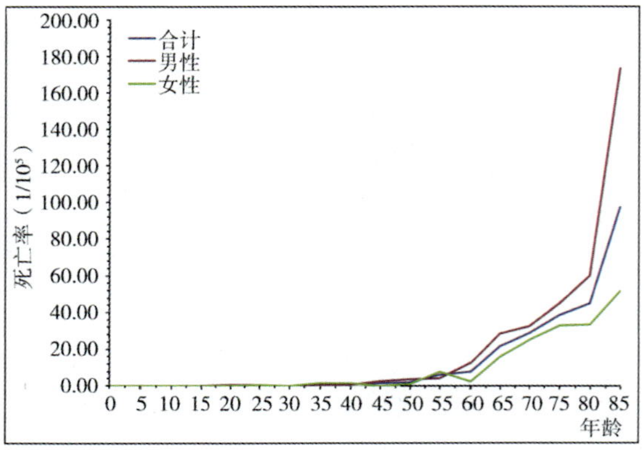

图 5-8e　城市肿瘤登记地区胰腺恶性肿瘤年龄别死亡率，2014

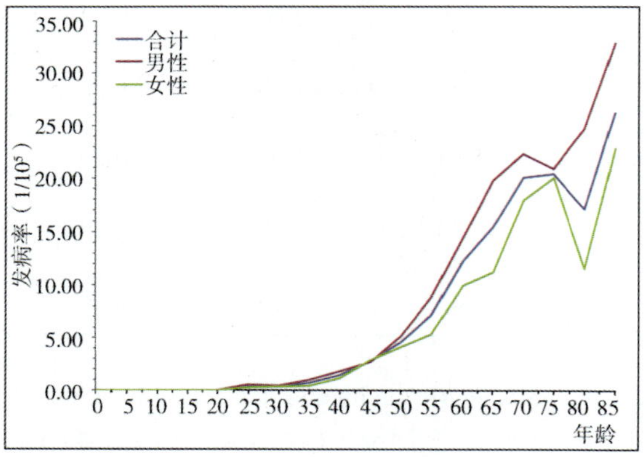

图 5-8c　农村肿瘤登记地区胰腺恶性肿瘤年龄别发病率，2014

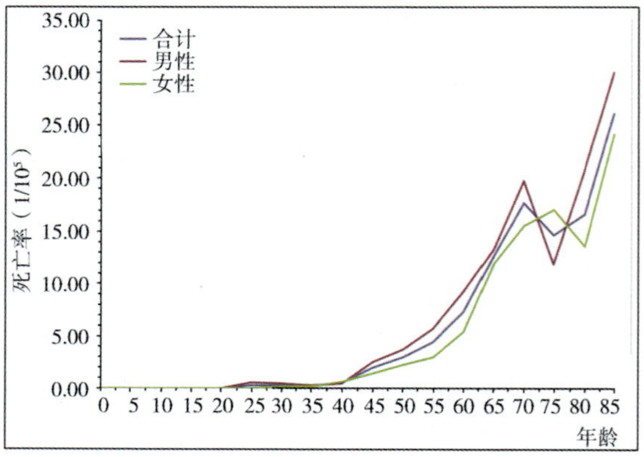

图 5-8f　农村肿瘤登记地区胰腺恶性肿瘤年龄别死亡率，2014

在 5 个城市肿瘤登记地区中，男性胰腺恶性肿瘤标化发病率最高的是洛阳市（8.98/10^5），其次是漯河市和三门峡市；女性发病率最高的是三门峡市（5.00/10^5），其次是洛阳市和鹤壁市。男性标化死亡率最高的是洛阳市（9.80/10^5），女性死亡率最高的是洛阳市（4.42/10^5）（图 5–8g）。

Among the 5 urban cancer registration areas, the ASR China incidence rate of pancreas cancer in males was the highest in Luoyang City (8.98/10^5), followed by Luohe City and Sanmenxia City. In females, it was the highest in Sanmenxia City (5.00/10^5), followed by Luoyang City and Hebi City. The highest ASR China mortality rates in both males (9.8/10^5) and females (4.42/10^5) were in Luoyang City (Figure 5–8g).

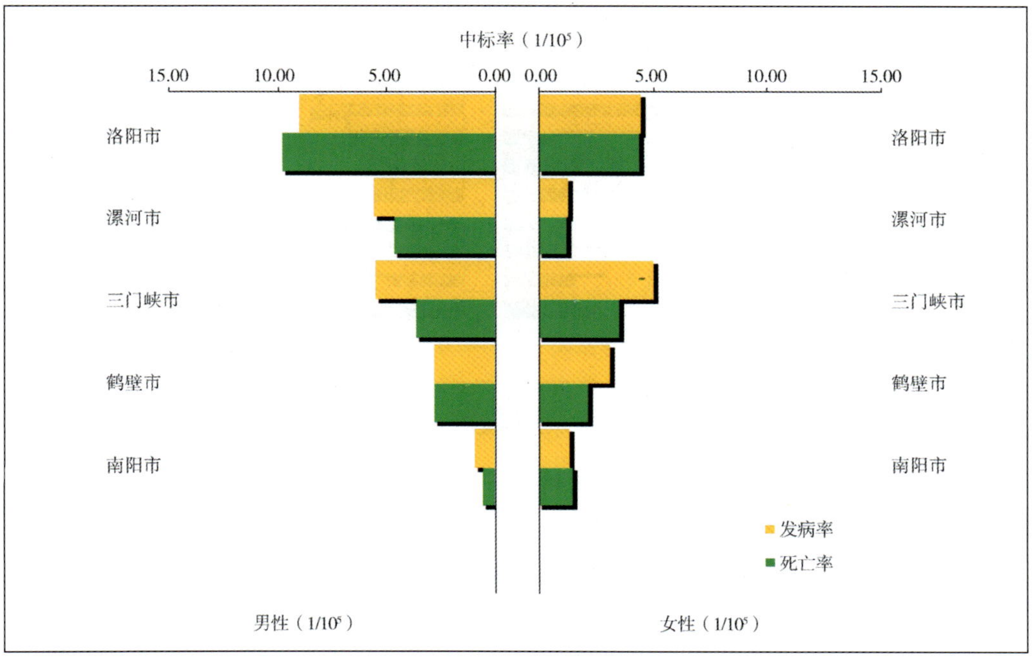

图 5–8g　城市肿瘤登记地区胰腺恶性肿瘤发病率与死亡率

在 22 个农村肿瘤登记地区中，男性胰腺恶性肿瘤标化发病率最高的是睢县（5.59/10^5），其次是济源市和罗山县；女性发病率最高的是汝阳县（3.74/10^5），其次是济源市和开封市祥符区。男性标化死亡率最高的是济源市（4.74/10^5），女性死亡率最高的是济源市（2.86/10^5）（图 5–8h）。

Among the 22 rural cancer registration areas, the ASR China incidence rate of pancreas cancer in males was the highest in Suixian County (5.59/10^5), followed by Jiyuan City and Luoshan County. For females, it was the highest in Ruyang County (3.74/10^5), followed by Jiyuan City and Xiangfu District, Kaifeng. The ASR China mortality were the highest in Jiyuan City for both males (4.74/10^5) and females (2.86/10^5) (Figure 5–8h).

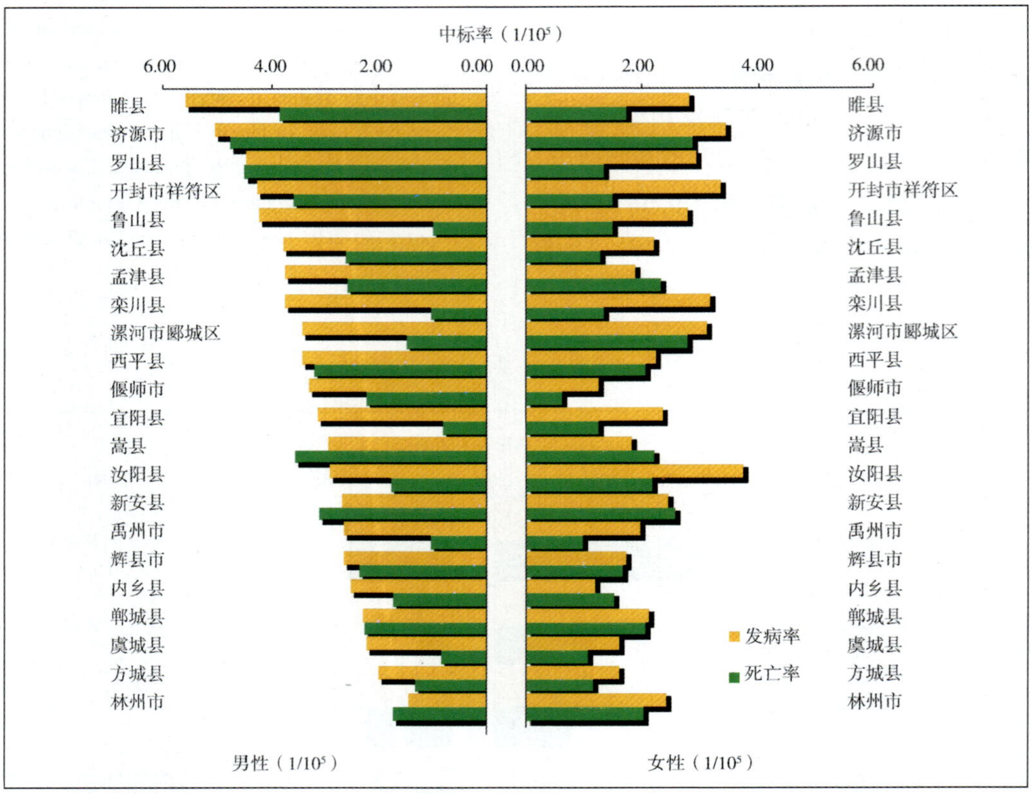

图 5-8h　农村肿瘤登记地区胰腺恶性肿瘤发病率与死亡率

2014 年肿瘤登记地区胰腺癌发病病例中有确切解剖学亚部位（C25.0~C25.4，C25.7，C25.8）信息的占 53.9%，亚部位未特指（C25.9）的占 46.1%。在有亚部位的胰腺癌病例中，发生在胰头（C25.0）的占 56.3%，胰体（C25.1）的占 17.9%，胰尾（C25.2）的占 6.1%，胰管（C25.3）的占 2.5%，内分泌的胰腺（C25.4）的占 15.2%，胰腺交搭跨越（C25.8）的占 2.0%（图 5–8i）。

Among all the reported pancreas cancer cases in 2014, 53.9% had specified subcategories (C25.0~C25.4, C25.7,C25.8) and the rest 46.1% had unspecified anatomic site (C25.9). The specified subcategories of pancreas cancer included the head of pancreas (C25.0) (56.3%), body (C25.1) (17.9%), tail (C25.2) (6.1%), pancreatic duct (C25.3) (2.5%), endocrine (C25.4) (15.2%) and overlapping (C25.8) (2.0%) (Figure 5–8i).

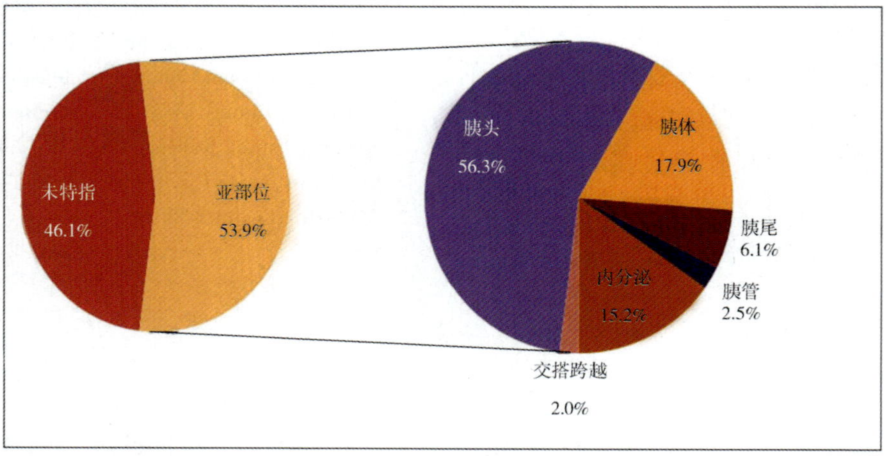

图 5-8i　河南省胰腺癌发病亚部位构成 (%)

九、气管、支气管、肺（C33–C34）

2013—2014 年，河南省肿瘤登记地区气管、支气管、肺恶性肿瘤的发病率为 48.28/10^5，中标率为 38.41/10^5，世标率为 38.42/10^5，占全部恶性肿瘤发病的 19.1%。其中男性发病率为 64.88/10^5，女性为 30.61/10^5。男性中标率为女性的 2.37 倍，城市为农村的 1.25 倍。同期气管、支气管、肺恶性肿瘤的死亡率为 36.3/10^5，中标率为 28.46/10^5，世标率为 28.46/10^5。其中男性死亡率为 49.61/10^5，女性为 22.14/10^5。气管、支气管、肺恶性肿瘤发病和死亡的 0~74 岁累积率分别为 4.75% 和 3.33%（表 5–9）。

9. Trachea, Bronchus & Lung (C33–C34)

In 2014, lung cancer cases accounted for 19.1% of all cancer cases in Henan cancer registration areas with the crude incidence of 48.28/10^5, ASR for China 38.41/10^5 and ASR for World 38.42/10^5. The incidence in males was 64.88/10^5, and 30.61/10^5 in females. The ASR China incidence was 2.37 times in males as high as that in females and it was 1.25 times in urban areas as that in rural areas. The crude mortality of lung cancer in 2014 was 36.3/10^5, ASR for China was 28.46/10^5 and ASR for World 28.46/10^5. The mortality in males was 49.61/10^5, and 22.14/10^5 in females. The cumulative rates of incidence and mortality from 0 to 74 years old were 4.75% and 3.33%, respectively (Table 5–9).

表 5–9　河南省肿瘤登记地区气管、支气管、肺恶性肿瘤发病与死亡

地区	性别	病例数	粗率（1/10^5）	构成（%）	中标率（1/10^5）	世标率（1/10^5）	累积率 0~74（%）
发病							
全省	合计	10 160	48.28	19.10	38.41	38.42	4.75
	男性	7 040	64.88	23.72	54.57	54.76	6.76
	女性	3 120	30.61	13.27	23.00	22.89	2.73
城市	合计	1 904	55.43	21.23	46.34	45.89	5.38
	男性	1 364	77.62	26.72	68.94	68.51	7.90
	女性	540	32.18	13.97	25.50	25.15	2.92
农村	合计	8 256	46.88	18.67	37.08	37.19	4.63
	男性	5 676	62.41	23.09	52.13	52.46	6.55
	女性	2 580	30.30	13.13	22.61	22.55	2.70
死亡							
全省	合计	7 640	36.30	23.19	28.46	28.46	3.33
	男性	5 383	49.61	26.37	41.90	41.98	4.88
	女性	2 257	22.14	18.00	15.98	15.97	1.78
城市	合计	1 412	41.10	25.90	34.45	34.20	3.66
	男性	1 029	58.56	30.08	52.79	52.74	5.46
	女性	383	22.82	18.86	17.99	17.72	1.90

续表

地区	性别	病例数	粗率（1/10^5）	构成（%）	中标率（1/10^5）	世标率（1/10^5）	累积率 0~74（%）
农村	合计	6 228	35.37	22.65	27.47	27.54	3.27
	男性	4 354	47.88	25.63	40.08	40.23	4.77
	女性	1 874	22.01	17.83	15.63	15.69	1.76

气管、支气管、肺恶性肿瘤年龄别发病率和死亡率在 0~49 岁年龄段处于较低水平，50 岁以后快速上升，在 80- 岁组达到高峰，男性高于女性。城乡和不同地区年龄别率的水平虽然有一定的差异，但总体趋势类同（图 5-9a ~ 图 5-9f）。

The age-specific incidence and mortality rates of lung cancer were relatively low before 49 years old and increased dramatically since 50 years old, reaching the peak at the age group 80 for both males and females. Incidence and mortality rates in males were generally higher than those in female. The age-specific incidence and mortality rates varied in urban and rural areas with similar curves (Figure 5-9a~Figure5-9f).

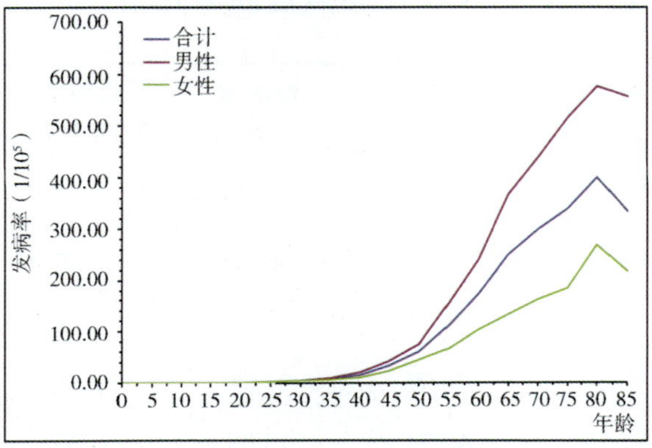

图 5-9a 河南省气管、支气管、肺恶性肿瘤年龄别发病率，2014

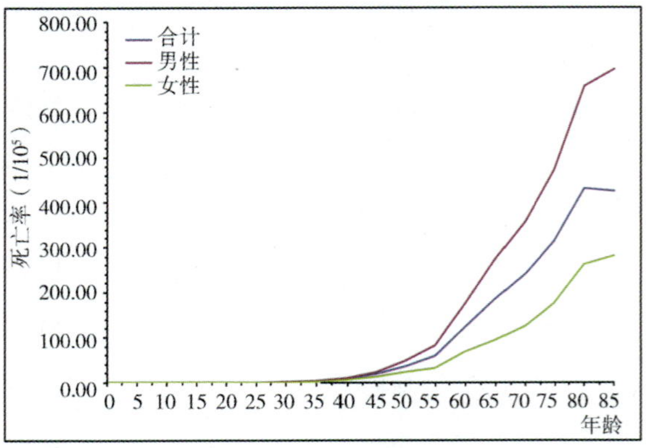

图 5-9d 河南省气管、支气管、肺恶性肿瘤年龄别死亡率，2014

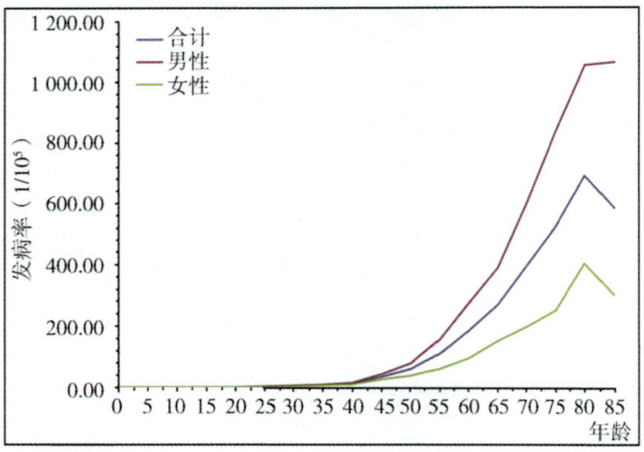

图 5-9b 城市肿瘤登记地区气管、支气管、肺恶性肿瘤年龄别发病率，2014

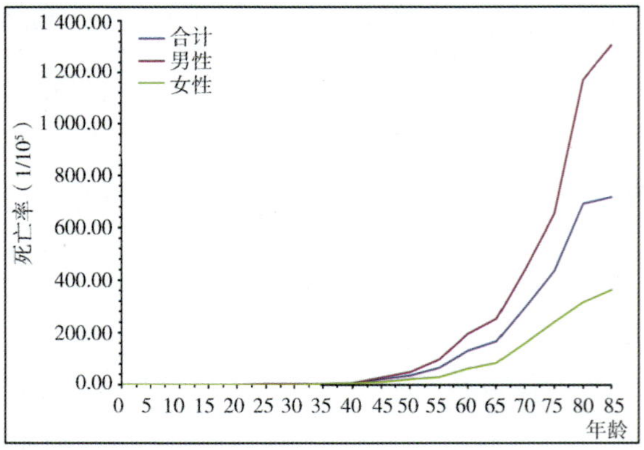

图 5-9e 城市肿瘤登记地区气管、支气管、肺恶性肿瘤年龄别死亡率，2014

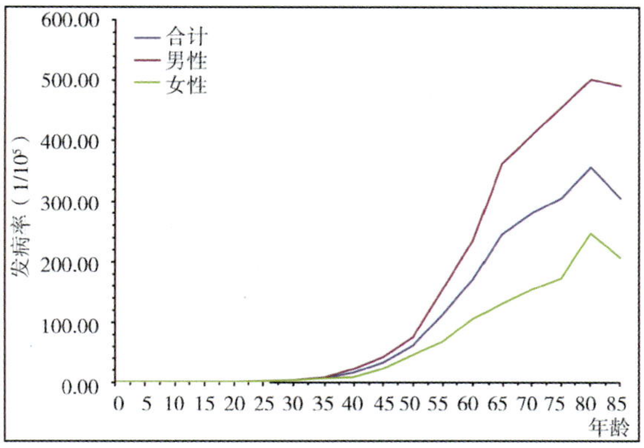

图 5-9c　农村肿瘤登记地区气管、支气管、肺恶性肿瘤年龄别发病率，2014

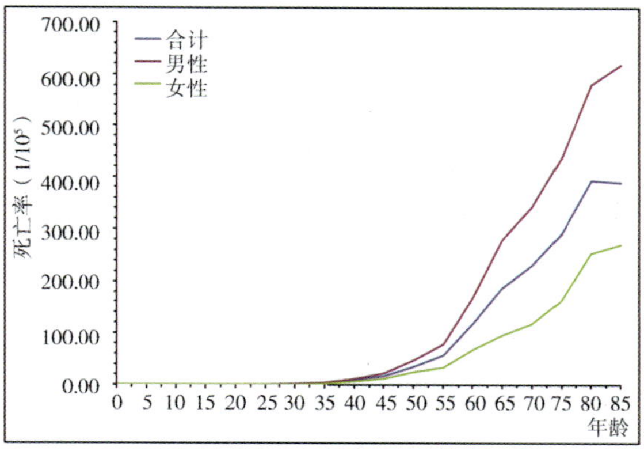

图 5-9f　农村肿瘤登记地区气管、支气管、肺恶性肿瘤年龄别死亡率，2014

在 5 个城市肿瘤登记地区中，男性气管、支气管、肺恶性肿瘤标化发病率最高的是洛阳市（89.06/10^5），其次是漯河市和南阳市；女性发病率最高的是洛阳市（32.23/10^5），其次是漯河市和南阳市。男性标化死亡率最高的是洛阳市（75.11/10^5），女性死亡率最高的是洛阳市（28.91/10^5）（图 5-9g）。

Among the 5 urban cancer registration areas, the age-specific incidence rate of lung cancer in males was the highest in Luoyang City (89.06/10^5), followed by Luohe City and Nanyang City. In females, it was the highest in Luoyang City (32.23/10^5), followed by Luohe City and Nanyang City. The highest age-specific mortality rates in both males (75.11/10^5) and female (28.91/10^5) were in Luoyang City (Figure 5-9g).

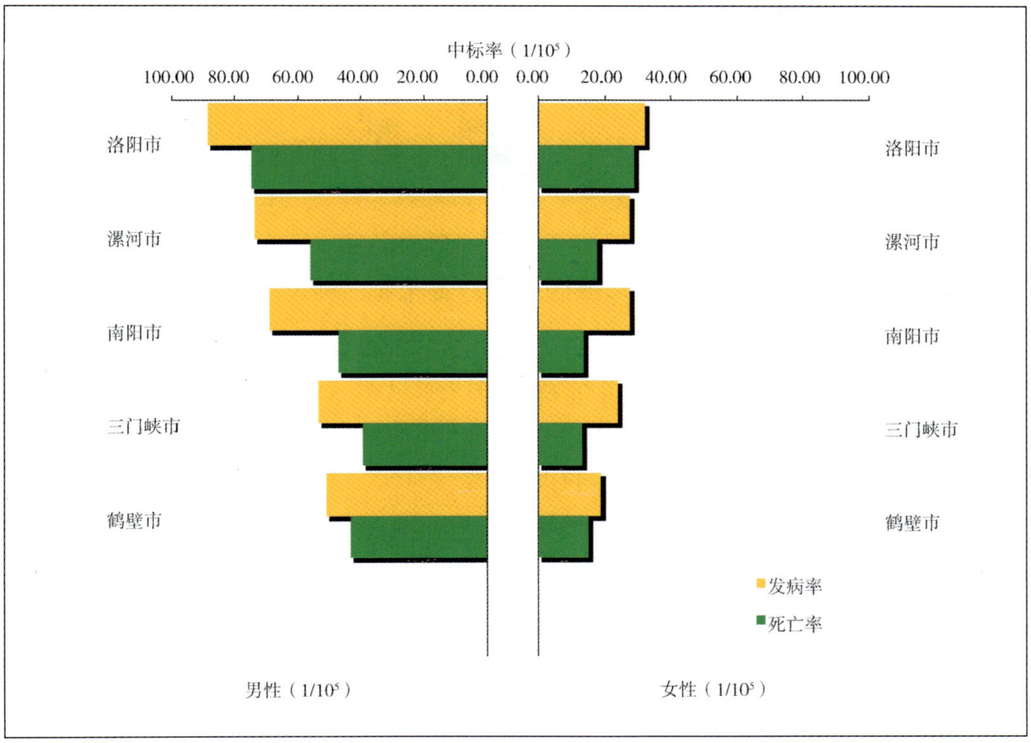

图 5-9g　城市肿瘤登记地区气管、支气管、肺恶性肿瘤发病率与死亡率

在 22 个农村肿瘤登记地区中，男性气管、支气管、肺恶性肿瘤标化发病率最高的是禹州市（$96.91/10^5$），其次是鲁山县和沈丘县；女性发病率最高的是沈丘县（$37.56/10^5$），其次是禹州市和虞城县。男性标化死亡率最高的是禹州市（$68.86/10^5$），女性死亡率最高的是沈丘县（$26.42/10^5$）（图 5-9h）。

Among the 22 rural cancer registration areas, the ASR China incidence rate of lung cancer in males was the highest in Yuzhou City ($96.91/10^5$), followed by Lushan County and Shenqiu County. For females, it was the highest in Shenqin City ($37.56/10^5$), followed by Yuzhou City and Yucheng County. The ASR China mortality was the highest in Yuzhou City for males ($68.86/10^5$) and Shenqiu County for females ($26.42/10^5$) (Figure 5-9h).

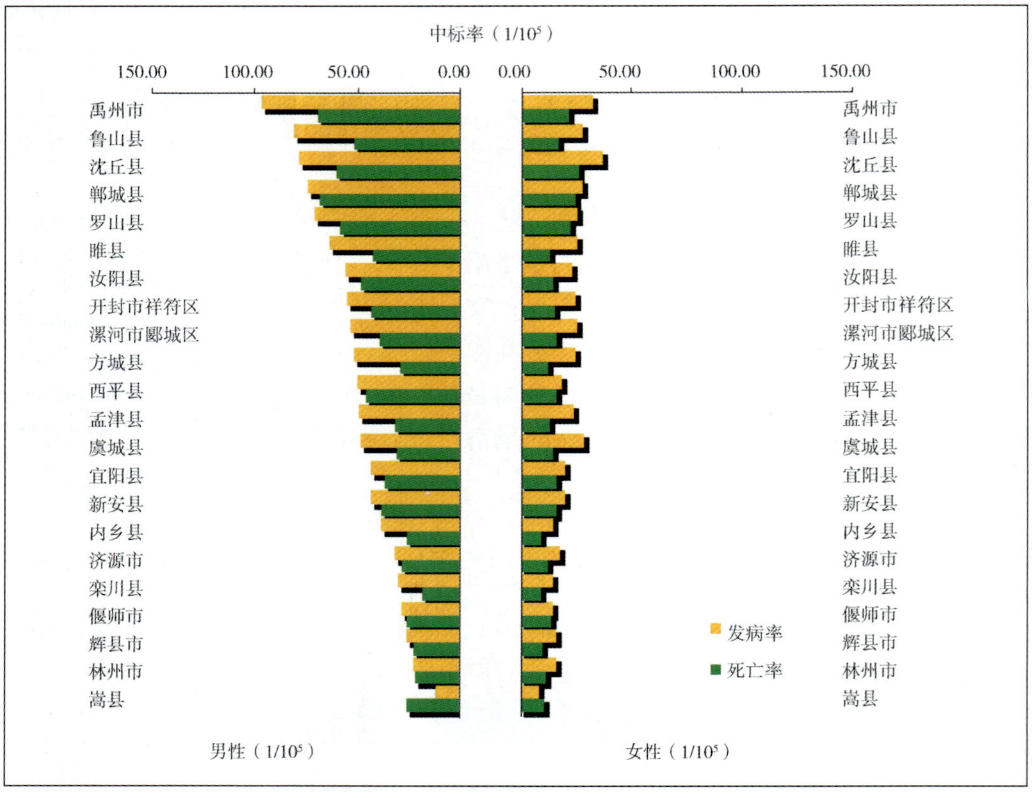

图 5-9h 农村肿瘤登记地区气管、支气管、肺恶性肿瘤发病率与死亡率

2014 年肿瘤登记地区肺癌发病病例中有确切解剖学亚部位（C33，C34.0–C34.3，C34.8）信息的占 50.8%，亚部位未特指（C34.9）的占 49.2%。在有亚部位的肺癌病例中，发生在气管（C33）的占 0.3%，主支气管（C34.0）的占 8.7%，肺上叶（C34.1）的占 37.3%，肺中叶（C34.2）的占 29.6%，肺下叶（C34.3）的占 22.6%，肺交搭跨越（C34.8）的占 1.5%（图 5-9i）。

Among all the reported lung cancer cases in 2014, 50.8% had specified subcategories (C33, C34.0–C34.3, C34.8) and the rest 49.2% had unspecified subcategory (C34.9). The specified subcategories of lung cancer included trachea (C33) (0.3%), main bronchus (C34.0) (8.7%), upper lobe(C34.1) (37.3%), middle lobe (C34.2) (29.6%), lower lobe (C34.3) (22.6%) and overlapping parts (C34.8) (1.5%) (Figure 5-9i).

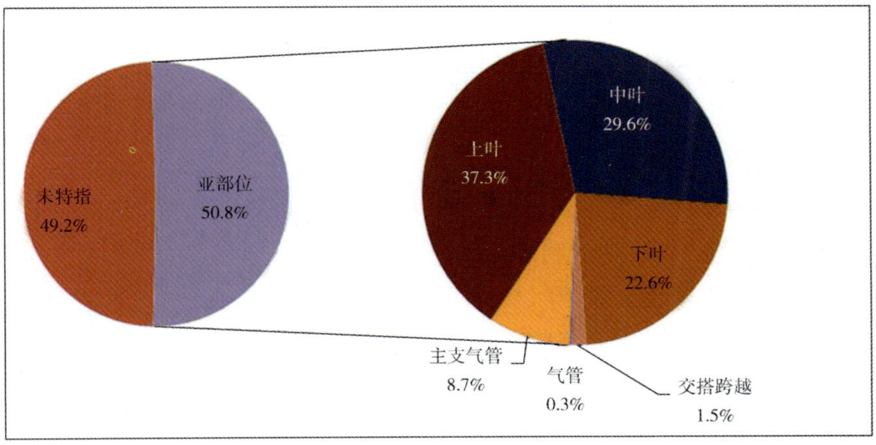

图 5-9i　河南省肺癌发病亚部位构成 (%)

2014 年肿瘤登记地区肺癌发病病例中有明确组织病理学分型的占 57.6%，组织学类型未特指的占 42.4%。在有组织病理学分型的肺癌病例中，鳞状细胞癌占 48.3%，腺癌占 42.6%，腺鳞癌占 0.4%，小细胞癌占 7.6%，大细胞癌占 0.1%，其他类型的肺癌占 1.1%（图 5-9j）。

Among all cases, 57.6% had specific pathological diagnostic information and the rest 42.4% had unspecified pathological type. Squamous cell carcinoma accounted for 48.3% of the cases with specified pathological diagnostic information, adenocarcinoma accounted for 42.6%, adenosquamous carcinoma 0.4%, small cell carcinoma 7.6%, big cell carcinoma 0.1% and other pathologic type 1.1% (Figure 5-9j).

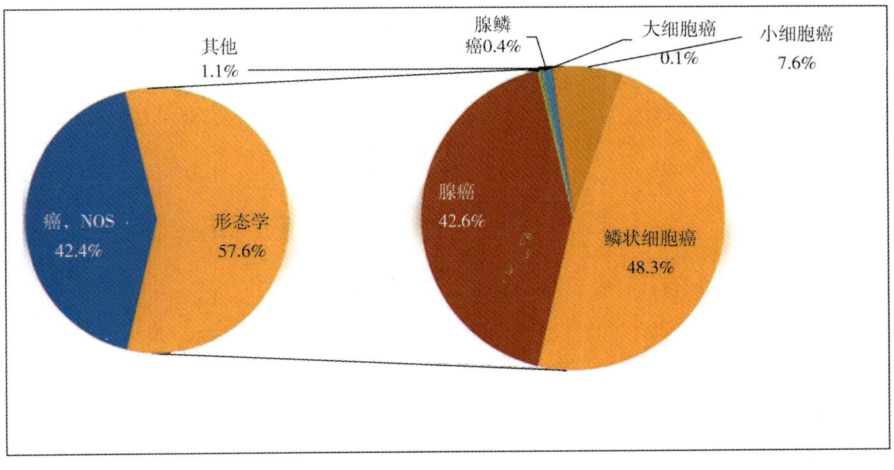

图 5-9j　河南省肺癌发病形态学构成 (%)

十、骨和关节软骨（C40–C41）

2014 年，河南省肿瘤登记地区骨恶性肿瘤的发病率为 2.54/10^5，中标率为 2.21/10^5，世标率为 2.14/10^5, 占全部恶性肿瘤发病的 1.01%。其中男性发病率为 2.79/10^5，女性为 2.28/10^5。男性中标率为女性的 1.34 倍，城市为农村的 0.82 倍。同期骨恶性肿瘤的死亡率为 1.27/10^5，中标率为 1.04/10^5，世标率为 1.03/10^5。其中男性死亡率为 1.46/10^5，女性为 1.08/10^5。骨恶性肿瘤发病和死亡的 0~74 岁累积率分别为 0.23% 和 0.12%（表 5–10）。

10. Bone，Joints and Articular Cartilage (C40–C41)

In 2014, malignant cancer cases of bone, joints and articular cartilage (bone cancer for short below) accounted for 1.01% of all cancer cases in Henan cancer registration areas with the crude incidence of 2.54/10^5, ASR for China 2.21/10^5 and ASR for World 2.14/10^5. The incidence in males was 2.79/10^5, and 2.28/10^5 in females. It was 1.34 times in males as high as that in females and it was 0.82 times in urban areas as that in rural areas. The crude mortality of bone cancer in 2014 was 1.27/10^5, ASR for China was 1.04/10^5 and ASR for World 1.03/10^5. The mortality in males was 1.46/10^5, and 1.08/10^5 in females. The cumulative rates of incidence and mortality from 0 to 74 years old were 0.23% and 0.12%, respectively (Table 5–10) .

表 5–10 河南省肿瘤登记地区骨恶性肿瘤发病与死亡

地区	性别	病例数	粗率（1/10^5）	构成（%）	中标率（1/10^5）	世标率（1/10^5）	累积率 0~74（%）
发病							
全省	合计	535	2.54	1.01	2.21	2.14	0.23
	男性	303	2.79	1.02	2.52	2.44	0.26
	女性	232	2.28	0.99	1.88	1.82	0.20
城市	合计	75	2.18	0.84	1.86	1.78	0.21
	男性	38	2.16	0.74	1.96	1.88	0.22
	女性	37	2.20	0.96	1.77	1.71	0.20
农村	合计	460	2.61	1.04	2.28	2.21	0.24
	男性	265	2.91	1.08	2.63	2.56	0.27
	女性	195	2.29	0.99	1.91	1.85	0.20
死亡							
全省	合计	268	1.27	0.81	1.04	1.03	0.12
	男性	158	1.46	0.77	1.25	1.25	0.14
	女性	110	1.08	0.88	0.83	0.82	0.09

续表

地区	性别	病例数	粗率 (1/10^5)	构成 (%)	中标率 (1/10^5)	世标率 (1/10^5)	累积率 0~74 (%)
城市	合计	49	1.43	0.90	1.22	1.19	0.13
	男性	28	1.59	0.82	1.50	1.46	0.15
	女性	21	1.25	1.03	0.95	0.96	0.11
农村	合计	219	1.24	0.80	1.01	1.00	0.12
	男性	130	1.43	0.77	1.21	1.22	0.14
	女性	89	1.05	0.85	0.81	0.80	0.09

骨恶性肿瘤年龄别发病率和死亡率在 0~44 岁年龄段处于较低水平，45 岁以后快速上升，在 80- 岁组达到高峰，男性稍高于女性。城乡和不同地区年龄别率的水平虽然有一定的差异，但总体趋势类同（图 5-10a ~ 图 5-10f）。

在 5 个城市肿瘤登记地区中，男性骨恶性肿瘤标化发病率最高的是漯河市（3.62/10^5），其次是南阳市和三门峡市；女性发病率最高的是南阳市（2.55/10^5），其次是洛阳市和三门峡市。男性标化死亡率最高的是三门峡市（2.78/10^5），女性死亡率最高的是南阳市（1.56/10^5）（图 5-10g）。

The age-specific incidence and mortality rates of bone cancer were relatively low before 44years old and increased dramatically since 45 years old. Incidence and mortality rates in males were slightly higher those in females.The ASR China incidence rate of bone cancer reaching the peak at the age group of 60 for males and at the age group of 80 for females. The ASR China mortality rate reached the peak at the age group of 85 for both males and females, increasing with fluctuation after 65 age group (Figure 5-10a~Figure 5-10f).

Among the 5 urban cancer registration areas, the ASR China incidence rate of bone cancer in males was the highest in Luohe City (3.62/10^5), followed by Nanyang City and Sanmenxia City. In females, it was the highest in Nanyang City (2.55/10^5), followed by Luoyang City and Sanmenxia City. The ASR China mortality were highest in Sanmenxia City for males (2.78/10^5) and Nanyang City for females (1.56/10^5) (Figure 5-10g).

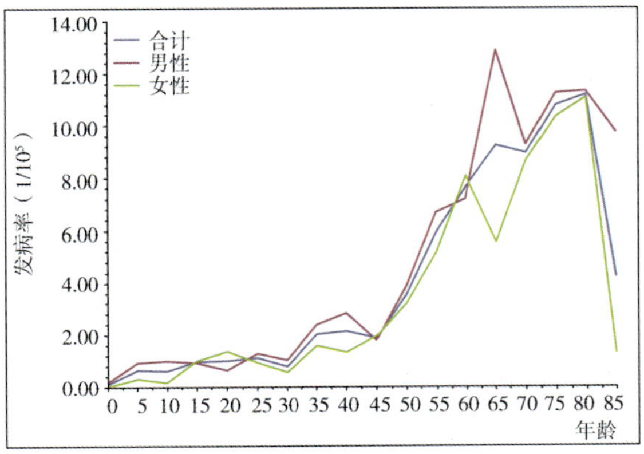

图 5-10a 河南省骨恶性肿瘤年龄别发病率，2014

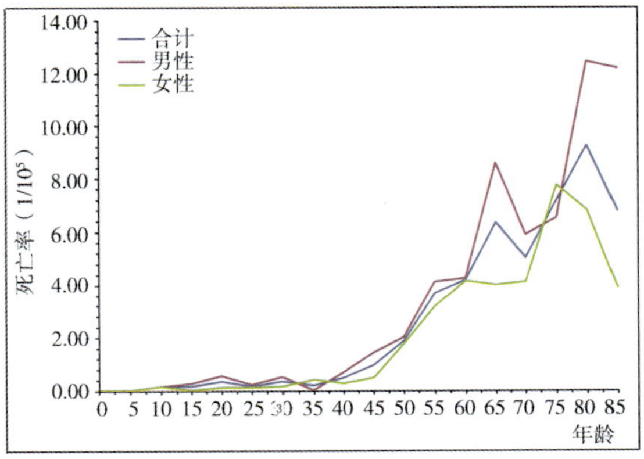

图 5-10d 河南省骨恶性肿瘤年龄别死亡率，2014

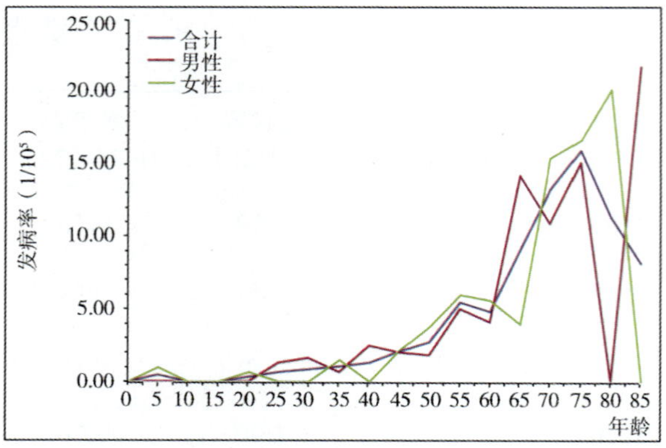

图 5-10b　城市肿瘤登记地区骨恶性肿瘤年龄别发病率，2014

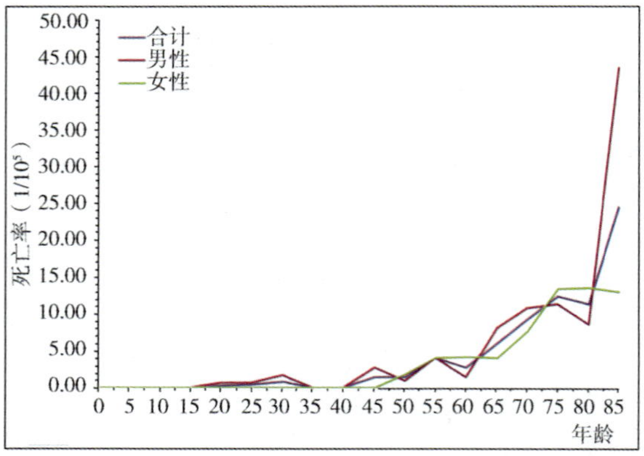

图 5-10e　城市肿瘤登记地区骨恶性肿瘤年龄别死亡率，2014

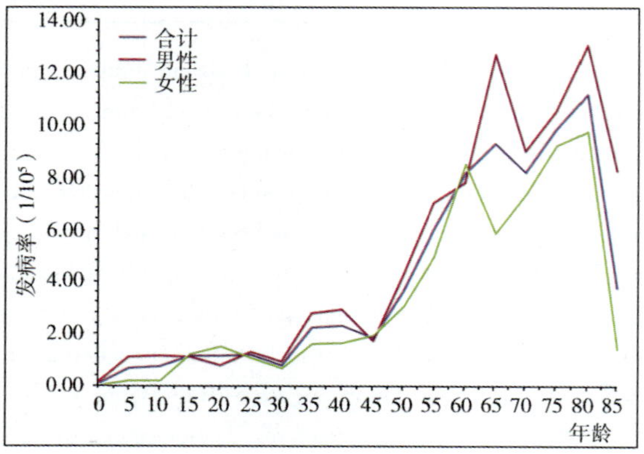

图 5-10c　农村肿瘤登记地区骨恶性肿瘤年龄别发病率，2014

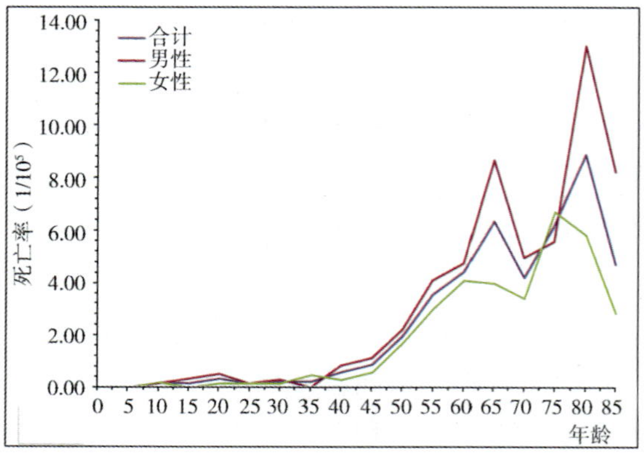

图 5-10f　农村肿瘤登记地区骨恶性肿瘤年龄别死亡率，2014

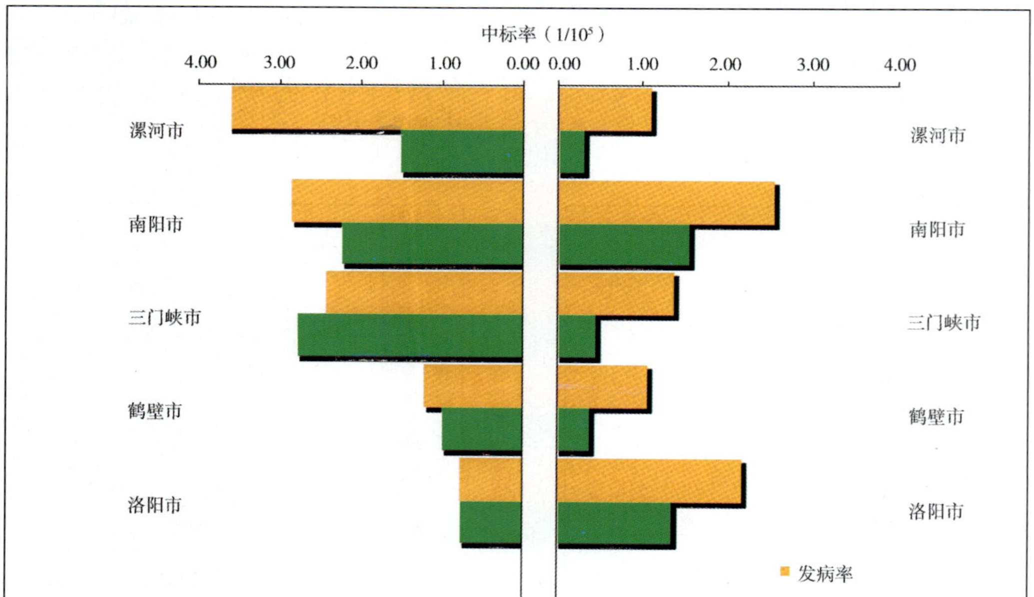

图 5-10g　城市肿瘤登记地区骨恶性肿瘤发病率与死亡率

在 22 个农村肿瘤登记地区中，男性骨恶性肿瘤标化发病率最高的是宜阳县（$6.51/10^5$），其次是栾川县和沈丘县；女性发病率最高的是栾川县（$3.8/10^5$），其次是宜阳县和沈丘县。男性标化死亡率最高的是济源市（$3.26/10^5$），女性死亡率最高的是济源市（$1.38/10^5$）（图 5-10h）。

Among the 22 rural cancer registration areas, the ASR China incidence rate of bone cancer in males was the highest in Yiyang County ($6.51/10^5$), followed by Luanchuan County and Shenqiu County. For females, it was the highest in Luanchuan County ($3.8/10^5$), followed by Yiyang County and Shenqiu County . The age-specific mortality rate was the highest in Jiyuan City for both males ($3.26/10^5$) and females ($1.38/10^5$) (Figure 5-10h).

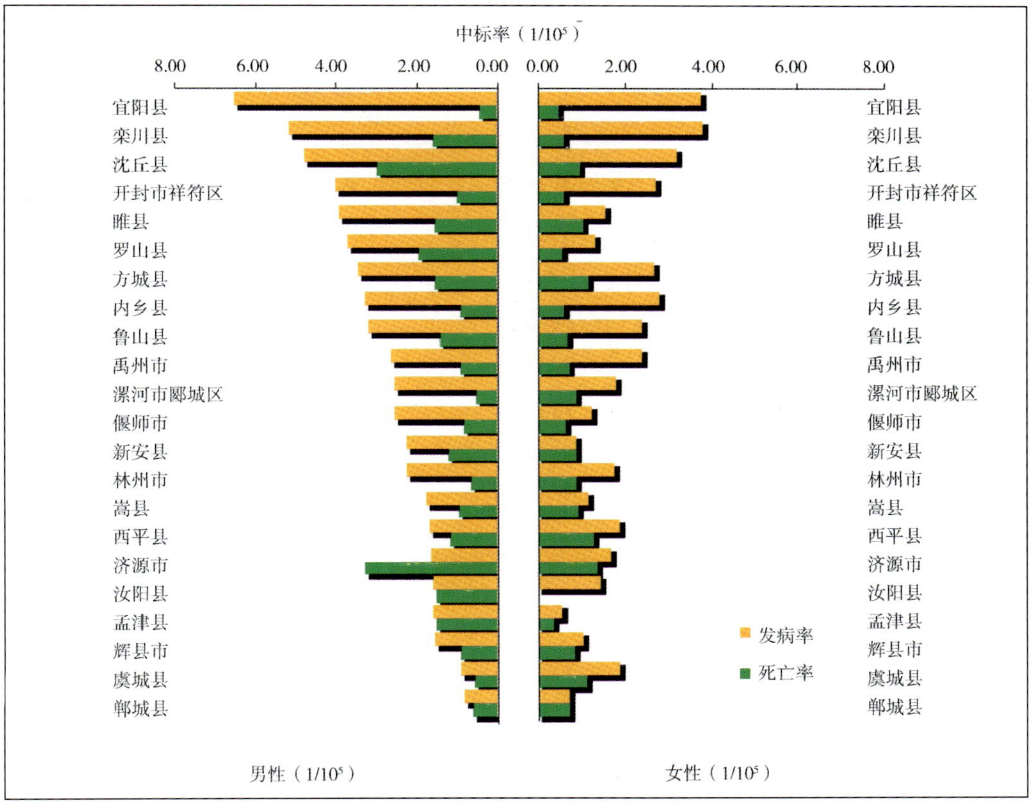

图 5-10h　农村肿瘤登记地区骨恶性肿瘤发病率与死亡率

十一、乳房（C50）

2014 年，河南省肿瘤登记地区女性乳房恶性肿瘤的发病率为 $36.39/10^5$，中标率为 $30.29/10^5$，世标率为 $28.52/10^5$，占全部恶性肿瘤发病的 6.97%。其中城市发病率为 $42.25/10^5$，农村为 $35.23/10^5$，城市中标率为农村的 1.2 倍。同期女性乳房恶性肿瘤的死亡率为 $10.46/10^5$，中标率为 $8.28/10^5$，世标率为 $8.08/10^5$。其中城市死亡率为 $13.88/10^5$，农村为 $9.78/10^5$。乳房恶性肿瘤发病和死亡的 0~74 岁累积率分别为 3.08% 和 0.92%（表 5-11）。

11. Breast (50)

In 2014, breast cancer cases accounted for 6.97% of all cancer cases in Henan cancer registration areas with the crude incidence of $36.39/10^5$, ASR for China $30.29/10^5$ and ASR for World $28.52/10^5$. The crude incidence in urban areas was $42.25/10^5$, and $35.23/10^5$ in rural areas. It was 1.2 times in urban areas as that in rural areas. The crude mortality of breast cancer in 2014 was $10.46/10^5$, ASR for China was $8.28/10^5$ and ASR for World $8.08/10^5$.The crude mortality in urban areas was $13.88/10^5$, and $9.78/10^5$ in rural areas. The cumulative rates of incidence and mortality from 0 to 74 years old were 3.08% and 0.92%, respectively (Table 5-11).

表 5-11 河南省肿瘤登记地区女性乳房恶性肿瘤发病与死亡

指标	地区	病例数	粗率 (1/10^5)	构成 (%)	中标率 (1/10^5)	世标率 (1/10^5)	累积率 0~74 (%)
发病	全省	3 709	36.39	6.97	30.29	28.52	3.08
	城市	709	42.25	7.91	34.50	32.44	3.51
	农村	3 000	35.23	6.78	29.48	27.76	3.00
死亡	全省	1 066	10.46	3.24	8.28	8.08	0.92
	城市	233	13.88	4.27	11.05	10.83	1.12
	农村	833	9.78	3.03	7.77	7.58	0.88

乳房恶性肿瘤年龄别发病率从 15 岁开始发病，30 岁开始迅速升高，60 岁达到高峰后逐渐下降。死亡率在 34 岁之前相对较低，在 60 岁达到高峰后，缓慢下降，于 80 岁达到最高值。农村地区和整体趋势相仿，城市地区的发病率分别在 60 岁、70 岁和 80 岁出现峰值，死亡率从 30 岁始开始升高，50~70 岁组出现震荡，尔后迅速升高，85 岁达到峰值（图 5-11a ~ 图 5-11b）。

The age-specific incidence rate of breast cancer emerged since 15 years old and increased dramatically since 30 years old, reaching the peak at the age group of 60 and then decreased gradually. The age-specific mortality rate of breast cancer was relatively low before 34 years old and increased dramatically since 35 years old, reaching a peak at the age group of 60, and reached the top at age group of 80. In rural areas, the age-specific incidence and mortality rates of breast cancer had the similar trends with the overall population. In the urban areas the age-specific incidence rate had three peaks at the age group of 60, 70 and 80 respectively, the mortality rate increased dramatically at the age group of 30, fluctuated between 50 and 70, then increased rapidly to the peak at age group of 85 (Figure 5-11a~Figure 5-11b).

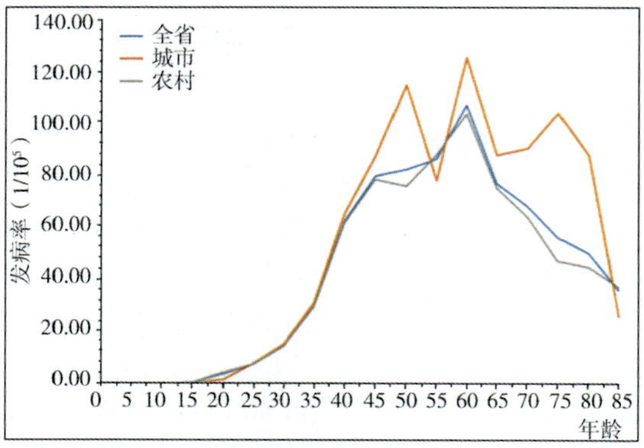

图 5-11a 河南省女性乳腺癌年龄别发病率，2014

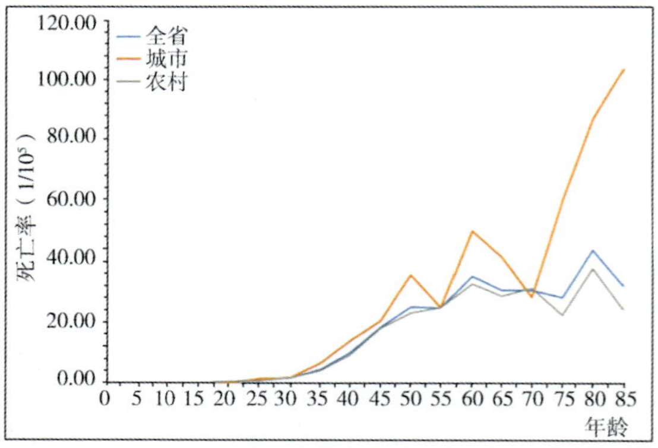

图 5-11b 河南省女性乳腺癌年龄别死亡率，2014

在 5 个城市肿瘤登记地区中，女性发病率最高的是漯河市（$44.73/10^5$），其次是洛阳市和三门峡市，标化死亡率最高的是漯河市（$15.77/10^5$）（图 5-11c）。

Among the 5 urban cancer registration areas, the ASR China incidence rate of breast cancer in was the highest in Luohe City ($44.73/10^5$), followed by Luoyang City and Sanmenxia City.The highest age-specific mortality was in Luohe City ($15.77/10^5$) for females (Figure 5-11c).

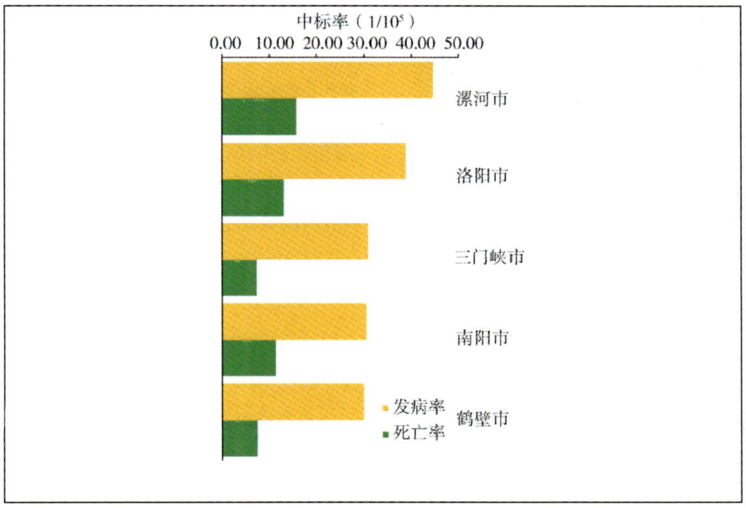

图 5-11c　城市肿瘤登记地区乳房恶性肿瘤发病率与死亡率

在 22 个农村肿瘤登记地区中，女性发病率最高的是郸城县（50.09/10^5），其次是方城县和睢县，女性死亡率最高的是郸城县（18.73/10^5）（图 5-11d）。

Among the 22 rural cancer registration areas, the ASR China incidence rate of breast cancer was the highest in Dancheng County (50.09/10^5), followed by Fangcheng County and Suixian County. The highest age-specific mortality of breast cancer was in Dancheng County (18.73/10^5) for females (Figure 5-11d).

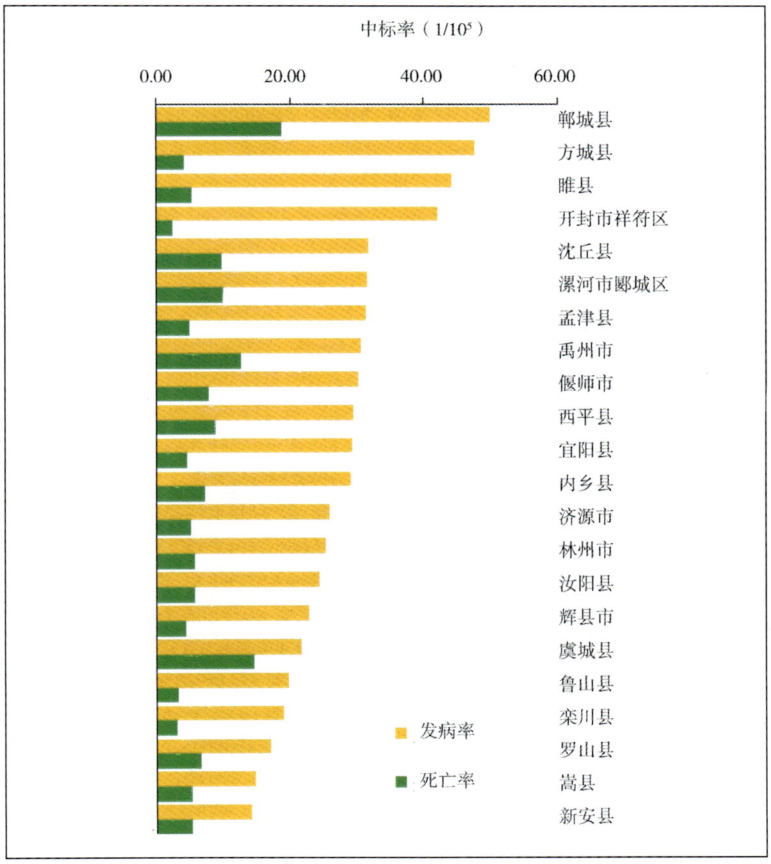

图 5-11d　农村肿瘤登记地区乳房恶性肿瘤发病率与死亡率

2014 年肿瘤登记地区女性乳腺癌发病病例中有确切解剖学亚部位（C50.0–C50.6，C50.8）信息的占 43.1%，亚部位未特指（C50.9）的占 56.9%。在有亚部位的乳腺癌病例中，发生在乳腺乳头和乳晕区（C50.0）的占 5.4%，乳腺中央部（C50.1）的占 10.4%，乳腺上内象限（C50.2）的占 27.1%，乳腺下内象限（C50.3）的占 15.3%，乳腺上外象限（C50.4）的占 28.7%，乳腺下外象限（C50.5）的占 8.6%，乳腺腋尾部（C50.6）的占 3.1%，乳腺交搭跨越（C50.8）的占 1.3%（图 5–11e）。

Among all the reported breast cancer cases in 2014, 43.1% had specified subcategories (C50.0–C50.6, C50.8) and the rest 56.9% had unspecified subcategory (C50.9). The specified subcategories of breast cancer included nipple and areola (C50.0) (5.4%), central portion (C50.1) (10.4%), upper inner (C50.2) (27.1%), lower inner (C50.3) (15.3%), upper outer (C50.4) (28.7%), lower outer (C50.5) (8.6%) and axillary tail (C50.6) (3.1%) and overlapping parts (C50.8) (1.3%) (Figure 5–11e).

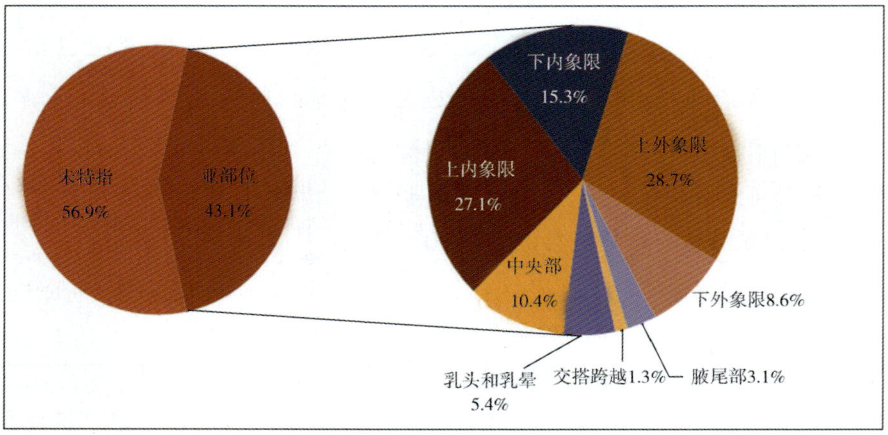

图 5–11e　河南省女性乳腺癌发病亚部位构成 (%)

2014 年肿瘤登记地区女性乳腺癌发病病例中有明确组织病理学分型的占 84.3%，组织学类型未特指的占 15.7%。在有组织病理学分型的乳腺癌病例中，导管内癌占 72.2%，小叶癌占 5.4%，髓样癌占 0.6%，佩吉特病占 0.5%，其他类型的乳腺癌占 21.3%（图 5–10f）。

Among all cases, 84.3% had specific pathological diagnostic information and the rest 15.7% had unspecified pathological type. Ductal carcinoma accounted for 72.2% of the cases with specific pathological diagnostic information, lobular carcinoma accounted for 5.4 %, medullary carcinoma 0.6%, Paget' s 0.5% and other histological breast type 21.3% (Figure 5–11f).

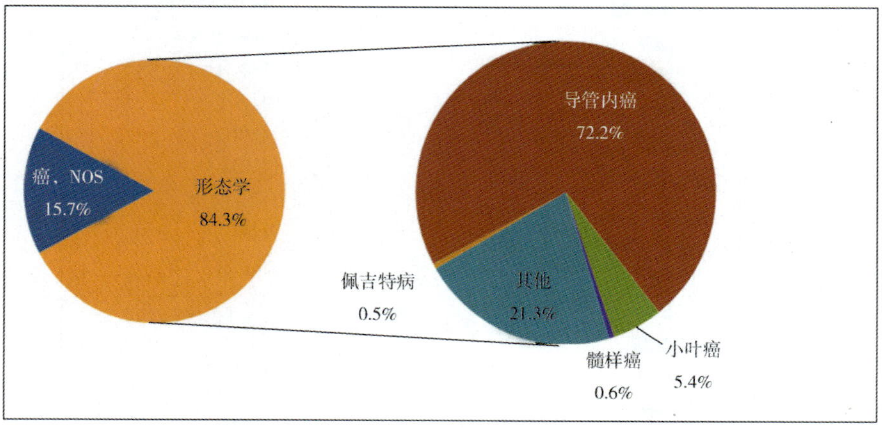

图 5–11f　河南省女性乳腺癌发病形态学构成 (%)

十二、子宫颈（C53）

2014 年，河南省肿瘤登记地区子宫颈恶性肿瘤的发病率为 17.07/10^5，中标率为 14.37/10^5，世标率为 13.36/10^5，占全部恶性肿瘤发病的 3.27%。其中城市发病率为 15.91/10^5，农村发病率为 17.30/10^5。同期子宫颈恶性肿瘤的死亡率为 5.15/10^5，中标率为 4.04/10^5，世标率为 3.96/10^5。子宫颈恶性肿瘤发病和死亡的 0~74 岁累积率分别为 1.45% 和 0.47%（表 5-12）。

12. Cervix (C53)

In 2014, cervical cancer cases accounted for 3.27% of all cancer cases in Henan cancer registration areas with the crude incidence of 17.07/10^5, ASR for China 14.37/10^5 and ASR for World 13.36/10^5. The crude incidence in urban areas was 15.91/10^5, and 17.30/10^5 in rural areas. It was 0.92times in urban areas as that in rural areas. The crude mortality of cervical cancer in 2014 was 5.15/10^5, ASR for China was 4.04/10^5 and ASR for World 3.96/10^5.The crude mortality in urban areas was 5.48/10^5, and 5.06/10^5 in rural areas. The cumulative rates of incidence and mortality from 0 to 74 years old were 1.45% and 0.47%, respectively (Table 5-12).

表 5-12　河南省肿瘤登记地区子宫颈恶性肿瘤发病与死亡

指标	地区	病例数	粗率（1/10^5）	构成（%）	中标率（1/10^5）	世标率（1/10^5）	累积率 0~74（%）
发病	**全省**	**1 740**	**17.07**	**3.27**	**14.37**	**13.36**	**1.45**
	城市	267	15.91	2.98	13.33	12.31	1.30
	农村	1 473	17.30	3.33	14.60	13.59	1.48
死亡	**全省**	**525**	**5.15**	**1.59**	**4.04**	**3.96**	**0.47**
	城市	92	5.48	1.69	4.45	4.10	0.43
	农村	433	5.08	1.57	3.94	3.90	0.48

子宫颈恶性肿瘤年龄别发病率和死亡率在 24 岁之前发病较低，25 岁以后快速上升，在 60- 岁组达到高峰。死亡率在 25 岁以后快速上升，在 80- 岁组达到高峰。农村地区和整体趋势一致。城市地区发病率在 50 岁和 80 岁组之间出现震荡，80 岁达到高峰，城市地区死亡率在 25~75 岁组之间缓慢上升， 75 岁以后快速升高，80 岁达到峰值后迅速回落（图 5-12a ~ 图 5-12b）。

The age-specific incidence rate of cervical cancer were relatively low before 24 years old and increased dramatically since 25 years old, reaching the peak at the age group of 60. The age-specific mortality rate increased dramatically since 25years old, reaching the peak at the age group of 80. In rural areas , the age-specific incidence and mortality rates had the similar trends with the whole population. In urban areas , the age-specific incidence rates fluctuated after 50, reaching the peak at age group of 80, the mortality rate increased gradually between 25 and 75, then increased rapidly, reaching the peak dramatically at age group of 80, then falling sharphy to the bottom (Figure 5-12a~Figure 5-12b).

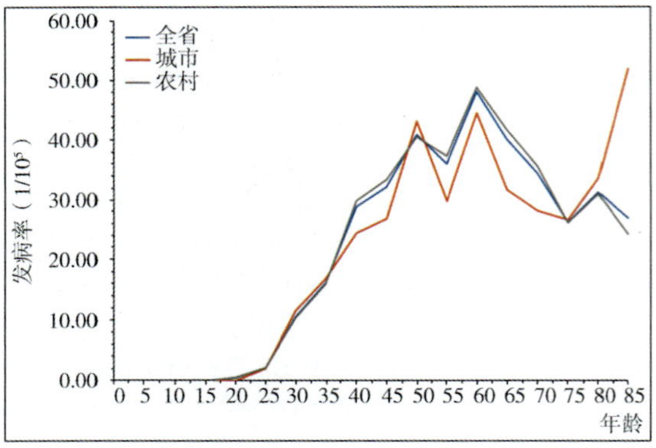

图 5-12a　河南省子宫颈恶性肿瘤年龄别发病率，2014

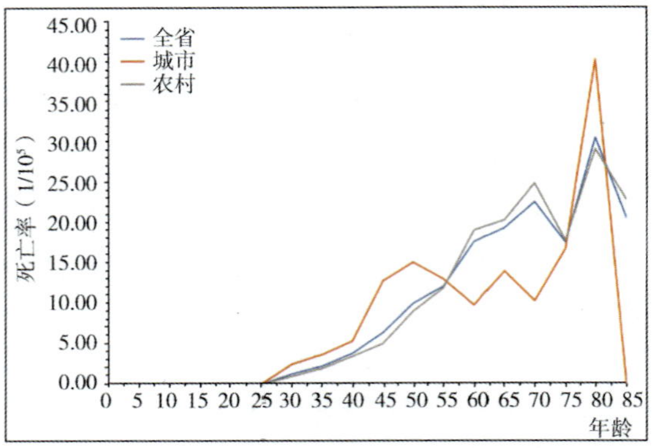

图 5-12b　河南省子宫颈恶性肿瘤年龄别死亡率，2014

在 5 个城市肿瘤登记地区中，女性发病率最高的是漯河市（$19.89/10^5$），其次是南阳市和三门峡市。女性死亡率最高的是南阳市（$8.05/10^5$）（图 5-12c）。

Among the 5 urban cancer registration areas, the ASR China incidence rate of cervical cancer was the highest in Luohe City ($19.89/10^5$), followed by Nanyang City and Sanmenxia City. The highest ASR China mortality in females was in Nanyang City ($8.05/10^5$) (Figure 5-12c).

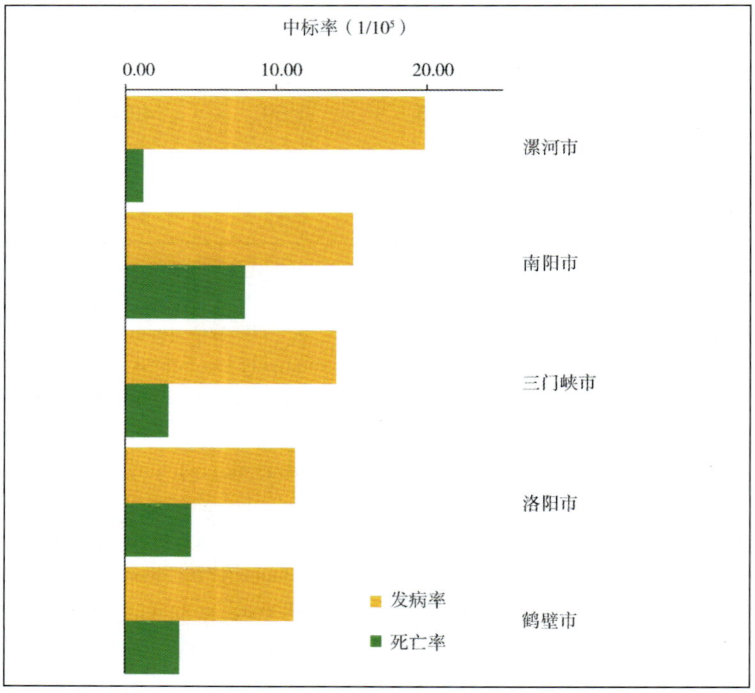

图 5-12c　城市肿瘤登记地区子宫颈恶性肿瘤发病率与死亡率

在 22 个农村肿瘤登记地区中，女性子宫颈癌发病率最高的是禹州市（$28.91/10^5$），其次是汝阳县和济源市。女性死亡率最高的是禹州市（$7.79/10^5$）（图 5-12d）。

Among the 22 rural cancer registration areas, the ASR China incidence rate of cervical cancer was the highest in Yuzhou City ($28.91/10^5$), followed by Ruyang County and Jiyuan City. The highest mortality was in Yuzhou County ($7.79/10^5$) (Figure 5-12d).

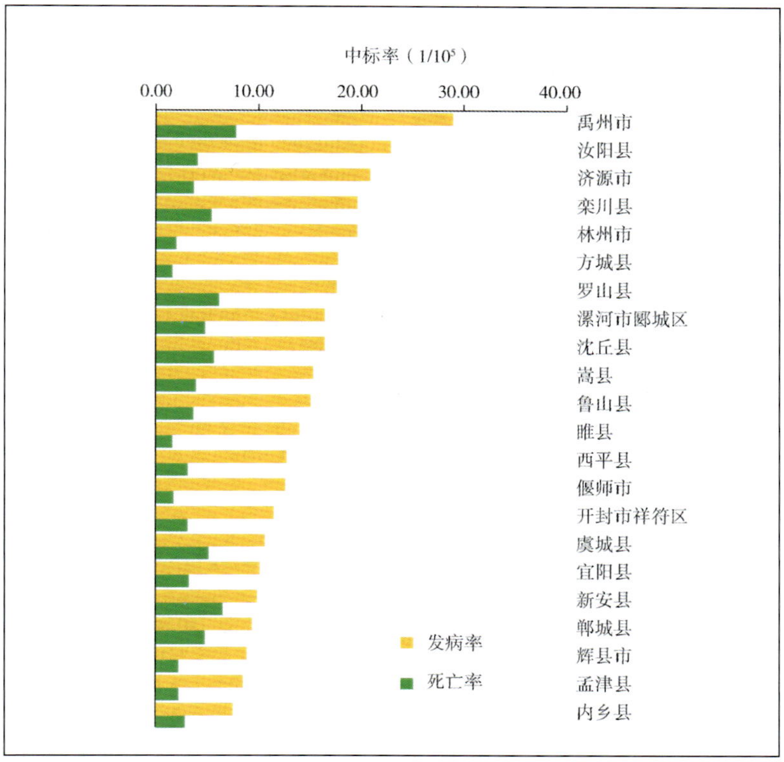

图 5-12d 农村肿瘤登记地区子宫颈恶性肿瘤发病率与死亡率

2014 年肿瘤登记地区子宫颈癌发病病例中有确切解剖学亚部位（C53.0，C53.1，C53.8）信息的占 40.1%，亚部位未特指（C53.9）的占 59.9%。在有亚部位的子宫颈癌病例中，发生在子宫颈内膜（C53.0）的占 68.1%，外宫颈（C53.1）的占 26.6%，子宫颈交搭跨越（C53.8）的占 5.3%（图 5-12e）。

Among all the reported cervical cancer cases in 2014, 40.1% had specified subcategories (C53.0, C53.1, C53.8) and the rest 59.9% had unspecified anatomic site (C53.9). The specified subcategories of cervical cancer included endometria (C53.0) (68.1%), exocervix (C53.1) (26.6%), and overlapping parts (C53.8) (5.3%) (Figure 5-12e).

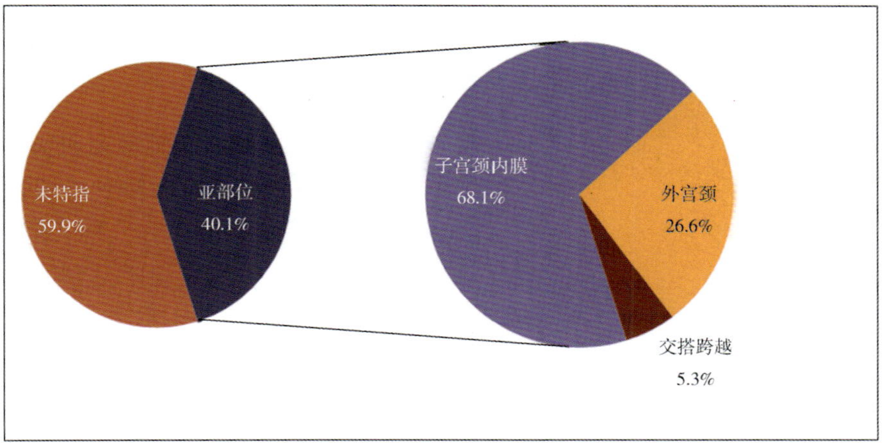

图 5-12e 河南省子宫颈癌发病亚部位构成 (%)

十三、子宫体（C54）

2014 年，河南省肿瘤登记地区子宫体恶性肿瘤的发病率为 6.60/10^5，中标率为 5.31/10^5，世标率为 5.17/10^5, 占全部恶性肿瘤发病的 1.27%。其中城市女性发病率为 6.44/10^5，农村女性为 6.64/10^5。城市为农村的 0.95 倍。同期子宫体恶性肿瘤的死亡率为 1.63/10^5，中标率为 1.26/10^5，世标率为 1.23/10^5。城市女性死亡率为 2.32/10^5，农村女性为 1.49/10^5。子宫体恶性肿瘤发病和死亡的 0~74 岁累积率分别为 0.57% 和 0.15%（表 5–13）。

13. Uterine Corpus (C54)

In 2014, uterine corpus cancer cases accounted for 1.27% of all cancer cases in Henan cancer registration areas with the crude incidence of 6.60/10^5, ASR for China 5.31/10^5 and ASR for World 5.17/10^5. The crude incidence in urban and rural areas were 6.44/10^5 and 6.64/10^5, respectively. It was 0.95 times in urban areas as that in rural areas. The crude mortality of uterine corpus cancer in 2014 was 1.63/10^5, ASR for China was 1.26/10^5 and ASR for World 1.23/10^5. The crude mortality in urban areas was 2.32/10^5, and 1.49/10^5 in rural areas. The cumulative rates of incidence and mortality from 0 to 74 years old were 0.57% and 0.15%, respectively (Table 5–13).

表 5–13　河南省肿瘤登记地区子宫体恶性肿瘤发病与死亡

指标	地区	病例数	粗率（1/10^5）	构成（%）	中标率（1/10^5）	世标率（1/10^5）	累积率 0~74（%）
发病	全省	673	6.60	1.27	5.31	5.17	0.57
	城市	108	6.44	1.20	5.11	5.05	0.62
	农村	565	6.64	1.28	5.36	5.21	0.57
死亡	全省	166	1.63	0.50	1.26	1.23	0.15
	城市	39	2.32	0.72	1.89	1.85	0.23
	农村	127	1.49	0.46	1.14	1.11	0.13

子宫体癌年龄别发病率在 29 岁之前处于较低水平，30 岁以后快速增加，在 60 岁组达到高峰，之后逐渐下降。死亡率在 0~39 岁年龄段处于较低水平，40 岁以后缓慢上升，在 80 岁组达到高峰。农村地区年龄别发病率和死亡率与全省趋势基本一致，城市地区年龄别发病率和死亡率均在 70 岁组达到高峰（图 5–13a ~ 图 5–13b）。

The age-specific China incidence rate of uterine corpus cancer were relatively low before 29 years old and increased dramatically since 30 years old, reaching the peak at the age group of 60 and then decreasing gradually. The age-specific mortality rates of uterine corpus cancer were relatively low before 39 years old and increased gradually since 40 years old, reaching the peak at the age group of 80. In the rural areas the age-specific incidence and mortality rates of uterine corpus cancer had the similar trends with the overall population, while in the urban areas the age-specific incidence and mortality rates reached the peak at the age group of 70 with fluctuations (Figure 5–13a~Figure 5–13b).

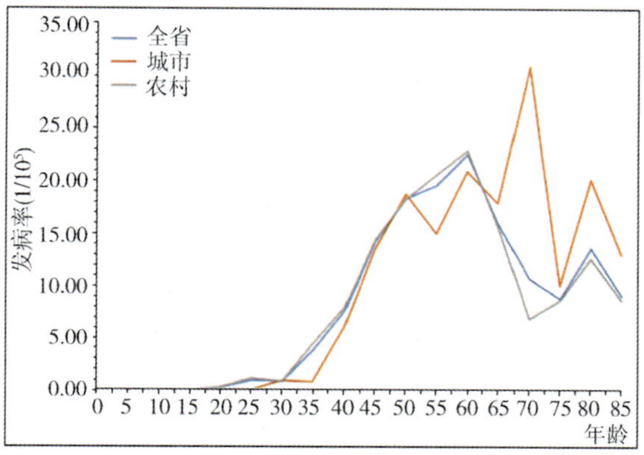

图 5-13a　河南省子宫体恶性肿瘤年龄别发病率，2014

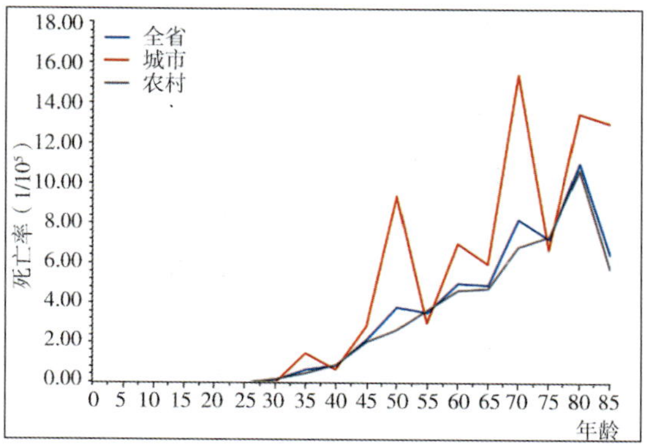

图 5-13b　河南省子宫体恶性肿瘤年龄别死亡率，2014

在 5 个城市肿瘤登记地区中，女性发病率最高的是漯河市（$6.89/10^5$），其次是三门峡市和洛阳市。女性死亡率最高的是洛阳市（$2.53/10^5$）（图 5-13c）。

Among the 5 urban cancer registration areas, the ASR China incidence rate of uterine corpus cancer was the highest in Luohe City ($6.89/10^5$), followed by Sanmenxia City and Luo yang City. The highest ASR China mortality was in Luoyang City ($2.53/10^5$) (Figure 5-13c).

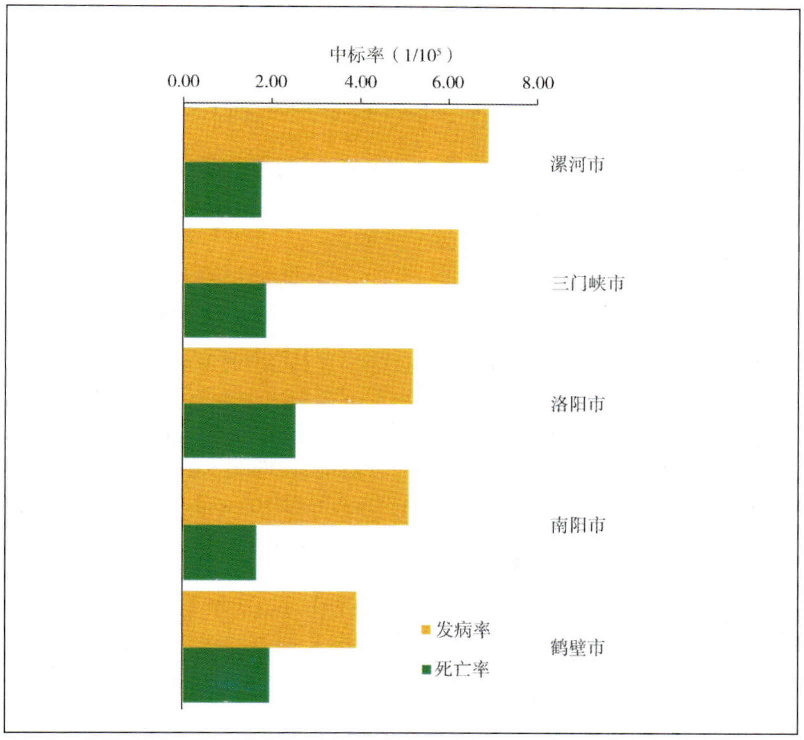

图 5-13c　城市肿瘤登记地区子宫体恶性肿瘤发病率与死亡率

在 22 个农村肿瘤登记地区中，女性发病率最高的是鲁山县（$27.3/10^5$），其次是睢县和漯河市郾城区。女性死亡率最高的是内乡县（$3.62/10^5$）（图 5-13d）。

Among the 22 rural cancer registration areas, the ASR China incidence rate of uterine corpus cancer was the highest in Lushan County ($27.3/10^5$), followed by Suixian County and Yancheng District, Luohe City. The highest ASR China mortality was in Neixiang County ($3.62/10^5$) (Figure 5-13d).

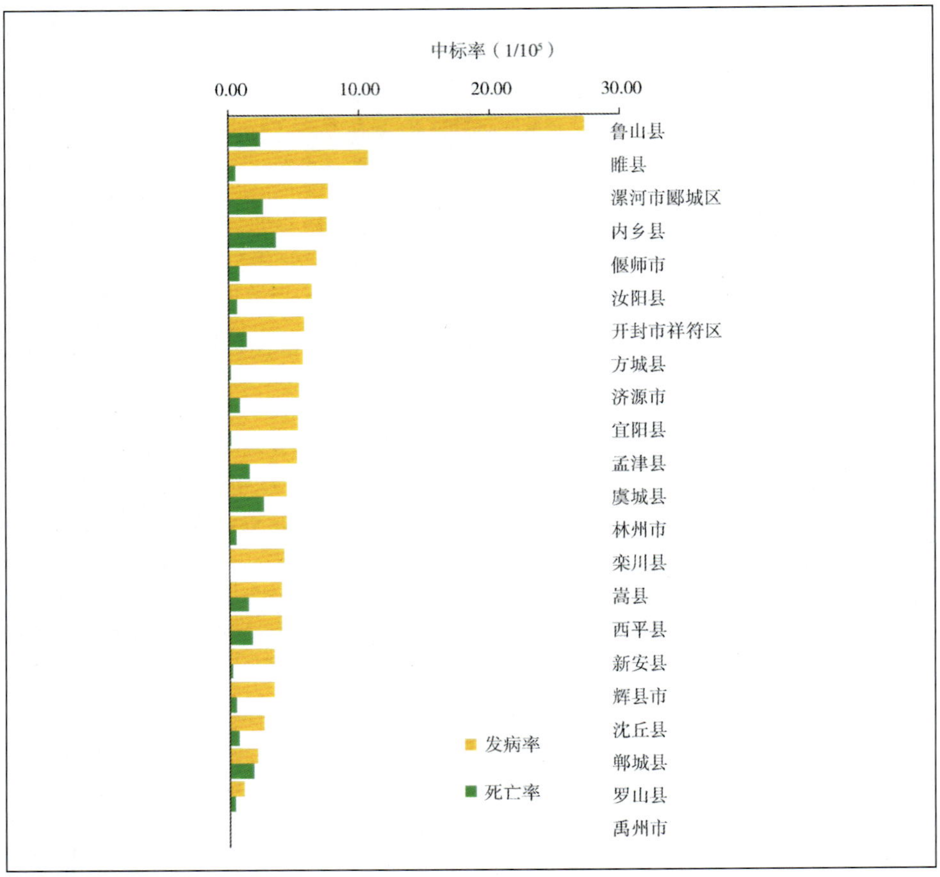

图 5-13d　农村肿瘤登记地区子宫体恶性肿瘤发病率与死亡率

十四、卵巢（C56）

2014 年，河南省肿瘤登记地区卵巢恶性肿瘤的发病率为 6.24/10^5，中标率为 5.17/10^5，世标率为 5.01/10^5，占全部恶性肿瘤发病的 1.20%。其中城市女性发病率为 6.67/10^5，农村女性为 6.15/10^5。城市为农村的 1.09 倍。同期卵巢恶性肿瘤的死亡率为 2.68/10^5，中标率为 2.1/10^5，世标率为 2.06/10^5。其中城市女性死亡率为 3.04/10^5，农村女性为 2.61/10^5。卵巢恶性肿瘤发病和死亡的 0~74 岁累积率分别为 0.56% 和 0.25%（表 5-14）。

14. Ovary (C56)

In 2014, ovary cancer cases accounted for 1.2% of all cancer cases in Henan cancer registration areas with the crude incidence of 6.24/10^5, ASR for China 5.17/10^5 and ASR for World 5.01/10^5. The crude incidence in urban areas was 6.67/10^5, and 6.15/10^5 in rural areas. It was 1.09 times in urban areas as that in rural areas. The crude mortality of ovary cancer in 2014 was 2.68/10^5, ASR for China was 2.1/10^5 and ASR for World 2.06/10^5. The crude mortality in urban areas was 3.04/10^5, and 2.61/10^5 in rural areas. The cumulative rates of incidence and mortality from 0 to 74 years old were 0.56% and 0.25%, respectively (Table 5-14).

表 5-14　河南省肿瘤登记地区卵巢恶性肿瘤发病与死亡

指标	地区	病例数	粗率（1/10⁵）	构成（%）	中标率（1/10⁵）	世标率（1/10⁵）	累积率 0~74（%）
发病	**全省**	636	6.24	1.20	5.17	5.01	0.56
	城市	112	6.67	1.25	5.57	5.29	0.62
	农村	524	6.15	1.18	5.09	4.96	0.54
死亡	**全省**	273	2.68	0.83	2.10	2.06	0.25
	城市	51	3.04	0.94	2.54	2.33	0.28
	农村	222	2.61	0.81	2.01	2.00	0.24

卵巢恶性肿瘤年龄别发病率和死亡率在0~29岁年龄段处于较低水平，30岁以后快速上升，在60-岁组和70-岁组分别达到高峰。城乡和不同地区年龄别率的水平虽然有一定的差异，但总体趋势类同，城市地区人群卵巢癌发病率波动起伏较大，70岁组达到高峰，80岁组发病率达到最低值。城市死亡率70岁达到高峰，85岁达到最低值（图5-14a ~ 图5-14b）。

The age-specific a incidence and mortality rate of ovarian cancer were relatively low before 29 years old and increased dramatically since 30 years old, reaching the peak at the age group of 60 and 70, respectively, then remained a relative high level. In rural areas the age-specific incidence and mortality rates of ovarian cancer had the similar trends with those of the overall population, while in the urban areas the age-specific incidence and mortality rates reached the peak at the age group of 70, then decreased with dramatic flctuations,incidence rate decreased to the lowest at 80 age group, and mortality rate decreased to the lowest at 85 age group (Figure 5-14a~Figure 5-14b).

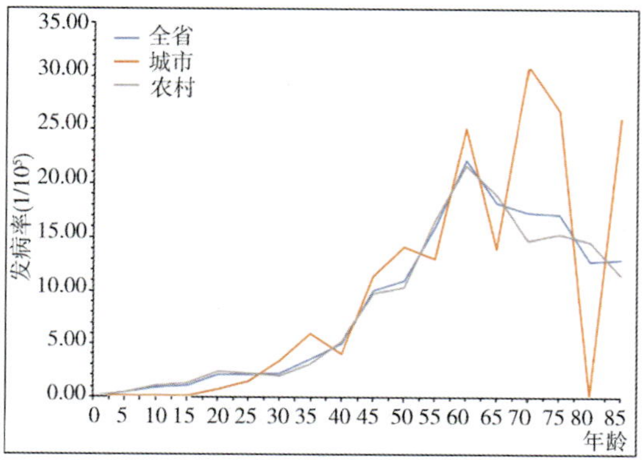

图 5-14a　河南省卵巢恶性肿瘤年龄别发病率，2014

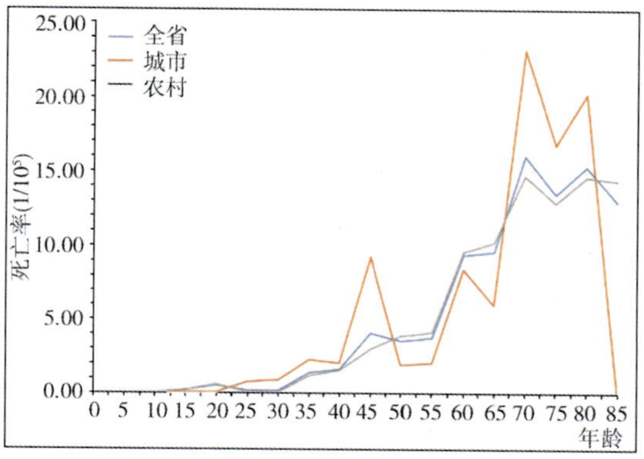

图 5-14d　河南省卵巢恶性肿瘤年龄别死亡率，2014

在 5 个城市肿瘤登记地区中，发病率最高的是漯河市（8.46/10^5），其次是洛阳市和南阳市。死亡率最高的是洛阳市（4.06/10^5）（图 5–14c）。

Among the 5 urban cancer registration areas, the ASR China incidence rate of ovarian cancer was the highest in Luohe City (8.46/10^5), followed by Luoyang City and Nanyang City. The highest ASR China mortality was in Luoyang City (4.06/10^5) (Figure 5–14c).

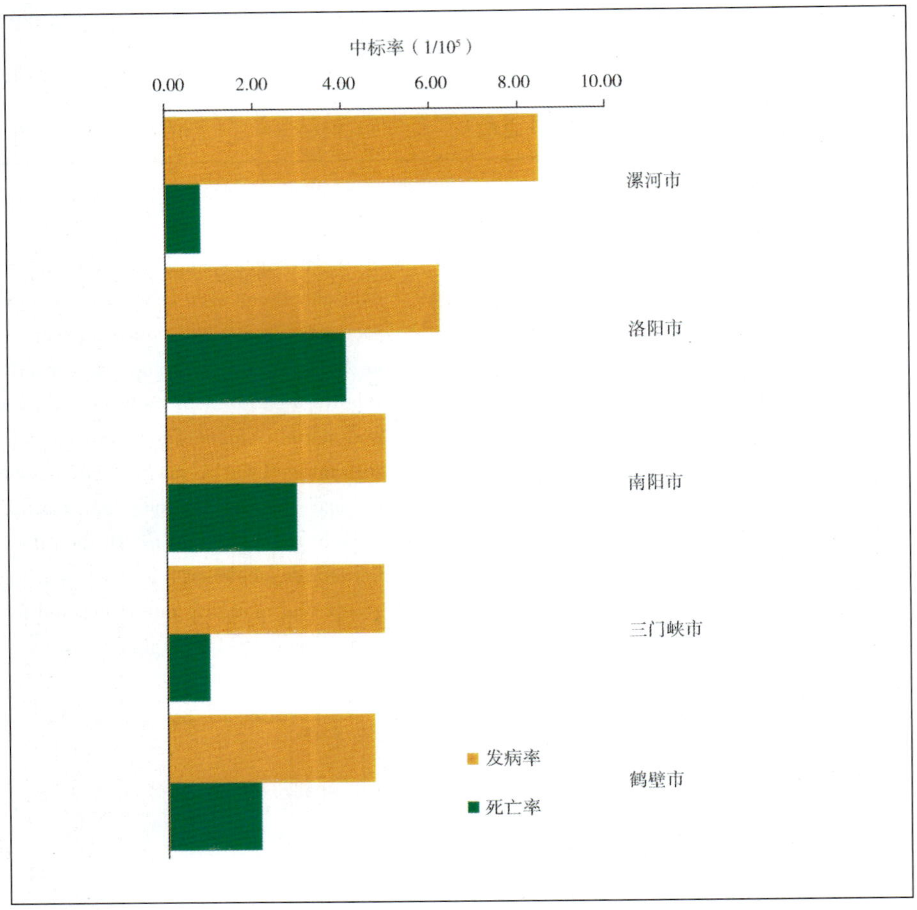

图 5–14c 城市肿瘤登记地区卵巢恶性肿瘤发病率与死亡率

在 22 个农村肿瘤登记地区中，发病率最高的是济源市（9.89/10^5），其次是开封市祥符区和虞城县。死亡率最高的是虞城县（6.49/10^5）（图 5–14d）。

Among the 22 rural cancer registration areas, the ASR China incidence rate of ovarian cancer was the highest in Jiyuan City (9.89/10^5), followed by Xiangfu District, Kaifeng and Yucheng County. The highest ASR China mortality of ovarian cancer was in Yucheng County (6.49/10^5) (Figure 5–14d).

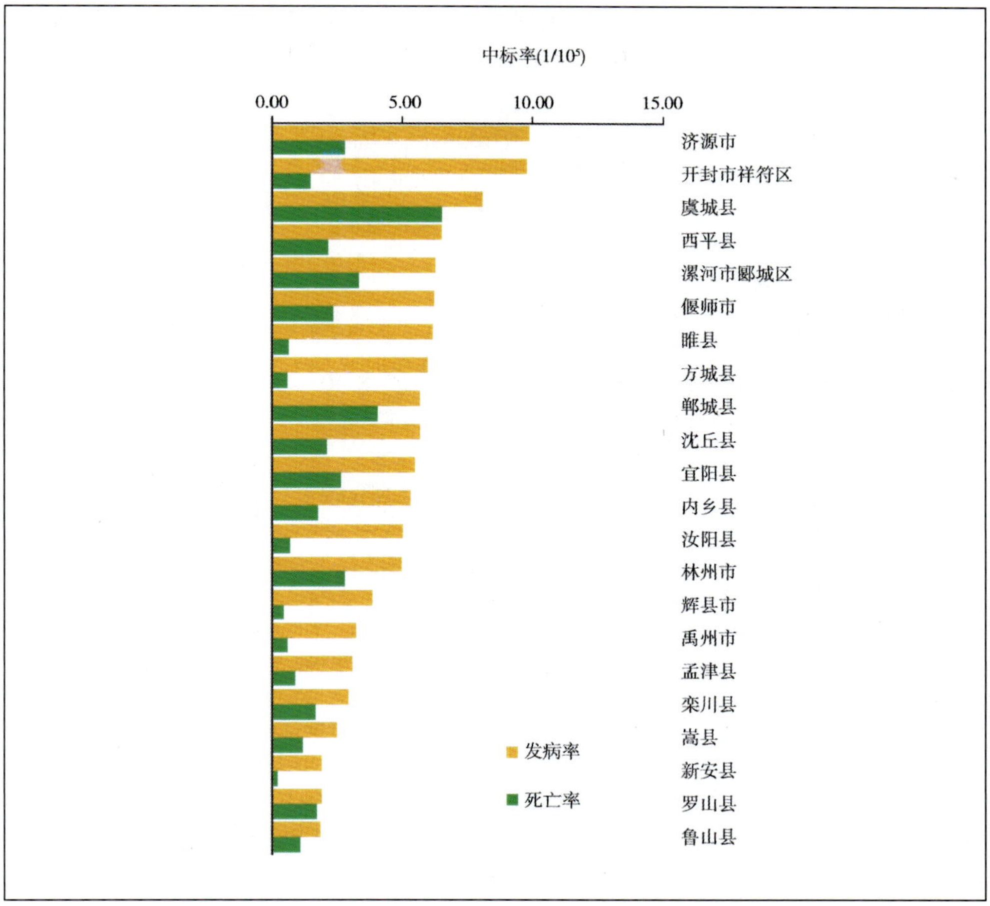

图 5-14d　农村肿瘤登记地区卵巢恶性肿瘤发病率与死亡率

十五、前列腺（C61）

2014 年，河南省肿瘤登记地区前列腺恶性肿瘤的发病率为 3.13/10^5，中标率为 2.66/10^5，世标率为 2.62/10^5，占全部恶性肿瘤发病的 0.64%。其中城市发病率为 5.92/10^5，农村发病率为 2.60/10^5。城市发病中标率为农村的 2.57 倍。同期前列腺恶性肿瘤的死亡率为 1.77/10^5，中标率为 1.49/10^5，世标率为 1.53/10^5。其中城市死亡率为 2.62/10^5，农村死亡率为 1.61/10^5。前列腺恶性肿瘤发病和死亡的 0~74 岁累积率分别为 0.26% 和 0.11%（表 5-15）。

15. Prostate (C61)

In 2014, prostate cancer cases accounted for 0.64% of all cancer cases in Henan cancer registration areas with the crude incidence of 3.13/10^5, ASR for China 2.66/10^5 and ASR for World 2.62/10^5. The crude incidence in urban areas was 5.92/10^5, and 2.60/10^5 in rural areas. It was 2.57 times in urban areas as that in rural areas. The crude mortality of prostate cancer in 2014 was 1.77/10^5, ASR for China was 1.49/10^5 and ASR for World 1.53/10^5. The crude mortality in urban areas was 2.62/10^5, and 1.61/10^5 in rural areas. The cumulative rates of incidence and mortality from 0 to 74 years old were 0.26% and 0.11%, respectively (Table 5-15).

表 5-15　河南省肿瘤登记地区前列腺恶性肿瘤发病与死亡

指标	地区	病例数	粗率（1/10⁵）	构成（%）	中标率（1/10⁵）	世标率（1/10⁵）	累积率 0~74（%）
发病	全省	340	3.13	0.64	2.66	2.62	0.26
	城市	104	5.92	1.16	5.63	5.52	0.43
	农村	236	2.60	0.53	2.19	2.16	0.23
死亡	全省	192	1.77	0.58	1.49	1.53	0.11
	城市	46	2.62	0.84	2.57	2.63	0.09
	农村	146	1.61	0.53	1.33	1.37	0.11

前列腺癌年龄别发病率在 0~54 岁年龄段处于较低水平，55 岁以后快速上升，农村地区和城市地区均在 80 岁组达到高峰。年龄别死亡率在 0~59 岁年龄段处于较低水平，60 岁以后快速上升，城市和农村地区均在 85 岁组达到高峰（图 5-15a ~图 5-15b）。

The age-specific incidence rate of prostate cancer was relatively low before 54 years old and increased dramatically since 55 years old, reaching the peak at the age group of 80. The age-specific mortality rate of prostate cancer was relatively low before 59 years old and increased dramatically since 60 years old, reaching the peak at the age group of 85 in both urban and rural areas (Figure 5-15a~Figure 5-15b).

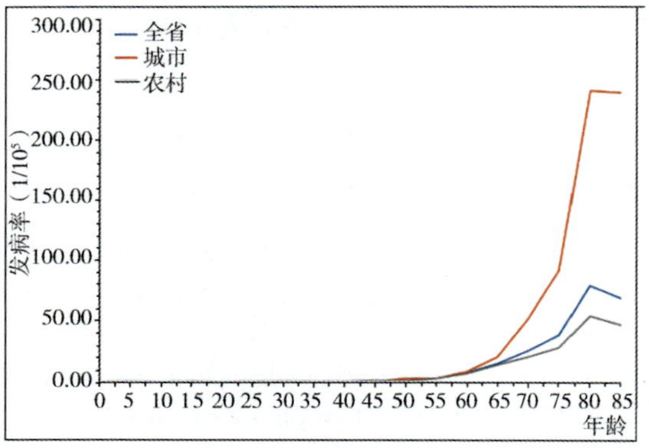

图 5-15a　河南省前列腺恶性肿瘤年龄别发病率，2014

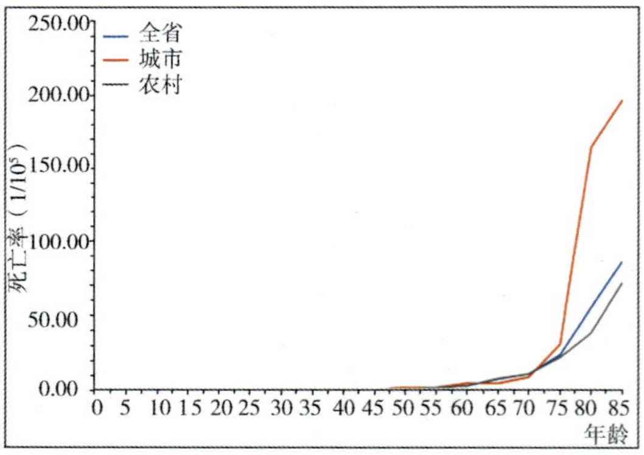

图 5-15b　河南省前列腺恶性肿瘤年龄别死亡率，2014

在 5 个城市肿瘤登记地区中，前列腺恶性肿瘤标化发病率最高的是洛阳市（9.90/10⁵），其次是三门峡市和漯河市。标化死亡率最高的是洛阳市（6.36/10⁵）（图 5-15c）。

Among the 5 urban cancer registration areas, the ASR China incidence rate of prostate cancer was the highest in Luoyang City (9.90/10⁵), followed by Sanmenxia City and Luohe City. The highest ASR China mortality was in Luoyang City (6.36/10⁵) (Figure 5-15c).

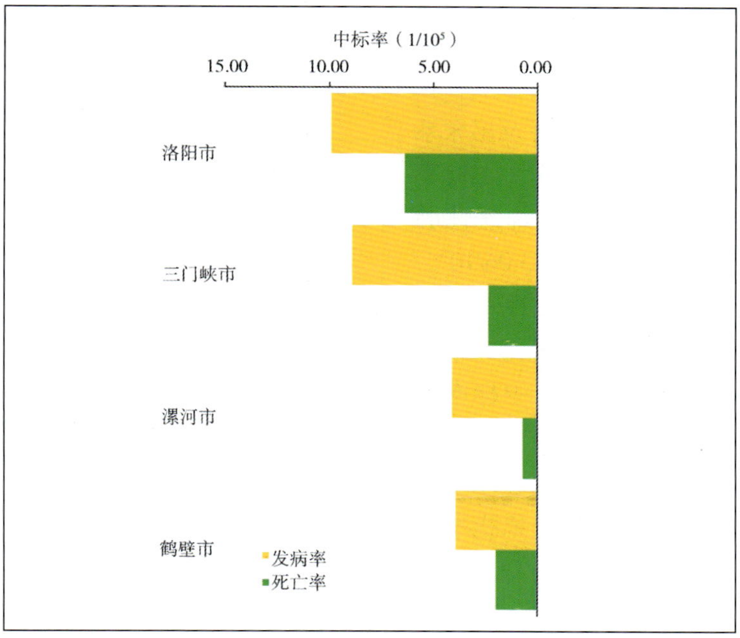

图 5-15c　城市肿瘤登记地区前列腺恶性肿瘤发病率与死亡率

在 22 个农村肿瘤登记地区中，前列腺恶性肿瘤标化发病率最高的是偃师市（5.63/10^5），其次是济源市和罗山县。标化死亡率最高的是罗山县（4.06/10^5）（图 5-15d）。

Among the 22 rural cancer registration areas, the ASR China incidence rate of prostate cancer was the highest in Yanshi County (5.63/10^5), followed by Jiyuan City and Luoshan County. The highest ASR China mortality of male prostate cancer was in Luoshan County (4.06/10^5) (Figure 5-15d).

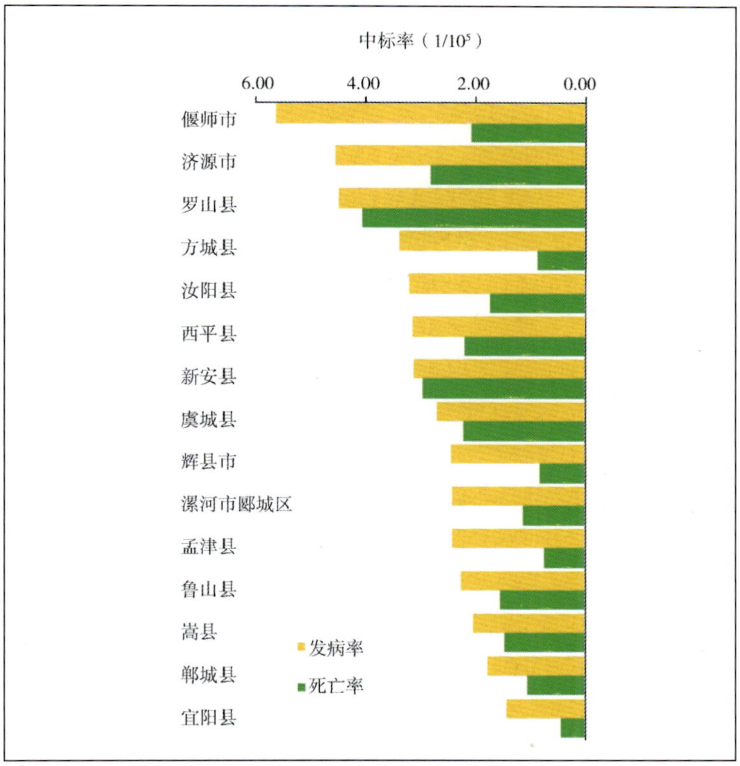

图 5-15d　农村肿瘤登记地区前列腺恶性肿瘤发病率与死亡率

十六、肾及泌尿系统部位不明（C64–C66，C68）

2014 年，河南省肿瘤登记地区肾及泌尿系统不明恶性肿瘤的发病率为 $2.50/10^5$，中标率为 $2.05/10^5$，世标率为 $2.08/10^5$, 占全部恶性肿瘤发病的 0.99%。其中男性发病率为 $3.06/10^5$，女性为 $1.90/10^5$。男性中标率为女性的 1.71 倍，城市为农村的 2.02 倍。同期肾及泌尿系统不明恶性肿瘤的死亡率为 $1.14/10^5$，中标率为 $0.90/10^5$，世标率为 $0.91/10^5$。其中男性死亡率为 1.54/10 万，女性为 $0.71/10^5$。肾及泌尿系统不明恶性肿瘤发病和死亡的 0~74 岁累积率分别为 0.24% 和 0.1%（表 5–16）。

16. Kidney & Unspecified Urinary Organs (C64–C66,C68)

In 2014, the cases of cancer of kidney and unspecified urinary organs (below named as kidney cancer) accounted for 0.99% of all cancer cases in Henan cancer registration areas with the crude incidence of $2.50/10^5$, ASR for China $2.05/10^5$ and ASR for World $2.08/10^5$. The incidence in males was $3.06/10^5$, and $1.90/10^5$ in females. It was 1.71 times in males as high as that in females and it was 2.02 times in urban areas as that in rural areas. The crude mortality of kidney cancer in 2014 was $1.14/10^5$, ASR for China was $0.90/10^5$ and ASR for World $0.91/10^5$. The mortality in males was$1.54/10^5$, and $0.71/10^5$ in females. The cumulative rates of incidence and mortality from 0 to 74 years old were 0.24% and 0.10%, respectively (Table 5–16).

表 5–16 河南省肿瘤登记地区肾及泌尿系统不明恶性肿瘤发病与死亡

地区	性别	病例数	粗率 ($1/10^5$)	构成 (%)	中标率 ($1/10^5$)	世标率 ($1/10^5$)	累积率 0~74 (%)
发病							
全省	合计	526	2.50	0.99	2.05	2.08	0.24
	男性	332	3.06	1.12	2.60	2.65	0.31
	女性	194	1.90	0.82	1.52	1.53	0.17
城市	合计	148	4.31	1.65	3.58	3.70	0.45
	男性	99	5.63	1.94	4.88	5.09	0.61
	女性	49	2.92	1.27	2.34	2.36	0.29
农村	合计	378	2.15	0.85	1.77	1.78	0.20
	男性	233	2.56	0.95	2.18	2.21	0.26
	女性	145	1.70	0.74	1.36	1.37	0.15
死亡							
全省	合计	239	1.14	0.73	0.90	0.91	0.10
	男性	167	1.54	0.82	1.30	1.31	0.15
	女性	72	0.71	0.57	0.52	0.53	0.06
城市	合计	73	2.13	1.34	1.80	1.81	0.21
	男性	50	2.85	1.46	2.54	2.61	0.32
	女性	23	1.37	1.13	1.12	1.09	0.11

续表

地区	性别	病例数	粗率（1/10⁵）	构成（%）	中标率（1/10⁵）	世标率（1/10⁵）	累积率 0~74（%）
农村	合计	166	0.94	0.60	0.74	0.74	0.08
	男性	117	1.29	0.69	1.08	1.09	0.12
	女性	49	0.58	0.47	0.42	0.42	0.05

前列腺癌年龄别发病率在0~44岁年龄段处于较低水平，45岁以后快速上升，65岁以后出现波动，在80岁组达到高峰。年龄别死亡率在0~59岁年龄段处于较低水平，60岁以后快速上升，城市和农村地区在80岁组和85岁组分别达到高峰（图5-16a～图5-16f）。

The age-specific incidence rate of kidney cancer was relatively low before 44 years old and increased dramatically since 45 years old, fluctuated after 65 and reached the peak at the age group of 80. The age-specific mortality rate of kidney cancer was relatively low before 59 years old and increased dramatically since 60 years old, reaching the peak at the age group of 80 in the urban areas and of 85 in the rural areas (Figure 5-16a~Figure 5-16f).

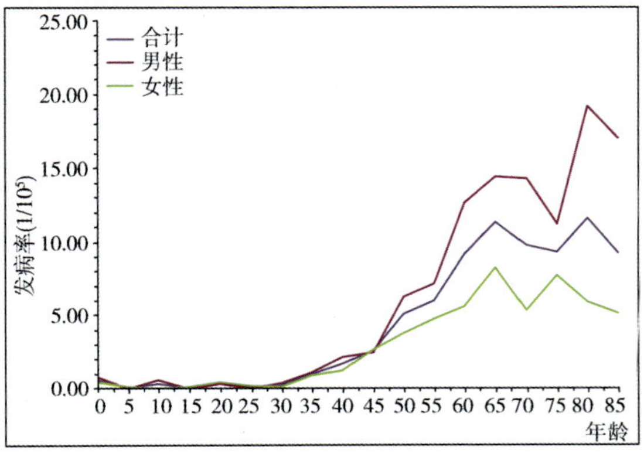

图5-16a　河南省肾及泌尿系统不明恶性肿瘤年龄别发病率，2014

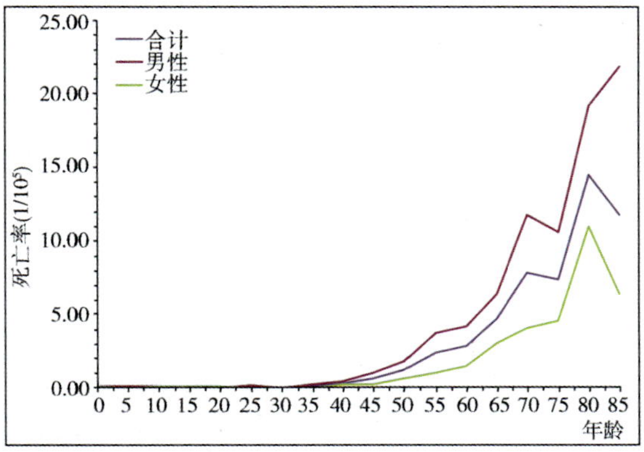

图5-16d　河南省肾及泌尿系统不明恶性肿瘤年龄别死亡率，2014

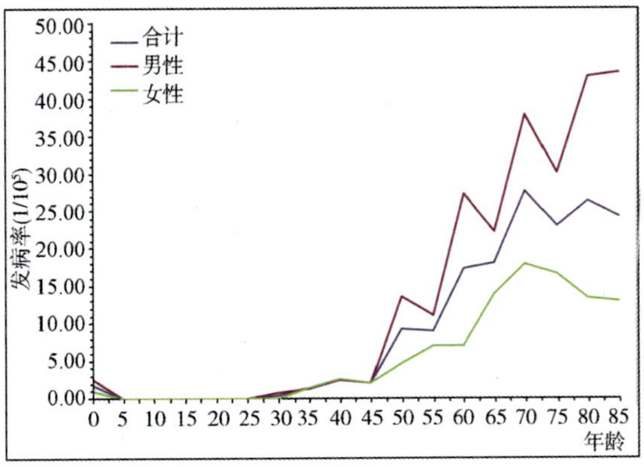

图5-16b　城市肿瘤登记地区肾及泌尿系统不明恶性肿瘤年龄别发病率，2014

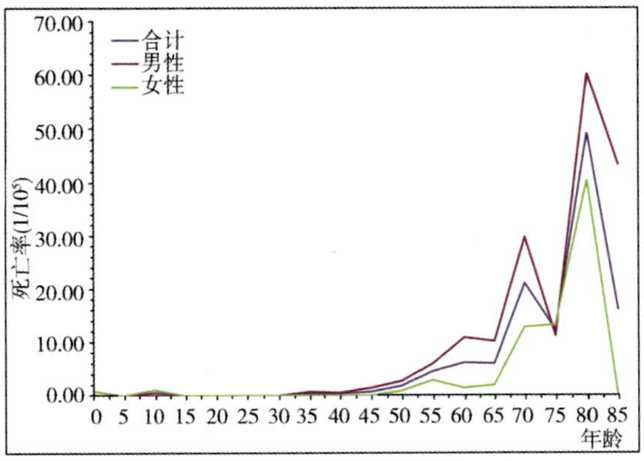

图5-16e　城市肿瘤登记地区肾及泌尿系统不明恶性肿瘤年龄别死亡率，2014

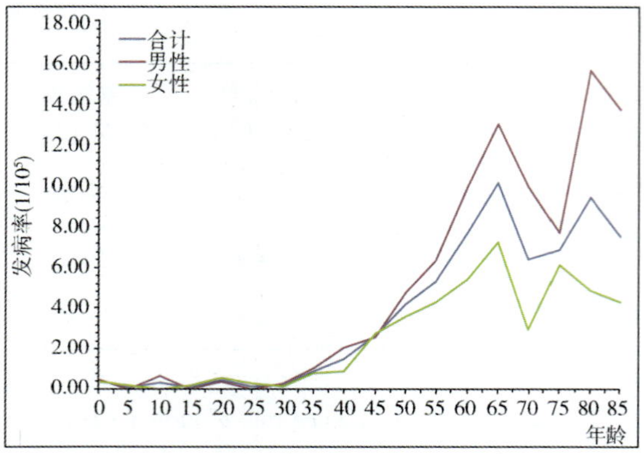

图 5-16c 农村肿瘤登记地区肾及泌尿系统不明恶性肿瘤年龄别发病率，2014

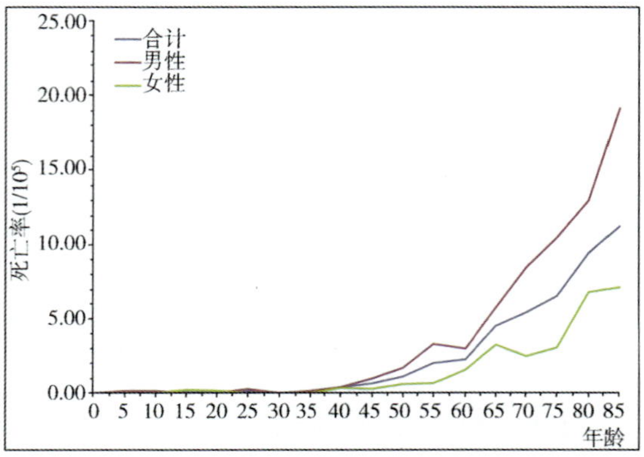

图 5-16f 农村肿瘤登记地区肾及泌尿系统不明恶性肿瘤年龄别死亡率，2014

在 5 个城市肿瘤登记地区中，男性肾及泌尿系统不明恶性肿瘤标化发病率最高的是洛阳市（9.30/10^5），其次是三门峡市和鹤壁市；女性发病率最高的是洛阳市（4.33/10^5），其次是鹤壁市和漯河市。男性标化死亡率最高的是洛阳市（4.34/10^5），女性死亡率最高的是洛阳市（2.25/10^5）（图 5-16g）。

Among the 5 urban cancer registration areas, the ASR China incidence rate of kidney cancer in males (9.30/10^5) was the highest in Luoyang City, followed by Sanmenxia City and Hebi City. In females, it was the highest in Luoyang City (4.33/10^5), followed by Hebi City and Luohe City. The ASR China mortality was the highest in Luoyang City for both males (4.34/10^5) and females (2.25/10^5) (Figure 5-16g).

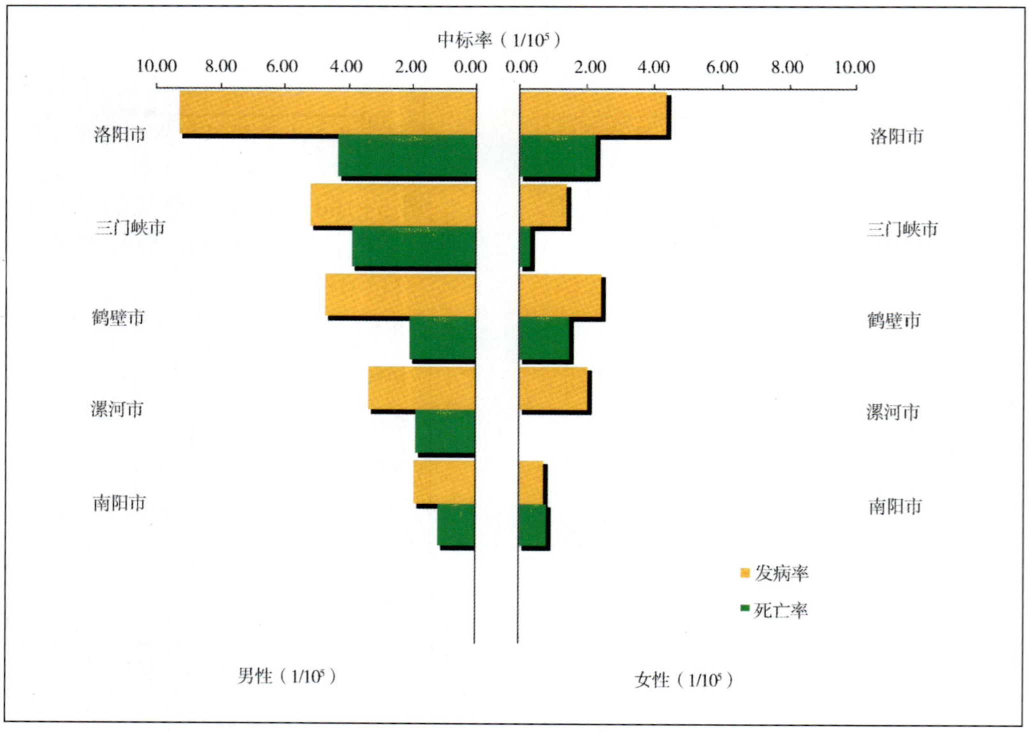

图 5-16g 城市肿瘤登记地区肾及泌尿系统不明恶性肿瘤发病率与死亡率

在 22 个农村肿瘤登记地区中，男性肾及泌尿系统不明恶性肿瘤标化发病率最高的是济源市（4.65/10^5），其次是偃师市和睢县；女性发病率最高的是济源市（2.76/10^5），其次是睢县和新安县。男性标化死亡率最高的是新安县（2.20/10^5），女性死亡率最高的是济源市（1.67/10 万）（图 5-16h）。

Among the 22 rural cancer registration areas, the ASR China incidence rate of kidney cancer in males was the highest in Jiyuan City (4.65/10^5), followed by Yanshi City and Suixian County. In females, it was the highest in Jiyuan City (2.76/10^5), followed by Suixian County and Xinan County. The age-specific mortality was the highest in Xin'an County for males (2.2/10^5) and Jiyuan City for females (1.67/10^5) (Figure 5-16h).

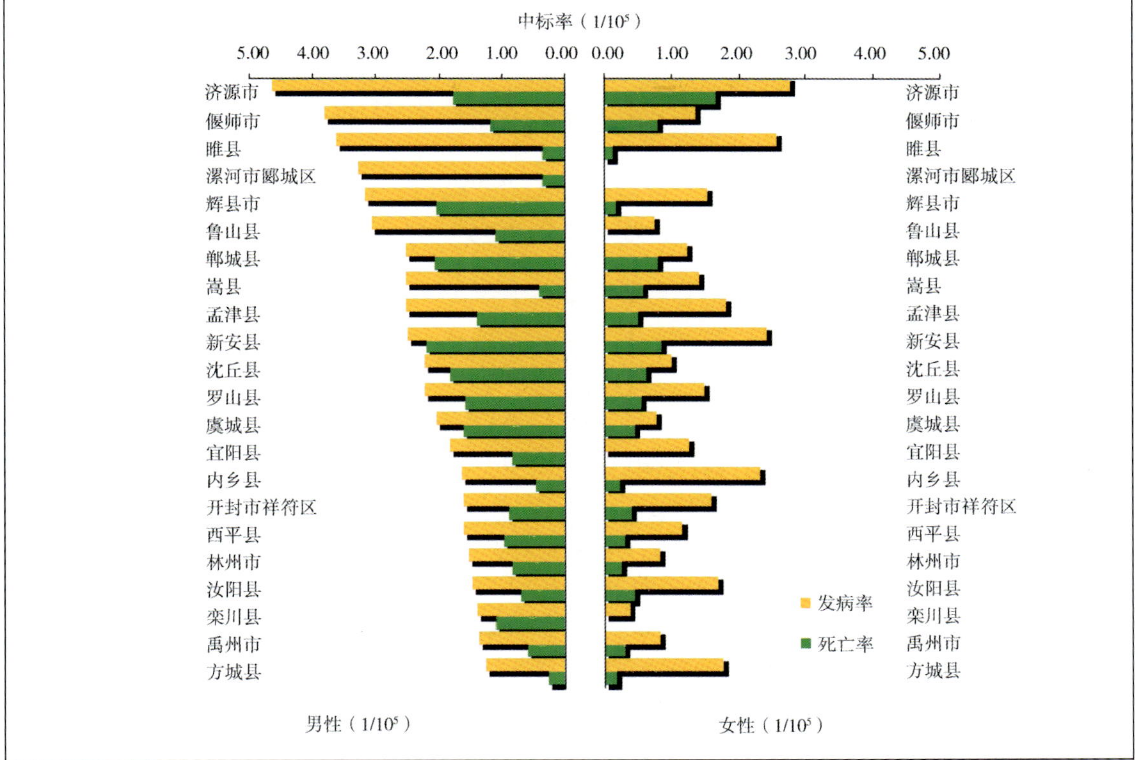

图 5-16h　农村肿瘤登记地区肾及泌尿系统不明恶性肿瘤发病率与死亡率

十七、膀胱（C67）

2014 年，河南省肿瘤登记地区膀胱恶性肿瘤的发病率为 2.72/10^5，中标率为 2.16/10^5，世标率为 2.16/10^5，占全部恶性肿瘤发病的 1.08%。其中男性发病率为 3.97/10^5，女性为 1.38/10^5。男性中标率为女性的 3.26 倍，城市为农村的 1.62 倍。同期膀胱恶性肿瘤的死亡率为 1.21/10^5，中标率为 0.95/10^5，世标率为 0.94/10^5。其中男性死亡率为 1.76/10^5，女性为 0.63/10^5。膀胱恶性肿瘤发病和死亡的 0~74 岁累积率分别为 0.25% 和 0.11%（表 5-17）。

17. Bladder (C67)

In 2014, bladder cancer cases accounted for 1.08% of all cancer cases in Henan cancer registration areas with the crude incidence of 2.72/10^5, ASR for China 2.16/10^{5}and ASR for World 2.16/10^5. The incidence in males was 3.97/10^5, and 1.38/10^5 in females. It was 3.26 times in males as high as that in females and it was 1.62 times in urban areas as that in rural areas. The crude mortality of bladder cancer in 2014 was 1.21/10^5, ASR for China was 0.95/10^5 and ASR for World 0.94/10^5. The mortality in males was1.76/10^5, and 0.63/10^5 in females. The cumulative rates of incidence and mortality from 0 to 74 years old were 0.25% and 0.11%, respectively (Table 5-17) .

表 5-17　河南省肿瘤登记地区膀胱恶性肿瘤发病与死亡

地区	性别	病例数	粗率（1/10^5）	构成（%）	中标率（1/10^5）	世标率（1/10^5）	累积率 0~74（%）
发病							
全省	合计	572	2.72	1.08	2.16	2.16	0.25
	男性	431	3.97	1.45	3.36	3.40	0.40
	女性	141	1.38	0.60	1.03	1.00	0.11
城市	合计	132	3.84	1.47	3.20	3.15	0.31
	男性	95	5.41	1.86	4.82	4.76	0.47
	女性	37	2.20	0.96	1.71	1.68	0.15
农村	合计	440	2.50	0.99	1.98	1.99	0.24
	男性	336	3.69	1.37	3.10	3.17	0.38
	女性	104	1.22	0.53	0.92	0.89	0.10
死亡							
全省	合计	255	1.21	0.77	0.95	0.94	0.11
	男性	191	1.76	0.94	1.49	1.49	0.16
	女性	64	0.63	0.51	0.46	0.47	0.05
城市	合计	56	1.63	1.03	1.37	1.39	0.12
	男性	41	2.33	1.20	2.22	2.27	0.19
	女性	15	0.89	0.74	0.67	0.68	0.05
农村	合计	199	1.13	0.72	0.88	0.88	0.10
	男性	150	1.65	0.88	1.39	1.38	0.15
	女性	49	0.58	0.47	0.43	0.44	0.05

膀胱恶性肿瘤年龄别发病率和死亡率在0~54岁年龄段处于较低水平，55岁以后快速上升，在85+或80-岁组达到高峰，男性高于女性。城乡和不同地区年龄别率的水平虽然有一定的差异，但总体趋势类同（图5-17a ~ 图5-17f）。

The age-specific incidence and mortality rates of bladder cancer were relatively low before 55 years old and increased rapidly since 55 years old, reaching the peak at the age group of 85 and 80, respectively. Incidence rates in males was generally higher than those in females. The age-specific incidence and mortality rates varied in urban and rural areas with similar curves（Figure 5-17a~Figure 5-17f）.

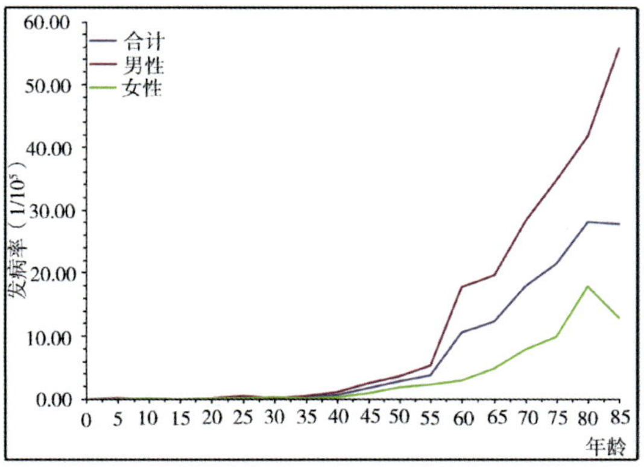

图 5-17a　河南省膀胱恶性肿瘤年龄别发病率，2014

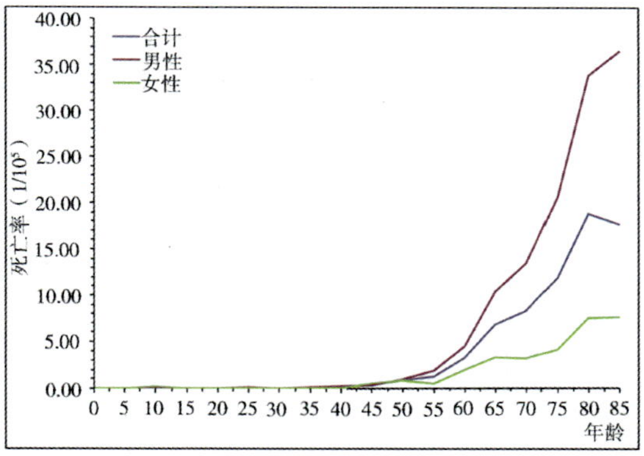

图 5-17d　河南省膀胱恶性肿瘤年龄别死亡率，2014

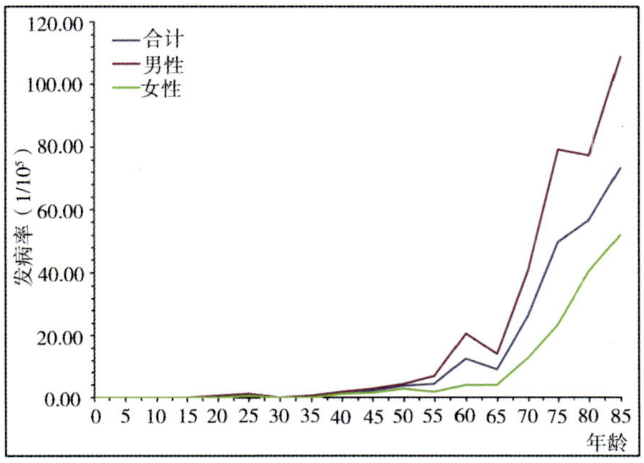

图 5-17b　城市肿瘤登记地区膀胱恶性肿瘤年龄别发病率，2014

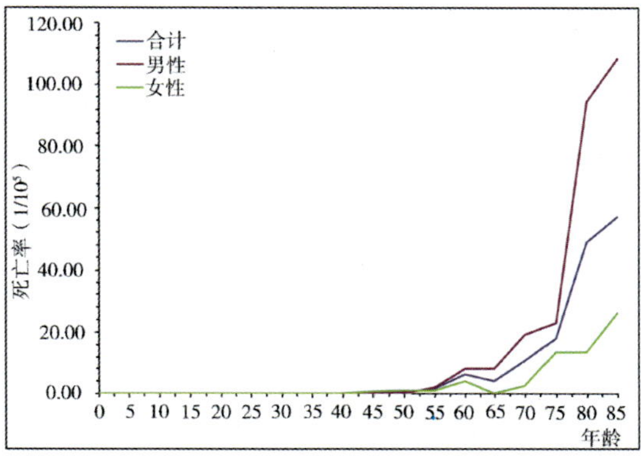

图 5-17e　城市肿瘤登记地区膀胱恶性肿瘤年龄别死亡率，2014

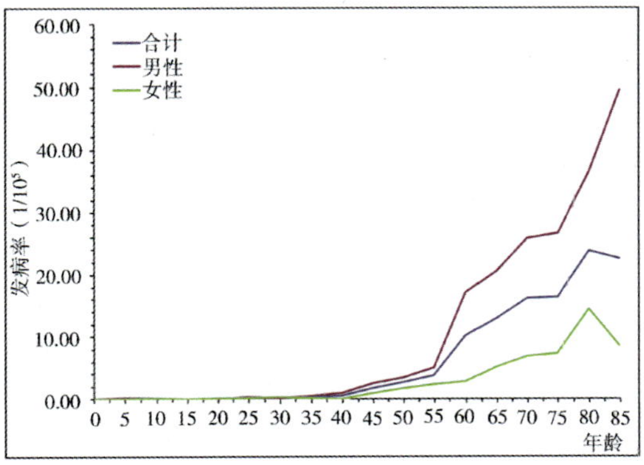

图 5-17c　农村肿瘤登记地区膀胱恶性肿瘤年龄别发病率，2014

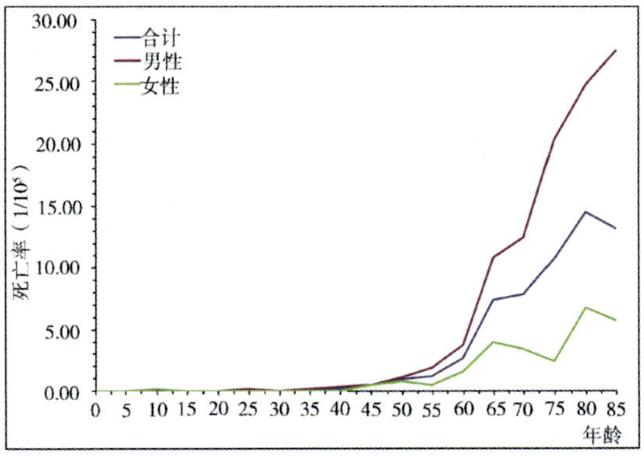

图 5-17f　农村肿瘤登记地区膀胱恶性肿瘤年龄别死亡率，2014

在 5 个城市肿瘤登记地区中，男性膀胱恶性肿瘤标化发病率最高的是洛阳市（9.82/10^5），其次是漯河市和三门峡市；女性发病率最高的是洛阳市（4.02/10^5），其次是漯河市和三门峡市。男性标化死亡率最高的是洛阳市（4.57/10^5），女性死亡率最高的是洛阳市（2.19/10^5）（图 5-17g）。

Among the 5 urban cancer registration areas, the ASR China incidence rate of bladder cancer in males was the highest in Luoyang City (9.82/10^5), followed by Luohe City and Sanmenxia City. In females, it was the highest in Luoyang City (4.02/10^5), followed by Luohe City and Sanmenxia City. The highest ASR China mortality were in Luoyang City for both males (4.57/10^5) and females (2.19/10^5)(Figure 5-17g).

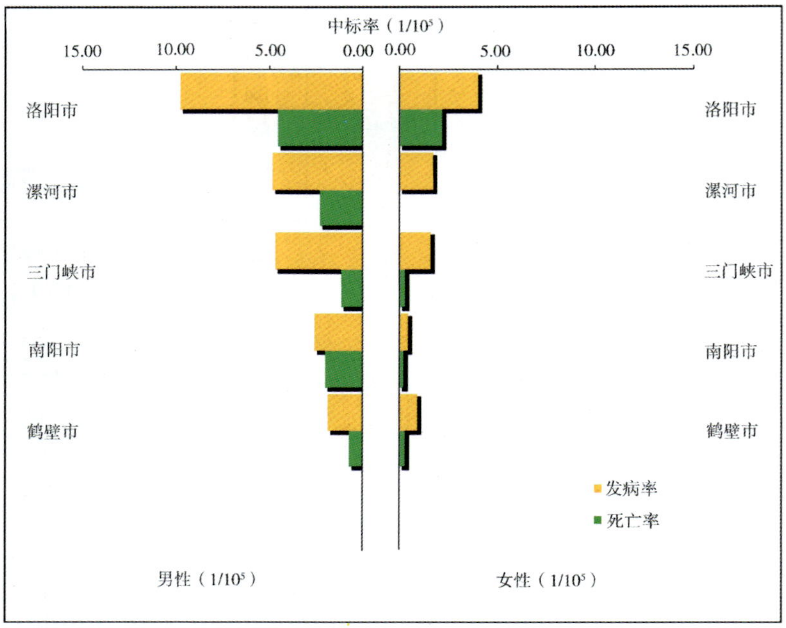

图 5-17g　城市肿瘤登记地区膀胱恶性肿瘤发病率与死亡率

在 22 个农村肿瘤登记地区中，男性膀胱恶性肿瘤标化发病率最高的是开封市祥符区（6.02/10^5），其次是宜阳县和济源市；女性发病率最高的是济源市（2.16/10^5），其次是宜阳县和虞城县。男性标化死亡率最高的是沈丘县（3.76/10^5），女性死亡率最高的是虞城县（1.12/10^5）（图 5-17h）。

2014 年肿瘤登记地区膀胱恶性肿瘤发病病例中有确切解剖学亚部位（C67.0–C67.7，C67.8）信息的占 37.8%，亚部位未特指（C67.9）的占 62.2%。在有亚部位的膀胱癌病例中，发生在膀胱三角区（C67.0）的占 49.1%，膀胱顶（C67.1）的占 10.2%，膀胱侧壁（C67.2）的占 8.8%，膀胱前壁（C67.3）的占 12.5%，膀胱后壁（C67.4）的占 7.4%，膀胱颈（C67.5）的占 6.9%，输尿管口（C67.6）的占 2.3%，脐尿管（C67.7）的占 1.9%，膀胱交搭跨越（C67.8）的占 0.9%（图 5-17i）。

Among the 22 rural cancer registration areas, the ASR China incidence rate of bladder cancer in males was the highest in Xiangfu District, Kaifeng (6.02/10^5), followed by Yiyang County and Jiyuan City. For females, it was the highest in Jiyuan City(2.16/10^5), followed by Yiyang County and Yucheng County. The ASR China mortality was the highest in Shenqiu County for males (3.76/10^5) and Yucheng County for females (1.12/10^5) (Figure 5-17h).

Among all the reported bladder cancer cases in 2014, 37.8% had specific anatomic site information (C67.0–C67.7, C67.8) and the rest 62.2% didn't have. The specific anatomic sites of kidney cancer included trigone (C67.0) (49.1%), dome (C67.1) (10.2%), lateral (C67.2) (8.8%), anterior (C67.3) (12.5%), posterior (C67.4) (7.4%), bladder neck (C67.5) (6.9%), ureteric orifice (C67.6) (2.3%), urachus (C67.7) (1.9%) and the overlapping part (C67.8) (0.9%) (Figure 5-17i).

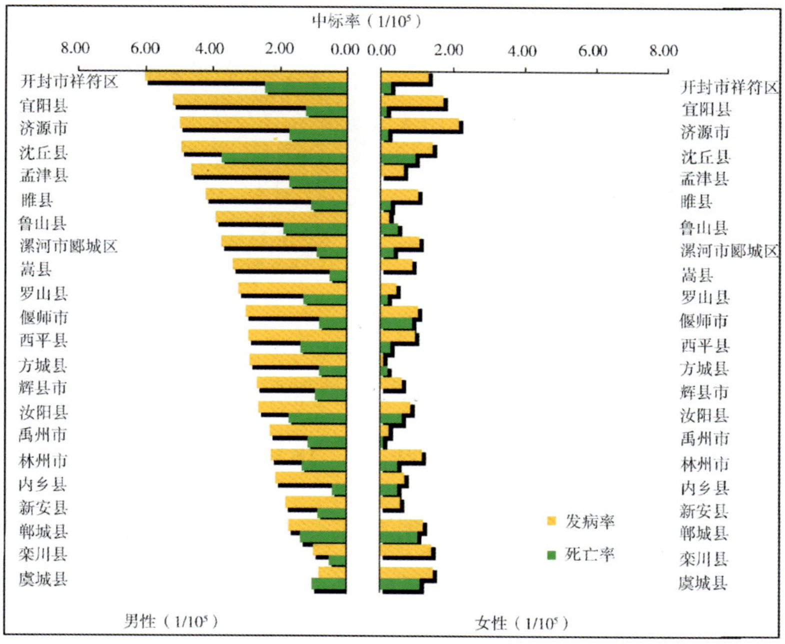

图 5-17h　农村肿瘤登记地区膀胱恶性肿瘤发病率与死亡率

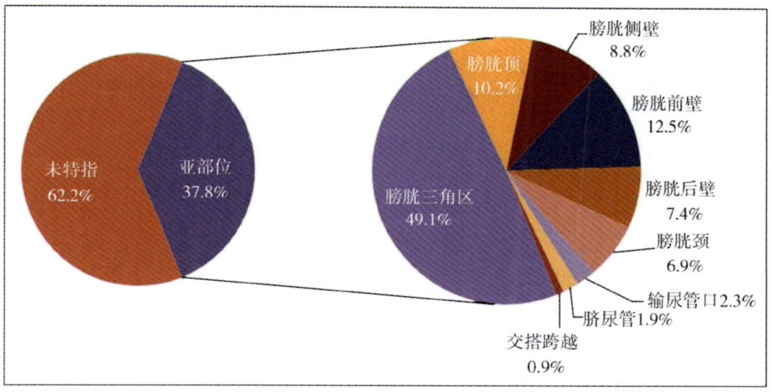

图 5-17i　河南省膀胱恶性肿瘤发病亚部位构成 (%)

2014 年肿瘤登记地区膀胱恶性肿瘤发病病例中有明确组织病理学分型的占 57.5%，组织学类型未特指的占 42.5%。在有组织病理学分型的膀胱癌病例中，鳞状细胞癌占 19.5%，移行细胞癌占 43.5%，腺癌占 23.4%，其他类型的膀胱癌占 13.7%（图 5-17j）。

Among all cases, 57.5% had specific pathological diagnostic information and the rest 42.5% didn't have. Squamous cell carcinoma accounted for 19.5% of the cases with specific pathological diagnostic information, transitional cell carcinoma accounted for 43.5%, adenocarcinoma 23.4% and other pathological type 13.7%(Figure 5-17j).

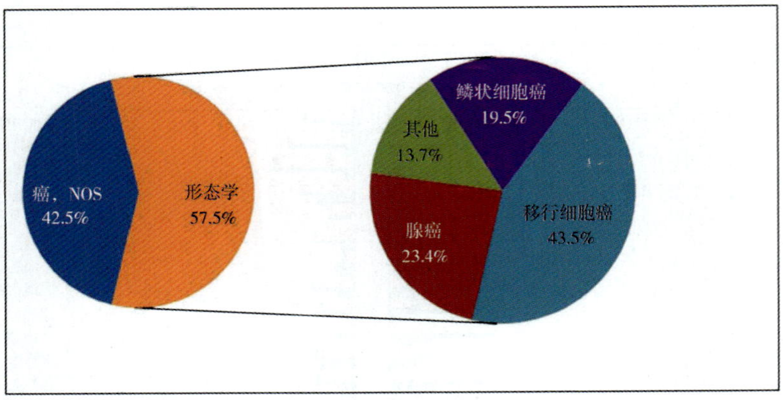

图 5-17j 河南省膀胱恶性肿瘤发病形态学构成 (%)

十八、脑及中枢神经系统 (C70-C72)

2014 年，河南省肿瘤登记地区脑及中枢神经系统恶性肿瘤的发病率为 6.69/10^5，中标率为 5.71/10^5，世标率为 5.67/10^5, 占全部恶性肿瘤发病的 2.65%。其中男性发病率为 6.5/10^5，女性为 6.9/10^5。男性中标率为女性的 1.01 倍，城市为农村的 0.93 倍。同期脑及中枢神经系统恶性肿瘤的死亡率为 3.93/10^5，中标率为 3.3/10^5，世标率为 3.26/10^5。其中男性死亡率为 4.2/10^5，女性为 3.64/10^5。脑及中枢神经系统恶性肿瘤发病和死亡的 0~74 岁累积率分别为 0.60% 和 0.34%（表 5-18）。

18.Brain & Central Nervous System (C70-C72)

In 2014, brain and central nervous system cancer (the following named as brain tumors) cases accounted for 2.65% of all cancer cases in Henan cancer registration areas with the crude incidence of 6.69/10^5, ASR for China 5.71/10^5 and ASR for World 5.67/10^5. The incidence in males was 6.5/10^5, and 6.9/10^5 in females. It was 1.01 times in males as high as that in females and it was 0.93 times in urban areas as that in rural areas. The crude mortality of brain tumors in 2014 was 3.93/10^5, ASR for China was 3.3/10^5 and ASR for World 3.26/10^5.The mortality in males was4.2/10^5, and 3.64/10^5 in females. The cumulative rates of incidence and mortality from 0 to 74 years old were 0.60% and 0.34%, respectively(Table 5-18).

表 5-18 河南省肿瘤登记地区脑及中枢神经系统恶性肿瘤发病与死亡

地区	性别	病例数	粗率 (1/10^5)	构成 (%)	中标率 (1/10^5)	世标率 (1/10^5)	累积率 0~74 (%)
发病							
全省	合计	1 408	6.69	2.65	5.71	5.67	0.60
	男性	705	6.50	2.38	5.75	5.72	0.58
	女性	703	6.90	2.99	5.68	5.63	0.61
城市	合计	217	6.32	2.42	5.40	5.23	0.53
	男性	115	6.54	2.25	5.82	5.60	0.52
	女性	102	6.08	2.64	5.06	4.94	0.53
	合计	1 191	6.76	2.69	5.78	5.77	0.61

续表

地区	性别	病例数	粗率(1/10⁵)	构成(%)	中标率(1/10⁵)	世标率(1/10⁵)	累积率0~74(%)
农村	男性	590	6.49	2.40	5.75	5.77	0.59
	女性	601	7.06	3.06	5.81	5.78	0.63
死亡							
	合计	827	3.93	2.51	3.30	3.26	0.34
全省	男性	456	4.20	2.23	3.73	3.67	0.37
	女性	371	3.64	2.96	2.89	2.89	0.31
	合计	110	3.20	2.02	2.76	2.77	0.26
城市	男性	66	3.76	1.93	3.39	3.39	0.30
	女性	44	2.62	2.17	2.19	2.23	0.21
	合计	717	4.07	2.61	3.42	3.38	0.36
农村	男性	390	4.29	2.30	3.81	3.75	0.38
	女性	327	3.84	3.11	3.04	3.04	0.33

脑及中枢神经系统恶性肿瘤年龄别发病率和死亡率在0~29岁年龄段处于较低水平，30岁以后快速上升，在80-岁或85+岁组达到高峰，男女差别不明显。城乡和不同地区年龄别率的水平虽然有一定的差异，但总体趋势类同（图5-18a ~图5-18f）。

The age-specific incidence and mortality rates of brain tumors were relatively low before 29 years old and increased dramatically since 30 years old, reaching the peak at the age group of 80 and 85 respectively. There were not significant differences between males and females. The age-specific incidence and mortality rates varied in urban and rural areas with similar curves(Figure 5-18a~Figure 5-18f).

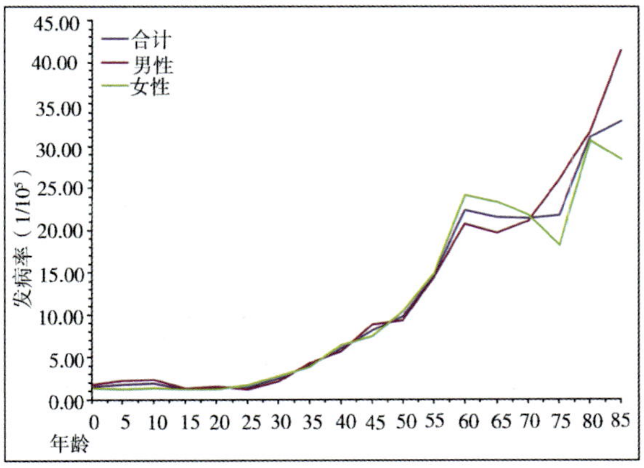

图5-18a 河南省脑及中枢神经系统恶性肿瘤年龄别发病率，2014

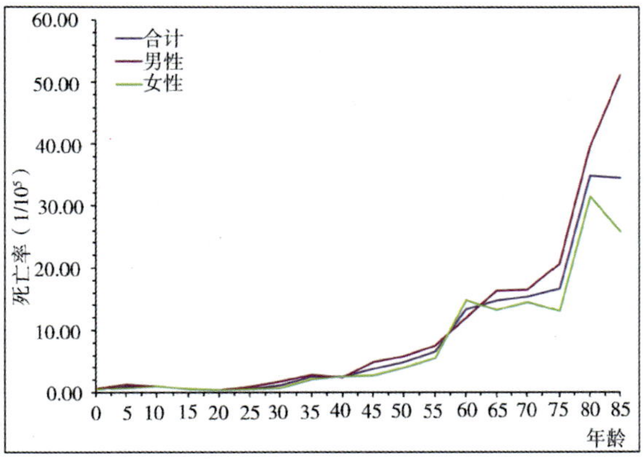

图5-18d 河南省脑及中枢神经系统恶性肿瘤年龄别死亡率，2014

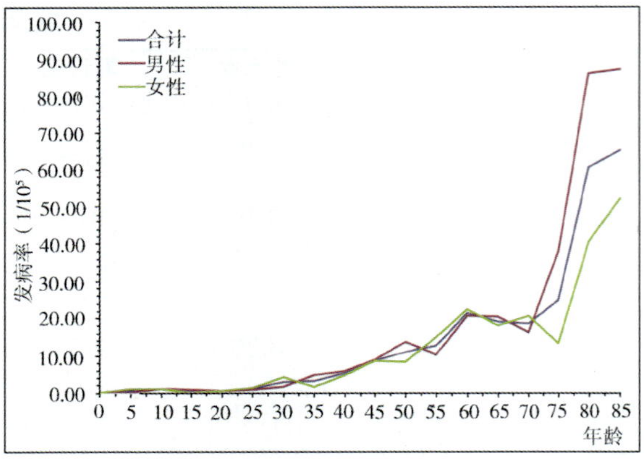

图 5-18b 城市肿瘤登记地区脑及中枢神经系统恶性肿瘤年龄别发病率，2014

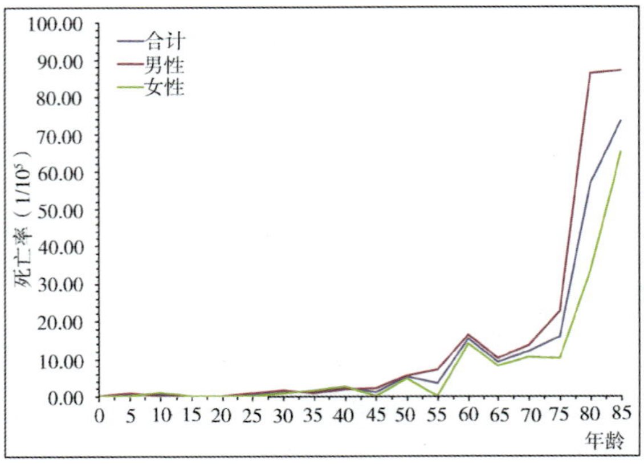

图 5-18e 城市肿瘤登记地区脑及中枢神经系统恶性肿瘤年龄别死亡率，2014

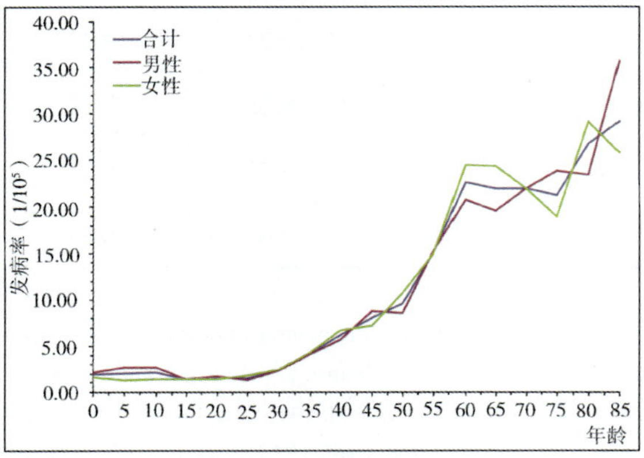

图 5-18c 农村肿瘤登记地区脑及中枢神经系统恶性肿瘤年龄别发病率，2014

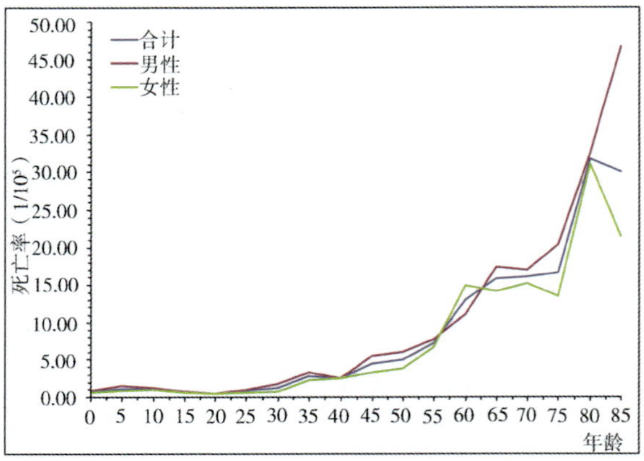

图 5-18f 农村肿瘤登记地区脑及中枢神经系统恶性肿瘤年龄别死亡率，2014

在 5 个城市肿瘤登记地区中，男性脑及中枢神经系统恶性肿瘤标化发病率最高的是南阳市（$7.82/10^5$），其次是鹤壁市和洛阳市；女性发病率最高的是洛阳市（$7.68/10^5$），其次是南阳市和三门峡市。男性标化死亡率最高的是鹤壁市（$4.81/10^5$），女性死亡率最高的是洛阳市（$3.47/10^5$）（图 5-18g）。

Among the 5 urban cancer registration areas, the ASR China incidence rate of brain tumors in males was the highest in Nanyang City ($7.82/10^5$), followed by Hebi City and Luoyang City. In females, it was the highest in Luoyang City ($7.68/10^5$), followed by Nanyang City and Sanmenxia City. The highest ASR China mortality were in Hebi City ($4.81/10^5$) for males and in Luoyang City ($3.47/10^5$) for females (Figure 5-18g).

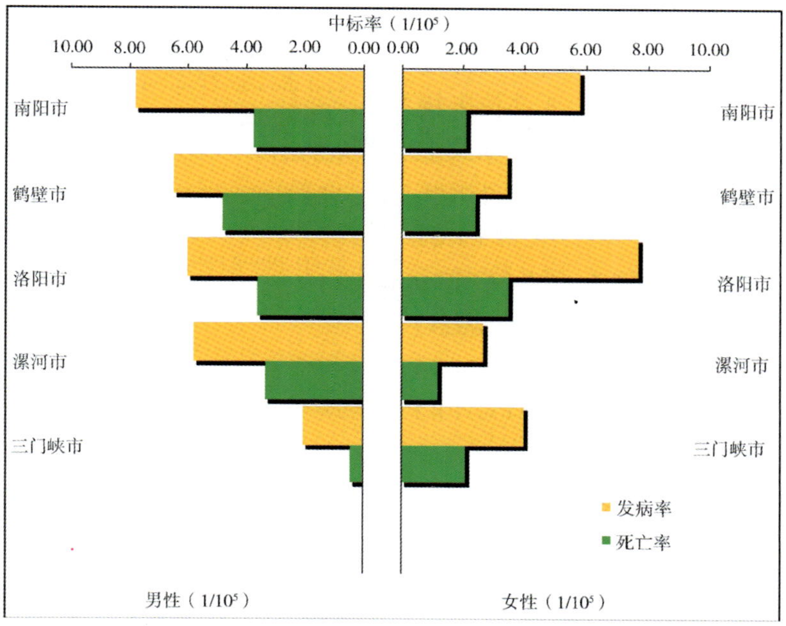

图 5-18g　城市肿瘤登记地区脑及中枢神经系统恶性肿瘤发病率与死亡率

在 22 个农村肿瘤登记地区中，男性脑及中枢神经系统恶性肿瘤标化发病率最高的是睢县（12.21/10^5），其次是沈丘县和偃师市；女性发病率最高的是沈丘县（13.63/10^5），其次是栾川县和孟津县。男性标化死亡率最高的是睢县(9.2/10^5),女性死亡率最高的是睢县(8.79/10^5)（图 5-18h）。

Among the 22 rural cancer registration rate,the ASR China incidence rate of brain tumors in males was the highest in Suixian County (12.21/10^5), followed by Shenqiu County and Yanshi City. For females, it was the highest in Shenqiu County (13.63/10^5), followed by Luanchuan County and Mengjin County. The ASR China mortality was the highest in Suixian County for males (9.2/10^5) and Suixian County for females (8.79/10^5) (Figure 5-18h).

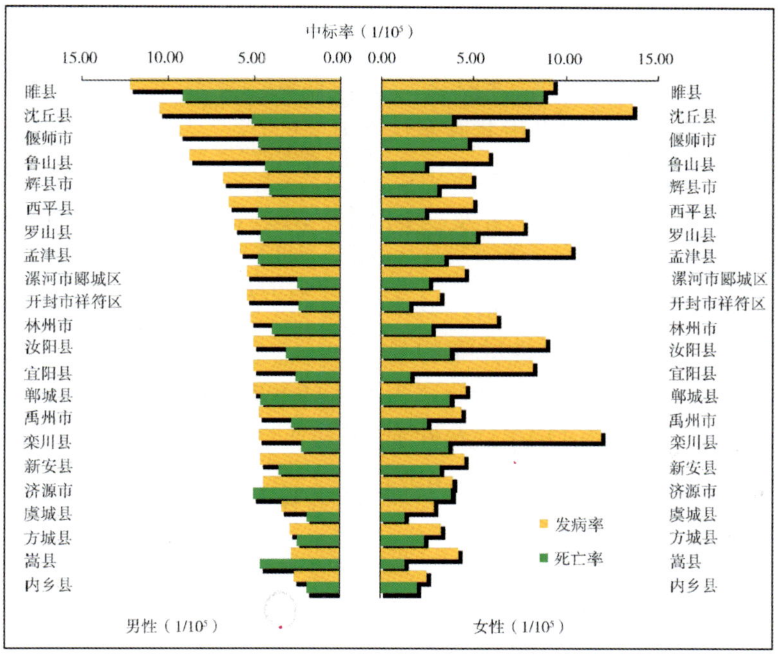

图 5-18h　农村肿瘤登记地区脑及中枢神经系统恶性肿瘤发病率与死亡率

2014 年肿瘤登记地区脑及中枢神经系统恶性肿瘤发病病例中有确切解剖学亚部位（C71.0–C71.8）信息的占 48.6%，亚部位未特指（C71.9）的占 51.4%。在有亚部位的脑及中枢神经系统癌病例中，发生在大脑，除外脑叶和脑室（C71.0）的占 44.1%，额叶（C71.1）的占 17.3%，颞叶（C71.2）的占 12.6%，顶叶（C71.3）的占 6.1%，枕叶（C71.4）的占 3.3%，脑室（C71.5）的占 3.8%，小脑（C71.6）的占 6.5%，脑干（C71.7）的占 5.8%，脑及中枢神经系统交搭跨越（C71.8）的占 0.5%（图 5–18i）。

Among all the reported brain tumor cases in 2014, 48.6% had specific anatomic site information (C71.0–C71.8) and the rest 51.4% didn' t have. The specific anatomic sites of brain tumors included cerebrum (C71.0) (44.1%), frontal (C71.1) (17.3%), temporal (C71.2) (12.6%), parietal (C71.3) (6.1%), occipital (C71.4) (3.3%), cerebral (C71.5) (3.8%), cerebellum (C71.6) (6.5%), brain stem (C71.7) (5.8%) and the overlapping part (C71.8) (0.5%) (Figure 5–18i).

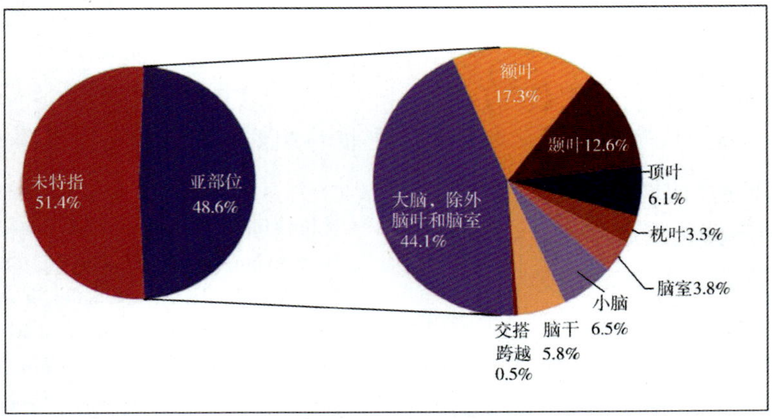

图 5–18i 河南省脑及中枢神经系统恶性肿瘤发病亚部位构成 (%)

十九、甲状腺 (C73)

2014 年，河南省肿瘤登记地区甲状腺恶性肿瘤的发病率为 3.81/10^5，中标率为 3.38/10^5，世标率为 3.07/10^5，占全部恶性肿瘤发病的 1.51%。其中男性发病率为 1.92/10^5，女性为 5.82/10^5。男性中标率为女性的 0.33 倍，城市为农村的 1.33 倍。同期甲状腺恶性肿瘤的死亡率为 0.62/10^5，中标率为 0.51/10^5，世标率为 0.50/10^5。其中男性死亡率为 0.47/10^5，女性为 0.78/10^5。甲状腺恶性肿瘤发病和死亡的 0~74 岁累积率分别为 0.31% 和 0.06%（表 5–19）。

19.Thyroid(C73)

In 2014, thyroid cancer cases accounted for 1.51% of all cancer cases in Henan cancer registration areas with the crude incidence of 3.81/10^5, ASR for China 3.38/10^5 and ASR for World 3.07/10^5. The incidence in males was 1.92/10^5, and 5.82/10^5 in females. It was 0.33 times in males as high as that in females and it was 1.33 times in urban areas as that in rural areas. The crude mortality of thyroid cancer in 2014 was 0.62/10^5, ASR for China was 0.51/10^5 and ASR for World 0.50/10^5. The mortality in males was 0.47/10^5, and 0.78/10^5 in females. The cumulative rates of incidence and mortality from 0 to 74 years old were 0.31% and 0.06%, respectively (Table 5–19).

表 5-19　河南省肿瘤登记地区甲状腺恶性肿瘤发病与死亡

地区	性别	病例数	粗率（1/10⁵）	构成（%）	中标率（1/10⁵）	世标率（1/10⁵）	累积率 0~74（%）
发病							
全省	**合计**	**801**	**3.81**	**1.51**	**3.38**	**3.07**	**0.31**
	男性	208	1.92	0.70	1.69	1.58	0.17
	女性	593	5.82	2.52	5.15	4.63	0.46
城市	**合计**	**165**	**4.80**	**1.84**	**4.27**	**3.81**	**0.40**
	男性	44	2.50	0.86	2.17	1.94	0.21
	女性	121	7.21	3.13	6.44	5.73	0.59
农村	**合计**	**636**	**3.61**	**1.44**	**3.20**	**2.92**	**0.30**
	男性	164	1.80	0.67	1.59	1.50	0.17
	女性	472	5.54	2.40	4.89	4.41	0.43
死亡							
全省	**合计**	**131**	**0.62**	**0.40**	**0.51**	**0.50**	**0.06**
	男性	51	0.47	0.25	0.40	0.38	0.05
	女性	80	0.78	0.64	0.61	0.62	0.07
城市	**合计**	**35**	**1.02**	**0.64**	**0.88**	**0.85**	**0.10**
	男性	8	0.46	0.23	0.40	0.37	0.05
	女性	27	1.61	1.33	1.35	1.33	0.16
农村	**合计**	**96**	**0.55**	**0.35**	**0.43**	**0.43**	**0.05**
	男性	43	0.47	0.25	0.40	0.38	0.04
	女性	53	0.62	0.50	0.47	0.47	0.05

甲状腺恶性肿瘤年龄别发病率在 0~49 岁年龄段处于上升状态，50 岁以后上下波动，75 岁以后呈下降趋势。女性发病率高于男性。甲状腺恶性肿瘤年龄别死亡率在 0~54 岁年龄段处于较低水平，55~75 年龄段呈快速上升趋势，之后呈现震荡态势，85+ 年龄组仍处于高位。其中，城市地区，50~60 岁死亡率上升，随后呈锯齿样震荡，女性死亡率明显高于男性；农村地区 75 岁之前死亡率持续上升，之后呈现震荡，男女死亡率除在 80 岁年龄组出现巨大反差外几乎相同（图 5-19a ~ 图 5-19f）。

The age-specific incidence rate of thyroid cancer increased by age before age years of 49, fluctuated between 50 and 74, and decreased after 75 years old. Incidence rate in females was generally higher than that in males. The age-specific mortality rate of thyroid cancer was relatively low before 54 years old, increased rapidly between 50 to 75 years old, and fluctuated between 75 to 85 with a relative high rate at age group of 85+. In urban areas, thyroid cancer mortality rate increased between 50 to 59 years old, fluctuated after 60 years, which was significantly higher in females than that in males. In rural areas, the mortality rate increased with age fluctuated after 75 years old. The mortality rates were similar betweeen females and males, except for a huge difference at 80 years old, where the males reached the peak and the females fell nearly to the lowest (Figure 5-19a~Figure 5-19f).

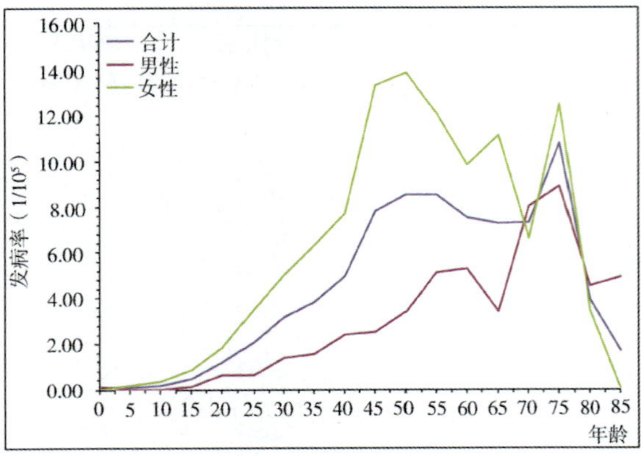

图 5-19a 河南省甲状腺恶性肿瘤年龄别发病率，2014

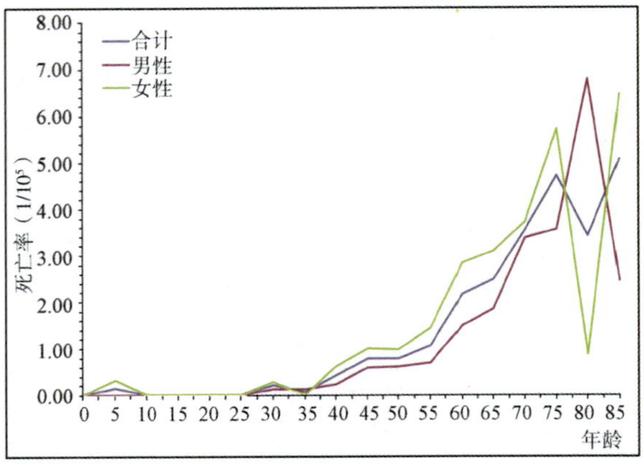

图 5-19d 河南省甲状腺恶性肿瘤年龄别死亡率，2014

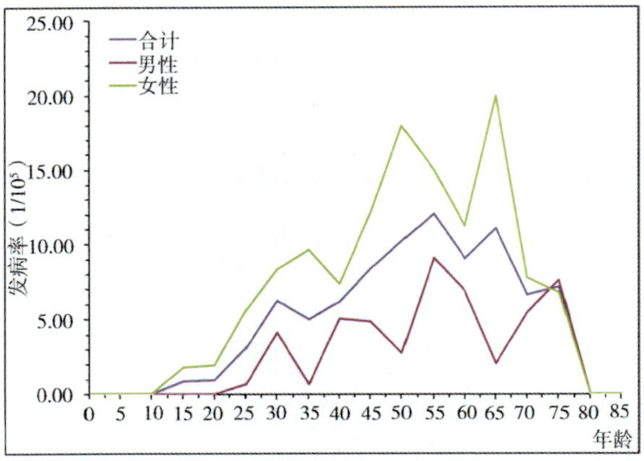

图 5-19b 城市肿瘤登记地区甲状腺恶性肿瘤年龄别发病率，2014

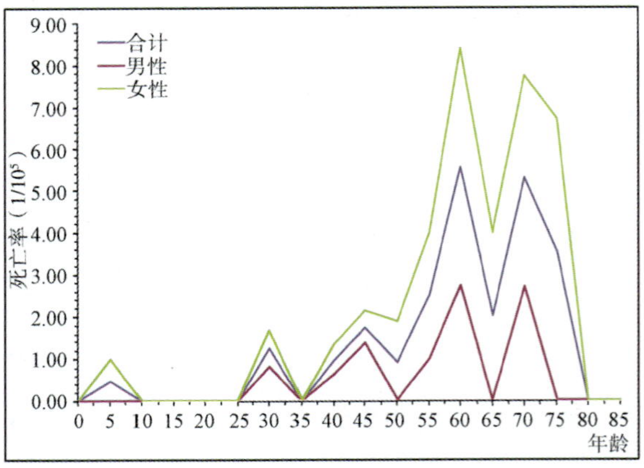

图 5-19e 城市肿瘤登记地区甲状腺恶性肿瘤年龄别死亡率，2014

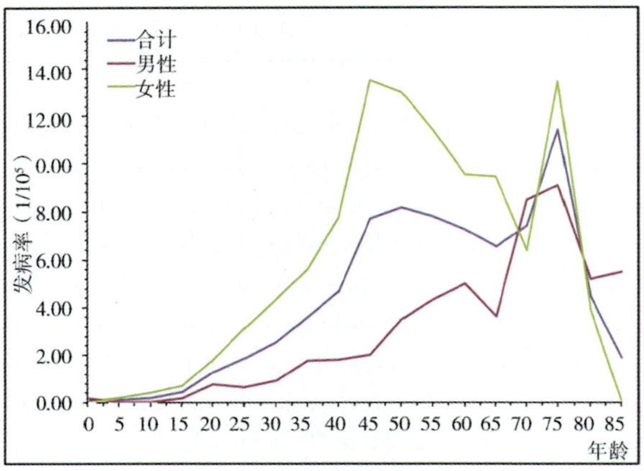

图 5-19c 农村肿瘤登记地区甲状腺恶性肿瘤年龄别发病率，2014

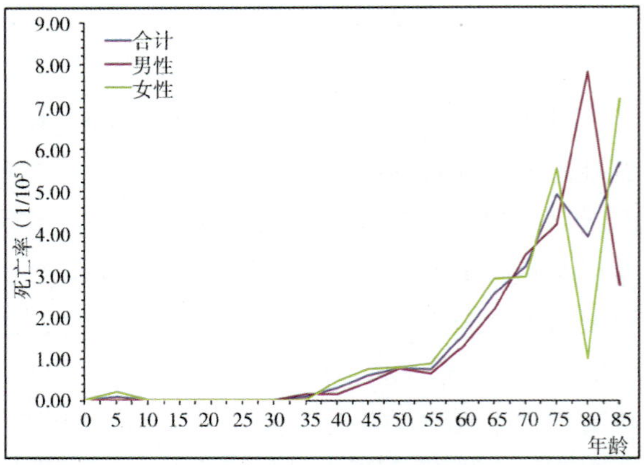

图 5-19f 农村肿瘤登记地区甲状腺恶性肿瘤年龄别死亡率，2014

在5个城市肿瘤登记地区中，男性甲状腺恶性肿瘤标化发病率最高的是三门峡市（$6.05/10^5$），其次是漯河市和洛阳市；女性发病率最高的是三门峡市（$15.86/10^5$），其次是洛阳市和漯河市。男性标化死亡率最高的是南阳市（$0.66/10^5$），女性死亡率最高的是南阳市（$2.17/10^5$）（图5-19g）。

Among the 5 urban cancer registration areas, the ASR China incidence rate of thyroid cancer in males was the highest in Sanmenxia City ($6.05/10^5$), followed by Luohe City and Luoyang City. In females, it was the highest in Sanmenxia City ($15.86/10^5$), followed by Luoyang City and Luohe City. The highest ASR China mortality in males was in Nanyang City ($0.66/10^5$) and in females it was in Nanyang City ($2.17/10^5$) (Figure 5-19g).

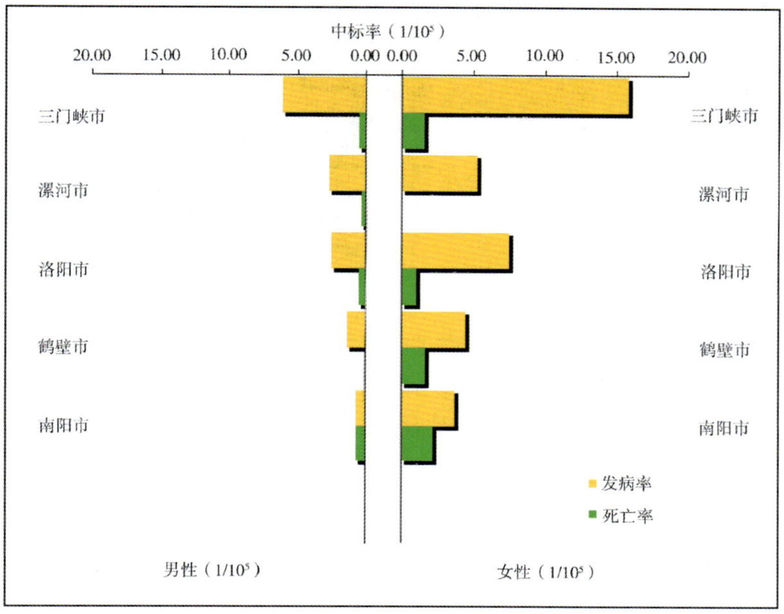

图5-19g 城市肿瘤登记地区甲状腺恶性肿瘤发病率与死亡率

在22个农村肿瘤登记地区中，男性甲状腺恶性肿瘤标化发病率最高的是睢县（$3.37/10^5$），其次是开封市祥符区和偃师市；女性发病率最高的是开封市祥符区（$13.3/10^5$），其次是罗山县和睢县。男性标化死亡率最高的是虞城县（$1.35/10^5$），女性死亡率最高的是虞城县（$1.55/10^5$）（图5-19h）。

Among the 22 rural cancer registration areas, the ASR China incidence rate of thyroid cancer in males was the highest in Suixian County ($3.37/10^5$), followed by Xiangfu District, Kaifeng City, and Yanshi County. For females, it was the highest in Xiangfu District ($13.3/10^5$), followed by Luoshan County and Suixian County. The ASR China mortality were the highest in Yucheng County for both males ($1.35/10^5$) and females ($1.55/10^5$)(Figure 5-19h).

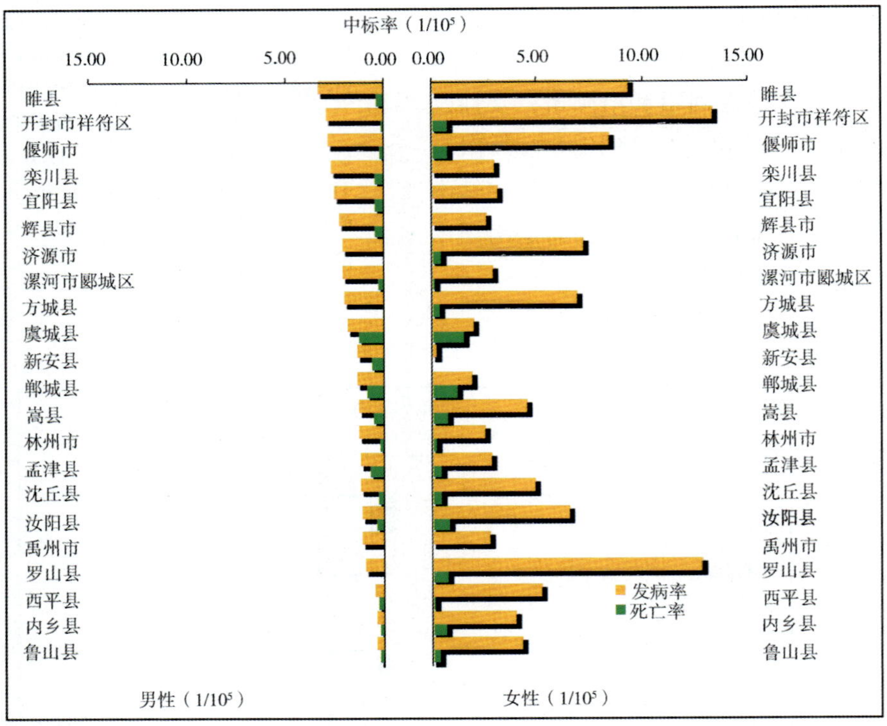

图 5-19h　农村肿瘤登记地区甲状腺恶性肿瘤发病率与死亡率

二十、恶性淋巴瘤 (C81–C85，C88，C90，C96)

2014 年，河南省肿瘤登记地区恶性淋巴瘤的发病率为 2.54/10^5，中标率为 2.13/10^5，世标率为 2.11/10^5，占全部恶性肿瘤发病的 1.01%。其中男性发病率为 2.80/10^5，女性为 2.27/10^5。男性中标率为女性的 1.31 倍，城市为农村的 1.07 倍。同期恶性淋巴瘤的死亡率为 1.48/10^5，中标率为 1.20/10^5，世标率为 1.19/10^5。其中男性死亡率为 1.83/10^5，女性为 1.10/10^5。恶性淋巴瘤发病和死亡的 0~74 岁累积率分别为 0.25% 和 0.14%（表 5–20）。

20. Lymphoma (C81–C85, C88, C90, C96)

In 2014, lymphomas cases accounted for 1.01% of all cancer cases in Henan cancer registration areas with the crude incidence of 2.54/10^5, ASR for China 2.13/10^5 and ASR for World 2.11/10^5. The incidence in males was 2.80/10^5, and 2.27/10^5 in females. It was 1.31 times in males as high as that in females and it was 1.07 times in urban areas as that in rural areas. The crude mortality of bladder cancer in 2014 was 1.48/10^5, ASR for China was 1.20/10^5 and ASR for World 1.19/10^5. The mortality in males was1.83/10^5, and 1.10/10^5 in females. The cumulative rates of incidence and mortality from 0 to 74 years old were 0.25% and 0.14%, respectively (Table 5–20).

表 5-20　河南省肿瘤登记地区恶性淋巴瘤发病与死亡

地区	性别	病例数	粗率（1/10^5）	构成（%）	中标率（1/10^5）	世标率（1/10^5）	累积率 0~74（%）
发病							
	合计	535	2.54	1.01	2.13	2.11	0.25
全省	男性	304	2.80	1.02	2.42	2.41	0.26
	女性	231	2.27	0.98	1.85	1.83	0.23
	合计	92	2.68	1.03	2.26	2.20	0.26
城市	男性	48	2.73	0.94	2.37	2.33	0.21
	女性	44	2.62	1.14	2.24	2.20	0.30
	合计	443	2.52	1.00	2.11	2.10	0.24
农村	男性	256	2.81	1.04	2.44	2.44	0.27
	女性	187	2.20	0.95	1.79	1.77	0.21
死亡							
	合计	311	1.48	0.94	1.20	1.19	0.14
全省	男性	199	1.83	0.97	1.55	1.55	0.17
	女性	112	1.10	0.89	0.86	0.86	0.11
	合计	46	1.34	0.84	1.15	1.12	0.12
城市	男性	30	1.71	0.88	1.55	1.52	0.14
	女性	16	0.95	0.79	0.80	0.79	0.10
	合计	265	1.50	0.96	1.21	1.21	0.14
农村	男性	169	1.86	0.99	1.56	1.57	0.18
	女性	96	1.13	0.91	0.88	0.87	0.11

恶性淋巴瘤年龄别发病率和死亡率在 0~44 岁年龄段处于较低水平，45 岁以后快速上升，在 80- 岁或 85+ 岁组达到高峰，男性高于女性。城乡和不同地区年龄别率的水平虽然有一定的差异，但总体趋势类同（图 5-20a ~ 图 5-20f）。

The ASR China incidence and mortality rates of lymphomas were relatively low before 44 years old and presented increase trends since 45 years old, reaching the peak at the age group of 80 or 85. The age-specific incidence and mortality rates varied in urban and rural areas with similar curve (Figure 5-20a~Figure 5-20f).

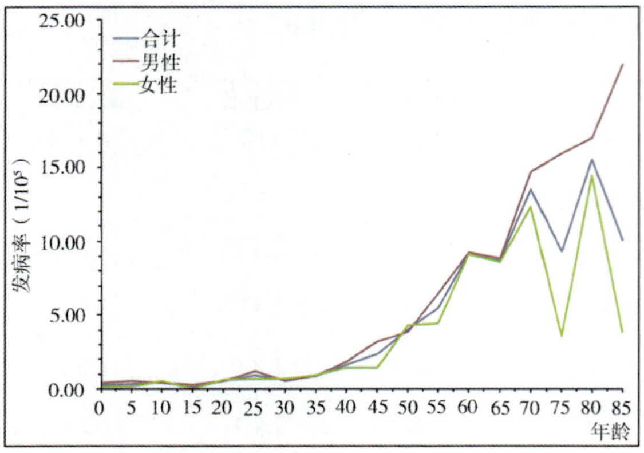

图 5-20a　河南省恶性淋巴瘤年龄别发病率，2014

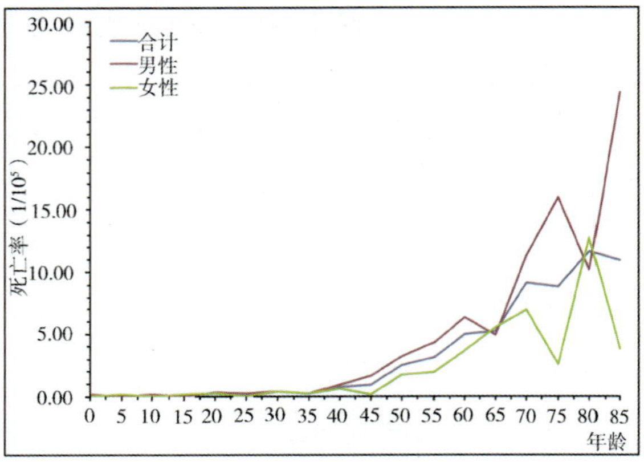

图 5-20d　河南省恶性淋巴瘤年龄别死亡率，2014

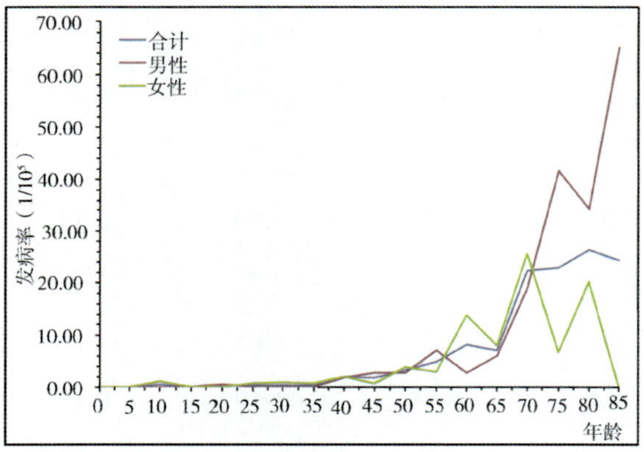

图 5-20b　城市肿瘤登记地区恶性淋巴瘤年龄别发病率， 2014

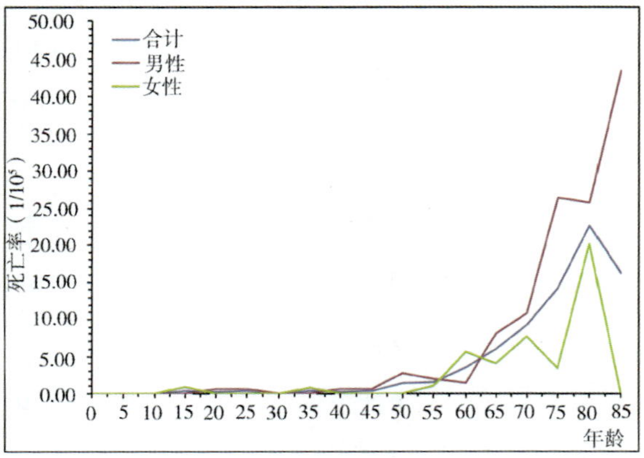

图 5-20e　城市肿瘤登记地区恶性淋巴瘤年龄别死亡率，2014

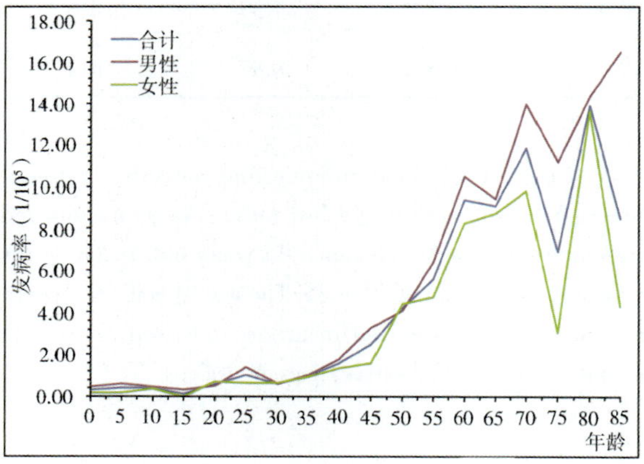

图 5-20c　农村肿瘤登记地区恶性淋巴瘤年龄别发病率，2014

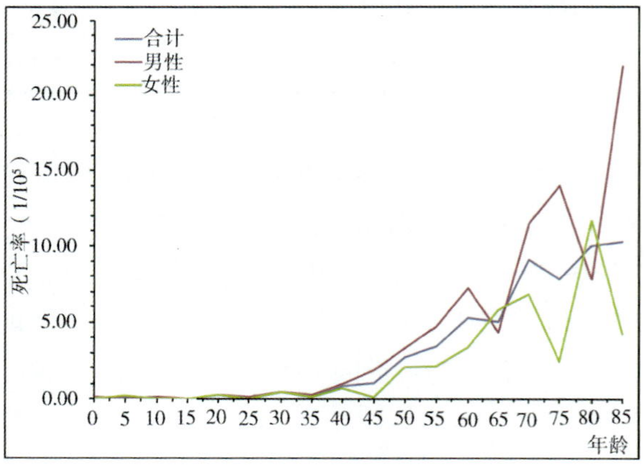

图 5-20f　农村肿瘤登记地区恶性淋巴瘤年龄别死亡率，2014

在 5 个城市肿瘤登记地区中，男性恶性淋巴瘤标化发病率最高的是洛阳市（4.78/10^5），其次是三门峡市和南阳市；女性发病率最高的是洛阳市（3.90/10^5），其次是三门峡市和南阳市。男性标化死亡率最高的是洛阳市（2.88/110^5），女性死亡率最高的是洛阳市（1.40/10^5）（图 5-20g）。

Among the 5 urban cancer registration areas, the ASR China incidence rate of lymphomas in Luoyang City was the highest in males (4.70/10^5) and females (3.90/10^5), followed by Sanmenxia City and Nanyang City. The age-specific mortality in Luoyang City was the highest in both males (2.88/10^5) and females (1.40/10^5)(Figure 5-20g).

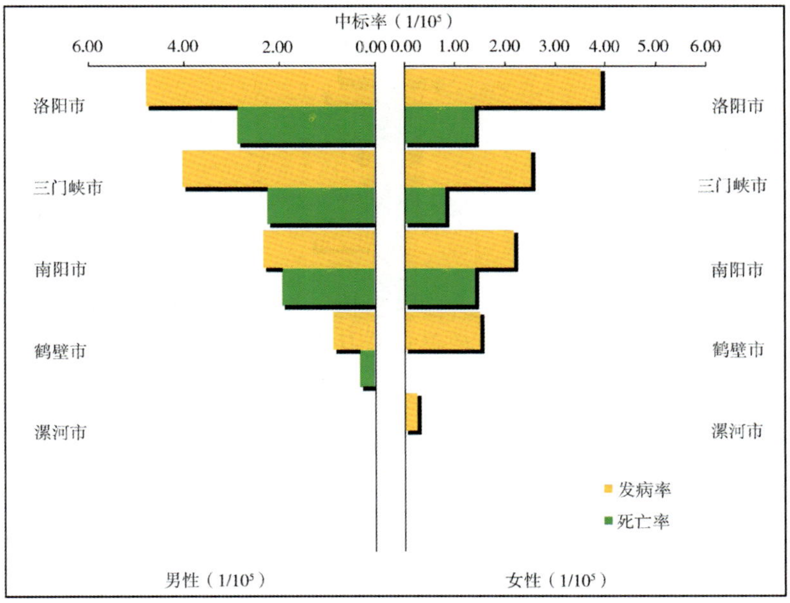

图 5-20g 城市肿瘤登记地区恶性淋巴瘤发病率与死亡率

在 22 个农村肿瘤登记地区中，男性恶性淋巴瘤标化发病率最高的是西平县（7.33/10^5），其次是孟津县和偃师市；女性发病率最高的是漯河市郾城区（5.04/10^5），其次是辉县市和偃师市。男性标化死亡率最高的是西平县（3.52/10^5），女性死亡率最高的是漯河市郾城区（2.27/10^5）（图 5-20h）。

Among the 22 rural cancer registration areas, the ASR China incidence rate of lymphomas in males was the highest in Xiping County (7.33/10^5), followed by Mengjin County and Yanshi County. For females, it was the highest in Yancheng District of Luohe City (5.04/10^5), followed by Huixian City and Yanshi City. The age-specific mortality was the highest in Xiping County for males (3.52/10^5) and Yancheng District of Luohe City for females (2.27/10^5)(Figure 5-20h).

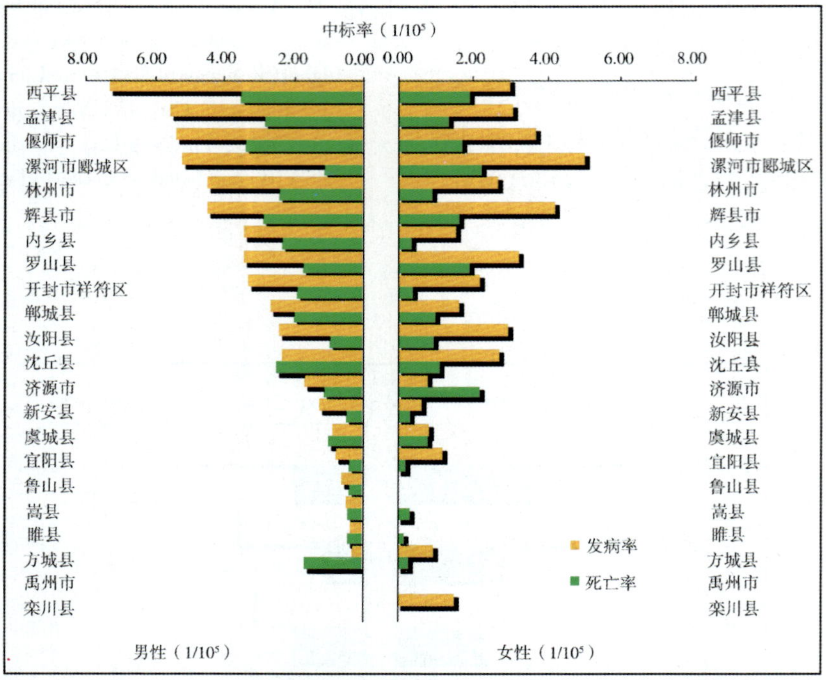

图 5-20h 农村肿瘤登记地区恶性淋巴瘤发病率与死亡率

二十一、白血病（C91–C95）

2014 年，河南省肿瘤登记地区白血病恶性肿瘤的发病率为 5.12/10^5，中标率为 4.70/10^5，世标率为 4.84/10^5，占全部恶性肿瘤发病的 2.03%。其中男性发病率为 5.63/10^5，女性为 4.58/10^5。男性中标率为女性的 1.28 倍，城市为农村的 1.21 倍。同期白血病的死亡率为 2.97/10^5，中标率为 2.65/10^5，世标率为 2.69/10^5。其中男性死亡率为 3.16/10^5，女性为 2.77/10^5。白血病发病和死亡的 0~74 岁累积率分别为 0.42% 和 0.25%（表 5-21）。

21. Leukemia (C91–C95)

In 2014, leukemia cases accounted for 2.03% of all cancer cases in Henan cancer registration areas with the crude incidence of 5.12/10^5, ASR for China 4.70/10^5 and ASR for World 4.84/10^5. The incidence in males was 5.63/10^5, and 4.58/10^5 in females. The ASR for China of leukemia incidence was 1.28 times in males as high as that in females and it was 1.21 times in urban areas as that in rural areas. The crude mortality of leukemia in 2014 was 2.97/10^5, ASR for China was 2.65/10^5 and ASR for World 2.69/10^5. The mortality in males was 3.16/10^5, and 2.77/10^5 in females. The cumulative rates of incidence and mortality from 0 to 74 years old were 0.42% and 0.25%, respectively(Table 5-21).

表 5-21 河南省肿瘤登记地区白血病恶性肿瘤发病与死亡

地区	性别	病例数	粗率（1/10^5）	构成（%）	中标率（1/10^5）	世标率（1/10^5）	累积率 0~74（%）
发病							
	合计	1 078	5.12	2.03	4.70	4.84	0.42
全省	男性	611	5.63	2.06	5.27	5.38	0.48
	女性	467	4.58	1.99	4.13	4.29	0.37
	合计	210	6.11	2.34	5.51	5.48	0.52
城市	男性	127	7.23	2.49	6.56	6.44	0.66
	女性	83	4.95	2.15	4.47	4.54	0.39
	合计	868	4.93	1.96	4.56	4.73	0.40

续表

地区	性别	病例数	粗率（1/10⁵）	构成（%）	中标率（1/10⁵）	世标率（1/10⁵）	累积率 0~74（%）
农村	男性	484	5.32	1.97	5.02	5.18	0.44
	女性	384	4.51	1.95	4.09	4.27	0.36
死亡							
	合计	**625**	**2.97**	**1.90**	**2.65**	**2.69**	**0.25**
全省	男性	343	3.16	1.68	2.97	2.95	0.28
	女性	282	2.77	2.25	2.31	2.41	0.21
	合计	**120**	**3.49**	**2.20**	**3.09**	**3.15**	**0.30**
城市	男性	66	3.76	1.93	3.45	3.46	0.37
	女性	54	3.22	2.66	2.73	2.85	0.23
	合计	**505**	**2.87**	**1.84**	**2.59**	**2.62**	**0.24**
农村	男性	277	3.05	1.63	2.90	2.87	0.26
	女性	228	2.68	2.17	2.25	2.35	0.21

白血病年龄别发病率和死亡率在0~44岁年龄段处于较低水平，45岁以后快速上升，在80-岁或85+岁组达到高峰，男性高于女性。城乡和不同地区年龄别率的水平虽然有一定的差异，但总体趋势类同（图5-21a ~ 5-21f）。

在5个城市肿瘤登记地区中，男性白血病恶性肿瘤标化发病率最高的是三门峡市（9.37/10⁵），其次是洛阳市和漯河市；女性发病率最高的是鹤壁市（7.29/10⁵），其次是三门峡市和洛阳市。男性标化死亡率最高的是洛阳市（5.58/10⁵），女性死亡率最高的是洛阳市（4.12/10⁵）（图5-21g）。

The age-specific incidence and mortality rates of leukemia were relatively low before 50 years old and increased dramatically since 50 years old, reaching the peak at the age group of 70 and 75 respectively. The age-specific incidence and mortality rates reached the peak at the age group of 80 and 70 in urban areas respectively and reached the peak at the age group of 60 and 75 in rural areas respectively (Figure 5-21a~Figure5-21f).

Among the 5 urban cancer registration areas, the ASR China incidence rate of leukemia in males was the highest in Sanmenxia City (9.37/10⁵), followed by Luoyang City and Luohe City. In females, it was the highest in He bi City (7.29/10⁵), followed by Sanmenxia City and Luoyang City. The age-specific mortality was the highest in Luoyang City for both males (5.58/10⁵) and females (4.12/10⁵) (Figure 5-21g).

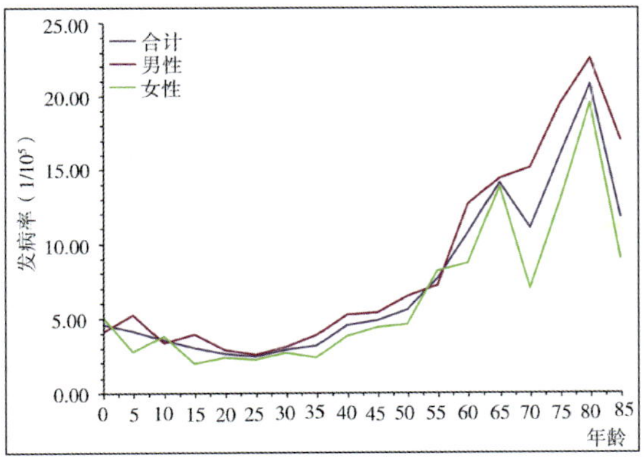

图 5-21a 河南省白血病恶性肿瘤年龄别发病率，2014

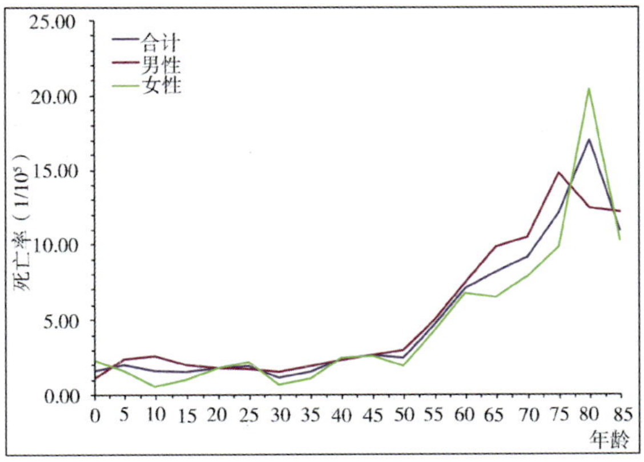

图 5-21d 河南省白血病恶性肿瘤年龄别死亡率，2014

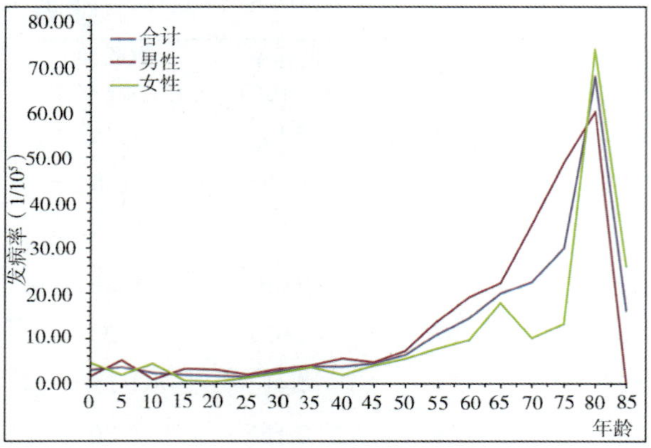

图 5-21b 城市肿瘤登记地区白血病恶性肿瘤年龄别发病率，2014

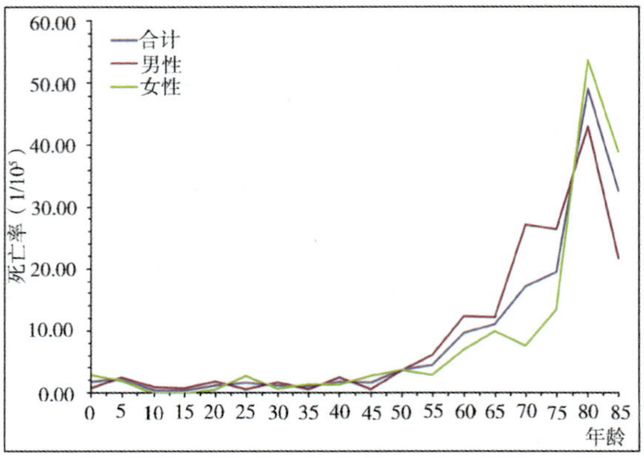

图 5-21e 城市肿瘤登记地区白血病恶性肿瘤年龄别死亡率，2014

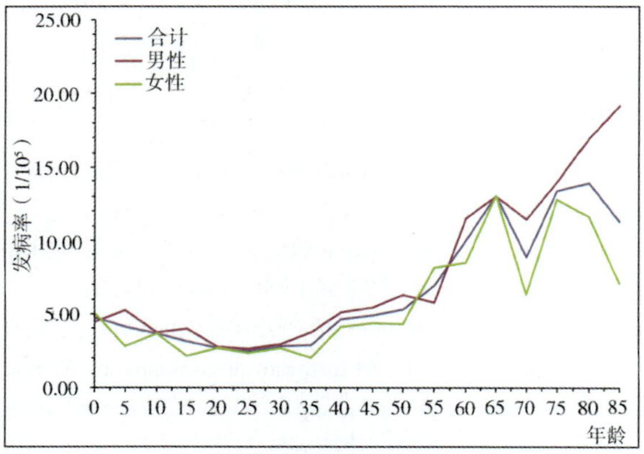

图 5-21c 农村肿瘤登记地区白血病恶性肿瘤年龄别发病率，2014

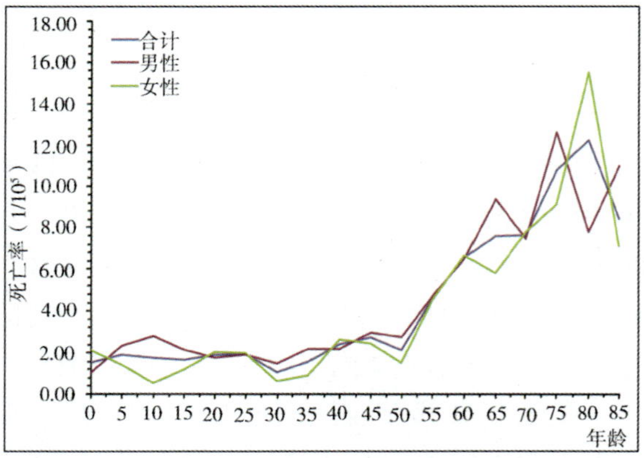

图 5-21f 农村肿瘤登记地区白血病恶性肿瘤年龄别死亡率，2014

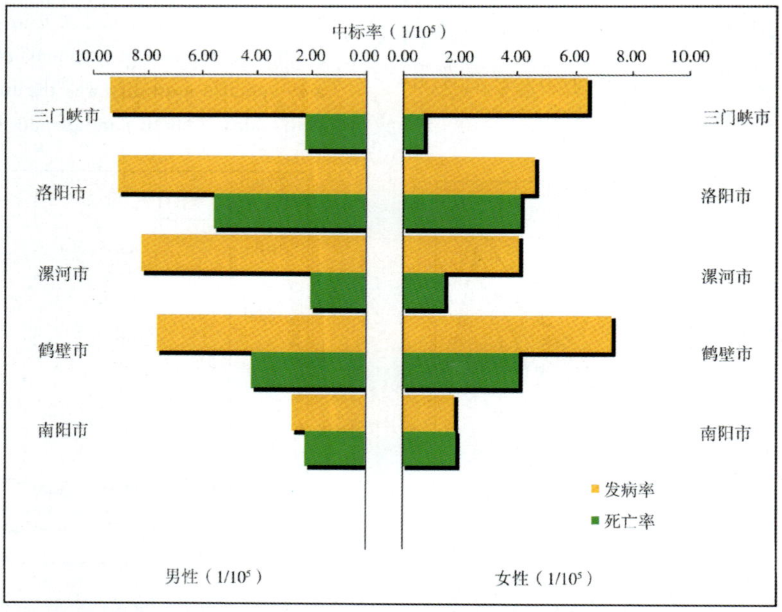

图 5-21g 城市肿瘤登记地区白血病恶性肿瘤发病率与死亡率

在 22 个农村肿瘤登记地区中，男性白血病标化发病率最高的是睢县（12.83/10^5），其次是郸城县和宜阳县；女性发病率最高的是睢县（8.85/10^5），其次是漯河市郾城区和沈丘县。男性标化死亡率最高的是郸城县（6.58/10^5），女性死亡率最高的是郸城县（4.66/10^5）（图 5-21h）。

Among the 22 rural cancer registration areas, the ASR China incidence rate of leukemia in males was the highest in Suixian County (12.83/10^5), followed by Dancheng County and Yiyang County. For females, it was the highest in Suixian County (8.85/10^5), followed by Yancheng District of Luohe City and shenqiu County. The age-specific mortality was the highest in Suixian County for both males (6.58/10^5) and females (4.66/10^5)(Figure 5-21h).

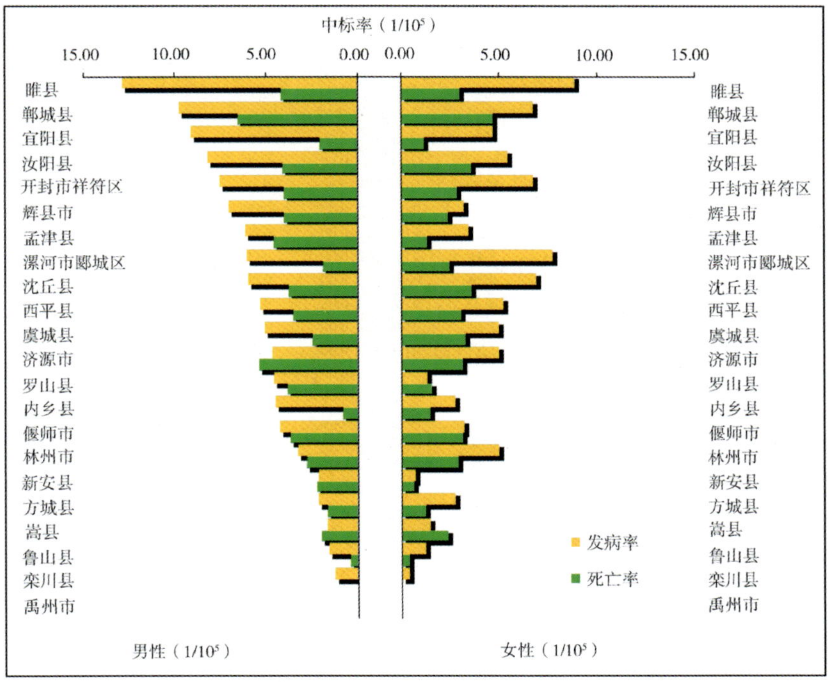

图 5-21h　农村肿瘤登记地区白血病恶性肿瘤发病率与死亡率

第六章 附 录

Chapter 6 Appendix

一、河南省肿瘤登记地区合计发病和死亡结果

1. Overall Incidences and Mortalities in Henan Cancer Registries

表 6-1-1 河南省全省肿瘤登记地区

部位		病例数	构成(%)	年龄组								
				0–	1–	5–	10–	15–	20–	25–	30–	35–
唇	C00	30	0.06	0.00	0.00	0.07	0.08	0.00	0.05	0.00	0.00	0.06
舌	C01–C02	89	0.17	0.00	0.17	0.00	0.00	0.00	0.00	0.11	0.13	0.31
口	C03–C06	145	0.27	0.00	0.08	0.07	0.15	0.00	0.11	0.00	0.20	0.37
唾液腺	C07–C08	109	0.20	0.00	0.00	0.00	0.15	0.07	0.05	0.16	0.46	0.31
扁桃体	C09	13	0.02	0.00	0.00	0.00	0.00	0.00	0.05	0.05	0.00	0.00
其他的口咽	C10	46	0.09	0.00	0.00	0.00	0.08	0.00	0.11	0.05	0.13	0.12
鼻咽	C11	273	0.51	0.00	0.00	0.07	0.15	0.00	0.16	0.66	0.91	0.62
喉咽	C12–C13	41	0.08	0.00	0.00	0.00	0.00	0.00	0.05	0.00	0.00	0.06
咽，部位不明	C14	42	0.08	0.00	0.00	0.00	0.00	0.00	0.00	0.00	0.00	0.06
食管	C15	8 010	15.06	0.00	0.00	0.00	0.00	0.00	0.16	0.33	0.91	1.43
胃	C16	8 274	15.55	0.00	0.00	0.14	0.00	0.20	0.65	1.59	2.80	4.80
小肠	C17	319	0.60	0.00	0.00	0.00	0.00	0.00	0.05	0.11	0.20	0.75
结肠	C18	1 495	2.81	0.00	0.00	0.00	0.08	0.00	0.33	0.60	0.85	1.87
直肠	C19–C20	1 813	3.41	0.00	0.00	0.00	0.00	0.00	0.11	0.71	1.30	2.31
肛门	C21	103	0.19	0.00	0.00	0.00	0.00	0.14	0.05	0.05	0.13	0.25
肝脏	C22	5 520	10.38	0.39	0.08	0.00	0.15	0.20	0.65	1.04	3.45	7.54
胆囊及其他	C23–C24	647	1.22	0.00	0.00	0.00	0.00	0.00	0.11	0.11	0.39	0.31
胰腺	C25	735	1.38	0.00	0.00	0.00	0.00	0.07	0.00	0.38	0.33	0.69
鼻、鼻窦及其他	C30–C31	75	0.14	0.00	0.00	0.07	0.08	0.00	0.00	0.11	0.13	0.25
喉	C32	307	0.58	0.00	0.08	0.00	0.00	0.00	0.00	0.11	0.07	0.06
气管、支气管、肺	C33–C34	10 160	19.10	0.00	0.00	0.00	0.00	0.20	0.43	1.21	3.78	6.98
其他的胸腔器官	C37–C38	144	0.27	0.00	0.08	0.07	0.00	0.07	0.00	0.22	0.13	0.25
骨	C40–C41	535	1.01	0.00	0.08	0.63	0.60	0.95	0.98	1.10	0.78	2.00
皮肤的黑色素瘤	C43	57	0.11	0.00	0.42	0.14	0.00	0.14	0.22	0.00	0.00	0.06
其他的皮肤	C44	245	0.46	0.00	0.00	0.00	0.00	0.41	0.05	0.33	0.20	0.50
间皮瘤	C45	9	0.02	0.00	0.00	0.00	0.00	0.00	0.00	0.05	0.00	0.00
卡波西肉瘤	C46	2	0.00	0.00	0.00	0.00	0.00	0.00	0.00	0.00	0.07	0.00
周围神经、其他结缔组织、软组织	C47;C49	89	0.17	0.00	0.17	0.07	0.15	0.14	0.11	0.16	0.07	0.00
乳房	C50	—	—	—	—	—	—	—	—	—	—	—
外阴	C51	—	—	—	—	—	—	—	—	—	—	—
阴道	C52	—	—	—	—	—	—	—	—	—	—	—
子宫颈	C53	—	—	—	—	—	—	—	—	—	—	—
子宫体	C54	—	—	—	—	—	—	—	—	—	—	—
子宫，部位不明	C55	—	—	—	—	—	—	—	—	—	—	—
卵巢	C56	—	—	—	—	—	—	—	—	—	—	—
其他的女性生殖器	C57	—	—	—	—	—	—	—	—	—	—	—
胎盘	C58	—	—	—	—	—	—	—	—	—	—	—
阴茎	C60	—	—	—	—	—	—	—	—	—	—	—
前列腺	C61	—	—	—	—	—	—	—	—	—	—	—
睾丸	C62	—	—	—	—	—	—	—	—	—	—	—
其他的男性生殖器	C63	—	—	—	—	—	—	—	—	—	—	—
肾	C64	403	0.76	1.17	0.50	0.07	0.23	0.07	0.33	0.11	0.20	0.75
肾盂	C65	56	0.11	0.00	0.00	0.00	0.08	0.00	0.00	0.00	0.00	0.19
输尿管	C66	43	0.08	0.00	0.00	0.00	0.00	0.00	0.00	0.00	0.07	0.06
膀胱	C67	572	1.08	0.00	0.00	0.07	0.08	0.00	0.11	0.33	0.20	0.31
其他的泌尿器官	C68	24	0.05	0.00	0.00	0.00	0.00	0.00	0.05	0.00	0.00	0.00
眼	C69	38	0.07	0.00	0.58	0.07	0.08	0.00	0.00	0.05	0.00	0.06
脑、神经系统	C70–C72	1 408	2.65	2.34	1.42	1.76	1.89	1.22	1.36	1.43	2.41	3.99
甲状腺	C73	801	1.51	0.00	0.08	0.07	0.15	0.48	1.19	2.03	3.13	3.80
肾上腺	C74	46	0.09	0.00	0.08	0.07	0.00	0.00	0.05	0.00	0.07	0.06
其他的内分泌腺	C75	59	0.11	0.00	0.00	0.00	0.00	0.07	0.05	0.16	0.13	0.19
霍奇金病	C81	99	0.19	0.00	0.00	0.07	0.00	0.20	0.22	0.38	0.33	0.31
非霍奇金淋巴瘤	C82–C85;C96	418	0.79	0.39	0.25	0.28	0.45	0.14	0.54	0.93	0.46	0.75
免疫增生性疾病	C88	2	0.00	0.00	0.00	0.00	0.00	0.00	0.00	0.00	0.00	0.00
多发性骨髓瘤	C90	115	0.22	0.00	0.00	0.07	0.00	0.00	0.00	0.00	0.13	0.12
淋巴样白血病	C91	179	0.34	0.39	1.17	1.06	0.60	0.82	0.43	0.22	0.46	0.44
髓样白血病	C92–C94	248	0.47	0.39	0.75	0.42	0.38	0.68	0.54	0.71	0.78	0.94
白血病，未特指	C95	651	1.22	1.56	3.09	2.61	2.57	1.50	1.63	1.48	1.63	1.75
其他的或未指明部位的	O&U	1 174	2.21	0.39	0.83	1.06	0.45	0.68	0.92	1.59	2.41	2.18
骨髓增殖性疾病	MPD	19	0.04	0.00	0.08	0.00	0.00	0.00	0.05	0.00	0.00	0.00
骨髓增生异常综合征	MDS	12	0.02	0.00	0.00	0.00	0.00	0.00	0.05	0.05	0.07	0.00
合计	ALL	53 200	100.00	7.03	10.10	9.24	9.14	9.39	15.56	25.43	44.11	74.63
所有部位除外 C44	ALL but C44	52 955	99.54	7.03	10.10	9.24	9.14	8.98	15.51	25.10	43.92	74.13

2014 年合计发病主要指标 $(1/10^5)$

40–	45–	50–	55–	60–	65–	70–	75–	80–	85–	粗率 $(1/10^5$ 万)	世标率 $(1/10^5$ 万)	累积率 (%) 0~64	累积率 (%) 0~74
0.12	0.12	0.08	0.35	0.43	0.61	0.83	0.83	0.00	1.68	0.14	0.12	0.01	0.01
0.12	0.60	0.54	0.95	1.93	1.23	1.66	2.20	2.42	0.84	0.42	0.35	0.02	0.04
0.76	0.48	0.70	1.39	2.57	2.45	2.28	4.41	5.82	4.21	0.69	0.55	0.03	0.06
0.41	1.02	1.25	1.39	1.39	1.23	0.42	1.65	1.45	1.68	0.52	0.42	0.03	0.04
0.00	0.00	0.08	0.17	0.21	0.15	0.21	0.55	0.48	0.84	0.06	0.05	0.00	0.00
0.00	0.18	0.16	0.43	0.96	0.77	0.83	1.10	1.94	1.68	0.22	0.18	0.01	0.02
1.23	1.92	2.57	2.95	3.96	4.14	3.11	5.78	3.88	2.53	1.30	1.05	0.08	0.11
0.12	0.24	0.23	0.52	0.43	1.07	0.62	1.10	2.91	0.00	0.19	0.15	0.01	0.02
0.00	0.18	0.31	0.69	1.07	1.07	0.42	0.83	0.97	1.68	0.20	0.16	0.01	0.02
5.27	16.96	36.58	84.34	157.66	225.90	247.69	270.41	331.51	289.70	38.06	30.56	1.52	3.89
12.29	23.97	43.51	90.93	164.73	210.41	234.20	264.62	300.01	229.06	39.32	31.53	1.73	3.95
0.64	1.44	2.41	2.69	5.35	7.97	9.55	7.71	9.21	7.58	1.52	1.23	0.07	0.16
4.92	6.59	10.59	16.57	24.08	31.90	34.67	39.38	61.55	36.21	7.10	5.62	0.33	0.67
4.98	7.91	10.82	19.87	29.54	40.18	46.51	53.70	61.07	61.48	8.61	6.86	0.39	0.82
0.29	0.66	0.78	1.21	1.39	2.45	2.08	2.20	2.42	0.84	0.49	0.40	0.02	0.05
16.04	24.99	40.71	64.81	104.79	118.09	123.12	132.45	172.06	142.32	26.23	21.03	1.32	2.53
1.05	1.80	2.18	7.72	11.45	13.19	16.82	26.43	27.14	34.53	3.07	2.41	0.13	0.28
1.46	2.76	4.59	7.29	11.77	17.18	23.25	23.13	20.84	30.32	3.49	2.81	0.15	0.35
0.23	0.24	0.54	0.61	1.07	1.69	1.66	2.48	1.45	1.68	0.36	0.29	0.02	0.03
0.29	0.96	2.96	3.12	5.99	7.67	8.51	10.19	8.72	4.21	1.46	1.18	0.07	0.15
14.52	32.60	59.78	111.41	172.32	249.06	297.52	338.14	398.88	332.65	48.28	38.42	2.02	4.75
0.70	0.78	1.01	1.04	3.64	2.61	1.66	1.93	3.39	6.74	0.68	0.57	0.04	0.06
2.11	1.86	3.50	5.90	7.60	9.20	8.93	10.74	11.15	4.21	2.54	2.14	0.14	0.23
0.06	0.12	0.47	0.52	0.21	1.53	1.25	1.65	1.45	0.84	0.27	0.25	0.01	0.03
0.76	0.36	0.93	1.82	2.57	3.22	6.23	9.64	15.99	21.90	1.16	0.91	0.04	0.09
0.00	0.06	0.23	0.09	0.00	0.15	0.00	0.28	0.48	0.00	0.04	0.03	0.00	0.00
0.00	0.06	0.00	0.00	0.00	0.00	0.00	0.00	0.00	0.00	0.01	0.01	0.00	0.00
0.64	0.60	0.78	1.04	1.50	0.46	1.45	1.38	1.45	0.84	0.42	0.36	0.03	0.04
—	—	—	—	—	—	—	—	—	—	—	—	—	—
—	—	—	—	—	—	—	—	—	—	—	—	—	—
—	—	—	—	—	—	—	—	—	—	—	—	—	—
—	—	—	—	—	—	—	—	—	—	—	—	—	—
—	—	—	—	—	—	—	—	—	—	—	—	—	—
—	—	—	—	—	—	—	—	—	—	—	—	—	—
—	—	—	—	—	—	—	—	—	—	—	—	—	—
—	—	—	—	—	—	—	—	—	—	—	—	—	—
—	—	—	—	—	—	—	—	—	—	—	—	—	—
—	—	—	—	—	—	—	—	—	—	—	—	—	—
—	—	—	—	—	—	—	—	—	—	—	—	—	—
—	—	—	—	—	—	—	—	—	—	—	—	—	—
—	—	—	—	—	—	—	—	—	—	—	—	—	—
1.40	1.92	3.81	4.77	6.21	9.35	7.89	6.06	9.21	6.74	1.91	1.61	0.10	0.19
0.23	0.48	0.54	0.61	1.07	0.92	0.62	1.10	0.97	0.84	0.27	0.22	0.02	0.02
0.00	0.12	0.54	0.52	0.96	0.61	1.25	1.10	0.48	1.68	0.20	0.17	0.01	0.02
0.70	1.74	2.80	3.82	10.49	12.27	17.86	21.48	28.11	27.79	2.72	2.16	0.10	0.25
0.06	0.06	0.16	0.09	0.96	0.46	0.00	1.10	0.97	0.00	0.11	0.09	0.01	0.01
0.18	0.12	0.39	0.17	0.43	0.46	0.42	0.28	1.94	0.84	0.18	0.18	0.01	0.01
5.97	8.09	9.81	14.58	22.37	21.47	21.39	21.75	31.02	32.84	6.69	5.67	0.38	0.60
4.92	7.79	8.48	8.50	7.49	7.21	7.27	10.74	3.88	1.68	3.81	3.07	0.24	0.31
0.18	0.36	0.47	0.61	0.75	0.46	0.42	0.55	2.42	0.00	0.22	0.18	0.01	0.02
0.29	0.48	0.62	0.87	0.64	0.31	1.04	0.55	0.97	0.84	0.28	0.23	0.02	0.02
0.18	0.66	0.70	0.61	0.96	1.23	2.70	2.20	1.45	2.53	0.47	0.39	0.02	0.04
1.40	1.56	3.42	3.56	7.06	6.75	11.21	6.61	12.12	6.74	1.99	1.67	0.10	0.19
0.00	0.00	0.00	0.00	0.00	0.00	0.00	0.28	0.00	0.84	0.01	0.01	0.00	0.00
0.23	0.78	0.62	1.91	2.14	1.99	2.28	2.48	3.39	2.53	0.55	0.44	0.03	0.05
0.64	1.02	0.86	1.04	1.50	2.45	1.04	2.20	2.91	2.53	0.85	0.85	0.05	0.07
1.17	1.62	1.01	2.00	2.57	3.07	2.49	4.13	5.33	1.68	1.18	1.04	0.07	0.10
2.69	2.22	3.66	4.60	6.64	8.59	7.47	9.64	12.60	7.58	3.09	2.95	0.18	0.26
3.57	5.39	7.63	11.02	19.27	21.47	24.29	33.32	28.60	17.69	5.58	4.60	0.28	0.51
0.18	0.06	0.39	0.09	0.43	0.15	0.21	0.00	0.00	0.84	0.09	0.08	0.01	0.01
0.00	0.12	0.00	0.26	0.11	0.00	0.42	0.00	0.48	0.00	0.06	0.05	0.00	0.01
144.71	234.09	353.75	572.49	918.46	1 146.37	1 267.95	1 422.80	1 698.74	1 423.23	252.79	203.78	12.10	24.17
143.95	233.73	352.82	570.66	915.89	1 143.15	1 261.72	1 413.16	1 682.75	1 401.33	251.63	202.88	12.06	24.09

表 6-1-2　河南省全省肿瘤登记地区

部位		病例数	构成 (%)	年龄组 0-	1-	5-	10-	15-	20-	25-	30-
唇	C00	18	0.06	0.00	0.00	0.13	0.14	0.00	0.11	0.00	0.00
舌	C01–C02	41	0.14	0.00	0.15	0.00	0.00	0.00	0.00	0.00	0.25
口	C03–C06	78	0.26	0.00	0.15	0.13	0.28	0.00	0.00	0.00	0.13
唾液腺	C07–C08	54	0.18	0.00	0.00	0.00	0.14	0.00	0.11	0.11	0.38
扁桃体	C09	7	0.02	0.00	0.00	0.00	0.00	0.00	0.00	0.00	0.00
其他的口咽	C10	35	0.12	0.00	0.00	0.00	0.14	0.00	0.21	0.00	0.00
鼻咽	C11	176	0.59	0.00	0.00	0.00	0.28	0.00	0.21	0.86	0.76
喉咽	C12–C13	32	0.11	0.00	0.00	0.00	0.00	0.00	0.11	0.00	0.00
咽，部位不明	C14	32	0.11	0.00	0.00	0.00	0.00	0.00	0.00	0.00	0.00
食管	C15	4 968	16.74	0.00	0.00	0.00	0.00	0.00	0.21	0.21	0.51
胃	C16	5 918	19.94	0.00	0.00	0.26	0.00	0.26	0.21	1.50	2.53
小肠	C17	193	0.65	0.00	0.00	0.00	0.00	0.00	0.11	0.00	0.00
结肠	C18	816	2.75	0.00	0.00	0.00	0.00	0.00	0.32	1.18	1.27
直肠	C19–C20	958	3.23	0.00	0.00	0.00	0.00	0.00	0.21	0.43	1.39
肛门	C21	54	0.18	0.00	0.00	0.00	0.00	0.13	0.00	0.00	0.25
肝脏	C22	3 796	12.79	0.73	0.00	0.00	0.28	0.39	0.63	1.18	4.82
胆囊及其他	C23–C24	272	0.92	0.00	0.00	0.00	0.00	0.00	0.11	0.21	0.38
胰腺	C25	424	1.43	0.00	0.00	0.00	0.00	0.00	0.00	0.43	0.38
鼻、鼻窦及其他	C30–C31	44	0.15	0.00	0.00	0.00	0.14	0.00	0.00	0.21	0.25
喉	C32	227	0.76	0.00	0.15	0.00	0.00	0.00	0.00	0.11	0.00
气管、支气管、肺	C33–C34	7 040	23.72	0.00	0.00	0.00	0.00	0.26	0.53	1.18	4.06
其他的胸腔器官	C37–C38	79	0.27	0.00	0.00	0.13	0.00	0.13	0.00	0.21	0.13
骨	C40–C41	303	1.02	0.00	0.15	0.92	0.98	0.92	0.63	1.28	1.01
皮肤的黑色素瘤	C43	27	0.09	0.00	0.31	0.13	0.00	0.13	0.21	0.00	0.00
其他的皮肤	C44	122	0.41	0.00	0.00	0.00	0.00	0.13	0.11	0.43	0.25
间皮瘤	C45	6	0.02	0.00	0.00	0.00	0.00	0.00	0.00	0.00	0.00
卡波西肉瘤	C46	1	0.00	0.00	0.00	0.00	0.00	0.00	0.00	0.00	0.00
周围神经、其他结缔组织、软组织	C47;C49	50	0.17	0.00	0.15	0.00	0.14	0.00	0.00	0.11	0.00
乳房	C50	—	—	—	—	—	—	—	—	—	—
外阴	C51	—	—	—	—	—	—	—	—	—	—
阴道	C52	—	—	—	—	—	—	—	—	—	—
子宫颈	C53	—	—	—	—	—	—	—	—	—	—
子宫体	C54	—	—	—	—	—	—	—	—	—	—
子宫，部位不明	C55	—	—	—	—	—	—	—	—	—	—
卵巢	C56	—	—	—	—	—	—	—	—	—	—
其他的女性生殖器	C57	—	—	—	—	—	—	—	—	—	—
胎盘	C58	—	—	—	—	—	—	—	—	—	—
阴茎	C60	57	0.19	0.00	0.00	0.00	0.14	0.00	0.00	0.00	0.13
前列腺	C61	340	1.15	0.00	0.00	0.13	0.00	0.13	0.00	0.11	0.13
睾丸	C62	43	0.14	0.00	0.15	0.00	0.00	0.13	0.32	0.54	0.38
其他的男性生殖器	C63	9	0.03	0.00	0.00	0.00	0.00	0.26	0.00	0.11	0.00
肾	C64	258	0.87	2.20	0.46	0.00	0.42	0.00	0.32	0.00	0.25
肾盂	C65	32	0.11	0.00	0.00	0.00	0.14	0.00	0.00	0.00	0.00
输尿管	C66	28	0.09	0.00	0.00	0.00	0.00	0.00	0.00	0.00	0.13
膀胱	C67	431	1.45	0.00	0.00	0.13	0.00	0.00	0.11	0.43	0.13
其他的泌尿器官	C68	14	0.05	0.00	0.00	0.00	0.00	0.00	0.00	0.00	0.00
眼	C69	26	0.09	0.00	0.77	0.13	0.14	0.00	0.00	0.00	0.00
脑、神经系统	C70–C72	705	2.38	2.94	1.53	2.23	2.37	1.31	1.47	1.18	2.15
甲状腺	C73	208	0.70	0.00	0.15	0.00	0.00	0.13	0.63	0.64	1.39
肾上腺	C74	34	0.11	0.00	0.15	0.13	0.00	0.00	0.00	0.00	0.13
其他的内分泌腺	C75	25	0.08	0.00	0.00	0.00	0.00	0.00	0.11	0.11	0.00
霍奇金病	C81	55	0.19	0.00	0.00	0.00	0.00	0.39	0.21	0.32	0.63
非霍奇金淋巴瘤	C82–C85;C96	232	0.78	0.00	0.46	0.52	0.42	0.26	0.53	1.18	0.38
免疫增生性疾病	C88	1	0.00	0.00	0.00	0.00	0.00	0.00	0.00	0.00	0.00
多发性骨髓瘤	C90	71	0.24	0.00	0.00	0.00	0.00	0.00	0.00	0.00	0.13
淋巴样白血病	C91	91	0.31	0.00	0.77	1.31	0.70	1.18	0.32	0.21	0.76
髓样白血病	C92–C94	158	0.53	0.00	1.07	0.52	0.42	0.92	0.42	0.64	0.89
白血病，未特指	C95	362	1.22	0.73	2.91	3.41	2.23	1.83	2.10	1.71	1.39
其他的或未指明部位的	O&U	674	2.27	0.73	0.77	1.57	0.56	0.52	1.16	1.93	2.41
骨髓增殖性疾病	MPD	6	0.02	0.00	0.00	0.00	0.00	0.00	0.00	0.00	0.00
骨髓增生异常综合征	MDS	7	0.02	0.00	0.00	0.00	0.00	0.00	0.00	0.11	0.00
合计	ALL	29 684	100.00	7.35	10.25	11.79	10.04	9.41	11.68	18.84	30.17
所有部位除外 C44	ALL but C44	29 562	99.59	7.35	10.25	11.79	10.04	9.28	11.57	18.41	29.91

2014 年男性发病主要指标 ($1/10^5$)

											粗率	世标率	累积率 (%)	
35–	40–	45–	50–	55–	60–	65–	70–	75–	80–	85–	($1/10^5$ 万)	($1/10^5$ 万)	0~64	0~74
0.12	0.00	0.24	0.00	0.51	0.21	1.23	1.26	0.00	0.00	2.43	0.17	0.16	0.01	0.02
0.12	0.11	0.47	0.61	1.02	1.90	0.92	2.10	1.77	2.26	0.00	0.38	0.32	0.02	0.04
0.36	1.02	0.59	0.77	1.19	2.53	2.76	3.36	5.31	5.65	2.43	0.72	0.61	0.04	0.07
0.12	0.34	0.83	1.07	1.36	1.90	1.53	0.00	2.95	2.26	2.43	0.50	0.41	0.03	0.04
0.00	0.00	0.00	0.00	0.17	0.42	0.31	0.00	0.59	1.13	2.43	0.06	0.06	0.00	0.00
0.24	0.00	0.24	0.31	0.51	1.69	1.23	1.26	1.18	4.52	4.87	0.32	0.28	0.02	0.03
1.08	1.36	3.08	3.37	3.41	4.01	6.13	4.20	9.44	2.26	4.87	1.62	1.35	0.09	0.14
0.12	0.00	0.36	0.46	1.02	0.84	1.23	1.26	1.18	5.65	0.00	0.29	0.24	0.01	0.03
0.12	0.00	0.12	0.61	1.36	1.69	1.53	0.84	1.18	1.13	0.00	0.29	0.25	0.02	0.03
1.67	6.00	23.08	47.00	108.01	199.94	281.15	315.21	336.98	449.75	423.40	45.78	39.05	1.93	4.91
5.26	15.61	33.25	65.21	131.35	239.21	319.17	351.78	383.01	462.18	362.57	54.54	46.23	2.47	5.83
0.84	0.57	2.49	2.91	3.58	6.12	9.20	12.61	8.85	13.56	7.30	1.78	1.50	0.08	0.19
2.03	4.87	7.57	11.18	17.72	25.76	34.03	39.93	45.44	79.10	38.93	7.52	6.23	0.36	0.73
2.27	5.66	7.10	11.18	21.64	32.51	44.76	53.38	55.47	70.06	70.57	8.83	7.43	0.41	0.90
0.24	0.23	0.71	0.92	1.02	1.90	2.76	1.68	2.36	2.26	2.43	0.50	0.42	0.03	0.05
11.95	24.21	39.88	62.15	89.10	143.15	167.71	155.08	174.09	209.06	197.10	34.98	29.37	1.89	3.50
0.60	0.79	1.07	1.53	6.64	9.92	10.73	19.33	17.70	27.12	34.07	2.51	2.13	0.11	0.26
0.96	1.58	2.96	5.20	9.03	14.36	22.08	24.80	24.79	29.38	38.93	3.91	3.33	0.17	0.41
0.36	0.34	0.24	0.77	0.85	1.06	1.84	2.10	1.18	2.26	2.43	0.41	0.35	0.02	0.04
0.00	0.45	1.42	4.75	4.60	8.66	10.73	13.03	16.52	15.82	4.87	2.09	1.75	0.10	0.22
8.24	19.91	42.72	75.01	155.04	240.27	365.78	438.36	515.20	575.19	554.80	64.88	54.76	2.74	6.76
0.48	0.45	0.59	0.92	1.36	4.43	2.76	2.10	1.77	4.52	12.17	0.73	0.64	0.04	0.07
2.39	2.83	1.78	3.83	6.64	7.18	12.88	9.25	11.21	11.30	9.73	2.79	2.44	0.15	0.26
0.00	0.11	0.00	0.46	0.85	0.21	1.53	1.26	1.77	0.00	0.00	0.25	0.23	0.01	0.03
0.24	0.79	0.36	0.77	1.70	2.96	3.37	7.57	13.57	13.56	21.90	1.12	0.94	0.04	0.09
0.00	0.00	0.00	0.31	0.17	0.00	0.31	0.00	0.59	1.13	0.00	0.06	0.04	0.00	0.00
0.00	0.00	0.12	0.00	0.00	0.00	0.00	0.00	0.00	0.00	0.00	0.01	0.01	0.00	0.00
0.00	1.13	0.95	0.77	0.85	1.48	0.31	1.68	2.36	2.26	2.43	0.46	0.38	0.03	0.04
—	—	—	—	—	—	—	—	—	—	—	—	—	—	—
—	—	—	—	—	—	—	—	—	—	—	—	—	—	—
—	—	—	—	—	—	—	—	—	—	—	—	—	—	—
—	—	—	—	—	—	—	—	—	—	—	—	—	—	—
—	—	—	—	—	—	—	—	—	—	—	—	—	—	—
—	—	—	—	—	—	—	—	—	—	—	—	—	—	—
—	—	—	—	—	—	—	—	—	—	—	—	—	—	—
—	—	—	—	—	—	—	—	—	—	—	—	—	—	—
—	—	—	—	—	—	—	—	—	—	—	—	—	—	—
0.36	0.23	0.12	0.31	1.19	2.11	3.99	0.84	5.31	5.65	2.43	0.53	0.44	0.02	0.05
0.36	0.11	0.71	1.07	2.73	7.18	14.72	25.22	37.77	77.97	68.13	3.13	2.62	0.06	0.26
0.00	0.68	0.47	0.61	0.17	0.63	0.61	1.26	1.77	4.52	0.00	0.40	0.33	0.02	0.03
0.00	0.00	0.00	0.15	0.34	0.00	0.61	0.00	0.59	0.00	0.00	0.08	0.08	0.00	0.01
0.84	1.81	2.01	4.90	5.96	8.23	11.96	12.61	7.08	14.69	9.73	2.38	2.07	0.13	0.25
0.12	0.34	0.36	0.92	0.17	1.48	1.23	0.84	0.59	2.26	2.43	0.29	0.26	0.02	0.03
0.12	0.00	0.12	0.31	0.85	1.69	0.61	0.84	1.77	1.13	4.87	0.26	0.22	0.02	0.02
0.48	1.13	2.49	3.67	5.28	17.74	19.62	28.16	34.82	41.81	55.97	3.97	3.40	0.16	0.40
0.00	0.00	0.00	0.15	0.17	1.27	0.61	0.00	1.77	1.13	0.00	0.13	0.11	0.01	0.01
0.12	0.23	0.12	0.61	0.34	0.63	0.31	0.84	0.00	2.26	2.43	0.24	0.25	0.01	0.02
4.18	5.66	8.76	9.34	14.31	20.69	19.62	21.01	25.97	31.64	41.37	6.50	5.72	0.38	0.58
1.55	2.38	2.49	3.37	5.11	5.28	3.37	7.99	8.85	4.52	4.87	1.92	1.58	0.12	0.17
0.12	0.23	0.36	0.77	0.85	1.06	0.61	0.84	0.59	5.65	0.00	0.31	0.26	0.02	0.03
0.12	0.00	0.83	0.31	0.85	0.42	0.31	1.26	0.59	1.13	0.00	0.23	0.19	0.01	0.02
0.24	0.00	0.71	0.31	0.51	1.27	1.23	3.36	4.13	1.13	7.30	0.51	0.45	0.02	0.05
0.84	1.47	1.89	3.37	3.92	6.33	7.36	13.03	11.21	11.30	14.60	2.14	1.87	0.11	0.21
0.00	0.00	0.00	0.00	0.00	0.00	0.00	0.00	0.59	0.00	0.00	0.01	0.01	0.00	0.00
0.00	0.34	1.30	0.46	2.56	2.96	1.53	1.68	4.13	5.65	7.30	0.65	0.54	0.04	0.05
0.36	0.68	0.59	0.92	0.85	1.48	2.15	1.68	2.36	3.39	2.43	0.84	0.85	0.05	0.07
1.19	1.47	2.13	1.84	2.39	3.59	3.68	4.62	4.13	4.52	4.87	1.46	1.33	0.09	0.13
2.27	3.06	2.60	3.67	3.92	7.60	8.58	8.83	12.98	14.69	9.73	3.34	3.21	0.19	0.28
2.15	3.73	5.44	8.42	12.10	20.27	27.90	33.20	41.90	30.51	31.63	6.21	5.36	0.31	0.61
0.00	0.11	0.12	0.31	0.17	0.21	0.00	0.00	0.00	0.00	0.00	0.06	0.04	0.00	0.00
0.00	0.00	0.00	0.00	0.34	0.21	0.00	0.84	0.00	1.13	0.00	0.06	0.05	0.00	0.01
55.43	112.25	206.39	348.43	637.01	1 067.28	1 441.65	1 633.64	1 846.58	2 265.72	2 080.49	273.55	232.51	12.64	28.02
55.19	111.45	206.03	347.66	635.30	1 064.32	1 438.27	1 626.07	1 833.01	2 252.16	2 058.59	272.42	231.56	12.60	27.93

表 6-1-3 河南省全省肿瘤登记地区

部位		病例数	构成(%)	年龄组							
				0–	1–	5–	10–	15–	20–	25–	30–
唇	C00	12	0.05	0.00	0.00	0.00	0.00	0.00	0.00	0.00	0.00
舌	C01–C02	48	0.20	0.00	0.18	0.00	0.00	0.00	0.00	0.22	0.00
口	C03–C06	67	0.28	0.00	0.00	0.00	0.00	0.00	0.22	0.00	0.27
唾液腺	C07–C08	55	0.23	0.00	0.00	0.00	0.16	0.14	0.00	0.22	0.54
扁桃体	C09	6	0.03	0.00	0.00	0.00	0.00	0.00	0.11	0.11	0.00
其他的口咽	C10	11	0.05	0.00	0.00	0.00	0.00	0.00	0.00	0.11	0.27
鼻咽	C11	97	0.41	0.00	0.00	0.15	0.00	0.00	0.11	0.45	1.07
喉咽	C12–C13	9	0.04	0.00	0.00	0.00	0.00	0.00	0.00	0.00	0.00
咽，部位不明	C14	10	0.04	0.00	0.00	0.00	0.00	0.00	0.00	0.00	0.00
食管	C15	3 042	12.94	0.00	0.00	0.00	0.00	0.00	0.11	0.45	1.34
胃	C16	2 356	10.02	0.00	0.00	0.00	0.00	0.14	1.12	1.69	3.08
小肠	C17	126	0.54	0.00	0.00	0.00	0.00	0.00	0.00	0.22	0.40
结肠	C18	679	2.89	0.00	0.00	0.00	0.16	0.00	0.34	0.00	0.40
直肠	C19–C20	855	3.64	0.00	0.00	0.00	0.00	0.00	0.00	1.01	1.21
肛门	C21	49	0.21	0.00	0.00	0.00	0.00	0.14	0.11	0.11	0.00
肝脏	C22	1 724	7.33	0.00	0.18	0.00	0.00	0.00	0.67	0.90	2.01
胆囊及其他	C23–C24	375	1.59	0.00	0.00	0.00	0.00	0.00	0.11	0.00	0.40
胰腺	C25	311	1.32	0.00	0.00	0.00	0.00	0.14	0.00	0.34	0.27
鼻、鼻窦及其他	C30–C31	31	0.13	0.00	0.00	0.15	0.00	0.00	0.00	0.00	0.00
喉	C32	80	0.34	0.00	0.00	0.00	0.00	0.00	0.00	0.11	0.13
气管、支气管、肺	C33–C34	3 120	13.27	0.00	0.00	0.00	0.00	0.14	0.34	1.24	3.49
其他的胸腔器官	C37–C38	65	0.28	0.00	0.18	0.00	0.00	0.00	0.00	0.22	0.13
骨	C40–C41	232	0.99	0.00	0.00	0.31	0.16	0.99	1.34	0.90	0.54
皮肤的黑色素瘤	C43	30	0.13	0.00	0.55	0.15	0.00	0.14	0.22	0.00	0.00
其他的皮肤	C44	123	0.52	0.00	0.00	0.00	0.00	0.71	0.00	0.22	0.13
间皮瘤	C45	3	0.01	0.00	0.00	0.00	0.00	0.00	0.00	0.11	0.00
卡波西肉瘤	C46	1	0.00	0.00	0.00	0.00	0.00	0.00	0.00	0.00	0.13
周围神经、其他结缔组织、软组织	C47;C49	39	0.17	0.00	0.18	0.15	0.16	0.28	0.22	0.22	0.13
乳房	C50	3 709	15.77	0.00	0.00	0.00	0.00	0.43	3.58	7.53	14.35
外阴	C51	25	0.11	0.00	0.00	0.00	0.00	0.00	0.11	0.00	0.00
阴道	C52	21	0.09	0.00	0.00	0.00	0.16	0.00	0.00	0.00	0.00
子宫颈	C53	1 740	7.40	0.00	0.00	0.00	0.00	0.00	0.45	2.13	10.59
子宫体	C54	673	2.86	0.00	0.00	0.00	0.00	0.00	0.22	0.90	0.80
子宫，部位不明	C55	171	0.73	0.00	0.00	0.00	0.00	0.00	0.34	0.11	0.54
卵巢	C56	636	2.70	0.00	0.00	0.31	0.82	0.99	2.01	2.02	2.15
其他的女性生殖器	C57	27	0.11	0.00	0.00	0.00	0.00	0.00	0.11	0.00	0.27
胎盘	C58	9	0.04	0.00	0.00	0.00	0.00	0.00	0.11	0.22	0.00
阴茎	C60	—	—	—	—	—	—	—	—	—	—
前列腺	C61	—	—	—	—	—	—	—	—	—	—
睾丸	C62	—	—	—	—	—	—	—	—	—	—
其他的男性生殖器	C63	—	—	—	—	—	—	—	—	—	—
肾	C64	145	0.62	0.00	0.55	0.15	0.00	0.14	0.34	0.22	0.13
肾盂	C65	24	0.10	0.00	0.00	0.00	0.00	0.00	0.00	0.00	0.00
输尿管	C66	15	0.06	0.00	0.00	0.00	0.00	0.00	0.00	0.00	0.00
膀胱	C67	141	0.60	0.00	0.00	0.00	0.16	0.00	0.11	0.22	0.27
其他的泌尿器官	C68	10	0.04	0.00	0.00	0.00	0.00	0.00	0.11	0.00	0.00
眼	C69	12	0.05	0.00	0.37	0.00	0.00	0.00	0.00	0.11	0.00
脑、神经系统	C70–C72	703	2.99	1.67	1.28	1.22	1.32	1.13	1.23	1.69	2.68
甲状腺	C73	593	2.52	0.00	0.00	0.15	0.33	0.85	1.79	3.48	4.96
肾上腺	C74	12	0.05	0.00	0.00	0.00	0.00	0.00	0.11	0.00	0.00
其他的内分泌腺	C75	34	0.14	0.00	0.00	0.00	0.00	0.14	0.00	0.22	0.27
霍奇金病	C81	44	0.19	0.00	0.00	0.15	0.00	0.00	0.22	0.45	0.00
非霍奇金淋巴瘤	C82–C85;C96	186	0.79	0.83	0.00	0.00	0.49	0.00	0.56	0.67	0.54
免疫增生性疾病	C88	1	0.00	0.00	0.00	0.00	0.00	0.00	0.00	0.00	0.00
多发性骨髓瘤	C90	44	0.19	0.00	0.00	0.15	0.00	0.00	0.00	0.00	0.13
淋巴样白血病	C91	88	0.37	0.83	1.65	0.76	0.49	0.43	0.56	0.22	0.13
髓样白血病	C92–C94	90	0.38	0.83	0.37	0.31	0.33	0.43	0.67	0.79	0.67
白血病，未特指	C95	289	1.23	2.50	3.30	1.68	2.96	1.13	1.12	1.24	1.88
其他的或未指明部位的	O&U	500	2.13	0.00	0.92	0.46	0.33	0.85	0.67	1.24	2.41
骨髓增殖性疾病	MPD	13	0.06	0.00	0.18	0.00	0.00	0.00	0.11	0.00	0.00
骨髓增生异常综合征	MDS	5	0.02	0.00	0.00	0.00	0.00	0.00	0.11	0.00	0.13
合计	ALL	23 516	100.00	6.67	9.91	6.26	8.07	9.36	19.70	32.36	58.87
所有部位除外 C44	ALL but C44	23 393	99.48	6.67	9.91	6.26	8.07	8.65	19.70	32.13	58.73

2014 年女性发病主要指标 ($1/10^5$)

											粗率	世标率	累积率 (%)	
35–	40–	45–	50–	55–	60–	65–	70–	75–	80–	85–	($1/10^5$ 万)	($1/10^5$ 万)	0~64	0~74
0.00	0.24	0.00	0.16	0.18	0.65	0.00	0.41	1.55	0.00	1.29	0.12	0.09	0.01	0.01
0.52	0.12	0.73	0.48	0.88	1.95	1.53	1.23	2.58	2.55	1.29	0.47	0.37	0.03	0.04
0.39	0.49	0.36	0.63	1.59	2.61	2.15	1.23	3.61	5.94	5.15	0.66	0.49	0.03	0.05
0.52	0.49	1.21	1.43	1.41	0.87	0.92	0.82	0.52	0.85	1.29	0.54	0.43	0.03	0.04
0.00	0.00	0.00	0.16	0.18	0.00	0.00	0.41	0.52	0.00	0.00	0.06	0.05	0.00	0.00
0.00	0.00	0.12	0.00	0.35	0.22	0.31	0.41	1.03	0.00	0.00	0.11	0.08	0.01	0.01
0.13	1.09	0.73	1.74	2.48	3.91	2.15	2.05	2.58	5.09	1.29	0.95	0.75	0.06	0.08
0.00	0.24	0.12	0.00	0.00	0.00	0.92	0.00	1.03	0.85	0.00	0.09	0.06	0.00	0.01
0.00	0.00	0.24	0.00	0.00	0.43	0.61	0.00	0.52	0.85	2.58	0.10	0.07	0.00	0.01
1.17	4.49	10.68	25.81	59.76	114.19	170.60	181.77	212.17	242.71	218.94	29.84	22.54	1.09	2.85
4.30	8.73	14.45	21.06	48.98	88.14	101.56	119.41	161.07	178.21	158.41	23.11	17.34	0.96	2.06
0.65	0.73	0.36	1.90	1.77	4.56	6.75	6.57	6.71	5.94	7.73	1.24	0.96	0.05	0.12
1.70	4.97	5.59	9.98	15.38	22.36	29.76	29.54	34.07	48.37	34.77	6.66	5.05	0.30	0.60
2.35	4.25	8.74	10.45	18.04	26.48	35.59	39.80	52.14	54.31	56.67	8.39	6.32	0.36	0.74
0.26	0.36	0.61	0.63	1.41	0.87	2.15	2.46	2.06	2.55	0.00	0.48	0.37	0.02	0.05
2.74	7.28	9.71	18.53	39.61	65.34	68.42	91.91	96.02	144.27	113.33	16.91	12.71	0.73	1.54
0.00	1.33	2.55	2.85	8.84	13.03	15.65	14.36	34.07	27.16	34.77	3.68	2.69	0.15	0.30
0.39	1.33	2.55	3.96	5.48	9.12	12.27	21.75	21.68	14.43	25.76	3.05	2.32	0.12	0.29
0.13	0.12	0.24	0.32	0.35	1.09	1.53	1.23	3.61	0.85	1.29	0.30	0.24	0.01	0.03
0.13	0.12	0.49	1.11	1.59	3.26	4.60	4.10	4.65	3.39	3.86	0.78	0.61	0.03	0.08
5.61	8.73	22.22	44.02	66.13	102.46	132.25	160.03	183.26	266.47	215.07	30.61	22.89	1.27	2.73
0.00	0.97	0.97	1.11	0.71	2.82	2.45	1.23	2.06	2.55	3.86	0.64	0.51	0.04	0.05
1.56	1.33	1.94	3.17	5.13	8.03	5.52	8.62	10.32	11.03	1.29	2.28	1.82	0.13	0.20
0.13	0.00	0.24	0.48	0.18	0.22	1.53	1.23	1.55	2.55	1.29	0.29	0.27	0.01	0.02
0.78	0.73	0.36	1.11	1.94	2.17	3.07	4.92	6.19	17.82	21.89	1.21	0.87	0.04	0.08
0.00	0.00	0.12	0.16	0.00	0.00	0.00	0.00	0.00	0.00	0.00	0.03	0.02	0.00	0.00
0.00	0.00	0.00	0.00	0.00	0.00	0.00	0.00	0.00	0.00	0.00	0.01	0.01	0.00	0.00
0.00	0.12	0.24	0.79	1.24	1.52	0.61	1.23	0.52	0.85	0.00	0.38	0.34	0.03	0.04
29.60	62.10	79.53	82.02	85.93	106.81	76.71	67.70	55.75	50.07	36.06	36.39	28.52	2.36	3.08
0.13	0.36	0.24	0.32	0.71	0.43	1.23	0.82	1.55	0.85	0.00	0.25	0.19	0.01	0.02
0.00	0.00	0.24	0.63	0.53	0.87	0.92	1.23	0.00	0.85	0.00	0.21	0.17	0.01	0.02
16.17	28.99	32.30	41.01	36.07	48.19	40.20	34.47	26.33	31.40	27.05	17.07	13.36	1.08	1.45
3.78	7.52	14.21	18.37	19.63	22.58	15.96	10.67	8.78	13.58	9.02	6.60	5.17	0.44	0.57
0.91	1.46	2.91	4.43	4.24	6.08	6.75	2.05	3.61	0.85	6.44	1.68	1.34	0.11	0.15
3.52	4.97	9.96	10.93	15.91	22.14	18.10	17.23	17.04	12.73	12.88	6.24	5.01	0.38	0.56
0.52	0.24	0.36	1.11	0.35	0.65	0.31	0.41	0.52	0.00	0.00	0.26	0.21	0.02	0.02
0.26	0.12	0.24	0.16	0.00	0.00	0.00	0.00	0.00	0.00	0.00	0.09	0.07	0.01	0.01
—	—	—	—	—	—	—	—	—	—	—	—	—	—	—
—	—	—	—	—	—	—	—	—	—	—	—	—	—	—
—	—	—	—	—	—	—	—	—	—	—	—	—	—	—
—	—	—	—	—	—	—	—	—	—	—	—	—	—	—
0.65	0.97	1.82	2.69	3.54	4.12	6.75	3.28	5.16	5.09	5.15	1.42	1.15	0.08	0.13
0.26	0.12	0.61	0.16	1.06	0.65	0.61	0.41	1.55	0.00	0.00	0.24	0.18	0.01	0.02
0.00	0.00	0.12	0.79	0.18	0.22	0.61	1.64	0.52	0.00	0.00	0.15	0.12	0.01	0.02
0.13	0.24	0.97	1.90	2.30	3.04	4.91	7.80	9.81	17.82	12.88	1.38	1.00	0.05	0.11
0.00	0.12	0.12	0.16	0.00	0.65	0.31	0.00	0.52	0.85	0.00	0.10	0.08	0.01	0.01
0.00	0.12	0.12	0.16	0.00	0.22	0.61	0.00	0.52	1.70	0.00	0.12	0.11	0.01	0.01
3.78	6.31	7.41	10.29	14.85	24.10	23.32	21.75	18.07	30.55	28.33	6.90	5.63	0.39	0.61
6.26	7.64	13.23	13.78	12.02	9.77	11.05	6.57	12.39	3.39	0.00	5.82	4.63	0.37	0.46
0.00	0.12	0.36	0.16	0.35	0.43	0.31	0.00	0.52	0.00	0.00	0.12	0.09	0.01	0.01
0.26	0.61	0.12	0.95	0.88	0.87	0.31	0.82	0.52	0.85	1.29	0.33	0.27	0.02	0.03
0.39	0.36	0.61	1.11	0.71	0.65	1.23	2.05	0.52	1.70	0.00	0.43	0.35	0.02	0.04
0.65	1.33	1.21	3.48	3.18	7.82	6.14	9.44	2.58	12.73	2.58	1.82	1.47	0.10	0.18
0.00	0.00	0.00	0.00	0.00	0.00	0.00	0.00	0.00	0.00	1.29	0.01	0.01	0.00	0.00
0.26	0.12	0.24	0.79	1.24	1.30	2.45	2.87	1.03	1.70	0.00	0.43	0.35	0.02	0.05
0.52	0.61	1.46	0.79	1.24	1.52	2.76	0.41	2.06	2.55	2.58	0.86	0.85	0.05	0.07
0.65	0.85	1.09	0.16	1.59	1.52	2.45	0.41	4.13	5.94	0.00	0.88	0.75	0.05	0.06
1.17	2.30	1.82	3.64	5.30	5.64	8.59	6.15	6.71	11.03	6.44	2.84	2.69	0.17	0.24
2.22	3.40	5.34	6.81	9.90	18.24	15.04	15.59	25.81	27.16	10.30	4.91	3.87	0.26	0.42
0.00	0.24	0.00	0.48	0.00	0.65	0.31	0.41	0.00	0.00	1.29	0.13	0.12	0.01	0.01
0.00	0.00	0.24	0.00	0.18	0.00	0.00	0.00	0.00	0.00	0.00	0.05	0.04	0.00	0.00
95.59	179.51	262.50	359.26	505.52	765.44	850.86	910.93	1 052.09	1 272.96	1 075.37	230.70	178.08	11.56	20.37
94.81	178.79	262.14	358.16	503.58	763.27	847.79	906.00	1 045.89	1 255.13	1 053.47	229.49	177.20	11.52	20.29

表 6-1-4 河南省城市肿瘤登记地区

部位		病例数	构成(%)	年龄组 0–	1–	5–	10–	15–	20–	25–	30–
唇	C00	1	0.01	0.00	0.00	0.00	0.00	0.00	0.00	0.00	0.00
舌	C01–C02	23	0.26	0.00	0.00	0.00	0.00	0.00	0.00	0.34	0.00
口	C03–C06	37	0.41	0.00	0.00	0.46	0.52	0.00	0.31	0.00	0.00
唾液腺	C07–C08	26	0.29	0.00	0.00	0.00	0.00	0.00	0.00	1.02	0.83
扁桃体	C09	0	0.00	0.00	0.00	0.00	0.00	0.00	0.00	0.00	0.00
其他的口咽	C10	6	0.07	0.00	0.00	0.00	0.00	0.00	0.00	0.00	0.00
鼻咽	C11	42	0.47	0.00	0.00	0.00	0.00	0.00	0.00	0.00	1.24
喉咽	C12–C13	10	0.11	0.00	0.00	0.00	0.00	0.00	0.00	0.00	0.00
咽，部位不明	C14	8	0.09	0.00	0.00	0.00	0.00	0.00	0.00	0.00	0.00
食管	C15	1 121	12.50	0.00	0.00	0.00	0.00	0.00	0.00	0.68	0.00
胃	C16	1 134	12.64	0.00	0.00	0.00	0.00	0.00	0.31	0.68	1.24
小肠	C17	41	0.46	0.00	0.00	0.00	0.00	0.00	0.00	0.00	0.00
结肠	C18	318	3.55	0.00	0.00	0.00	0.52	0.00	0.00	0.34	0.41
直肠	C19–C20	371	4.14	0.00	0.00	0.00	0.00	0.00	0.00	1.35	0.41
肛门	C21	14	0.16	0.00	0.00	0.00	0.00	0.00	0.00	0.00	0.00
肝脏	C22	894	9.97	2.50	0.00	0.00	0.00	0.00	0.63	1.35	3.30
胆囊及其他	C23–C24	104	1.16	0.00	0.00	0.00	0.00	0.00	0.00	0.34	0.00
胰腺	C25	149	1.66	0.00	0.00	0.00	0.00	0.43	0.00	0.34	0.00
鼻、鼻窦及其他	C30–C31	11	0.12	0.00	0.00	0.00	0.00	0.00	0.00	0.00	0.00
喉	C32	32	0.36	0.00	0.00	0.00	0.00	0.00	0.00	0.00	0.00
气管、支气管、肺	C33–C34	1 904	21.23	0.00	0.00	0.00	0.00	0.00	0.00	1.35	4.13
其他的胸腔器官	C37–C38	37	0.41	0.00	0.00	0.00	0.00	0.00	0.00	0.34	0.00
骨	C40–C41	75	0.84	0.00	0.00	0.46	0.00	0.00	0.31	0.68	0.83
皮肤的黑色素瘤	C43	7	0.08	0.00	0.00	0.00	0.00	0.00	0.00	0.00	0.00
其他的皮肤	C44	44	0.49	0.00	0.00	0.00	0.00	0.00	0.00	0.34	0.41
间皮瘤	C45	3	0.03	0.00	0.00	0.00	0.00	0.00	0.00	0.00	0.00
卡波西肉瘤	C46	0	0.00	0.00	0.00	0.00	0.00	0.00	0.00	0.00	0.00
周围神经、其他结缔组织、软组织	C47;C49	21	0.23	0.00	0.00	0.00	0.00	0.00	0.00	0.68	0.00
乳房	C50	—	—	—	—	—	—	—	—	—	—
外阴	C51	—	—	—	—	—	—	—	—	—	—
阴道	C52	—	—	—	—	—	—	—	—	—	—
子宫颈	C53	—	—	—	—	—	—	—	—	—	—
子宫体	C54	—	—	—	—	—	—	—	—	—	—
子宫，部位不明	C55	—	—	—	—	—	—	—	—	—	—
卵巢	C56	—	—	—	—	—	—	—	—	—	—
其他的女性生殖器	C57	—	—	—	—	—	—	—	—	—	—
胎盘	C58	—	—	—	—	—	—	—	—	—	—
阴茎	C60	—	—	—	—	—	—	—	—	—	—
前列腺	C61	—	—	—	—	—	—	—	—	—	—
睾丸	C62	—	—	—	—	—	—	—	—	—	—
其他的男性生殖器	C63	—	—	—	—	—	—	—	—	—	—
肾	C64	105	1.17	5.00	1.11	0.00	0.00	0.00	0.00	0.00	0.41
肾盂	C65	14	0.16	0.00	0.00	0.00	0.00	0.00	0.00	0.00	0.00
输尿管	C66	16	0.18	0.00	0.00	0.00	0.00	0.00	0.00	0.00	0.00
膀胱	C67	132	1.47	0.00	0.00	0.00	0.00	0.00	0.31	1.02	0.00
其他的泌尿器官	C68	13	0.14	0.00	0.00	0.00	0.00	0.00	0.00	0.00	0.00
眼	C69	8	0.09	0.00	0.56	0.00	0.00	0.00	0.00	0.00	0.00
脑、神经系统	C70–C72	217	2.42	0.00	0.00	0.46	1.03	0.43	0.63	1.02	2.89
甲状腺	C73	165	1.84	0.00	0.00	0.00	0.00	0.86	0.94	3.05	6.19
肾上腺	C74	9	0.10	0.00	0.00	0.00	0.00	0.00	0.31	0.00	0.00
其他的内分泌腺	C75	11	0.12	0.00	0.00	0.00	0.00	0.00	0.00	0.00	0.00
霍奇金病	C81	27	0.30	0.00	0.00	0.46	0.00	0.86	0.00	0.34	0.00
非霍奇金淋巴瘤	C82–C85;C96	72	0.80	0.00	0.00	0.00	0.52	0.00	0.31	0.34	0.41
免疫增生性疾病	C88	1	0.01	0.00	0.00	0.00	0.00	0.00	0.00	0.00	0.00
多发性骨髓瘤	C90	19	0.21	0.00	0.00	0.00	0.00	0.00	0.00	0.00	0.00
淋巴样白血病	C91	51	0.57	0.00	2.22	0.92	1.55	0.86	0.31	0.00	0.00
髓样白血病	C92–C94	58	0.65	0.00	0.00	1.84	0.00	1.29	0.63	1.02	1.65
白血病，未特指	C95	101	1.13	2.50	1.11	0.92	1.03	0.00	0.94	0.68	1.24
其他的或未指明部位的	O&U	140	1.56	0.00	0.00	0.92	1.03	0.43	1.26	0.68	2.48
骨髓增殖性疾病	MPD	5	0.06	0.00	0.00	0.00	0.00	0.00	0.00	0.00	0.00
骨髓增生异常综合征	MDS	5	0.06	0.00	0.00	0.00	0.00	0.00	0.00	0.34	0.00
合计	ALL	8 969	100.00	10.00	5.00	6.43	6.70	5.15	8.79	24.37	44.16
所有部位除外 C44	ALL but C44	8 925	99.51	10.00	5.00	6.43	6.70	5.15	8.79	24.03	43.75

2014 年合计发病主要指标 ($1/10^5$)

											粗率	世标率	累积率 (%)	
35–	40–	45–	50–	55–	60–	65–	70–	75–	80–	85–	($1/10^5$ 万)	($1/10^5$ 万)	0~64	0~74
0.00	0.00	0.00	0.00	0.00	0.00	1.00	0.00	0.00	0.00	0.00	0.03	0.03	0.00	0.01
0.71	0.00	1.04	0.92	2.50	2.07	1.00	2.64	1.77	7.54	8.13	0.67	0.54	0.04	0.06
0.35	0.00	1.39	1.38	1.50	2.07	7.02	2.64	10.62	18.86	0.00	1.08	0.90	0.04	0.09
0.35	0.00	1.39	3.22	1.00	1.38	0.00	0.00	5.31	3.77	8.13	0.76	0.60	0.05	0.05
0.00	0.00	0.00	0.00	0.00	0.00	0.00	0.00	0.00	0.00	0.00	0.00	0.00	0.00	0.00
0.00	0.00	0.00	0.00	0.50	1.38	1.00	0.00	1.77	0.00	8.13	0.17	0.16	0.01	0.01
1.06	0.97	1.04	0.46	4.00	4.84	5.01	5.28	7.08	0.00	8.13	1.22	1.00	0.07	0.12
0.00	0.00	0.35	0.46	0.00	0.69	3.01	1.32	3.54	3.77	0.00	0.29	0.24	0.01	0.03
0.00	0.00	0.00	0.00	0.00	2.76	0.00	0.00	1.77	7.54	8.13	0.23	0.21	0.01	0.01
1.41	1.61	10.44	25.33	66.96	135.40	191.43	244.04	246.12	467.62	455.25	32.63	27.92	1.21	3.39
3.53	9.34	15.66	37.77	56.97	134.71	180.40	218.98	283.31	377.12	382.08	33.01	27.84	1.30	3.30
0.00	0.32	1.39	1.38	2.00	5.53	7.02	3.96	8.85	22.63	0.00	1.19	0.96	0.05	0.11
2.47	2.90	3.48	10.59	21.99	22.11	41.09	55.40	81.45	181.02	105.68	9.26	7.51	0.32	0.81
3.88	4.51	5.22	15.66	24.99	32.47	42.09	60.68	93.85	120.68	178.85	10.80	8.94	0.44	0.96
0.00	0.32	0.35	0.46	0.00	0.69	1.00	6.60	5.31	3.77	0.00	0.41	0.32	0.01	0.05
6.35	15.45	17.75	37.31	62.97	94.64	124.28	135.87	166.44	241.35	268.27	26.02	21.61	1.20	2.50
0.35	0.97	0.70	3.22	3.50	13.13	13.03	11.87	44.27	37.71	56.91	3.03	2.52	0.11	0.24
0.35	1.29	2.44	4.15	8.00	8.98	26.06	39.57	37.18	45.25	65.04	4.34	3.69	0.13	0.46
0.35	0.32	0.00	0.92	0.00	0.00	0.00	3.96	7.08	0.00	0.00	0.32	0.24	0.01	0.03
0.00	0.00	0.35	0.92	3.00	1.38	6.01	7.91	8.85	11.31	8.13	0.93	0.77	0.03	0.10
7.05	12.23	34.79	58.49	107.94	185.14	269.60	395.74	525.89	690.12	585.32	55.43	45.89	2.06	5.38
0.35	0.64	1.04	0.92	2.00	4.14	4.01	3.96	5.31	11.31	40.65	1.08	0.95	0.05	0.09
1.06	1.29	2.09	2.76	5.50	4.84	9.02	13.19	15.94	11.31	8.13	2.18	1.78	0.10	0.21
0.35	0.00	0.00	0.92	0.50	0.00	2.00	0.00	1.77	0.00	0.00	0.20	0.17	0.01	0.02
0.71	0.64	0.35	3.22	2.00	2.76	3.01	1.32	15.94	18.86	32.52	1.28	1.04	0.05	0.07
0.00	0.00	0.35	0.92	0.00	0.00	0.00	0.00	0.00	0.00	0.00	0.09	0.07	0.01	0.01
0.00	0.00	0.00	0.00	0.00	0.00	0.00	0.00	0.00	0.00	0.00	0.00	0.00	0.00	0.00
0.00	0.64	1.04	1.38	0.00	2.76	2.00	1.32	5.31	3.77	0.00	0.61	0.49	0.03	0.05
—	—	—	—	—	—	—	—	—	—	—	—	—	—	—
—	—	—	—	—	—	—	—	—	—	—	—	—	—	—
—	—	—	—	—	—	—	—	—	—	—	—	—	—	—
—	—	—	—	—	—	—	—	—	—	—	—	—	—	—
—	—	—	—	—	—	—	—	—	—	—	—	—	—	—
—	—	—	—	—	—	—	—	—	—	—	—	—	—	—
—	—	—	—	—	—	—	—	—	—	—	—	—	—	—
—	—	—	—	—	—	—	—	—	—	—	—	—	—	—
—	—	—	—	—	—	—	—	—	—	—	—	—	—	—
—	—	—	—	—	—	—	—	—	—	—	—	—	—	—
—	—	—	—	—	—	—	—	—	—	—	—	—	—	—
—	—	—	—	—	—	—	—	—	—	—	—	—	—	—
—	—	—	—	—	—	—	—	—	—	—	—	—	—	—
0.71	1.61	1.74	6.45	7.50	11.05	14.03	18.47	14.17	18.86	16.26	3.06	2.66	0.16	0.32
0.35	0.64	0.00	0.92	0.50	0.69	3.01	3.96	0.00	3.77	0.00	0.41	0.34	0.02	0.05
0.35	0.00	0.35	1.38	0.50	2.07	0.00	5.28	3.54	0.00	8.13	0.47	0.40	0.02	0.05
0.35	1.61	2.09	3.68	4.50	12.43	9.02	26.38	49.58	56.57	73.16	3.84	3.15	0.13	0.31
0.00	0.32	0.00	0.46	0.50	3.45	1.00	0.00	5.31	3.77	0.00	0.38	0.30	0.02	0.03
0.00	0.00	0.35	0.46	0.50	0.00	1.00	0.00	0.00	7.54	8.13	0.23	0.23	0.01	0.01
3.17	5.15	8.70	11.05	12.49	21.41	19.04	18.47	24.79	60.34	65.04	6.32	5.23	0.34	0.53
4.94	6.12	8.35	10.13	11.99	8.98	11.02	6.60	7.08	0.00	0.00	4.80	3.81	0.31	0.40
0.00	0.00	0.00	0.00	1.00	1.38	1.00	1.32	1.77	3.77	0.00	0.26	0.21	0.01	0.03
0.00	0.32	0.35	0.92	1.00	0.69	2.00	2.64	0.00	0.00	0.00	0.32	0.27	0.02	0.04
0.00	0.32	1.04	0.92	2.00	0.00	3.01	3.96	8.85	0.00	16.26	0.79	0.70	0.03	0.06
0.35	1.61	1.04	2.76	4.50	6.22	4.01	19.79	15.94	18.86	16.26	2.10	1.72	0.09	0.21
0.00	0.00	0.00	0.00	0.00	0.00	0.00	0.00	1.77	0.00	0.00	0.03	0.02	0.00	0.00
0.00	0.32	0.70	0.46	0.50	2.07	3.01	2.64	5.31	7.54	8.13	0.55	0.46	0.02	0.05
0.71	0.32	1.74	1.38	2.50	4.14	8.02	2.64	7.08	7.54	8.13	1.48	1.50	0.08	0.13
1.06	1.29	2.09	1.38	3.50	2.07	4.01	6.60	7.08	11.31	0.00	1.69	1.47	0.09	0.14
2.12	2.25	0.70	3.68	5.00	8.29	8.02	13.19	15.94	49.03	8.13	2.94	2.52	0.14	0.25
0.71	2.90	2.44	4.61	8.00	13.13	17.04	21.11	26.56	30.17	32.52	4.08	3.48	0.19	0.38
0.00	0.32	0.00	0.92	0.00	0.00	0.00	1.32	0.00	0.00	8.13	0.15	0.13	0.01	0.01
0.00	0.00	0.00	0.00	1.00	0.00	0.00	2.64	0.00	0.00	0.00	0.15	0.12	0.01	0.02
72.64	128.14	204.94	363.39	520.22	875.94	1 142.55	1 494.58	1 921.17	2 760.49	2 674.58	261.09	216.64	11.33	24.52
71.94	127.49	204.59	360.17	518.22	873.18	1 139.54	1 493.27	1 905.23	2 741.64	2 642.06	259.80	215.60	11.28	24.45

表 6-1-5 河南省城市肿瘤登记地区

部位		病例数	构成 (%)	年龄组							
				0–	1–	5–	10–	15–	20–	25–	30–
唇	C00	1	0.02	0.00	0.00	0.00	0.00	0.00	0.00	0.00	0.00
舌	C01–C02	8	0.16	0.00	0.00	0.00	0.00	0.00	0.00	0.00	0.00
口	C03–C06	20	0.39	0.00	0.00	0.85	0.95	0.00	0.00	0.00	0.00
唾液腺	C07–C08	15	0.29	0.00	0.00	0.00	0.00	0.00	0.00	0.66	0.00
扁桃体	C09	0	0.00	0.00	0.00	0.00	0.00	0.00	0.00	0.00	0.00
其他的口咽	C10	6	0.12	0.00	0.00	0.00	0.00	0.00	0.00	0.00	0.00
鼻咽	C11	28	0.55	0.00	0.00	0.00	0.00	0.00	0.00	0.00	1.65
喉咽	C12–C13	6	0.12	0.00	0.00	0.00	0.00	0.00	0.00	0.00	0.00
咽，部位不明	C14	4	0.08	0.00	0.00	0.00	0.00	0.00	0.00	0.00	0.00
食管	C15	732	14.34	0.00	0.00	0.00	0.00	0.00	0.00	0.66	0.00
胃	C16	814	15.95	0.00	0.00	0.00	0.00	0.00	0.62	0.00	0.82
小肠	C17	20	0.39	0.00	0.00	0.00	0.00	0.00	0.00	0.00	0.00
结肠	C18	177	3.47	0.00	0.00	0.00	0.00	0.00	0.00	0.66	0.82
直肠	C19–C20	207	4.06	0.00	0.00	0.00	0.00	0.00	0.00	0.66	0.82
肛门	C21	6	0.12	0.00	0.00	0.00	0.00	0.00	0.00	0.00	0.00
肝脏	C22	644	12.62	4.75	0.00	0.00	0.00	0.00	0.62	1.99	5.77
胆囊及其他	C23–C24	44	0.86	0.00	0.00	0.00	0.00	0.00	0.00	0.66	0.00
胰腺	C25	88	1.72	0.00	0.00	0.00	0.00	0.00	0.00	0.00	0.00
鼻、鼻窦及其他	C30–C31	7	0.14	0.00	0.00	0.00	0.00	0.00	0.00	0.00	0.00
喉	C32	27	0.53	0.00	0.00	0.00	0.00	0.00	0.00	0.00	0.00
气管、支气管、肺	C33–C34	1364	26.72	0.00	0.00	0.00	0.00	0.00	0.00	1.99	5.77
其他的胸腔器官	C37–C38	24	0.47	0.00	0.00	0.00	0.00	0.00	0.00	0.66	0.00
骨	C40–C41	38	0.74	0.00	0.00	0.00	0.00	0.00	0.00	1.33	1.65
皮肤的黑色素瘤	C43	5	0.10	0.00	0.00	0.00	0.00	0.00	0.00	0.00	0.00
其他的皮肤	C44	21	0.41	0.00	0.00	0.00	0.00	0.00	0.00	0.66	0.00
间皮瘤	C45	1	0.02	0.00	0.00	0.00	0.00	0.00	0.00	0.00	0.00
卡波西肉瘤	C46	0	0.00	0.00	0.00	0.00	0.00	0.00	0.00	0.00	0.00
周围神经、其他结缔组织、软组织	C47;C49	13	0.25	0.00	0.00	0.00	0.00	0.00	0.00	0.66	0.00
乳房	C50	—	—	—	—	—	—	—	—	—	—
外阴	C51	—	—	—	—	—	—	—	—	—	—
阴道	C52	—	—	—	—	—	—	—	—	—	—
子宫颈	C53	—	—	—	—	—	—	—	—	—	—
子宫体	C54	—	—	—	—	—	—	—	—	—	—
子宫，部位不明	C55	—	—	—	—	—	—	—	—	—	—
卵巢	C56	—	—	—	—	—	—	—	—	—	—
其他的女性生殖器	C57	—	—	—	—	—	—	—	—	—	—
胎盘	C58	—	—	—	—	—	—	—	—	—	—
阴茎	C60	7	0.14	0.00	0.00	0.00	0.00	0.00	0.00	0.00	0.00
前列腺	C61	104	2.04	0.00	0.00	0.00	0.00	0.00	0.00	0.00	0.00
睾丸	C62	10	0.20	0.00	0.00	0.00	0.00	0.00	0.62	1.33	0.82
其他的男性生殖器	C63	1	0.02	0.00	0.00	0.00	0.00	0.00	0.00	0.00	0.00
肾	C64	71	1.39	9.49	1.04	0.00	0.00	0.00	0.00	0.00	0.82
肾盂	C65	9	0.18	0.00	0.00	0.00	0.00	0.00	0.00	0.00	0.00
输尿管	C66	9	0.18	0.00	0.00	0.00	0.00	0.00	0.00	0.00	0.00
膀胱	C67	95	1.86	0.00	0.00	0.00	0.00	0.00	0.62	1.33	0.00
其他的泌尿器官	C68	10	0.20	0.00	0.00	0.00	0.00	0.00	0.00	0.00	0.00
眼	C69	4	0.08	0.00	0.00	0.00	0.00	0.00	0.00	0.00	0.00
脑、神经系统	C70–C72	115	2.25	0.00	0.00	0.00	0.95	0.85	0.62	0.66	1.65
甲状腺	C73	44	0.86	0.00	0.00	0.00	0.00	0.00	0.00	0.66	4.12
肾上腺	C74	4	0.08	0.00	0.00	0.00	0.00	0.00	0.00	0.00	0.00
其他的内分泌腺	C75	5	0.10	0.00	0.00	0.00	0.00	0.00	0.00	0.00	0.00
霍奇金病	C81	17	0.33	0.00	0.00	0.00	0.00	1.70	0.00	0.00	0.00
非霍奇金淋巴瘤	C82–C85;C96	36	0.71	0.00	0.00	0.00	0.00	0.00	0.62	0.00	0.00
免疫增生性疾病	C88	1	0.02	0.00	0.00	0.00	0.00	0.00	0.00	0.00	0.00
多发性骨髓瘤	C90	11	0.22	0.00	0.00	0.00	0.00	0.00	0.00	0.00	0.00
淋巴样白血病	C91	29	0.57	0.00	2.07	0.85	0.95	1.70	0.62	0.00	0.00
髓样白血病	C92–C94	39	0.76	0.00	0.00	2.56	0.00	1.70	0.62	1.33	1.65
白血病，未特指	C95	59	1.16	0.00	0.00	1.71	0.00	0.00	1.85	0.66	1.65
其他的或未指明部位的	O&U	85	1.67	0.00	0.00	1.71	1.90	0.00	0.62	0.66	4.12
骨髓增殖性疾病	MPD	2	0.04	0.00	0.00	0.00	0.00	0.00	0.00	0.00	0.00
骨髓增生异常综合征	MDS	4	0.08	0.00	0.00	0.00	0.00	0.00	0.00	0.66	0.00
合计	ALL	5 104	100.00	14.24	3.11	7.69	4.76	5.95	7.40	17.89	32.13
所有部位除外 C44	ALL but C44	5 083	99.59	14.24	3.11	7.69	4.76	5.95	7.40	17.23	32.13

2014 年男性发病主要指标 ($1/10^5$)

											粗率	世标率	累积率 (%)	
35–	40–	45–	50–	55–	60–	65–	70–	75–	80–	85–	($1/10^5$ 万)	($1/10^5$ 万)	0~64	0~74
0.00	0.00	0.00	0.00	0.00	0.00	2.02	0.00	0.00	0.00	0.00	0.06	0.06	0.00	0.01
0.68	0.00	0.68	1.81	2.01	1.37	2.02	0.00	0.00	0.00	0.00	0.46	0.37	0.03	0.04
0.00	0.00	2.05	1.81	2.01	1.37	10.12	2.71	7.54	17.18	0.00	1.14	1.04	0.05	0.11
0.68	0.00	0.68	3.62	1.00	2.74	0.00	0.00	11.31	8.59	21.72	0.85	0.73	0.05	0.05
0.00	0.00	0.00	0.00	0.00	0.00	0.00	0.00	0.00	0.00	0.00	0.00	0.00	0.00	0.00
0.00	0.00	0.00	0.00	1.00	2.74	2.02	0.00	3.77	0.00	21.72	0.34	0.36	0.02	0.03
1.36	1.25	2.05	0.90	6.02	4.11	6.07	8.13	7.54	0.00	21.72	1.59	1.36	0.09	0.16
0.00	0.00	0.00	0.90	0.00	1.37	2.02	2.71	3.77	8.59	0.00	0.34	0.30	0.01	0.04
0.00	0.00	0.00	0.00	0.00	4.11	0.00	0.00	0.00	8.59	0.00	0.23	0.21	0.02	0.02
2.72	3.13	18.48	39.80	91.29	176.71	259.09	314.43	320.59	695.76	456.13	41.66	37.25	1.66	4.53
3.40	13.77	23.95	59.70	75.24	194.52	269.21	330.70	414.88	609.86	673.33	46.32	41.60	1.86	4.86
0.00	0.00	1.37	1.81	3.01	5.48	8.10	2.71	3.77	25.77	0.00	1.14	0.98	0.06	0.11
0.00	5.01	2.74	12.66	22.07	28.77	36.43	73.19	98.06	240.51	152.04	10.07	8.73	0.36	0.91
1.36	6.26	3.42	18.09	30.10	39.73	60.72	65.05	94.29	163.20	238.92	11.78	10.54	0.50	1.13
0.00	0.00	0.68	0.00	0.00	0.00	2.02	2.71	7.54	8.59	0.00	0.34	0.27	0.00	0.03
12.22	21.29	30.79	59.70	96.30	120.55	198.36	176.19	214.98	360.76	499.57	36.65	32.10	1.75	3.62
0.68	1.25	0.68	2.71	5.02	13.70	8.10	8.13	26.40	34.36	65.16	2.50	2.26	0.12	0.20
0.68	0.63	4.11	5.43	10.03	13.70	34.41	37.95	45.26	60.13	86.88	5.01	4.52	0.17	0.53
0.68	0.63	0.00	1.81	0.00	0.00	0.00	5.42	3.77	0.00	0.00	0.40	0.31	0.02	0.04
0.00	0.00	0.68	1.81	5.02	1.37	8.10	16.26	18.86	25.77	0.00	1.54	1.27	0.04	0.17
8.83	14.40	45.17	78.69	155.49	273.98	390.66	604.47	837.29	1 056.52	1 064.29	77.62	68.51	2.92	7.90
0.68	0.00	0.68	1.81	2.01	6.85	4.05	5.42	7.54	17.18	86.88	1.37	1.41	0.06	0.11
0.68	2.50	2.05	1.81	5.02	4.11	14.17	10.84	15.09	0.00	21.72	2.16	1.88	0.10	0.22
0.00	0.00	0.00	0.90	1.00	0.00	4.05	0.00	3.77	0.00	0.00	0.28	0.24	0.01	0.03
0.00	1.25	0.00	2.71	2.01	2.74	6.07	2.71	18.86	8.59	21.72	1.20	1.03	0.05	0.09
0.00	0.00	0.00	0.90	0.00	0.00	0.00	0.00	0.00	0.00	0.00	0.06	0.05	0.00	0.00
0.00	0.00	0.00	0.00	0.00	0.00	0.00	0.00	0.00	0.00	0.00	0.00	0.00	0.00	0.00
0.00	1.25	2.05	0.90	0.00	2.74	0.00	2.71	11.31	0.00	0.00	0.74	0.57	0.04	0.05
—	—	—	—	—	—	—	—	—	—	—	—	—	—	—
—	—	—	—	—	—	—	—	—	—	—	—	—	—	—
—	—	—	—	—	—	—	—	—	—	—	—	—	—	—
—	—	—	—	—	—	—	—	—	—	—	—	—	—	—
—	—	—	—	—	—	—	—	—	—	—	—	—	—	—
—	—	—	—	—	—	—	—	—	—	—	—	—	—	—
—	—	—	—	—	—	—	—	—	—	—	—	—	—	—
—	—	—	—	—	—	—	—	—	—	—	—	—	—	—
—	—	—	—	—	—	—	—	—	—	—	—	—	—	—
0.00	0.00	0.68	0.00	1.00	0.00	4.05	0.00	11.31	0.00	0.00	0.40	0.32	0.01	0.03
0.00	0.00	0.00	2.71	3.01	8.22	20.24	51.50	90.52	240.51	238.92	5.92	5.52	0.07	0.43
0.00	1.25	0.00	0.90	0.00	0.00	2.02	0.00	3.77	8.59	0.00	0.57	0.47	0.02	0.03
0.00	0.00	0.00	0.00	0.00	0.00	0.00	0.00	3.77	0.00	0.00	0.06	0.04	0.00	0.00
0.68	1.88	2.05	9.04	9.03	17.81	18.22	29.82	15.09	25.77	21.72	4.04	3.69	0.22	0.46
0.00	0.63	0.00	1.81	1.00	1.37	2.02	5.42	0.00	8.59	0.00	0.51	0.44	0.02	0.06
0.68	0.00	0.00	1.81	0.00	4.11	0.00	2.71	3.77	0.00	21.72	0.51	0.50	0.03	0.05
0.68	1.88	2.74	4.52	7.02	20.55	14.17	40.66	79.20	77.31	108.60	5.41	4.76	0.20	0.47
0.00	0.00	0.00	0.90	1.00	4.11	2.02	0.00	11.31	8.59	0.00	0.57	0.47	0.03	0.04
0.00	0.00	0.00	0.90	1.00	0.00	0.00	0.00	0.00	8.59	21.72	0.23	0.24	0.01	0.01
4.75	5.63	8.90	13.57	10.03	20.55	20.24	16.26	37.72	85.90	86.88	6.54	5.60	0.34	0.52
0.68	5.01	4.79	2.71	9.03	6.85	2.02	5.42	7.54	0.00	0.00	2.50	1.94	0.17	0.21
0.00	0.00	0.00	0.00	1.00	0.00	0.00	2.71	3.77	8.59	0.00	0.23	0.18	0.01	0.02
0.00	0.00	0.00	0.00	1.00	1.37	2.02	5.42	0.00	0.00	0.00	0.28	0.26	0.01	0.05
0.00	0.00	0.68	0.90	2.01	0.00	4.05	5.42	18.86	0.00	43.44	0.97	0.96	0.03	0.07
0.00	1.88	1.37	1.81	7.02	1.37	4.05	16.26	26.40	25.77	43.44	2.05	1.73	0.07	0.17
0.00	0.00	0.00	0.00	0.00	0.00	0.00	0.00	3.77	0.00	0.00	0.06	0.04	0.00	0.00
0.00	0.00	1.37	0.90	0.00	1.37	2.02	2.71	11.31	8.59	21.72	0.63	0.56	0.02	0.04
0.68	0.63	1.37	1.81	2.01	5.48	10.12	5.42	11.31	0.00	0.00	1.65	1.65	0.09	0.17
0.68	1.25	2.74	2.71	5.02	4.11	6.07	13.55	11.31	0.00	0.00	2.22	2.01	0.12	0.22
2.72	3.76	0.68	2.71	7.02	9.59	6.07	16.26	26.40	60.13	0.00	3.36	2.77	0.16	0.27
1.36	2.50	2.05	4.52	11.03	15.07	28.34	24.40	30.17	42.95	43.44	4.84	4.39	0.23	0.49
0.00	0.63	0.00	0.90	0.00	0.00	0.00	0.00	0.00	0.00	0.00	0.11	0.08	0.01	0.01
0.00	0.00	0.00	0.00	1.00	0.00	0.00	5.42	0.00	0.00	0.00	0.23	0.20	0.01	0.04
47.54	100.17	173.13	358.17	595.88	1 024.67	1 477.61	1 921.83	2 587.31	3 976.98	4 126.85	290.47	257.44	11.90	28.90
47.54	98.92	173.13	355.46	593.88	1 021.93	1 471.54	1 919.12	2 568.45	3 968.39	4 105.13	289.27	256.41	11.86	28.81

表 6-1-6 河南省城市肿瘤登记地区

部位		病例数	构成(%)	年龄组 0–	1–	5–	10–	15–	20–	25–	30–
唇	C00	0	0.00	0.00	0.00	0.00	0.00	0.00	0.00	0.00	0.00
舌	C01–C02	15	0.39	0.00	0.00	0.00	0.00	0.00	0.00	0.69	0.00
口	C03–C06	17	0.44	0.00	0.00	0.00	0.00	0.00	0.64	0.00	0.00
唾液腺	C07–C08	11	0.28	0.00	0.00	0.00	0.00	0.00	0.00	1.38	1.65
扁桃体	C09	0	0.00	0.00	0.00	0.00	0.00	0.00	0.00	0.00	0.00
其他的口咽	C10	0	0.00	0.00	0.00	0.00	0.00	0.00	0.00	0.00	0.00
鼻咽	C11	14	0.36	0.00	0.00	0.00	0.00	0.00	0.00	0.00	0.83
喉咽	C12–C13	4	0.10	0.00	0.00	0.00	0.00	0.00	0.00	0.00	0.00
咽，部位不明	C14	4	0.10	0.00	0.00	0.00	0.00	0.00	0.00	0.00	0.00
食管	C15	389	10.06	0.00	0.00	0.00	0.00	0.00	0.00	0.69	0.00
胃	C16	320	8.28	0.00	0.00	0.00	0.00	0.00	0.00	1.38	1.65
小肠	C17	21	0.54	0.00	0.00	0.00	0.00	0.00	0.00	0.00	0.00
结肠	C18	141	3.65	0.00	0.00	0.00	1.12	0.00	0.00	0.00	0.00
直肠	C19–C20	164	4.24	0.00	0.00	0.00	0.00	0.00	0.00	2.08	0.00
肛门	C21	8	0.21	0.00	0.00	0.00	0.00	0.00	0.00	0.00	0.00
肝脏	C22	250	6.47	0.00	0.00	0.00	0.00	0.00	0.64	0.69	0.83
胆囊及其他	C23–C24	60	1.55	0.00	0.00	0.00	0.00	0.00	0.00	0.00	0.00
胰腺	C25	61	1.58	0.00	0.00	0.00	0.00	0.87	0.00	0.69	0.00
鼻、鼻窦及其他	C30–C31	4	0.10	0.00	0.00	0.00	0.00	0.00	0.00	0.00	0.00
喉	C32	5	0.13	0.00	0.00	0.00	0.00	0.00	0.00	0.00	0.00
气管、支气管、肺	C33–C34	540	13.97	0.00	0.00	0.00	0.00	0.00	0.00	0.69	2.48
其他的胸腔器官	C37–C38	13	0.34	0.00	0.00	0.00	0.00	0.00	0.00	0.00	0.00
骨	C40–C41	37	0.96	0.00	0.00	0.99	0.00	0.00	0.64	0.00	0.00
皮肤的黑色素瘤	C43	2	0.05	0.00	0.00	0.00	0.00	0.00	0.00	0.00	0.00
其他的皮肤	C44	23	0.60	0.00	0.00	0.00	0.00	0.00	0.00	0.00	0.83
间皮瘤	C45	2	0.05	0.00	0.00	0.00	0.00	0.00	0.00	0.00	0.00
卡波西肉瘤	C46	0	0.00	0.00	0.00	0.00	0.00	0.00	0.00	0.00	0.00
周围神经、其他结缔组织、软组织	C47;C49	8	0.21	0.00	0.00	0.00	0.00	0.00	0.00	0.69	0.00
乳房	C50	709	18.34	0.00	0.00	0.00	0.00	0.00	1.28	7.61	14.89
外阴	C51	2	0.05	0.00	0.00	0.00	0.00	0.00	0.00	0.00	0.00
阴道	C52	2	0.05	0.00	0.00	0.00	1.12	0.00	0.00	0.00	0.00
子宫颈	C53	267	6.91	0.00	0.00	0.00	0.00	0.00	0.00	2.08	11.58
子宫体	C54	108	2.79	0.00	0.00	0.00	0.00	0.00	0.00	0.00	0.83
子宫，部位不明	C55	27	0.70	0.00	0.00	0.00	0.00	0.00	0.64	0.00	0.83
卵巢	C56	112	2.90	0.00	0.00	0.00	0.00	0.00	0.64	1.38	3.31
其他的女性生殖器	C57	5	0.13	0.00	0.00	0.00	0.00	0.00	0.00	0.00	0.00
胎盘	C58	0	0.00	0.00	0.00	0.00	0.00	0.00	0.00	0.00	0.00
阴茎	C60	—	—	—	—	—	—	—	—	—	—
前列腺	C61	—	—	—	—	—	—	—	—	—	—
睾丸	C62	—	—	—	—	—	—	—	—	—	—
其他的男性生殖器	C63	—	—	—	—	—	—	—	—	—	—
肾	C64	34	0.88	0.00	1.20	0.00	0.00	0.00	0.00	0.00	0.00
肾盂	C65	5	0.13	0.00	0.00	0.00	0.00	0.00	0.00	0.00	0.00
输尿管	C66	7	0.18	0.00	0.00	0.00	0.00	0.00	0.00	0.00	0.00
膀胱	C67	37	0.96	0.00	0.00	0.00	0.00	0.00	0.00	0.69	0.00
其他的泌尿器官	C68	3	0.08	0.00	0.00	0.00	0.00	0.00	0.00	0.00	0.00
眼	C69	4	0.10	0.00	1.20	0.00	0.00	0.00	0.00	0.00	0.00
脑、神经系统	C70–C72	102	2.64	0.00	0.00	0.99	1.12	0.00	0.64	1.38	4.14
甲状腺	C73	121	3.13	0.00	0.00	0.00	0.00	1.74	1.92	5.53	8.27
肾上腺	C74	5	0.13	0.00	0.00	0.00	0.00	0.00	0.64	0.00	0.00
其他的内分泌腺	C75	6	0.16	0.00	0.00	0.00	0.00	0.00	0.00	0.00	0.00
霍奇金病	C81	10	0.26	0.00	0.00	0.99	0.00	0.00	0.00	0.69	0.00
非霍奇金淋巴瘤	C82–C85;C96	36	0.93	0.00	0.00	0.00	1.12	0.00	0.00	0.69	0.83
免疫增生性疾病	C88	0	0.00	0.00	0.00	0.00	0.00	0.00	0.00	0.00	0.00
多发性骨髓瘤	C90	8	0.21	0.00	0.00	0.00	0.00	0.00	0.00	0.00	0.00
淋巴样白血病	C91	22	0.57	0.00	2.40	0.99	2.25	0.00	0.00	0.00	0.00
髓样白血病	C92–C94	19	0.49	0.00	0.00	0.99	0.00	0.87	0.64	0.69	1.65
白血病，未特指	C95	42	1.09	5.28	2.40	0.00	2.25	0.00	0.00	0.69	0.83
其他的或未指明部位的	O&U	55	1.42	0.00	0.00	0.00	0.00	0.87	1.92	0.69	0.83
骨髓增殖性疾病	MPD	3	0.08	0.00	0.00	0.00	0.00	0.00	0.00	0.00	0.00
骨髓增生异常综合征	MDS	1	0.03	0.00	0.00	0.00	0.00	0.00	0.00	0.00	0.00
合计	ALL	3 865	100.00	5.28	7.19	4.96	9.00	4.34	10.23	31.13	56.24
所有部位除外 C44	ALL but C44	3 842	99.40	5.28	7.19	4.96	9.00	4.34	10.23	31.13	55.41

2014 年女性发病主要指标 (1/10^5)

											粗率	世标率	累积率 (%)	
35–	40–	45–	50–	55–	60–	65–	70–	75–	80–	85–	(1/10^5 万)	(1/10^5 万)	0~64	0~74
0.00	0.00	0.00	0.00	0.00	0.00	0.00	0.00	0.00	0.00	0.00	0.00	0.00	0.00	0.00
0.73	0.00	1.42	0.00	2.99	2.79	0.00	5.14	3.34	13.45	12.99	0.89	0.68	0.04	0.07
0.73	0.00	0.71	0.94	1.00	2.79	3.97	2.57	13.35	20.17	0.00	1.01	0.74	0.03	0.07
0.00	0.00	2.12	2.82	1.00	0.00	0.00	0.00	0.00	0.00	0.00	0.66	0.52	0.04	0.04
0.00	0.00	0.00	0.00	0.00	0.00	0.00	0.00	0.00	0.00	0.00	0.00	0.00	0.00	0.00
0.00	0.00	0.00	0.00	0.00	0.00	0.00	0.00	0.00	0.00	0.00	0.00	0.00	0.00	0.00
0.73	0.66	0.00	0.00	1.99	5.57	3.97	2.57	6.68	0.00	0.00	0.83	0.67	0.05	0.08
0.00	0.00	0.71	0.00	0.00	0.00	3.97	0.00	3.34	0.00	0.00	0.24	0.19	0.00	0.02
0.00	0.00	0.00	0.00	0.00	1.39	0.00	0.00	3.34	6.72	12.99	0.24	0.19	0.01	0.01
0.00	0.00	2.12	10.32	42.82	93.37	125.07	177.31	180.23	289.08	454.72	23.18	18.97	0.75	2.26
3.67	4.64	7.08	15.02	38.84	73.86	93.30	113.07	166.88	194.96	207.87	19.07	15.13	0.73	1.76
0.00	0.66	1.42	0.94	1.00	5.57	5.96	5.14	13.35	20.17	0.00	1.25	0.95	0.05	0.10
5.14	0.66	4.25	8.45	21.91	15.33	45.66	38.55	66.75	134.45	77.95	8.40	6.49	0.28	0.71
6.60	2.65	7.08	13.14	19.92	25.08	23.82	56.53	93.45	87.39	142.91	9.77	7.53	0.38	0.78
0.00	0.66	0.00	0.94	0.00	1.39	0.00	10.28	3.34	0.00	0.00	0.48	0.38	0.01	0.07
0.00	9.28	4.25	14.08	29.87	68.28	51.61	97.65	123.49	147.90	129.92	14.90	11.72	0.64	1.39
0.00	0.66	0.71	3.75	1.99	12.54	17.87	15.42	60.08	40.34	51.97	3.58	2.76	0.10	0.26
0.00	1.99	0.71	2.82	5.97	4.18	17.87	41.12	30.04	33.61	51.97	3.64	2.93	0.09	0.38
0.00	0.00	0.00	0.00	0.00	0.00	0.00	2.57	10.01	0.00	0.00	0.24	0.15	0.00	0.01
0.00	0.00	0.00	0.00	1.00	1.39	3.97	0.00	0.00	0.00	12.99	0.30	0.28	0.01	0.03
5.14	9.94	24.07	37.54	60.74	94.76	150.87	197.87	250.32	403.36	298.82	32.18	25.15	1.18	2.92
0.00	1.33	1.42	0.00	1.99	1.39	3.97	2.57	3.34	6.72	12.99	0.77	0.60	0.03	0.06
1.47	0.00	2.12	3.75	5.97	5.57	3.97	15.42	16.69	20.17	0.00	2.20	1.71	0.10	0.20
0.73	0.00	0.00	0.94	0.00	0.00	0.00	0.00	0.00	0.00	0.00	0.12	0.09	0.01	0.01
1.47	0.00	0.71	3.75	1.99	2.79	0.00	0.00	13.35	26.89	38.98	1.37	1.02	0.06	0.06
0.00	0.00	0.71	0.94	0.00	0.00	0.00	0.00	0.00	0.00	0.00	0.12	0.09	0.01	0.01
0.00	0.00	0.00	0.00	0.00	0.00	0.00	0.00	0.00	0.00	0.00	0.00	0.00	0.00	0.00
0.00	0.00	0.00	1.88	0.00	2.79	3.97	0.00	0.00	6.72	0.00	0.48	0.41	0.03	0.05
30.81	64.95	87.07	114.49	77.67	125.42	87.35	89.94	103.46	87.39	25.98	42.25	32.44	2.62	3.51
0.00	0.00	0.71	0.94	0.00	0.00	0.00	0.00	0.00	0.00	0.00	0.12	0.09	0.01	0.01
0.00	0.00	0.00	0.00	0.00	0.00	1.99	0.00	0.00	0.00	0.00	0.12	0.16	0.01	0.02
16.87	24.52	26.90	43.17	29.87	44.59	31.76	28.27	26.70	33.61	51.97	15.91	12.31	1.00	1.30
0.73	5.96	13.45	18.77	14.94	20.90	17.87	30.84	10.01	20.17	12.99	6.44	5.05	0.38	0.62
1.47	0.66	1.42	2.82	8.96	2.79	5.96	7.71	0.00	0.00	0.00	1.61	1.26	0.10	0.17
5.87	3.98	11.33	14.08	12.95	25.08	13.90	30.84	26.70	0.00	25.98	6.67	5.29	0.39	0.62
0.73	0.00	0.71	0.94	0.00	2.79	0.00	0.00	0.00	0.00	0.00	0.30	0.24	0.03	0.03
0.00	0.00	0.00	0.00	0.00	0.00	0.00	0.00	0.00	0.00	0.00	0.00	0.00	0.00	0.00
—	—	—	—	—	—	—	—	—	—	—	—	—	—	—
—	—	—	—	—	—	—	—	—	—	—	—	—	—	—
—	—	—	—	—	—	—	—	—	—	—	—	—	—	—
—	—	—	—	—	—	—	—	—	—	—	—	—	—	—
0.73	1.33	1.42	3.75	5.97	4.18	9.93	7.71	13.35	13.45	12.99	2.03	1.64	0.09	0.18
0.73	0.66	0.00	0.00	0.00	0.00	3.97	2.57	0.00	0.00	0.00	0.30	0.25	0.01	0.04
0.00	0.00	0.71	0.94	1.00	0.00	0.00	7.71	3.34	0.00	0.00	0.42	0.32	0.01	0.05
0.00	1.33	1.42	2.82	1.99	4.18	3.97	12.85	23.36	40.34	51.97	2.20	1.68	0.06	0.15
0.00	0.66	0.00	0.00	0.00	2.79	0.00	0.00	0.00	0.00	0.00	0.18	0.15	0.02	0.02
0.00	0.00	0.71	0.00	0.00	0.00	1.99	0.00	0.00	6.72	0.00	0.24	0.25	0.01	0.02
1.47	4.64	8.49	8.45	14.94	22.30	17.87	20.56	13.35	40.34	51.97	6.08	4.94	0.34	0.53
9.54	7.29	12.03	17.83	14.94	11.15	19.85	7.71	6.68	0.00	0.00	7.21	5.73	0.45	0.59
0.00	0.00	0.00	0.00	1.00	2.79	1.99	0.00	0.00	0.00	0.00	0.30	0.26	0.02	0.03
0.00	0.66	0.71	1.88	1.00	0.00	1.99	0.00	0.00	0.00	0.00	0.36	0.28	0.02	0.03
0.00	0.66	1.42	0.94	1.99	0.00	1.99	2.57	0.00	0.00	0.00	0.60	0.52	0.03	0.06
0.73	1.33	0.71	3.75	1.99	11.15	3.97	23.13	6.68	13.45	0.00	2.15	1.80	0.11	0.25
0.00	0.00	0.00	0.00	0.00	0.00	0.00	0.00	0.00	0.00	0.00	0.00	0.00	0.00	0.00
0.00	0.66	0.00	0.00	1.00	2.79	3.97	2.57	0.00	6.72	0.00	0.48	0.40	0.02	0.05
0.73	0.00	2.12	0.94	2.99	2.79	5.96	0.00	3.34	13.45	12.99	1.31	1.33	0.07	0.10
1.47	1.33	1.42	0.00	1.99	0.00	1.99	0.00	3.34	20.17	0.00	1.13	0.91	0.06	0.07
1.47	0.66	0.71	4.69	2.99	6.97	9.93	10.28	6.68	40.34	12.99	2.50	2.30	0.12	0.22
0.00	3.31	2.83	4.69	4.98	11.15	5.96	17.99	23.36	20.17	25.98	3.28	2.59	0.16	0.28
0.00	0.00	0.00	0.94	0.00	0.00	0.00	2.57	0.00	0.00	12.99	0.18	0.16	0.00	0.02
0.00	0.00	0.00	0.00	1.00	0.00	0.00	0.00	0.00	0.00	0.00	0.06	0.04	0.00	0.00
99.77	157.74	237.84	368.81	445.12	724.64	813.93	1 089.55	1 331.69	1 808.40	1 805.90	230.32	181.75	10.78	20.30
98.30	157.74	237.13	365.06	443.13	721.85	813.93	1 089.55	1 318.34	1 781.51	1 766.92	228.95	180.73	10.73	20.24

表 6-1-7 河南省农村肿瘤登记地区

部位		病例数	构成 (%)	年龄组							
				0–	1–	5–	10–	15–	20–	25–	30–
唇	C00	29	0.07	0.00	0.00	0.08	0.09	0.00	0.07	0.00	0.00
舌	C01–C02	66	0.15	0.00	0.20	0.00	0.00	0.00	0.00	0.07	0.15
口	C03–C06	108	0.24	0.00	0.10	0.00	0.09	0.00	0.07	0.00	0.23
唾液腺	C07–C08	83	0.19	0.00	0.00	0.00	0.18	0.08	0.07	0.00	0.39
扁桃体	C09	13	0.03	0.00	0.00	0.00	0.00	0.00	0.07	0.07	0.00
其他的口咽	C10	40	0.09	0.00	0.00	0.00	0.09	0.00	0.13	0.07	0.15
鼻咽	C11	231	0.52	0.00	0.00	0.08	0.18	0.00	0.20	0.78	0.85
喉咽	C12–C13	31	0.07	0.00	0.00	0.00	0.00	0.00	0.07	0.00	0.00
咽，部位不明	C14	34	0.08	0.00	0.00	0.00	0.00	0.00	0.00	0.00	0.00
食管	C15	6 889	15.58	0.00	0.00	0.00	0.00	0.00	0.20	0.26	1.08
胃	C16	7 140	16.14	0.00	0.00	0.17	0.00	0.24	0.72	1.77	3.09
小肠	C17	278	0.63	0.00	0.00	0.00	0.00	0.00	0.07	0.13	0.23
结肠	C18	1 177	2.66	0.00	0.00	0.00	0.00	0.00	0.39	0.65	0.93
直肠	C19–C20	1 442	3.26	0.00	0.00	0.00	0.00	0.00	0.13	0.59	1.47
肛门	C21	89	0.20	0.00	0.00	0.00	0.00	0.16	0.07	0.07	0.15
肝脏	C22	4 626	10.46	0.00	0.10	0.00	0.18	0.24	0.66	0.98	3.48
胆囊及其他	C23–C24	543	1.23	0.00	0.00	0.00	0.00	0.00	0.13	0.07	0.46
胰腺	C25	586	1.32	0.00	0.00	0.00	0.00	0.00	0.00	0.39	0.39
鼻、鼻窦及其他	C30–C31	64	0.14	0.00	0.00	0.08	0.09	0.00	0.00	0.13	0.15
喉	C32	275	0.62	0.00	0.10	0.00	0.00	0.00	0.00	0.13	0.08
气管、支气管、肺	C33–C34	8 256	18.67	0.00	0.00	0.00	0.00	0.24	0.52	1.18	3.71
其他的胸腔器官	C37–C38	107	0.24	0.00	0.10	0.08	0.00	0.08	0.00	0.20	0.15
骨	C40–C41	460	1.04	0.00	0.10	0.67	0.71	1.13	1.11	1.18	0.77
皮肤的黑色素瘤	C43	50	0.11	0.00	0.49	0.17	0.00	0.16	0.26	0.00	0.00
其他的皮肤	C44	201	0.45	0.00	0.00	0.00	0.00	0.48	0.07	0.33	0.15
间皮瘤	C45	6	0.01	0.00	0.00	0.00	0.00	0.00	0.00	0.07	0.00
卡波西肉瘤	C46	2	0.00	0.00	0.00	0.00	0.00	0.00	0.00	0.00	0.08
周围神经、其他结缔组织、软组织	C47;C49	68	0.15	0.00	0.20	0.08	0.18	0.16	0.13	0.07	0.08
乳房	C50	—	—	—	—	—	—	—	—	—	—
外阴	C51	—	—	—	—	—	—	—	—	—	—
阴道	C52	—	—	—	—	—	—	—	—	—	—
子宫颈	C53	—	—	—	—	—	—	—	—	—	—
子宫体	C54	—	—	—	—	—	—	—	—	—	—
子宫，部位不明	C55	—	—	—	—	—	—	—	—	—	—
卵巢	C56	—	—	—	—	—	—	—	—	—	—
其他的女性生殖器	C57	—	—	—	—	—	—	—	—	—	—
胎盘	C58	—	—	—	—	—	—	—	—	—	—
阴茎	C60	—	—	—	—	—	—	—	—	—	—
前列腺	C61	—	—	—	—	—	—	—	—	—	—
睾丸	C62	—	—	—	—	—	—	—	—	—	—
其他的男性生殖器	C63	—	—	—	—	—	—	—	—	—	—
肾	C64	298	0.67	0.46	0.39	0.08	0.27	0.08	0.39	0.13	0.15
肾盂	C65	42	0.09	0.00	0.00	0.00	0.09	0.00	0.00	0.00	0.00
输尿管	C66	27	0.06	0.00	0.00	0.00	0.00	0.00	0.00	0.00	0.08
膀胱	C67	440	0.99	0.00	0.00	0.08	0.09	0.00	0.07	0.20	0.23
其他的泌尿器官	C68	11	0.02	0.00	0.00	0.00	0.00	0.00	0.07	0.00	0.00
眼	C69	30	0.07	0.00	0.59	0.08	0.09	0.00	0.00	0.07	0.00
脑、神经系统	C70–C72	1 191	2.69	2.78	1.67	2.00	2.03	1.37	1.51	1.50	2.32
甲状腺	C73	636	1.44	0.00	0.10	0.08	0.18	0.40	1.25	1.83	2.55
肾上腺	C74	37	0.08	0.00	0.10	0.08	0.00	0.00	0.00	0.00	0.08
其他的内分泌腺	C75	48	0.11	0.00	0.00	0.00	0.00	0.08	0.07	0.20	0.15
霍奇金病	C81	72	0.16	0.00	0.00	0.00	0.00	0.08	0.26	0.39	0.39
非霍奇金淋巴瘤	C82–C85;C96	346	0.78	0.46	0.29	0.33	0.44	0.16	0.59	1.05	0.46
免疫增生性疾病	C88	1	0.00	0.00	0.00	0.00	0.00	0.00	0.00	0.00	0.00
多发性骨髓瘤	C90	96	0.22	0.00	0.00	0.08	0.00	0.00	0.00	0.00	0.15
淋巴样白血病	C91	128	0.29	0.46	0.98	1.08	0.44	0.81	0.46	0.26	0.54
髓样白血病	C92–C94	190	0.43	0.46	0.88	0.17	0.44	0.57	0.52	0.65	0.62
白血病，未特指	C95	550	1.24	1.39	3.44	2.91	2.83	1.78	1.77	1.64	1.70
其他的或未指明部位的	O&U	1 034	2.34	0.46	0.98	1.08	0.35	0.73	0.85	1.77	2.40
骨髓增殖性疾病	MPD	14	0.03	0.00	0.10	0.00	0.00	0.00	0.07	0.00	0.00
骨髓增生异常综合征	MDS	7	0.02	0.00	0.00	0.00	0.00	0.00	0.07	0.00	0.08
合计	ALL	44 231	100.00	6.48	11.00	9.74	9.55	10.18	16.98	25.64	44.10
所有部位除外 C44	ALL but C44	44 030	99.55	6.48	11.00	9.74	9.55	9.70	16.92	25.31	43.95

2014 年合计发病主要指标 ($1/10^5$)

											粗率	世标率	累积率 (%)	
35–	40–	45–	50–	55–	60–	65–	70–	75–	80–	85–	($1/10^5$ 万)	($1/10^5$ 万)	0~64	0~74
0.08	0.14	0.14	0.09	0.42	0.51	0.54	0.99	0.98	0.00	1.88	0.16	0.14	0.01	0.02
0.23	0.14	0.51	0.47	0.63	1.90	1.27	1.48	2.28	1.67	0.00	0.37	0.31	0.02	0.04
0.38	0.93	0.29	0.56	1.36	2.66	1.63	2.22	3.26	3.89	4.70	0.61	0.49	0.03	0.05
0.30	0.50	0.94	0.84	1.47	1.39	1.45	0.49	0.98	1.11	0.94	0.47	0.39	0.03	0.04
0.00	0.00	0.00	0.09	0.21	0.25	0.18	0.25	0.65	0.56	0.94	0.07	0.06	0.00	0.01
0.15	0.00	0.22	0.19	0.42	0.89	0.72	0.99	0.98	2.22	0.94	0.23	0.18	0.01	0.02
0.53	1.29	2.10	3.00	2.73	3.80	3.98	2.71	5.54	4.45	1.88	1.31	1.06	0.08	0.11
0.08	0.14	0.22	0.19	0.63	0.38	0.72	0.49	0.65	2.78	0.00	0.18	0.13	0.01	0.01
0.08	0.00	0.22	0.37	0.84	0.76	1.27	0.49	0.65	0.00	0.94	0.19	0.16	0.01	0.02
1.44	6.08	18.32	38.87	87.99	161.74	232.13	248.38	274.88	311.44	270.57	39.12	31.17	1.58	3.98
5.07	12.95	25.70	44.68	98.07	170.23	215.83	237.04	261.18	288.63	211.38	40.55	32.34	1.81	4.08
0.91	0.72	1.45	2.62	2.83	5.32	8.15	10.60	7.50	7.23	8.46	1.58	1.28	0.07	0.17
1.74	5.37	7.24	10.58	15.43	24.45	30.24	30.80	31.63	43.93	28.18	6.68	5.32	0.33	0.64
1.97	5.08	8.47	9.83	18.79	29.00	39.83	43.86	46.30	52.28	47.91	8.19	6.52	0.38	0.80
0.30	0.29	0.72	0.84	1.47	1.52	2.72	1.23	1.63	2.22	0.94	0.51	0.41	0.03	0.05
7.80	16.17	26.50	41.40	65.20	106.65	116.97	120.74	126.19	161.84	127.77	26.27	20.99	1.35	2.54
0.30	1.07	2.03	1.97	8.61	11.15	13.22	17.74	23.15	25.58	31.94	3.08	2.41	0.13	0.28
0.76	1.50	2.82	4.68	7.14	12.29	15.57	20.21	20.54	17.24	26.31	3.33	2.67	0.15	0.33
0.23	0.21	0.29	0.47	0.73	1.27	1.99	1.23	1.63	1.67	1.88	0.36	0.30	0.02	0.03
0.08	0.36	1.09	3.37	3.15	6.84	7.97	8.62	10.43	8.34	3.76	1.56	1.26	0.08	0.16
6.97	15.03	32.15	60.04	112.14	169.98	245.35	279.18	303.57	355.93	303.45	46.88	37.19	2.01	4.63
0.23	0.72	0.72	1.03	0.84	3.55	2.35	1.23	1.30	2.22	2.82	0.61	0.51	0.04	0.06
2.20	2.29	1.81	3.65	5.98	8.11	9.23	8.13	9.78	11.12	3.76	2.61	2.21	0.15	0.24
0.00	0.07	0.14	0.37	0.52	0.25	1.45	1.48	1.63	1.67	0.94	0.28	0.27	0.01	0.03
0.45	0.79	0.36	0.47	1.78	2.53	3.26	7.15	8.48	15.57	20.67	1.14	0.88	0.04	0.09
0.00	0.00	0.00	0.09	0.10	0.00	0.18	0.00	0.33	0.56	0.00	0.03	0.03	0.00	0.00
0.00	0.00	0.07	0.00	0.00	0.00	0.00	0.00	0.00	0.00	0.00	0.01	0.01	0.00	0.00
0.00	0.64	0.51	0.66	1.26	1.27	0.18	1.48	0.65	1.11	0.94	0.39	0.33	0.03	0.03
—	—	—	—	—	—	—	—	—	—	—	—	—	—	—
—	—	—	—	—	—	—	—	—	—	—	—	—	—	—
—	—	—	—	—	—	—	—	—	—	—	—	—	—	—
—	—	—	—	—	—	—	—	—	—	—	—	—	—	—
—	—	—	—	—	—	—	—	—	—	—	—	—	—	—
—	—	—	—	—	—	—	—	—	—	—	—	—	—	—
—	—	—	—	—	—	—	—	—	—	—	—	—	—	—
—	—	—	—	—	—	—	—	—	—	—	—	—	—	—
—	—	—	—	—	—	—	—	—	—	—	—	—	—	—
—	—	—	—	—	—	—	—	—	—	—	—	—	—	—
—	—	—	—	—	—	—	—	—	—	—	—	—	—	—
—	—	—	—	—	—	—	—	—	—	—	—	—	—	—
—	—	—	—	—	—	—	—	—	—	—	—	—	—	—
0.76	1.36	1.95	3.28	4.20	5.32	8.51	5.91	4.56	7.79	5.64	1.69	1.41	0.09	0.16
0.15	0.14	0.58	0.47	0.63	1.14	0.54	0.00	1.30	0.56	0.94	0.24	0.19	0.02	0.02
0.00	0.00	0.07	0.37	0.52	0.76	0.72	0.49	0.65	0.56	0.94	0.15	0.12	0.01	0.02
0.30	0.50	1.67	2.62	3.67	10.13	12.86	16.26	16.30	23.91	22.55	2.50	1.99	0.10	0.24
0.00	0.00	0.07	0.09	0.00	0.51	0.36	0.00	0.33	0.56	0.00	0.06	0.05	0.00	0.01
0.08	0.21	0.07	0.37	0.10	0.51	0.36	0.49	0.33	1.11	0.00	0.17	0.17	0.01	0.01
4.17	6.15	7.96	9.55	15.01	22.55	21.91	21.93	21.19	26.69	29.12	6.76	5.77	0.39	0.61
3.56	4.65	7.67	8.15	7.77	7.22	6.52	7.39	11.41	4.45	1.88	3.61	2.92	0.23	0.30
0.08	0.21	0.43	0.56	0.52	0.63	0.36	0.25	0.33	2.22	0.00	0.21	0.17	0.01	0.02
0.23	0.29	0.51	0.56	0.84	0.63	0.00	0.74	0.65	1.11	0.94	0.27	0.22	0.02	0.02
0.38	0.14	0.58	0.66	0.31	1.14	0.91	2.46	0.98	1.67	0.94	0.41	0.34	0.02	0.04
0.83	1.36	1.67	3.56	3.36	7.22	7.24	9.61	4.89	11.12	5.64	1.96	1.66	0.11	0.19
0.00	0.00	0.00	0.00	0.00	0.00	0.00	0.00	0.00	0.00	0.94	0.01	0.00	0.00	0.00
0.15	0.21	0.80	0.66	2.20	2.15	1.81	2.22	1.96	2.78	1.88	0.55	0.44	0.03	0.05
0.38	0.72	0.87	0.75	0.73	1.01	1.45	0.74	1.30	2.22	1.88	0.73	0.73	0.04	0.06
0.91	1.14	1.52	0.94	1.68	2.66	2.90	1.72	3.59	4.45	1.88	1.08	0.96	0.06	0.09
1.67	2.79	2.53	3.65	4.51	6.33	8.69	6.41	8.48	7.23	7.52	3.12	3.03	0.19	0.26
2.50	3.72	6.01	8.24	11.65	20.39	22.27	24.89	34.56	28.36	15.97	5.87	4.83	0.30	0.54
0.00	0.14	0.07	0.28	0.10	0.51	0.18	0.00	0.00	0.00	0.00	0.08	0.07	0.01	0.01
0.00	0.00	0.14	0.00	0.10	0.13	0.00	0.00	0.00	0.56	0.00	0.04	0.03	0.00	0.00
75.06	148.40	240.15	351.79	583.47	926.26	1 147.06	1 225.62	1 331.02	1 542.17	1 278.62	251.18	202.16	12.26	24.12
74.60	147.61	239.79	351.32	581.68	923.72	1 143.80	1 218.47	1 322.54	1 526.59	1 257.95	250.03	201.28	12.22	24.03

表 6-1-8 河南省农村肿瘤登记地区

部位		病例数	构成(%)	年龄组							
				0–	1–	5–	10–	15–	20–	25–	30–
唇	C00	17	0.07	0.00	0.00	0.15	0.16	0.00	0.13	0.00	0.00
舌	C01–C02	33	0.13	0.00	0.18	0.00	0.00	0.00	0.00	0.00	0.30
口	C03–C06	58	0.24	0.00	0.18	0.00	0.16	0.00	0.00	0.00	0.15
唾液腺	C07–C08	39	0.16	0.00	0.00	0.00	0.16	0.00	0.13	0.00	0.45
扁桃体	C09	7	0.03	0.00	0.00	0.00	0.00	0.00	0.00	0.00	0.00
其他的口咽	C10	29	0.12	0.00	0.00	0.00	0.16	0.00	0.25	0.00	0.00
鼻咽	C11	148	0.60	0.00	0.00	0.00	0.33	0.00	0.25	1.02	0.60
喉咽	C12–C13	26	0.11	0.00	0.00	0.00	0.00	0.00	0.13	0.00	0.00
咽，部位不明	C14	28	0.11	0.00	0.00	0.00	0.00	0.00	0.00	0.00	0.00
食管	C15	4 236	17.23	0.00	0.00	0.00	0.00	0.00	0.25	0.13	0.60
胃	C16	5 104	20.76	0.00	0.00	0.31	0.00	0.31	0.13	1.79	2.85
小肠	C17	173	0.70	0.00	0.00	0.00	0.00	0.00	0.13	0.00	0.00
结肠	C18	639	2.60	0.00	0.00	0.00	0.00	0.00	0.38	1.28	1.35
直肠	C19–C20	751	3.06	0.00	0.00	0.00	0.00	0.00	0.25	0.38	1.50
肛门	C21	48	0.20	0.00	0.00	0.00	0.00	0.15	0.00	0.00	0.30
肝脏	C22	3 152	12.82	0.00	0.00	0.00	0.33	0.46	0.63	1.02	4.64
胆囊及其他	C23–C24	228	0.93	0.00	0.00	0.00	0.00	0.00	0.13	0.13	0.45
胰腺	C25	336	1.37	0.00	0.00	0.00	0.00	0.00	0.00	0.51	0.45
鼻、鼻窦及其他	C30–C31	37	0.15	0.00	0.00	0.00	0.16	0.00	0.00	0.26	0.30
喉	C32	200	0.81	0.00	0.18	0.00	0.00	0.00	0.00	0.13	0.00
气管、支气管、肺	C33–C34	5 676	23.09	0.00	0.00	0.00	0.00	0.31	0.63	1.02	3.74
其他的胸腔器官	C37–C38	55	0.22	0.00	0.00	0.15	0.00	0.15	0.00	0.13	0.15
骨	C40–C41	265	1.08	0.00	0.18	1.08	1.14	1.08	0.76	1.28	0.90
皮肤的黑色素瘤	C43	22	0.09	0.00	0.36	0.15	0.00	0.15	0.25	0.00	0.00
其他的皮肤	C44	101	0.41	0.00	0.00	0.00	0.00	0.15	0.13	0.38	0.30
间皮瘤	C45	5	0.02	0.00	0.00	0.00	0.00	0.00	0.00	0.00	0.00
卡波西肉瘤	C46	1	0.00	0.00	0.00	0.00	0.00	0.00	0.00	0.00	0.00
周围神经、其他结缔组织、软组织	C47;C49	37	0.15	0.00	0.18	0.00	0.16	0.00	0.00	0.00	0.00
乳房	C50	—	—	—	—	—	—	—	—	—	—
外阴	C51	—	—	—	—	—	—	—	—	—	—
阴道	C52	—	—	—	—	—	—	—	—	—	—
子宫颈	C53	—	—	—	—	—	—	—	—	—	—
子宫体	C54	—	—	—	—	—	—	—	—	—	—
子宫，部位不明	C55	—	—	—	—	—	—	—	—	—	—
卵巢	C56	—	—	—	—	—	—	—	—	—	—
其他的女性生殖器	C57	—	—	—	—	—	—	—	—	—	—
胎盘	C58	—	—	—	—	—	—	—	—	—	—
阴茎	C60	50	0.20	0.00	0.00	0.00	0.16	0.00	0.00	0.00	0.15
前列腺	C61	236	0.96	0.00	0.00	0.15	0.00	0.15	0.00	0.13	0.15
睾丸	C62	33	0.13	0.00	0.18	0.00	0.00	0.15	0.25	0.38	0.30
其他的男性生殖器	C63	8	0.03	0.00	0.00	0.00	0.00	0.31	0.00	0.13	0.00
肾	C64	187	0.76	0.87	0.36	0.00	0.49	0.00	0.38	0.00	0.15
肾盂	C65	23	0.09	0.00	0.00	0.00	0.16	0.00	0.00	0.00	0.00
输尿管	C66	19	0.08	0.00	0.00	0.00	0.00	0.00	0.00	0.00	0.15
膀胱	C67	336	1.37	0.00	0.00	0.15	0.00	0.00	0.00	0.26	0.15
其他的泌尿器官	C68	4	0.02	0.00	0.00	0.00	0.00	0.00	0.00	0.00	0.00
眼	C69	22	0.09	0.00	0.90	0.15	0.16	0.00	0.00	0.00	0.00
脑、神经系统	C70–C72	590	2.40	3.48	1.80	2.63	2.61	1.39	1.65	1.28	2.25
甲状腺	C73	164	0.67	0.00	0.18	0.00	0.00	0.15	0.76	0.64	0.90
肾上腺	C74	30	0.12	0.00	0.18	0.15	0.00	0.00	0.00	0.00	0.15
其他的内分泌腺	C75	20	0.08	0.00	0.00	0.00	0.00	0.00	0.13	0.13	0.00
霍奇金病	C81	38	0.15	0.00	0.00	0.00	0.00	0.15	0.25	0.38	0.75
非霍奇金淋巴瘤	C82–C85;C96	196	0.80	0.00	0.54	0.62	0.49	0.31	0.51	1.40	0.45
免疫增生性疾病	C88	0	0.00	0.00	0.00	0.00	0.00	0.00	0.00	0.00	0.00
多发性骨髓瘤	C90	60	0.24	0.00	0.00	0.00	0.00	0.00	0.00	0.00	0.15
淋巴样白血病	C91	62	0.25	0.00	0.54	1.39	0.65	1.08	0.25	0.26	0.90
髓样白血病	C92–C94	119	0.48	0.00	1.26	0.15	0.49	0.77	0.38	0.51	0.75
白血病，未特指	C95	303	1.23	0.87	3.41	3.71	2.61	2.16	2.16	1.91	1.35
其他的或未指明部位的	O&U	589	2.40	0.87	0.90	1.55	0.33	0.62	1.27	2.17	2.10
骨髓增殖性疾病	MPD	4	0.02	0.00	0.00	0.00	0.00	0.00	0.00	0.00	0.00
骨髓增生异常综合征	MDS	3	0.01	0.00	0.00	0.00	0.00	0.00	0.00	0.00	0.00
合计	ALL	24 580	100.00	6.08	11.49	12.54	10.94	10.04	12.56	19.02	29.81
所有部位除外 C44	ALL but C44	24 479	99.59	6.08	11.49	12.54	10.94	9.89	12.43	18.63	29.51

2014 年男性发病主要指标 (1/10^5)

											粗率	世标率	累积率 (%)	
35–	40–	45–	50–	55–	60–	65–	70–	75–	80–	85–	(1/10^5 万)	(1/10^5 万)	0~64	0~74
0.14	0.00	0.29	0.00	0.62	0.25	1.08	1.49	0.00	0.00	2.74	0.19	0.18	0.01	0.02
0.00	0.14	0.43	0.37	0.82	2.00	0.72	2.49	2.10	2.60	0.00	0.36	0.31	0.02	0.04
0.43	1.24	0.29	0.55	1.03	2.75	1.45	3.48	4.90	3.90	2.74	0.64	0.53	0.03	0.06
0.00	0.41	0.86	0.55	1.44	1.75	1.81	0.00	1.40	1.30	0.00	0.43	0.36	0.03	0.04
0.00	0.00	0.00	0.00	0.21	0.50	0.36	0.00	0.70	1.30	2.74	0.08	0.07	0.00	0.01
0.29	0.00	0.29	0.37	0.41	1.50	1.08	1.49	0.70	5.20	2.74	0.32	0.27	0.02	0.03
1.01	1.38	3.29	3.87	2.87	3.99	6.14	3.48	9.79	2.60	2.74	1.63	1.36	0.09	0.14
0.14	0.00	0.43	0.37	1.23	0.75	1.08	0.99	0.70	5.20	0.00	0.29	0.23	0.02	0.03
0.14	0.00	0.14	0.74	1.64	1.25	1.81	0.99	1.40	0.00	0.00	0.31	0.26	0.02	0.03
1.45	6.63	24.04	48.46	111.43	204.18	285.09	315.36	340.02	412.49	419.27	46.58	39.46	1.99	4.99
5.65	16.02	35.20	66.34	142.83	247.36	328.09	355.65	377.10	439.81	323.36	56.12	47.26	2.59	6.01
1.01	0.69	2.72	3.13	3.69	6.24	9.39	14.42	9.79	11.71	8.22	1.90	1.60	0.09	0.21
2.46	4.83	8.59	10.87	16.83	25.21	33.60	33.82	35.68	54.65	24.66	7.03	5.83	0.36	0.70
2.46	5.52	7.87	9.77	19.91	31.20	41.91	51.23	48.27	55.95	49.33	8.26	6.92	0.39	0.86
0.29	0.28	0.72	1.11	1.23	2.25	2.89	1.49	1.40	1.30	2.74	0.53	0.45	0.03	0.05
11.89	24.86	41.78	62.65	87.63	147.27	162.24	151.21	166.51	186.07	158.94	34.66	29.00	1.92	3.48
0.58	0.69	1.14	1.29	6.98	9.24	11.20	21.39	16.09	26.02	30.14	2.51	2.11	0.10	0.27
1.01	1.80	2.72	5.16	8.82	14.48	19.87	22.38	20.99	24.72	32.88	3.69	3.13	0.17	0.39
0.29	0.28	0.29	0.55	1.03	1.25	2.17	1.49	0.70	2.60	2.74	0.41	0.35	0.02	0.04
0.00	0.55	1.57	5.34	4.51	9.98	11.20	12.44	16.09	14.31	5.48	2.20	1.85	0.11	0.23
8.12	21.13	42.21	74.26	154.94	234.13	361.34	407.87	455.45	502.27	490.52	62.41	52.46	2.70	6.55
0.43	0.55	0.57	0.74	1.23	3.99	2.53	1.49	0.70	2.60	2.74	0.60	0.53	0.04	0.06
2.75	2.90	1.72	4.24	6.98	7.74	12.65	8.95	10.49	13.01	8.22	2.91	2.56	0.16	0.27
0.00	0.14	0.00	0.37	0.82	0.25	1.08	1.49	1.40	0.00	0.00	0.24	0.23	0.01	0.03
0.29	0.69	0.43	0.37	1.64	3.00	2.89	8.46	12.59	14.31	21.92	1.11	0.92	0.04	0.09
0.00	0.00	0.00	0.18	0.21	0.00	0.36	0.00	0.70	1.30	0.00	0.05	0.04	0.00	0.00
0.00	0.00	0.14	0.00	0.00	0.00	0.00	0.00	0.00	0.00	0.00	0.01	0.01	0.00	0.00
0.00	1.10	0.72	0.74	1.03	1.25	0.36	1.49	0.70	2.60	2.74	0.41	0.34	0.03	0.03
—	—	—	—	—	—	—	—	—	—	—	—	—	—	—
—	—	—	—	—	—	—	—	—	—	—	—	—	—	—
—	—	—	—	—	—	—	—	—	—	—	—	—	—	—
—	—	—	—	—	—	—	—	—	—	—	—	—	—	—
—	—	—	—	—	—	—	—	—	—	—	—	—	—	—
—	—	—	—	—	—	—	—	—	—	—	—	—	—	—
—	—	—	—	—	—	—	—	—	—	—	—	—	—	—
—	—	—	—	—	—	—	—	—	—	—	—	—	—	—
—	—	—	—	—	—	—	—	—	—	—	—	—	—	—
0.43	0.28	0.00	0.37	1.23	2.50	3.97	0.99	4.20	6.51	2.74	0.55	0.46	0.03	0.05
0.43	0.14	0.86	0.74	2.67	6.99	13.73	20.39	27.98	53.35	46.59	2.60	2.16	0.06	0.23
0.00	0.55	0.57	0.55	0.21	0.75	0.36	1.49	1.40	3.90	0.00	0.36	0.31	0.02	0.03
0.00	0.00	0.00	0.18	0.41	0.00	0.72	0.00	0.00	0.00	0.00	0.09	0.09	0.01	0.01
0.87	1.80	2.00	4.05	5.34	6.49	10.84	9.45	5.60	13.01	8.22	2.06	1.77	0.11	0.21
0.14	0.28	0.43	0.74	0.00	1.50	1.08	0.00	0.70	1.30	2.74	0.25	0.22	0.02	0.02
0.00	0.00	0.14	0.00	1.03	1.25	0.72	0.50	1.40	1.30	2.74	0.21	0.17	0.01	0.02
0.43	0.97	2.43	3.50	4.93	17.22	20.60	25.87	26.59	36.43	49.33	3.69	3.17	0.15	0.38
0.00	0.00	0.00	0.00	0.00	0.75	0.36	0.00	0.00	0.00	0.00	0.04	0.04	0.00	0.01
0.14	0.28	0.14	0.55	0.21	0.75	0.36	0.99	0.00	1.30	0.00	0.24	0.26	0.02	0.02
4.06	5.66	8.73	8.48	15.19	20.72	19.51	21.89	23.79	23.42	35.62	6.49	5.77	0.38	0.59
1.74	1.80	2.00	3.50	4.31	4.99	3.61	8.46	9.10	5.20	5.48	1.80	1.50	0.10	0.17
0.14	0.28	0.43	0.92	0.82	1.25	0.72	0.50	0.00	5.20	0.00	0.33	0.28	0.02	0.03
0.14	0.00	1.00	0.37	0.82	0.25	0.00	0.50	0.70	1.30	0.00	0.22	0.17	0.01	0.02
0.29	0.00	0.72	0.18	0.21	1.50	0.72	2.98	1.40	1.30	2.74	0.42	0.36	0.02	0.04
1.01	1.38	2.00	3.69	3.28	7.24	7.95	12.44	8.40	9.11	10.96	2.16	1.91	0.11	0.22
0.00	0.00	0.00	0.00	0.00	0.00	0.00	0.00	0.00	0.00	0.00	0.00	0.00	0.00	0.00
0.00	0.41	1.29	0.37	3.08	3.24	1.45	1.49	2.80	5.20	5.48	0.66	0.54	0.04	0.06
0.29	0.69	0.43	0.74	0.62	0.75	0.72	0.99	0.70	3.90	2.74	0.68	0.70	0.04	0.05
1.30	1.52	2.00	1.66	1.85	3.49	3.25	2.98	2.80	5.20	5.48	1.31	1.20	0.08	0.11
2.17	2.90	3.00	3.87	3.28	7.24	9.03	7.46	10.49	7.81	10.96	3.33	3.28	0.20	0.28
2.32	4.01	6.15	9.21	12.31	21.22	27.82	34.82	44.08	28.63	30.14	6.48	5.56	0.32	0.63
0.00	0.00	0.14	0.18	0.21	0.25	0.00	0.00	0.00	0.00	0.00	0.04	0.04	0.00	0.00
0.00	0.00	0.00	0.00	0.21	0.25	0.00	0.00	0.00	1.30	0.00	0.03	0.02	0.00	0.00
57.11	114.91	213.34	346.44	645.42	1 075.04	1 435.23	1 580.76	1 709.18	2 006.48	1 822.32	270.28	228.89	12.79	27.87
56.82	114.22	212.91	346.07	643.78	1 072.05	1 432.33	1 572.30	1 696.59	1 992.17	1 800.39	269.17	227.97	12.75	27.77

表 6-1-9 河南省农村肿瘤登记地区

部位		病例数	构成 (%)	年龄组							
				0-	1-	5-	10-	15-	20-	25-	30-
唇	C00	12	0.06	0.00	0.00	0.00	0.00	0.00	0.00	0.00	0.00
舌	C01–C02	33	0.17	0.00	0.22	0.00	0.00	0.00	0.00	0.13	0.00
口	C03–C06	50	0.25	0.00	0.00	0.00	0.00	0.00	0.14	0.00	0.32
唾液腺	C07–C08	44	0.22	0.00	0.00	0.00	0.19	0.17	0.00	0.00	0.32
扁桃体	C09	6	0.03	0.00	0.00	0.00	0.00	0.00	0.14	0.13	0.00
其他的口咽	C10	11	0.06	0.00	0.00	0.00	0.00	0.00	0.00	0.13	0.32
鼻咽	C11	83	0.42	0.00	0.00	0.18	0.00	0.00	0.14	0.54	1.12
喉咽	C12–C13	5	0.03	0.00	0.00	0.00	0.00	0.00	0.00	0.00	0.00
咽，部位不明	C14	6	0.03	0.00	0.00	0.00	0.00	0.00	0.00	0.00	0.00
食管	C15	2 653	13.50	0.00	0.00	0.00	0.00	0.00	0.14	0.40	1.60
胃	C16	2 036	10.36	0.00	0.00	0.00	0.00	0.17	1.36	1.74	3.36
小肠	C17	105	0.53	0.00	0.00	0.00	0.00	0.00	0.00	0.27	0.48
结肠	C18	538	2.74	0.00	0.00	0.00	0.00	0.00	0.41	0.00	0.48
直肠	C19–C20	691	3.52	0.00	0.00	0.00	0.00	0.00	0.00	0.80	1.44
肛门	C21	41	0.21	0.00	0.00	0.00	0.00	0.17	0.14	0.13	0.00
肝脏	C22	1 474	7.50	0.00	0.22	0.00	0.00	0.00	0.68	0.94	2.24
胆囊及其他	C23–C24	315	1.60	0.00	0.00	0.00	0.00	0.00	0.14	0.00	0.48
胰腺	C25	250	1.27	0.00	0.00	0.00	0.00	0.00	0.00	0.27	0.32
鼻、鼻窦及其他	C30–C31	27	0.14	0.00	0.00	0.18	0.00	0.00	0.00	0.00	0.00
喉	C32	75	0.38	0.00	0.00	0.00	0.00	0.00	0.00	0.13	0.16
气管、支气管、肺	C33–C34	2 580	13.13	0.00	0.00	0.00	0.00	0.17	0.41	1.34	3.68
其他的胸腔器官	C37–C38	52	0.26	0.00	0.22	0.00	0.00	0.00	0.00	0.27	0.16
骨	C40–C41	195	0.99	0.00	0.00	0.18	0.19	1.19	1.49	1.07	0.64
皮肤的黑色素瘤	C43	28	0.14	0.00	0.65	0.18	0.00	0.17	0.27	0.00	0.00
其他的皮肤	C44	100	0.51	0.00	0.00	0.00	0.00	0.85	0.00	0.27	0.00
间皮瘤	C45	1	0.01	0.00	0.00	0.00	0.00	0.00	0.00	0.13	0.00
卡波西肉瘤	C46	1	0.01	0.00	0.00	0.00	0.00	0.00	0.00	0.00	0.16
周围神经、其他结缔组织、软组织	C47;C49	31	0.16	0.00	0.22	0.18	0.19	0.34	0.27	0.13	0.16
乳房	C50	3 000	15.27	0.00	0.00	0.00	0.00	0.51	4.07	7.51	14.24
外阴	C51	23	0.12	0.00	0.00	0.00	0.00	0.00	0.14	0.00	0.00
阴道	C52	19	0.10	0.00	0.00	0.00	0.00	0.00	0.00	0.00	0.00
子宫颈	C53	1473	7.50	0.00	0.00	0.00	0.00	0.00	0.54	2.15	10.40
子宫体	C54	565	2.88	0.00	0.00	0.00	0.00	0.00	0.27	1.07	0.80
子宫，部位不明	C55	144	0.73	0.00	0.00	0.00	0.00	0.00	0.27	0.13	0.48
卵巢	C56	524	2.67	0.00	0.00	0.36	0.96	1.19	2.31	2.15	1.92
其他的女性生殖器	C57	22	0.11	0.00	0.00	0.00	0.00	0.00	0.14	0.00	0.32
胎盘	C58	9	0.05	0.00	0.00	0.00	0.00	0.00	0.14	0.27	0.00
阴茎	C60	—	—	—	—	—	—	—	—	—	—
前列腺	C61	—	—	—	—	—	—	—	—	—	—
睾丸	C62	—	—	—	—	—	—	—	—	—	—
其他的男性生殖器	C63	—	—	—	—	—	—	—	—	—	—
肾	C64	111	0.56	0.00	0.43	0.18	0.00	0.17	0.41	0.27	0.16
肾盂	C65	19	0.10	0.00	0.00	0.00	0.00	0.00	0.00	0.00	0.00
输尿管	C66	8	0.04	0.00	0.00	0.00	0.00	0.00	0.00	0.00	0.00
膀胱	C67	104	0.53	0.00	0.00	0.00	0.19	0.00	0.14	0.13	0.32
其他的泌尿器官	C68	7	0.04	0.00	0.00	0.00	0.00	0.00	0.14	0.00	0.00
眼	C69	8	0.04	0.00	0.22	0.00	0.00	0.00	0.00	0.13	0.00
脑、神经系统	C70–C72	601	3.06	1.98	1.52	1.26	1.35	1.36	1.36	1.74	2.40
甲状腺	C73	472	2.40	0.00	0.00	0.18	0.39	0.68	1.76	3.08	4.32
肾上腺	C74	7	0.04	0.00	0.00	0.00	0.00	0.00	0.00	0.00	0.00
其他的内分泌腺	C75	28	0.14	0.00	0.00	0.00	0.00	0.17	0.00	0.27	0.32
霍奇金病	C81	34	0.17	0.00	0.00	0.00	0.00	0.00	0.27	0.40	0.00
非霍奇金淋巴瘤	C82–C85;C96	150	0.76	0.99	0.00	0.00	0.39	0.00	0.68	0.67	0.48
免疫增生性疾病	C88	1	0.01	0.00	0.00	0.00	0.00	0.00	0.00	0.00	0.00
多发性骨髓瘤	C90	36	0.18	0.00	0.00	0.18	0.00	0.00	0.00	0.00	0.16
淋巴样白血病	C91	66	0.34	0.99	1.52	0.72	0.19	0.51	0.68	0.27	0.16
髓样白血病	C92–C94	71	0.36	0.99	0.43	0.18	0.39	0.34	0.68	0.80	0.48
白血病，未特指	C95	247	1.26	1.98	3.47	1.98	3.09	1.36	1.36	1.34	2.08
其他的或未指明部位的	O&U	445	2.26	0.00	1.08	0.54	0.39	0.85	0.41	1.34	2.72
骨髓增殖性疾病	MPD	10	0.05	0.00	0.22	0.00	0.00	0.00	0.14	0.00	0.00
骨髓增生异常综合征	MDS	4	0.02	0.00	0.00	0.00	0.00	0.00	0.14	0.00	0.16
合计	ALL	19 651	100.00	6.93	10.40	6.49	7.91	10.33	21.71	32.59	59.37
所有部位除外 C44	ALL but C44	19 551	99.49	6.93	10.40	6.49	7.91	9.49	21.71	32.32	59.37

2014 年女性发病主要指标 ($1/10^5$)

											粗率	世标率	累积率 (%)	
35–	40–	45–	50–	55–	60–	65–	70–	75–	80–	85–	($1/10^5$ 万)	($1/10^5$ 万)	0~64	0~74
0.00	0.30	0.00	0.19	0.21	0.77	0.00	0.49	1.83	0.00	1.43	0.14	0.10	0.01	0.01
0.48	0.15	0.59	0.57	0.43	1.80	1.81	0.49	2.44	0.97	0.00	0.39	0.32	0.02	0.03
0.32	0.59	0.29	0.57	1.72	2.57	1.81	0.98	1.83	3.88	5.72	0.59	0.44	0.03	0.05
0.63	0.59	1.03	1.14	1.50	1.03	1.09	0.98	0.61	0.97	1.43	0.52	0.42	0.03	0.04
0.00	0.00	0.00	0.19	0.21	0.00	0.00	0.49	0.61	0.00	0.00	0.07	0.06	0.00	0.01
0.00	0.00	0.15	0.00	0.43	0.26	0.36	0.49	1.22	0.00	0.00	0.13	0.10	0.01	0.01
0.00	1.19	0.88	2.10	2.58	3.60	1.81	1.95	1.83	5.83	1.43	0.97	0.76	0.06	0.08
0.00	0.30	0.00	0.00	0.00	0.00	0.36	0.00	0.61	0.97	0.00	0.06	0.04	0.00	0.00
0.00	0.00	0.29	0.00	0.00	0.26	0.73	0.00	0.00	0.00	1.43	0.07	0.06	0.00	0.01
1.43	5.49	12.46	28.95	63.42	118.03	178.93	182.62	218.02	236.01	192.99	31.16	23.35	1.16	2.97
4.44	9.65	15.97	22.29	51.17	90.77	103.07	120.61	160.00	175.79	152.96	23.91	17.81	1.00	2.12
0.79	0.74	0.15	2.10	1.93	4.37	6.90	6.84	5.50	3.88	8.58	1.23	0.97	0.05	0.12
0.95	5.94	5.86	10.29	13.97	23.66	26.86	27.83	28.09	35.94	30.02	6.32	4.82	0.31	0.58
1.43	4.60	9.09	9.90	17.63	26.74	37.75	36.62	44.58	49.53	47.18	8.11	6.12	0.36	0.73
0.32	0.30	0.73	0.57	1.72	0.77	2.54	0.98	1.83	2.91	0.00	0.48	0.37	0.02	0.04
3.33	6.83	10.85	19.43	41.71	64.80	71.50	90.82	90.99	143.74	111.51	17.31	12.92	0.75	1.57
0.00	1.48	2.93	2.67	10.32	13.11	15.24	14.16	29.31	25.25	32.88	3.70	2.70	0.16	0.30
0.48	1.19	2.93	4.19	5.37	10.03	11.25	18.07	20.15	11.65	22.87	2.94	2.22	0.12	0.27
0.16	0.15	0.29	0.38	0.43	1.29	1.81	0.98	2.44	0.97	1.43	0.32	0.25	0.01	0.03
0.16	0.15	0.59	1.33	1.72	3.60	4.72	4.88	5.50	3.88	2.86	0.88	0.68	0.04	0.09
5.71	8.46	21.84	45.33	67.29	103.89	128.84	152.84	170.99	246.70	205.86	30.30	22.55	1.29	2.70
0.00	0.89	0.88	1.33	0.43	3.09	2.18	0.98	1.83	1.94	2.86	0.61	0.49	0.04	0.05
1.59	1.63	1.91	3.05	4.94	8.49	5.81	7.32	9.16	9.71	1.43	2.29	1.85	0.13	0.20
0.00	0.00	0.29	0.38	0.21	0.26	1.81	1.46	1.83	2.91	1.43	0.33	0.30	0.01	0.03
0.63	0.89	0.29	0.57	1.93	2.06	3.63	5.86	4.89	16.51	20.01	1.17	0.85	0.04	0.08
0.00	0.00	0.00	0.00	0.00	0.00	0.00	0.00	0.00	0.00	0.00	0.01	0.01	0.00	0.00
0.00	0.00	0.00	0.00	0.00	0.00	0.00	0.00	0.00	0.00	0.00	0.01	0.01	0.00	0.00
0.00	0.15	0.29	0.57	1.50	1.29	0.00	1.46	0.61	0.00	0.00	0.36	0.33	0.03	0.03
29.34	61.46	77.97	75.43	87.72	103.37	74.76	63.48	47.02	44.68	37.17	35.23	27.76	2.31	3.00
0.16	0.45	0.15	0.19	0.86	0.51	1.45	0.98	1.83	0.97	0.00	0.27	0.21	0.01	0.02
0.00	0.00	0.29	0.76	0.64	1.03	0.73	1.46	0.00	0.97	0.00	0.22	0.18	0.01	0.02
16.02	29.99	33.41	40.57	37.41	48.86	41.74	35.65	26.26	31.08	24.30	17.30	13.59	1.10	1.48
4.44	7.87	14.36	18.29	20.64	22.89	15.61	6.84	8.55	12.63	8.58	6.64	5.21	0.45	0.57
0.79	1.63	3.22	4.76	3.22	6.69	6.90	0.98	4.27	0.97	7.15	1.69	1.34	0.11	0.15
3.01	5.20	9.67	10.29	16.55	21.60	18.87	14.65	15.27	14.57	11.44	6.15	4.96	0.38	0.54
0.48	0.30	0.29	1.14	0.43	0.26	0.36	0.49	0.61	0.00	0.00	0.26	0.21	0.02	0.02
0.32	0.15	0.29	0.19	0.00	0.00	0.00	0.00	0.00	0.00	0.00	0.11	0.09	0.01	0.01
—	—	—	—	—	—	—	—	—	—	—	—	—	—	—
—	—	—	—	—	—	—	—	—	—	—	—	—	—	—
—	—	—	—	—	—	—	—	—	—	—	—	—	—	—
—	—	—	—	—	—	—	—	—	—	—	—	—	—	—
0.63	0.89	1.91	2.48	3.01	4.11	6.17	2.44	3.66	3.88	4.29	1.30	1.07	0.07	0.12
0.16	0.00	0.73	0.19	1.29	0.77	0.00	0.00	1.83	0.00	0.00	0.22	0.16	0.02	0.02
0.00	0.00	0.00	0.76	0.00	0.26	0.73	0.49	0.00	0.00	0.00	0.09	0.08	0.01	0.01
0.16	0.00	0.88	1.71	2.36	2.83	5.08	6.84	7.33	14.57	8.58	1.22	0.89	0.04	0.10
0.00	0.00	0.15	0.19	0.00	0.26	0.36	0.00	0.61	0.97	0.00	0.08	0.06	0.00	0.01
0.00	0.15	0.00	0.19	0.00	0.26	0.36	0.00	0.61	0.97	0.00	0.09	0.08	0.00	0.01
4.28	6.68	7.18	10.67	14.83	24.43	24.32	21.97	18.93	29.14	25.73	7.06	5.78	0.40	0.63
5.55	7.72	13.48	12.95	11.39	9.51	9.44	6.35	13.44	3.88	0.00	5.54	4.41	0.36	0.43
0.00	0.15	0.44	0.19	0.21	0.00	0.00	0.00	0.61	0.00	0.00	0.08	0.06	0.00	0.00
0.32	0.59	0.00	0.76	0.86	1.03	0.00	0.98	0.61	0.97	1.43	0.33	0.26	0.02	0.03
0.48	0.30	0.44	1.14	0.43	0.77	1.09	1.95	0.61	1.94	0.00	0.40	0.32	0.02	0.04
0.63	1.34	1.32	3.43	3.44	7.20	6.53	6.84	1.83	12.63	2.86	1.76	1.42	0.10	0.17
0.00	0.00	0.00	0.00	0.00	0.00	0.00	0.00	0.00	0.00	1.43	0.01	0.01	0.00	0.00
0.32	0.00	0.29	0.95	1.29	1.03	2.18	2.93	1.22	0.97	0.00	0.42	0.35	0.02	0.05
0.48	0.74	1.32	0.76	0.86	1.29	2.18	0.49	1.83	0.97	1.43	0.78	0.77	0.05	0.06
0.48	0.74	1.03	0.19	1.50	1.80	2.54	0.49	4.27	3.88	0.00	0.83	0.72	0.05	0.06
1.11	2.67	2.05	3.43	5.80	5.40	8.35	5.37	6.72	6.80	5.72	2.90	2.78	0.17	0.24
2.70	3.41	5.86	7.24	10.96	19.54	16.69	15.14	26.26	28.17	8.58	5.23	4.13	0.28	0.44
0.00	0.30	0.00	0.38	0.00	0.77	0.36	0.00	0.00	0.00	0.00	0.12	0.11	0.01	0.01
0.00	0.00	0.29	0.00	0.00	0.00	0.00	0.00	0.00	0.00	0.00	0.05	0.04	0.00	0.00
94.69	184.39	267.61	357.33	518.56	772.97	857.61	876.98	1 000.93	1 195.60	994.98	230.77	177.93	11.72	20.39
94.06	183.50	267.32	356.75	516.63	770.92	853.98	871.12	996.04	1 179.09	974.97	229.60	177.08	11.68	20.31

表 6-1-10 河南省肿瘤登记地区

部位		病例数	构成 (%)	年龄组 0–	1–	5–	10–	15–	20–	25–	30–
唇	C00	11	0.03	0.00	0.00	0.00	0.00	0.00	0.00	0.00	0.00
舌	C01–C02	41	0.12	0.00	0.00	0.00	0.00	0.00	0.00	0.05	0.00
口	C03–C06	66	0.20	0.00	0.00	0.00	0.00	0.00	0.00	0.00	0.00
唾液腺	C07–C08	26	0.08	0.00	0.00	0.00	0.00	0.00	0.00	0.11	0.07
扁桃体	C09	10	0.03	0.00	0.00	0.00	0.00	0.00	0.00	0.00	0.00
其他的口咽	C10	27	0.08	0.00	0.00	0.00	0.00	0.00	0.00	0.00	0.00
鼻咽	C11	126	0.38	0.00	0.00	0.07	0.00	0.00	0.11	0.05	0.26
喉咽	C12–C13	23	0.07	0.00	0.00	0.00	0.00	0.00	0.00	0.00	0.00
咽，部位不明	C14	36	0.11	0.00	0.00	0.00	0.00	0.00	0.00	0.00	0.00
食管	C15	5 502	16.70	0.00	0.00	0.00	0.00	0.00	0.11	0.16	0.59
胃	C16	5 946	18.04	0.00	0.00	0.00	0.00	0.00	0.33	1.04	1.69
小肠	C17	135	0.41	0.00	0.00	0.00	0.00	0.00	0.00	0.05	0.07
结肠	C18	700	2.12	0.00	0.00	0.00	0.00	0.00	0.11	0.38	0.39
直肠	C19–C20	963	2.92	0.00	0.00	0.00	0.00	0.00	0.00	0.22	0.52
肛门	C21	54	0.16	0.00	0.00	0.00	0.00	0.00	0.00	0.00	0.07
肝脏	C22	4 622	14.03	0.39	0.00	0.00	0.23	0.14	0.22	0.66	2.15
胆囊及其他	C23–C24	431	1.31	0.00	0.00	0.00	0.00	0.00	0.05	0.00	0.07
胰腺	C25	554	1.68	0.00	0.00	0.00	0.00	0.00	0.05	0.33	0.26
鼻、鼻窦及其他	C30–C31	32	0.10	0.00	0.00	0.00	0.08	0.00	0.00	0.05	0.26
喉	C32	159	0.48	0.00	0.00	0.00	0.00	0.00	0.00	0.00	0.07
气管、支气管、肺	C33–C34	7 640	23.19	0.00	0.00	0.00	0.00	0.00	0.11	0.71	1.76
其他的胸腔器官	C37–C38	73	0.22	0.39	0.00	0.00	0.15	0.00	0.05	0.11	0.13
骨	C40–C41	268	0.81	0.00	0.00	0.00	0.15	0.14	0.33	0.16	0.33
皮肤的黑色素瘤	C43	25	0.08	0.00	0.08	0.00	0.00	0.00	0.05	0.00	0.00
其他的皮肤	C44	116	0.35	0.00	0.00	0.00	0.00	0.14	0.00	0.00	0.07
间皮瘤	C45	7	0.02	0.00	0.00	0.00	0.00	0.00	0.00	0.00	0.00
卡波西肉瘤	C46	0	0.00	0.00	0.00	0.00	0.00	0.00	0.00	0.00	0.00
周围神经、其他结缔组织、软组织	C47;C49	26	0.08	0.00	0.08	0.00	0.00	0.00	0.00	0.00	0.13
乳房	C50	—	—	—	—	—	—	—	—	—	—
外阴	C51	—	—	—	—	—	—	—	—	—	—
阴道	C52	—	—	—	—	—	—	—	—	—	—
子宫颈	C53	—	—	—	—	—	—	—	—	—	—
子宫体	C54	—	—	—	—	—	—	—	—	—	—
子宫，部位不明	C55	—	—	—	—	—	—	—	—	—	—
卵巢	C56	—	—	—	—	—	—	—	—	—	—
其他的女性生殖器	C57	—	—	—	—	—	—	—	—	—	—
胎盘	C58	—	—	—	—	—	—	—	—	—	—
阴茎	C60	—	—	—	—	—	—	—	—	—	—
前列腺	C61	—	—	—	—	—	—	—	—	—	—
睾丸	C62	—	—	—	—	—	—	—	—	—	—
其他的男性生殖器	C63	—	—	—	—	—	—	—	—	—	—
肾	C64	172	0.52	0.00	0.17	0.07	0.08	0.07	0.05	0.11	0.00
肾盂	C65	28	0.08	0.00	0.00	0.00	0.00	0.00	0.00	0.00	0.00
输尿管	C66	29	0.09	0.00	0.00	0.00	0.08	0.00	0.00	0.00	0.00
膀胱	C67	255	0.77	0.00	0.00	0.00	0.08	0.00	0.00	0.05	0.00
其他的泌尿器官	C68	10	0.03	0.00	0.00	0.00	0.00	0.00	0.00	0.00	0.00
眼	C69	9	0.03	0.00	0.00	0.07	0.08	0.00	0.00	0.00	0.00
脑、神经系统	C70–C72	827	2.51	0.39	0.58	0.99	0.98	0.48	0.33	0.66	1.17
甲状腺	C73	131	0.40	0.00	0.00	0.14	0.00	0.00	0.00	0.00	0.20
肾上腺	C74	23	0.07	0.00	0.08	0.14	0.00	0.00	0.00	0.00	0.07
其他的内分泌腺	C75	15	0.05	0.00	0.00	0.00	0.00	0.00	0.00	0.00	0.00
霍奇金病	C81	50	0.15	0.00	0.00	0.00	0.08	0.00	0.00	0.00	0.07
非霍奇金淋巴瘤	C82–C85;C96	246	0.75	0.00	0.08	0.07	0.08	0.07	0.22	0.11	0.33
免疫增生性疾病	C88	2	0.01	0.00	0.00	0.00	0.00	0.00	0.00	0.00	0.00
多发性骨髓瘤	C90	63	0.19	0.00	0.00	0.00	0.00	0.00	0.05	0.00	0.07
淋巴样白血病	C91	121	0.37	0.39	0.25	0.21	0.38	0.41	0.71	0.38	0.26
髓样白血病	C92–C94	134	0.41	0.00	0.42	0.28	0.15	0.20	0.22	0.38	0.26
白血病，未特指	C95	370	1.12	0.00	1.17	1.48	1.06	0.88	0.87	1.15	0.59
其他的或未指明部位的	O&U	434	1.32	0.39	0.25	0.21	0.23	0.20	0.49	0.44	0.39
骨髓增殖性疾病	MPD	4	0.01	0.00	0.00	0.00	0.00	0.00	0.00	0.00	0.00
骨髓增生异常综合征	MDS	17	0.05	0.00	0.00	0.00	0.00	0.00	0.00	0.00	0.00
合计	ALL	32 952	100.00	1.95	3.17	3.81	3.85	2.86	4.88	8.00	13.88
所有部位除外 C44	ALL but C44	32 836	99.65	1.95	3.17	3.81	3.85	2.72	4.88	8.00	13.81

2014 年合计死亡主要指标 (1/10^5^)

35–	40–	45–	50–	55–	60–	65–	70–	75–	80–	85–	粗率 (1/10^5^ 万)	世标率 (1/10^5^ 万)	累积率 (%) 0~64	累积率 (%) 0~74
0.00	0.06	0.06	0.00	0.09	0.21	0.15	0.00	0.83	0.48	0.84	0.05	0.04	0.00	0.00
0.06	0.12	0.24	0.16	0.35	0.75	1.07	0.83	1.38	1.45	0.84	0.19	0.16	0.01	0.02
0.12	0.18	0.12	0.16	0.35	0.96	1.69	1.45	3.30	4.36	4.21	0.31	0.24	0.01	0.03
0.06	0.00	0.18	0.23	0.17	0.54	0.46	0.21	1.10	0.00	0.84	0.12	0.10	0.01	0.01
0.00	0.00	0.00	0.00	0.00	0.32	0.31	0.00	0.55	0.97	0.84	0.05	0.04	0.00	0.00
0.00	0.12	0.18	0.00	0.26	0.43	0.46	0.42	1.10	1.45	2.53	0.13	0.10	0.00	0.01
0.06	0.47	0.60	1.25	1.21	1.71	3.68	1.87	2.20	3.88	3.37	0.60	0.49	0.03	0.06
0.00	0.00	0.18	0.08	0.26	0.43	0.46	0.42	0.83	1.45	0.84	0.11	0.08	0.00	0.01
0.06	0.00	0.12	0.39	0.69	0.43	0.61	0.83	0.83	1.45	1.68	0.17	0.13	0.01	0.02
0.87	2.22	6.95	18.68	41.13	88.20	151.06	178.56	228.55	347.99	327.60	26.14	20.53	0.79	2.44
1.87	6.91	10.97	22.26	45.99	97.62	143.55	182.29	251.41	361.07	306.54	28.25	22.06	0.94	2.57
0.12	0.35	0.42	0.54	1.04	1.71	2.76	3.94	5.23	7.27	10.11	0.64	0.50	0.02	0.06
0.25	1.11	2.40	3.58	5.90	10.06	15.49	17.65	25.33	46.04	34.53	3.33	2.58	0.12	0.29
0.75	1.40	3.66	4.98	8.24	14.45	18.40	27.61	36.90	49.92	58.95	4.58	3.57	0.17	0.40
0.12	0.23	0.24	0.70	0.52	0.64	1.07	1.25	0.83	1.45	2.53	0.26	0.21	0.01	0.02
4.86	12.23	18.94	33.94	50.24	82.84	102.60	104.43	123.64	175.45	161.69	21.96	17.51	1.03	2.07
0.19	0.12	1.14	1.48	3.21	6.32	7.82	14.95	20.65	23.75	36.21	2.05	1.59	0.06	0.18
0.37	0.59	1.92	2.88	4.69	7.39	14.11	19.52	18.45	20.36	33.69	2.63	2.11	0.09	0.26
0.00	0.06	0.06	0.16	0.35	0.32	0.92	0.42	0.55	1.45	1.68	0.15	0.13	0.01	0.01
0.06	0.06	0.30	0.93	1.82	2.35	3.53	6.44	5.78	7.75	4.21	0.76	0.60	0.03	0.08
3.49	8.43	17.74	35.18	57.44	120.31	182.96	238.56	312.26	429.90	421.92	36.30	28.46	1.23	3.33
0.00	0.29	0.18	0.47	0.69	0.96	0.77	1.87	1.93	2.91	5.90	0.35	0.28	0.02	0.03
0.19	0.47	0.96	1.87	3.64	4.17	6.29	4.98	7.16	9.21	6.74	1.27	1.03	0.06	0.12
0.06	0.00	0.18	0.00	0.00	0.54	0.46	1.25	0.28	0.48	2.53	0.12	0.11	0.00	0.01
0.12	0.06	0.36	0.47	0.87	1.07	1.23	2.70	4.13	7.27	22.74	0.55	0.43	0.02	0.04
0.00	0.00	0.12	0.08	0.00	0.11	0.15	0.00	0.00	0.97	0.00	0.03	0.02	0.00	0.00
0.00	0.00	0.00	0.00	0.00	0.00	0.00	0.00	0.00	0.00	0.00	0.00	0.00	0.00	0.00
0.00	0.12	0.18	0.16	0.09	0.43	0.31	0.62	0.83	0.97	0.84	0.12	0.10	0.01	0.01
—	—	—	—	—	—	—	—	—	—	—	—	—	—	—
—	—	—	—	—	—	—	—	—	—	—	—	—	—	—
—	—	—	—	—	—	—	—	—	—	—	—	—	—	—
—	—	—	—	—	—	—	—	—	—	—	—	—	—	—
—	—	—	—	—	—	—	—	—	—	—	—	—	—	—
—	—	—	—	—	—	—	—	—	—	—	—	—	—	—
—	—	—	—	—	—	—	—	—	—	—	—	—	—	—
—	—	—	—	—	—	—	—	—	—	—	—	—	—	—
—	—	—	—	—	—	—	—	—	—	—	—	—	—	—
—	—	—	—	—	—	—	—	—	—	—	—	—	—	—
—	—	—	—	—	—	—	—	—	—	—	—	—	—	—
—	—	—	—	—	—	—	—	—	—	—	—	—	—	—
—	—	—	—	—	—	—	—	—	—	—	—	—	—	—
0.06	0.18	0.48	1.09	1.82	1.93	3.68	5.61	5.51	10.66	5.05	0.82	0.65	0.03	0.08
0.06	0.18	0.12	0.08	0.26	0.21	0.46	0.83	0.55	2.42	1.68	0.13	0.10	0.00	0.01
0.00	0.00	0.06	0.08	0.26	0.32	0.61	1.45	1.10	0.48	3.37	0.14	0.12	0.00	0.01
0.06	0.12	0.42	0.86	1.21	3.21	6.90	8.30	11.84	18.90	17.69	1.21	0.94	0.03	0.11
0.00	0.00	0.00	0.00	0.09	0.43	0.00	0.00	0.28	0.97	1.68	0.05	0.04	0.00	0.00
0.00	0.00	0.00	0.00	0.09	0.32	0.15	0.21	0.00	0.00	0.84	0.04	0.04	0.00	0.00
2.43	2.46	3.78	4.90	6.51	13.27	14.72	15.36	16.52	34.90	34.53	3.93	3.26	0.19	0.34
0.06	0.41	0.78	0.78	1.04	2.14	2.45	3.53	4.68	3.39	5.05	0.62	0.50	0.03	0.06
0.00	0.00	0.06	0.23	0.17	0.11	0.31	0.62	0.83	0.97	1.68	0.11	0.10	0.00	0.01
0.06	0.00	0.06	0.16	0.09	0.11	0.15	0.42	0.83	1.45	0.00	0.07	0.05	0.00	0.01
0.19	0.06	0.24	0.16	0.35	0.75	0.92	2.08	1.10	1.94	2.53	0.24	0.19	0.01	0.02
0.25	0.59	0.54	2.26	2.52	3.64	3.68	7.47	6.61	10.66	8.42	1.17	0.94	0.05	0.11
0.00	0.00	0.00	0.00	0.00	0.00	0.15	0.00	0.00	0.00	0.84	0.01	0.01	0.00	0.00
0.00	0.18	0.36	0.23	0.61	1.39	1.38	1.66	2.20	0.97	1.68	0.30	0.24	0.01	0.03
0.37	0.53	0.60	0.39	0.61	0.86	1.23	1.87	2.48	2.42	2.53	0.57	0.52	0.03	0.05
0.50	0.59	0.66	0.54	1.48	1.50	1.53	1.25	3.30	4.36	0.84	0.64	0.55	0.04	0.05
0.62	1.23	1.32	1.48	2.52	4.71	5.37	6.02	6.33	10.18	7.58	1.76	1.62	0.09	0.15
0.75	1.05	1.56	2.02	3.73	6.21	7.36	10.17	15.14	21.33	16.00	2.06	1.65	0.09	0.18
0.00	0.00	0.00	0.08	0.00	0.00	0.00	0.42	0.28	0.00	0.00	0.02	0.01	0.00	0.00
0.00	0.00	0.00	0.16	0.09	0.32	0.31	0.00	0.83	1.45	2.53	0.08	0.06	0.00	0.00
23.69	51.40	96.31	168.28	275.74	523.40	753.00	928.90	1 186.81	1 725.88	1 653.14	156.58	123.80	5.90	14.30
23.57	51.34	95.95	167.81	274.88	522.33	751.77	926.20	1 182.68	1 718.61	1 630.40	156.03	123.37	5.88	14.27

表 6-1-11 河南省肿瘤登记地区

部位		病例数	构成 (%)	年龄组 0–	1–	5–	10–	15–	20–	25–	30–
唇	C00	6	0.03	0.00	0.00	0.00	0.00	0.00	0.00	0.00	0.00
舌	C01–C02	18	0.09	0.00	0.00	0.00	0.00	0.00	0.00	0.00	0.00
口	C03–C06	32	0.16	0.00	0.00	0.00	0.00	0.00	0.00	0.00	0.00
唾液腺	C07–C08	15	0.07	0.00	0.00	0.00	0.00	0.00	0.00	0.21	0.00
扁桃体	C09	7	0.03	0.00	0.00	0.00	0.00	0.00	0.00	0.00	0.00
其他的口咽	C10	17	0.08	0.00	0.00	0.00	0.00	0.00	0.00	0.00	0.00
鼻咽	C11	73	0.36	0.00	0.00	0.00	0.00	0.00	0.11	0.11	0.13
喉咽	C12–C13	19	0.09	0.00	0.00	0.00	0.00	0.00	0.00	0.00	0.00
咽，部位不明	C14	26	0.13	0.00	0.00	0.00	0.00	0.00	0.00	0.00	0.00
食管	C15	3 447	16.89	0.00	0.00	0.00	0.00	0.00	0.11	0.11	0.38
胃	C16	4 203	20.59	0.00	0.00	0.00	0.00	0.00	0.32	0.96	1.27
小肠	C17	78	0.38	0.00	0.00	0.00	0.00	0.00	0.00	0.00	0.00
结肠	C18	396	1.94	0.00	0.00	0.00	0.00	0.00	0.11	0.43	0.38
直肠	C19–C20	558	2.73	0.00	0.00	0.00	0.00	0.00	0.00	0.11	0.51
肛门	C21	28	0.14	0.00	0.00	0.00	0.00	0.00	0.00	0.00	0.13
肝脏	C22	3 201	15.68	0.73	0.00	0.00	0.00	0.26	0.21	0.86	3.04
胆囊及其他	C23–C24	177	0.87	0.00	0.00	0.00	0.00	0.00	0.11	0.00	0.00
胰腺	C25	314	1.54	0.00	0.00	0.00	0.00	0.00	0.11	0.54	0.38
鼻、鼻窦及其他	C30–C31	13	0.06	0.00	0.00	0.00	0.14	0.00	0.00	0.11	0.38
喉	C32	117	0.57	0.00	0.00	0.00	0.00	0.00	0.00	0.00	0.00
气管、支气管、肺	C33–C34	5 383	26.37	0.00	0.00	0.00	0.00	0.00	0.21	0.86	2.53
其他的胸腔器官	C37–C38	43	0.21	0.73	0.00	0.00	0.28	0.00	0.00	0.00	0.25
骨	C40–C41	158	0.77	0.00	0.00	0.00	0.14	0.26	0.53	0.21	0.51
皮肤的黑色素瘤	C43	12	0.06	0.00	0.15	0.00	0.00	0.00	0.00	0.00	0.00
其他的皮肤	C44	63	0.31	0.00	0.00	0.00	0.00	0.00	0.00	0.00	0.13
间皮瘤	C45	4	0.02	0.00	0.00	0.00	0.00	0.00	0.00	0.00	0.00
卡波西肉瘤	C46	0	0.00	0.00	0.00	0.00	0.00	0.00	0.00	0.00	0.00
周围神经、其他结缔组织、软组织	C47;C49	19	0.09	0.00	0.15	0.00	0.00	0.00	0.00	0.00	0.25
乳房	C50	—	—	—	—	—	—	—	—	—	—
外阴	C51	—	—	—	—	—	—	—	—	—	—
阴道	C52	—	—	—	—	—	—	—	—	—	—
子宫颈	C53	—	—	—	—	—	—	—	—	—	—
子宫体	C54	—	—	—	—	—	—	—	—	—	—
子宫，部位不明	C55	—	—	—	—	—	—	—	—	—	—
卵巢	C56	—	—	—	—	—	—	—	—	—	—
其他的女性生殖器	C57	—	—	—	—	—	—	—	—	—	—
胎盘	C58	—	—	—	—	—	—	—	—	—	—
阴茎	C60	15	0.07	0.00	0.00	0.00	0.00	0.00	0.00	0.00	0.00
前列腺	C61	192	0.94	0.00	0.00	0.13	0.00	0.13	0.00	0.00	0.00
睾丸	C62	20	0.10	0.00	0.00	0.00	0.00	0.00	0.00	0.11	0.00
其他的男性生殖器	C63	5	0.02	0.00	0.00	0.00	0.00	0.00	0.00	0.00	0.00
肾	C64	120	0.59	0.00	0.15	0.13	0.14	0.00	0.00	0.21	0.00
肾盂	C65	20	0.10	0.00	0.00	0.00	0.00	0.00	0.00	0.00	0.00
输尿管	C66	22	0.11	0.00	0.00	0.00	0.00	0.00	0.00	0.00	0.00
膀胱	C67	191	0.94	0.00	0.00	0.00	0.00	0.00	0.00	0.11	0.00
其他的泌尿器官	C68	5	0.02	0.00	0.00	0.00	0.00	0.00	0.00	0.00	0.00
眼	C69	5	0.02	0.00	0.00	0.13	0.00	0.00	0.00	0.00	0.00
脑、神经系统	C70–C72	456	2.23	0.73	0.61	1.31	0.98	0.52	0.32	0.86	1.65
甲状腺	C73	51	0.25	0.00	0.00	0.00	0.00	0.00	0.00	0.00	0.13
肾上腺	C74	15	0.07	0.00	0.15	0.00	0.00	0.00	0.00	0.00	0.13
其他的内分泌腺	C75	9	0.04	0.00	0.00	0.00	0.00	0.00	0.00	0.00	0.00
霍奇金病	C81	31	0.15	0.00	0.00	0.00	0.14	0.00	0.00	0.00	0.13
非霍奇金淋巴瘤	C82–C85;C96	155	0.76	0.00	0.15	0.00	0.14	0.00	0.21	0.21	0.25
免疫增生性疾病	C88	0	0.00	0.00	0.00	0.00	0.00	0.00	0.00	0.00	0.00
多发性骨髓瘤	C90	44	0.22	0.00	0.00	0.00	0.00	0.00	0.11	0.00	0.13
淋巴样白血病	C91	66	0.32	0.00	0.31	0.26	0.70	0.65	0.63	0.43	0.51
髓样白血病	C92–C94	78	0.38	0.00	0.31	0.26	0.28	0.26	0.21	0.32	0.25
白血病，未特指	C95	199	0.97	0.00	0.61	1.83	1.53	1.05	0.95	0.96	0.76
其他的或未指明部位的	O&U	259	1.27	0.73	0.31	0.26	0.14	0.13	0.63	0.54	0.51
骨髓增殖性疾病	MPD	2	0.01	0.00	0.00	0.00	0.00	0.00	0.00	0.00	0.00
骨髓增生异常综合征	MDS	12	0.06	0.00	0.00	0.00	0.00	0.00	0.00	0.00	0.00
合计	ALL	20 412	100.00	2.94	2.91	4.32	4.60	3.27	4.84	8.24	14.70
所有部位除外 C44	ALL but C44	20 349	99.69	2.94	2.91	4.32	4.60	3.27	4.84	8.24	14.58

2014 年男性死亡主要指标 (1/10^5)

35-	40-	45-	50-	55-	60-	65-	70-	75-	80-	85-	粗率 (1/10^5万)	世标率 (1/10^5万)	累积率 (%) 0~64	0~74
0.00	0.00	0.12	0.00	0.17	0.00	0.31	0.00	0.59	1.13	2.43	0.06	0.05	0.00	0.00
0.12	0.11	0.24	0.00	0.51	0.42	1.53	0.42	1.18	1.13	0.00	0.17	0.14	0.01	0.02
0.24	0.23	0.12	0.15	0.34	0.63	2.15	1.26	2.95	4.52	4.87	0.29	0.25	0.01	0.03
0.00	0.00	0.00	0.15	0.17	0.63	0.92	0.00	2.36	0.00	2.43	0.14	0.12	0.01	0.01
0.00	0.00	0.00	0.00	0.00	0.42	0.61	0.00	0.59	1.13	2.43	0.06	0.06	0.00	0.01
0.00	0.23	0.12	0.00	0.34	0.63	0.31	0.42	1.18	2.26	7.30	0.16	0.14	0.01	0.01
0.12	0.45	0.83	1.38	1.02	1.69	5.21	2.52	2.36	5.65	7.30	0.67	0.58	0.03	0.07
0.00	0.00	0.24	0.15	0.51	0.84	0.31	0.84	1.77	3.39	0.00	0.18	0.14	0.01	0.01
0.12	0.00	0.24	0.46	1.19	0.42	1.23	0.84	1.77	1.13	2.43	0.24	0.20	0.01	0.02
0.72	2.94	9.70	24.49	55.03	118.02	199.60	224.43	290.94	479.13	447.73	31.77	27.01	1.06	3.18
2.27	10.07	14.67	32.61	67.13	143.36	210.64	269.82	374.75	567.28	479.37	38.73	32.55	1.36	3.77
0.12	0.34	0.83	0.77	1.19	1.90	3.68	5.88	5.31	7.91	9.73	0.72	0.61	0.03	0.07
0.36	0.79	3.08	3.98	6.13	11.61	17.78	19.75	31.87	64.41	46.23	3.65	3.03	0.13	0.32
0.84	1.70	3.91	5.51	9.03	17.31	25.14	34.04	47.21	63.28	68.13	5.14	4.32	0.19	0.49
0.12	0.11	0.24	0.77	0.34	0.63	1.53	1.68	0.00	1.13	7.30	0.26	0.23	0.01	0.03
7.53	19.58	29.94	52.51	70.70	114.43	144.72	136.17	162.88	227.14	248.20	29.50	24.83	1.50	2.90
0.36	0.00	0.95	0.92	3.41	5.28	6.13	13.45	14.16	22.60	43.80	1.63	1.41	0.06	0.15
0.36	0.45	2.60	3.67	5.45	9.71	15.64	21.85	17.11	25.99	46.23	2.89	2.51	0.12	0.30
0.00	0.00	0.12	0.15	0.17	0.21	0.31	0.42	0.00	1.13	2.43	0.12	0.11	0.01	0.01
0.12	0.11	0.47	1.38	2.21	3.59	5.21	9.67	10.62	13.56	4.87	1.08	0.89	0.04	0.11
4.54	11.09	23.67	47.46	82.12	172.50	273.80	357.24	471.53	656.55	693.50	49.61	41.98	1.72	4.88
0.00	0.23	0.24	0.61	0.85	1.48	0.92	1.68	2.36	3.39	9.73	0.40	0.36	0.02	0.03
0.00	0.68	1.42	1.99	4.09	4.22	8.58	5.88	6.49	12.43	12.17	1.46	1.25	0.07	0.14
0.00	0.00	0.24	0.00	0.00	0.63	0.31	1.26	0.00	0.00	4.87	0.11	0.11	0.00	0.01
0.00	0.11	0.12	0.61	1.36	1.06	0.61	4.20	7.08	7.91	29.20	0.58	0.51	0.02	0.04
0.00	0.00	0.12	0.15	0.00	0.00	0.31	0.00	0.00	1.13	0.00	0.04	0.03	0.00	0.00
0.00	0.00	0.00	0.00	0.00	0.00	0.00	0.00	0.00	0.00	0.00	0.00	0.00	0.00	0.00
0.00	0.11	0.36	0.15	0.17	0.42	0.31	0.84	1.77	2.26	0.00	0.18	0.14	0.01	0.01
—	—	—	—	—	—	—	—	—	—	—	—	—	—	—
—	—	—	—	—	—	—	—	—	—	—	—	—	—	—
—	—	—	—	—	—	—	—	—	—	—	—	—	—	—
—	—	—	—	—	—	—	—	—	—	—	—	—	—	—
—	—	—	—	—	—	—	—	—	—	—	—	—	—	—
—	—	—	—	—	—	—	—	—	—	—	—	—	—	—
—	—	—	—	—	—	—	—	—	—	—	—	—	—	—
—	—	—	—	—	—	—	—	—	—	—	—	—	—	—
—	—	—	—	—	—	—	—	—	—	—	—	—	—	—
0.12	0.00	0.00	0.00	0.17	0.00	0.92	1.26	2.36	2.26	2.43	0.14	0.11	0.00	0.01
0.00	0.00	0.36	0.15	1.02	2.53	6.75	10.09	23.02	54.24	85.17	1.77	1.53	0.02	0.11
0.00	0.00	0.24	0.46	0.00	0.63	0.61	1.26	1.18	4.52	0.00	0.18	0.15	0.01	0.02
0.00	0.00	0.00	0.15	0.00	0.00	0.31	0.00	0.59	1.13	2.43	0.05	0.04	0.00	0.00
0.12	0.11	0.83	1.53	3.07	2.74	5.21	8.41	7.67	13.56	7.30	1.11	0.94	0.05	0.11
0.12	0.34	0.12	0.15	0.00	0.42	0.61	1.68	0.59	3.39	4.87	0.18	0.16	0.01	0.02
0.00	0.00	0.12	0.15	0.51	0.42	0.61	1.68	2.36	1.13	9.73	0.20	0.18	0.01	0.02
0.12	0.23	0.36	0.92	1.87	4.43	10.42	13.45	20.66	33.90	36.50	1.76	1.49	0.04	0.16
0.00	0.00	0.00	0.00	0.17	0.63	0.00	0.00	0.00	1.13	0.00	0.05	0.04	0.00	0.00
0.00	0.00	0.00	0.00	0.17	0.42	0.31	0.00	0.00	0.00	0.00	0.05	0.05	0.00	0.01
2.75	2.38	4.85	5.82	7.50	11.82	16.25	16.39	20.66	39.55	51.10	4.20	3.67	0.21	0.37
0.12	0.23	0.59	0.61	0.68	1.48	1.84	3.36	3.54	6.78	2.43	0.47	0.38	0.02	0.05
0.00	0.00	0.12	0.46	0.34	0.21	0.31	0.00	1.18	2.26	2.43	0.14	0.12	0.01	0.01
0.00	0.00	0.12	0.15	0.17	0.00	0.31	0.84	0.00	3.39	0.00	0.08	0.06	0.00	0.01
0.00	0.00	0.12	0.31	0.51	1.06	1.53	2.94	1.77	1.13	4.87	0.29	0.26	0.01	0.03
0.24	0.68	1.07	2.76	3.24	4.86	3.68	9.25	11.21	10.17	19.47	1.43	1.21	0.07	0.13
0.00	0.00	0.00	0.00	0.00	0.00	0.00	0.00	0.00	0.00	0.00	0.00	0.00	0.00	0.00
0.00	0.23	0.59	0.46	1.02	1.48	1.23	2.10	4.72	0.00	4.87	0.41	0.34	0.02	0.04
0.36	0.57	0.47	0.46	0.85	0.84	1.84	2.10	1.77	0.00	0.00	0.61	0.58	0.03	0.05
0.72	0.57	0.83	0.77	1.36	1.69	2.45	2.52	4.13	2.26	2.43	0.72	0.64	0.04	0.06
0.84	1.13	1.30	1.68	2.73	4.86	5.52	5.88	8.85	10.17	9.73	1.83	1.73	0.10	0.16
0.84	1.47	1.66	1.84	4.43	7.81	9.20	12.61	20.07	24.86	29.20	2.39	2.04	0.10	0.21
0.00	0.00	0.00	0.15	0.00	0.00	0.00	0.42	0.00	0.00	0.00	0.02	0.02	0.00	0.00
0.00	0.00	0.00	0.31	0.17	0.63	0.31	0.00	0.59	2.26	4.87	0.11	0.10	0.01	0.01
24.25	57.37	108.87	199.32	343.63	661.06	998.30	1 211.68	1 595.77	2 397.93	2 467.39	188.10	159.47	7.19	18.24
24.25	57.25	108.76	198.71	342.27	660.00	997.69	1 207.47	1 588.69	2 390.02	2 438.19	187.52	158.96	7.17	18.20

表 6-1-12 河南省肿瘤登记地区

部位		病例数	构成	年龄组							
			(%)	0–	1–	5–	10–	15–	20–	25–	30–
唇	C00	5	0.04	0.00	0.00	0.00	0.00	0.00	0.00	0.00	0.00
舌	C01–C02	23	0.18	0.00	0.00	0.00	0.00	0.00	0.00	0.11	0.00
口	C03–C06	34	0.27	0.00	0.00	0.00	0.00	0.00	0.00	0.00	0.00
唾液腺	C07–C08	11	0.09	0.00	0.00	0.00	0.00	0.00	0.00	0.00	0.13
扁桃体	C09	3	0.02	0.00	0.00	0.00	0.00	0.00	0.00	0.00	0.00
其他的口咽	C10	10	0.08	0.00	0.00	0.00	0.00	0.00	0.00	0.00	0.00
鼻咽	C11	53	0.42	0.00	0.00	0.15	0.00	0.00	0.11	0.00	0.40
喉咽	C12–C13	4	0.03	0.00	0.00	0.00	0.00	0.00	0.00	0.00	0.00
咽，部位不明	C14	10	0.08	0.00	0.00	0.00	0.00	0.00	0.00	0.00	0.00
食管	C15	2 055	16.39	0.00	0.00	0.00	0.00	0.00	0.11	0.22	0.80
胃	C16	1 743	13.90	0.00	0.00	0.00	0.00	0.00	0.34	1.12	2.15
小肠	C17	57	0.45	0.00	0.00	0.00	0.00	0.00	0.00	0.11	0.13
结肠	C18	304	2.42	0.00	0.00	0.00	0.00	0.00	0.11	0.34	0.40
直肠	C19–C20	405	3.23	0.00	0.00	0.00	0.00	0.00	0.00	0.34	0.54
肛门	C21	26	0.21	0.00	0.00	0.00	0.00	0.00	0.00	0.00	0.00
肝脏	C22	1 421	11.33	0.00	0.00	0.00	0.49	0.00	0.22	0.45	1.21
胆囊及其他	C23–C24	254	2.03	0.00	0.00	0.00	0.00	0.00	0.00	0.00	0.13
胰腺	C25	240	1.91	0.00	0.00	0.00	0.00	0.00	0.00	0.11	0.13
鼻、鼻窦及其他	C30–C31	19	0.15	0.00	0.00	0.00	0.00	0.00	0.00	0.00	0.13
喉	C32	42	0.33	0.00	0.00	0.00	0.00	0.00	0.00	0.00	0.13
气管、支气管、肺	C33–C34	2 257	18.00	0.00	0.00	0.00	0.00	0.00	0.00	0.56	0.94
其他的胸腔器官	C37–C38	30	0.24	0.00	0.00	0.00	0.00	0.00	0.11	0.22	0.00
骨	C40–C41	110	0.88	0.00	0.00	0.00	0.16	0.00	0.11	0.11	0.13
皮肤的黑色素瘤	C43	13	0.10	0.00	0.00	0.00	0.00	0.00	0.11	0.00	0.00
其他的皮肤	C44	53	0.42	0.00	0.00	0.00	0.00	0.28	0.00	0.00	0.00
间皮瘤	C45	3	0.02	0.00	0.00	0.00	0.00	0.00	0.00	0.00	0.00
卡波西肉瘤	C46	0	0.00	0.00	0.00	0.00	0.00	0.00	0.00	0.00	0.00
周围神经、其他结缔组织、软组织	C47;C49	7	0.06	0.00	0.00	0.00	0.00	0.00	0.00	0.00	0.00
乳房	C50	1 066	8.50	0.00	0.00	0.00	0.00	0.00	0.45	0.90	1.74
外阴	C51	8	0.06	0.00	0.00	0.00	0.00	0.00	0.00	0.00	0.00
阴道	C52	12	0.10	0.00	0.00	0.00	0.00	0.00	0.00	0.00	0.00
子宫颈	C53	525	4.19	0.00	0.00	0.00	0.00	0.00	0.00	0.00	1.21
子宫体	C54	166	1.32	0.00	0.00	0.00	0.00	0.00	0.00	0.00	0.13
子宫，部位不明	C55	85	0.68	0.00	0.00	0.00	0.00	0.00	0.00	0.11	0.00
卵巢	C56	273	2.18	0.00	0.00	0.00	0.00	0.14	0.45	0.11	0.13
其他的女性生殖器	C57	11	0.09	0.00	0.00	0.00	0.00	0.00	0.00	0.00	0.00
胎盘	C58	2	0.02	0.00	0.00	0.00	0.00	0.00	0.00	0.00	0.13
阴茎	C60	—	—	—	—	—	—	—	—	—	—
前列腺	C61	—	—	—	—	—	—	—	—	—	—
睾丸	C62	—	—	—	—	—	—	—	—	—	—
其他的男性生殖器	C63	—	—	—	—	—	—	—	—	—	—
肾	C64	52	0.41	0.00	0.18	0.00	0.00	0.14	0.11	0.00	0.00
肾盂	C65	8	0.06	0.00	0.00	0.00	0.00	0.00	0.00	0.00	0.00
输尿管	C66	7	0.06	0.00	0.00	0.00	0.16	0.00	0.00	0.00	0.00
膀胱	C67	64	0.51	0.00	0.00	0.00	0.16	0.00	0.00	0.00	0.00
其他的泌尿器官	C68	5	0.04	0.00	0.00	0.00	0.00	0.00	0.00	0.00	0.00
眼	C69	4	0.03	0.00	0.00	0.00	0.16	0.00	0.00	0.00	0.00
脑、神经系统	C70–C72	371	2.96	0.00	0.55	0.61	0.99	0.43	0.34	0.45	0.67
甲状腺	C73	80	0.64	0.00	0.00	0.31	0.00	0.00	0.00	0.00	0.27
肾上腺	C74	8	0.06	0.00	0.00	0.31	0.00	0.00	0.00	0.00	0.00
其他的内分泌腺	C75	6	0.05	0.00	0.00	0.00	0.00	0.00	0.00	0.00	0.00
霍奇金病	C81	19	0.15	0.00	0.00	0.00	0.00	0.00	0.00	0.00	0.00
非霍奇金淋巴瘤	C82–C85;C96	91	0.73	0.00	0.00	0.15	0.00	0.14	0.22	0.00	0.40
免疫增生性疾病	C88	2	0.02	0.00	0.00	0.00	0.00	0.00	0.00	0.00	0.00
多发性骨髓瘤	C90	19	0.15	0.00	0.00	0.00	0.00	0.00	0.00	0.00	0.00
淋巴样白血病	C91	55	0.44	0.83	0.18	0.15	0.00	0.14	0.78	0.34	0.00
髓样白血病	C92–C94	56	0.45	0.00	0.55	0.31	0.00	0.14	0.22	0.45	0.27
白血病，未特指	C95	171	1.36	0.00	1.84	1.07	0.49	0.71	0.78	1.35	0.40
其他的或未指明部位的	O&U	175	1.40	0.00	0.18	0.15	0.33	0.28	0.34	0.34	0.27
骨髓增殖性疾病	MPD	2	0.02	0.00	0.00	0.00	0.00	0.00	0.00	0.00	0.00
骨髓增生异常综合征	MDS	5	0.04	0.00	0.00	0.00	0.00	0.00	0.00	0.00	0.00
合计	ALL	12 540	100.00	0.83	3.49	3.20	2.96	2.41	4.93	7.75	13.01
所有部位除外 C44	ALL but C44	12 487	99.58	0.83	3.49	3.20	2.96	2.13	4.93	7.75	13.01

2014 年女性死亡主要指标 (1/10^5)

											粗率	世标率	累积率 (%)	
35–	40–	45–	50–	55–	60–	65–	70–	75–	80–	85–	(1/10^{5}万)	(1/10^{5}万)	0~64	0~74
0.00	0.12	0.00	0.00	0.00	0.43	0.00	0.00	1.03	0.00	0.00	0.05	0.03	0.00	0.00
0.00	0.12	0.24	0.32	0.18	1.09	0.61	1.23	1.55	1.70	1.29	0.23	0.17	0.01	0.02
0.00	0.12	0.12	0.16	0.35	1.30	1.23	1.64	3.61	4.24	3.86	0.33	0.24	0.01	0.02
0.13	0.00	0.36	0.32	0.18	0.43	0.00	0.41	0.00	0.00	0.00	0.11	0.09	0.01	0.01
0.00	0.00	0.00	0.00	0.00	0.22	0.00	0.00	0.52	0.85	0.00	0.03	0.02	0.00	0.00
0.00	0.00	0.24	0.00	0.18	0.22	0.61	0.41	1.03	0.85	0.00	0.10	0.07	0.00	0.01
0.00	0.49	0.36	1.11	1.41	1.74	2.15	1.23	2.06	2.55	1.29	0.52	0.41	0.03	0.05
0.00	0.00	0.12	0.00	0.00	0.00	0.61	0.00	0.00	0.00	1.29	0.04	0.03	0.00	0.00
0.00	0.00	0.00	0.32	0.18	0.43	0.00	0.82	0.00	1.70	1.29	0.10	0.07	0.00	0.01
1.04	1.46	4.13	12.67	26.70	57.53	102.48	133.77	173.97	249.50	264.01	20.16	14.53	0.52	1.70
1.43	3.52	7.16	11.56	24.05	50.58	76.40	96.84	143.51	206.22	215.07	17.10	12.31	0.51	1.38
0.13	0.36	0.00	0.32	0.88	1.52	1.84	2.05	5.16	6.79	10.30	0.56	0.39	0.02	0.04
0.13	1.46	1.70	3.17	5.66	8.47	13.19	15.59	19.62	32.25	28.33	2.98	2.19	0.11	0.25
0.65	1.09	3.40	4.43	7.43	11.51	11.66	21.34	27.88	39.89	54.09	3.97	2.87	0.15	0.31
0.13	0.36	0.24	0.63	0.71	0.65	0.61	0.82	1.55	1.70	0.00	0.26	0.19	0.01	0.02
1.96	4.37	7.65	14.73	29.00	50.36	60.45	73.45	89.31	136.63	115.91	13.94	10.36	0.55	1.22
0.00	0.24	1.34	2.06	3.01	7.38	9.51	16.41	26.33	24.61	32.20	2.49	1.78	0.07	0.20
0.39	0.73	1.21	2.06	3.89	4.99	12.58	17.23	19.62	16.12	27.05	2.35	1.75	0.07	0.22
0.00	0.12	0.00	0.16	0.53	0.43	1.53	0.41	1.03	1.70	1.29	0.19	0.14	0.01	0.02
0.00	0.00	0.12	0.48	1.41	1.09	1.84	3.28	1.55	3.39	3.86	0.41	0.31	0.02	0.04
2.35	5.58	11.66	22.48	31.83	66.65	92.05	122.69	172.94	259.68	278.18	22.14	15.97	0.71	1.78
0.00	0.36	0.12	0.32	0.53	0.43	0.61	2.05	1.55	2.55	3.86	0.29	0.22	0.01	0.02
0.39	0.24	0.49	1.74	3.18	4.12	3.99	4.10	7.74	6.79	3.86	1.08	0.82	0.05	0.09
0.13	0.00	0.12	0.00	0.00	0.43	0.61	1.23	0.52	0.85	1.29	0.13	0.10	0.00	0.01
0.26	0.00	0.61	0.32	0.35	1.09	1.84	1.23	1.55	6.79	19.32	0.52	0.38	0.01	0.03
0.00	0.00	0.12	0.00	0.00	0.22	0.00	0.00	0.00	0.85	0.00	0.03	0.02	0.00	0.00
0.00	0.00	0.00	0.00	0.00	0.00	0.00	0.00	0.00	0.00	0.00	0.00	0.00	0.00	0.00
0.00	0.12	0.00	0.16	0.00	0.43	0.31	0.41	0.00	0.00	1.29	0.07	0.06	0.00	0.01
4.56	10.19	18.46	25.18	24.93	35.38	30.68	30.77	28.39	44.13	32.20	10.46	8.08	0.61	0.92
0.00	0.00	0.24	0.00	0.00	0.65	0.00	0.41	1.03	0.00	0.00	0.08	0.06	0.00	0.01
0.00	0.00	0.00	0.32	0.18	0.22	0.61	1.64	0.00	1.70	0.00	0.12	0.09	0.00	0.01
2.22	3.76	6.31	9.98	12.02	17.58	19.33	22.57	17.55	30.55	20.61	5.15	3.96	0.27	0.47
0.65	0.85	2.19	3.80	3.54	4.99	4.91	8.21	7.23	11.03	6.44	1.63	1.23	0.08	0.15
0.39	0.61	1.58	1.11	1.41	2.82	4.30	2.46	2.58	4.24	6.44	0.83	0.65	0.04	0.07
1.30	1.58	4.01	3.48	3.71	9.33	9.51	16.00	13.42	15.28	12.88	2.68	2.06	0.12	0.25
0.26	0.00	0.24	0.32	0.00	0.22	0.31	0.82	0.52	0.00	0.00	0.11	0.09	0.01	0.01
0.00	0.00	0.00	0.16	0.00	0.00	0.00	0.00	0.00	0.00	0.00	0.02	0.02	0.00	0.00
—	—	—	—	—	—	—	—	—	—	—	—	—	—	—
—	—	—	—	—	—	—	—	—	—	—	—	—	—	—
—	—	—	—	—	—	—	—	—	—	—	—	—	—	—
—	—	—	—	—	—	—	—	—	—	—	—	—	—	—
0.00	0.24	0.12	0.63	0.53	1.09	2.15	2.87	3.61	8.49	3.86	0.51	0.38	0.02	0.04
0.00	0.00	0.12	0.00	0.53	0.00	0.31	0.00	0.52	1.70	0.00	0.08	0.05	0.00	0.00
0.00	0.00	0.00	0.00	0.00	0.22	0.61	1.23	0.00	0.00	0.00	0.07	0.07	0.00	0.01
0.00	0.00	0.49	0.79	0.53	1.95	3.38	3.28	4.13	7.64	7.73	0.63	0.47	0.02	0.05
0.00	0.00	0.00	0.00	0.00	0.22	0.00	0.00	0.52	0.85	2.58	0.05	0.03	0.00	0.00
0.00	0.00	0.00	0.00	0.00	0.22	0.00	0.41	0.00	0.00	1.29	0.04	0.04	0.00	0.00
2.09	2.55	2.67	3.96	5.48	14.76	13.19	14.36	12.91	31.40	25.76	3.64	2.89	0.18	0.31
0.00	0.61	0.97	0.95	1.41	2.82	3.07	3.69	5.68	0.85	6.44	0.78	0.62	0.04	0.07
0.00	0.00	0.00	0.00	0.00	0.00	0.31	1.23	0.52	0.00	1.29	0.08	0.08	0.00	0.01
0.13	0.00	0.00	0.16	0.00	0.22	0.00	0.00	1.55	0.00	0.00	0.06	0.04	0.00	0.00
0.39	0.12	0.36	0.00	0.18	0.43	0.31	1.23	0.52	2.55	1.29	0.19	0.14	0.01	0.02
0.26	0.49	0.00	1.74	1.77	2.39	3.68	5.74	2.58	11.03	2.58	0.89	0.69	0.04	0.08
0.00	0.00	0.00	0.00	0.00	0.00	0.31	0.00	0.00	0.00	1.29	0.02	0.02	0.00	0.00
0.00	0.12	0.12	0.00	0.18	1.30	1.53	1.23	0.00	1.70	0.00	0.19	0.15	0.01	0.02
0.39	0.49	0.73	0.32	0.35	0.87	0.61	1.64	3.10	4.24	3.86	0.54	0.44	0.02	0.04
0.26	0.61	0.49	0.32	1.59	1.30	0.61	0.00	2.58	5.94	0.00	0.55	0.45	0.03	0.04
0.39	1.33	1.34	1.27	2.30	4.56	5.22	6.15	4.13	10.18	6.44	1.68	1.52	0.09	0.14
0.65	0.61	1.46	2.22	3.01	4.56	5.52	7.80	10.84	18.67	9.02	1.72	1.30	0.07	0.14
0.00	0.00	0.00	0.00	0.00	0.00	0.00	0.41	0.52	0.00	0.00	0.02	0.01	0.00	0.00
0.00	0.00	0.00	0.00	0.00	0.00	0.31	0.00	1.03	0.85	1.29	0.05	0.03	0.00	0.00
23.08	45.00	83.41	136.17	205.29	381.85	507.51	652.83	829.07	1 221.19	1 222.18	123.02	91.13	4.56	10.36
22.82	45.00	82.81	135.85	204.93	380.77	505.67	651.60	827.53	1 214.40	1 202.86	122.50	90.76	4.55	10.33

表 6-1-13 河南省城市肿瘤登记地区

部位		病例数	构成	年龄组							
			(%)	0–	1–	5–	10–	15–	20–	25–	30–
唇	C00	0	0.00	0.00	0.00	0.00	0.00	0.00	0.00	0.00	0.00
舌	C01–C02	14	0.26	0.00	0.00	0.00	0.00	0.00	0.00	0.34	0.00
口	C03–C06	18	0.33	0.00	0.00	0.00	0.00	0.00	0.00	0.00	0.00
唾液腺	C07–C08	5	0.09	0.00	0.00	0.00	0.00	0.00	0.00	0.34	0.00
扁桃体	C09	0	0.00	0.00	0.00	0.00	0.00	0.00	0.00	0.00	0.00
其他的口咽	C10	5	0.09	0.00	0.00	0.00	0.00	0.00	0.00	0.00	0.00
鼻咽	C11	21	0.39	0.00	0.00	0.00	0.00	0.00	0.00	0.00	0.41
喉咽	C12–C13	3	0.06	0.00	0.00	0.00	0.00	0.00	0.00	0.00	0.00
咽，部位不明	C14	8	0.15	0.00	0.00	0.00	0.00	0.00	0.00	0.00	0.00
食管	C15	726	13.32	0.00	0.00	0.00	0.00	0.00	0.31	0.00	0.83
胃	C16	742	13.61	0.00	0.00	0.00	0.00	0.00	0.00	0.34	1.24
小肠	C17	24	0.44	0.00	0.00	0.00	0.00	0.00	0.00	0.00	0.00
结肠	C18	188	3.45	0.00	0.00	0.00	0.00	0.00	0.31	1.02	0.00
直肠	C19–C20	213	3.91	0.00	0.00	0.00	0.00	0.00	0.00	0.34	0.41
肛门	C21	6	0.11	0.00	0.00	0.00	0.00	0.00	0.00	0.00	0.00
肝脏	C22	697	12.78	2.50	0.00	0.00	0.52	0.00	0.00	0.34	1.65
胆囊及其他	C23–C24	65	1.19	0.00	0.00	0.00	0.00	0.00	0.00	0.00	0.00
胰腺	C25	131	2.40	0.00	0.00	0.00	0.00	0.00	0.31	0.68	0.00
鼻、鼻窦及其他	C30–C31	2	0.04	0.00	0.00	0.00	0.00	0.00	0.00	0.00	0.00
喉	C32	24	0.44	0.00	0.00	0.00	0.00	0.00	0.00	0.00	0.00
气管、支气管、肺	C33–C34	1 412	25.90	0.00	0.00	0.00	0.00	0.00	0.63	1.35	2.06
其他的胸腔器官	C37–C38	20	0.37	0.00	0.00	0.00	0.00	0.00	0.00	0.00	0.00
骨	C40–C41	49	0.90	0.00	0.00	0.00	0.00	0.00	0.31	0.34	0.83
皮肤的黑色素瘤	C43	5	0.09	0.00	0.00	0.00	0.00	0.00	0.00	0.00	0.00
其他的皮肤	C44	21	0.39	0.00	0.00	0.00	0.00	0.00	0.00	0.00	0.00
间皮瘤	C45	3	0.06	0.00	0.00	0.00	0.00	0.00	0.00	0.00	0.00
卡波西肉瘤	C46	0	0.00	0.00	0.00	0.00	0.00	0.00	0.00	0.00	0.00
周围神经、其他结缔组织、软组织	C47;C49	5	0.09	0.00	0.00	0.00	0.00	0.00	0.00	0.00	0.41
乳房	C50	—	—	—	—	—	—	—	—	—	—
外阴	C51	—	—	—	—	—	—	—	—	—	—
阴道	C52	—	—	—	—	—	—	—	—	—	—
子宫颈	C53	—	—	—	—	—	—	—	—	—	—
子宫体	C54	—	—	—	—	—	—	—	—	—	—
子宫，部位不明	C55	—	—	—	—	—	—	—	—	—	—
卵巢	C56	—	—	—	—	—	—	—	—	—	—
其他的女性生殖器	C57	—	—	—	—	—	—	—	—	—	—
胎盘	C58	—	—	—	—	—	—	—	—	—	—
阴茎	C60	—	—	—	—	—	—	—	—	—	—
前列腺	C61	—	—	—	—	—	—	—	—	—	—
睾丸	C62	—	—	—	—	—	—	—	—	—	—
其他的男性生殖器	C63	—	—	—	—	—	—	—	—	—	—
肾	C64	52	0.95	0.00	1.11	0.00	0.00	0.00	0.00	0.00	0.00
肾盂	C65	5	0.09	0.00	0.00	0.00	0.00	0.00	0.00	0.00	0.00
输尿管	C66	11	0.20	0.00	0.00	0.00	0.52	0.00	0.00	0.00	0.00
膀胱	C67	56	1.03	0.00	0.00	0.00	0.00	0.00	0.00	0.00	0.00
其他的泌尿器官	C68	5	0.09	0.00	0.00	0.00	0.00	0.00	0.00	0.00	0.00
眼	C69	1	0.02	0.00	0.00	0.00	0.52	0.00	0.00	0.00	0.00
脑、神经系统	C70–C72	110	2.02	0.00	0.00	0.46	0.52	0.00	0.00	0.34	1.24
甲状腺	C73	35	0.64	0.00	0.00	0.46	0.00	0.00	0.00	0.00	1.24
肾上腺	C74	3	0.06	0.00	0.00	0.46	0.00	0.00	0.00	0.00	0.00
其他的内分泌腺	C75	2	0.04	0.00	0.00	0.00	0.00	0.00	0.00	0.00	0.00
霍奇金病	C81	18	0.33	0.00	0.00	0.00	0.00	0.00	0.00	0.00	0.00
非霍奇金淋巴瘤	C82–C85;C96	40	0.73	0.00	0.00	0.00	0.00	0.43	0.31	0.34	0.00
免疫增生性疾病	C88	0	0.00	0.00	0.00	0.00	0.00	0.00	0.00	0.00	0.00
多发性骨髓瘤	C90	6	0.11	0.00	0.00	0.00	0.00	0.00	0.00	0.00	0.00
淋巴样白血病	C91	28	0.51	0.00	0.56	0.00	0.00	0.43	0.31	0.34	0.00
髓样白血病	C92–C94	21	0.39	0.00	0.56	0.92	0.00	0.00	0.00	0.68	0.00
白血病，未特指	C95	71	1.30	0.00	1.11	1.38	0.52	0.00	0.94	0.68	1.24
其他的或未指明部位的	O&U	83	1.52	0.00	0.00	0.46	0.52	0.00	0.94	1.02	0.00
骨髓增殖性疾病	MPD	1	0.02	0.00	0.00	0.00	0.00	0.00	0.00	0.00	0.00
骨髓增生异常综合征	MDS	5	0.09	0.00	0.00	0.00	0.00	0.00	0.00	0.00	0.00
合计	ALL	5 452	100.00	2.50	3.34	4.13	3.09	0.86	4.39	10.15	14.03
所有部位除外 C44	ALL but C44	5 431	99.61	2.50	3.34	4.13	3.09	0.86	4.39	10.15	14.03

2014 年合计死亡主要指标 ($1/10^5$)

											粗率	世标率	累积率 (%)	
35–	40–	45–	50–	55–	60–	65–	70–	75–	80–	85–	($1/10^5$ 万)	($1/10^5$ 万)	0~64	0~74
0.00	0.00	0.00	0.00	0.00	0.00	0.00	0.00	0.00	0.00	0.00	0.00	0.00	0.00	0.00
0.00	0.32	0.70	0.46	0.50	2.07	3.01	0.00	1.77	0.00	8.13	0.41	0.36	0.02	0.04
0.00	0.00	0.35	0.92	0.00	0.69	4.01	2.64	7.08	11.31	8.13	0.52	0.44	0.01	0.04
0.00	0.00	0.35	0.00	0.00	0.00	0.00	0.00	3.54	0.00	8.13	0.15	0.12	0.00	0.00
0.00	0.00	0.00	0.00	0.00	0.00	0.00	0.00	0.00	0.00	0.00	0.00	0.00	0.00	0.00
0.00	0.00	0.35	0.00	0.00	0.00	1.00	0.00	3.54	0.00	8.13	0.15	0.13	0.00	0.01
0.35	0.32	0.70	0.92	1.00	0.00	8.02	0.00	3.54	3.77	8.13	0.61	0.53	0.02	0.06
0.00	0.00	0.35	0.00	0.00	0.00	1.00	0.00	0.00	3.77	0.00	0.09	0.07	0.00	0.01
0.00	0.00	0.00	0.00	1.50	0.69	0.00	0.00	1.77	7.54	8.13	0.23	0.18	0.01	0.01
0.35	1.29	5.57	10.59	33.98	64.24	115.26	147.74	208.94	433.68	471.51	21.13	17.99	0.59	1.90
1.41	4.83	5.57	18.42	28.48	65.63	124.28	126.64	233.73	418.60	390.21	21.60	18.14	0.63	1.88
0.00	0.32	0.35	0.46	1.00	0.00	3.01	6.60	8.85	11.31	24.39	0.70	0.59	0.01	0.06
0.35	0.97	1.04	5.53	10.49	6.91	26.06	29.02	72.60	113.13	121.94	5.47	4.48	0.13	0.41
1.06	2.58	2.44	6.45	6.50	22.11	26.06	36.94	61.97	90.51	170.72	6.20	5.33	0.21	0.52
0.00	0.00	0.00	0.00	0.50	0.00	0.00	3.96	1.77	3.77	0.00	0.17	0.14	0.00	0.02
4.23	11.27	14.61	25.33	45.98	69.08	90.20	117.40	138.11	230.04	292.66	20.29	16.95	0.87	1.91
0.00	0.32	0.70	1.38	3.00	7.60	8.02	14.51	17.71	33.94	32.52	1.89	1.59	0.06	0.18
1.06	0.97	1.39	2.30	6.00	7.60	22.05	29.02	38.95	45.25	97.55	3.81	3.29	0.10	0.36
0.00	0.00	0.00	0.00	0.00	0.00	0.00	1.32	1.77	0.00	0.00	0.06	0.04	0.00	0.01
0.00	0.00	0.35	0.46	2.00	0.69	2.00	3.96	12.39	15.08	8.13	0.70	0.53	0.02	0.05
4.58	7.73	20.53	35.92	63.97	130.56	168.38	296.81	435.58	690.12	715.39	41.10	34.20	1.34	3.66
0.00	0.32	0.35	0.92	1.50	0.69	1.00	2.64	5.31	3.77	40.65	0.58	0.53	0.02	0.04
0.00	0.00	1.39	1.38	4.00	2.76	6.01	9.23	12.39	11.31	24.39	1.43	1.19	0.06	0.13
0.35	0.00	0.00	0.00	0.00	1.38	1.00	0.00	0.00	0.00	8.13	0.15	0.15	0.01	0.01
0.35	0.00	1.04	1.38	1.00	0.69	1.00	2.64	7.08	0.00	32.52	0.61	0.54	0.02	0.04
0.00	0.00	0.70	0.00	0.00	0.00	0.00	0.00	0.00	3.77	0.00	0.09	0.06	0.00	0.00
0.00	0.00	0.00	0.00	0.00	0.00	0.00	0.00	0.00	0.00	0.00	0.00	0.00	0.00	0.00
0.00	0.00	0.35	0.00	0.00	0.00	1.00	0.00	3.54	0.00	0.00	0.15	0.11	0.00	0.01
—	—	—	—	—	—	—	—	—	—	—	—	—	—	—
—	—	—	—	—	—	—	—	—	—	—	—	—	—	—
—	—	—	—	—	—	—	—	—	—	—	—	—	—	—
—	—	—	—	—	—	—	—	—	—	—	—	—	—	—
—	—	—	—	—	—	—	—	—	—	—	—	—	—	—
—	—	—	—	—	—	—	—	—	—	—	—	—	—	—
—	—	—	—	—	—	—	—	—	—	—	—	—	—	—
—	—	—	—	—	—	—	—	—	—	—	—	—	—	—
—	—	—	—	—	—	—	—	—	—	—	—	—	—	—
—	—	—	—	—	—	—	—	—	—	—	—	—	—	—
—	—	—	—	—	—	—	—	—	—	—	—	—	—	—
—	—	—	—	—	—	—	—	—	—	—	—	—	—	—
—	—	—	—	—	—	—	—	—	—	—	—	—	—	—
0.35	0.00	0.35	1.38	4.00	4.14	5.01	15.83	10.62	30.17	0.00	1.51	1.27	0.06	0.16
0.00	0.32	0.00	0.00	0.00	0.00	0.00	2.64	0.00	7.54	0.00	0.15	0.11	0.00	0.01
0.00	0.00	0.35	0.46	0.00	0.69	1.00	2.64	1.77	3.77	16.26	0.32	0.32	0.01	0.03
0.00	0.00	0.35	0.46	1.50	6.22	4.01	10.55	17.71	49.03	56.91	1.63	1.39	0.04	0.12
0.00	0.00	0.00	0.00	0.50	1.38	0.00	0.00	0.00	7.54	0.00	0.15	0.11	0.01	0.01
0.00	0.00	0.00	0.00	0.00	0.00	0.00	0.00	0.00	0.00	0.00	0.03	0.05	0.00	0.00
1.06	2.25	1.04	5.07	3.50	15.20	9.02	11.87	15.94	56.57	73.16	3.20	2.77	0.15	0.26
0.00	0.97	1.74	0.92	2.50	5.53	2.00	5.28	3.54	0.00	0.00	1.02	0.85	0.07	0.10
0.00	0.00	0.00	0.00	0.00	0.69	0.00	1.32	0.00	0.00	0.00	0.09	0.10	0.01	0.01
0.00	0.00	0.00	0.46	0.00	0.00	1.00	0.00	0.00	0.00	0.00	0.06	0.05	0.00	0.01
0.35	0.00	1.04	0.46	0.50	0.00	4.01	5.28	5.31	0.00	8.13	0.52	0.45	0.01	0.06
0.35	0.32	0.35	1.38	1.50	2.07	5.01	7.91	12.39	22.63	8.13	1.16	0.95	0.04	0.10
0.00	0.00	0.00	0.00	0.00	0.00	0.00	0.00	0.00	0.00	0.00	0.00	0.00	0.00	0.00
0.00	0.00	0.00	0.00	0.00	1.38	1.00	1.32	1.77	0.00	8.13	0.17	0.17	0.01	0.02
0.35	0.64	0.35	0.92	1.50	2.07	5.01	2.64	3.54	7.54	8.13	0.82	0.73	0.04	0.08
0.35	0.00	0.00	0.92	1.00	1.38	1.00	3.96	3.54	11.31	0.00	0.61	0.56	0.03	0.05
0.35	1.29	1.39	1.84	2.00	6.22	5.01	10.55	12.39	30.17	24.39	2.07	1.86	0.09	0.17
0.71	1.93	1.04	1.84	2.50	7.60	5.01	17.15	21.25	33.94	40.65	2.42	2.04	0.09	0.20
0.00	0.00	0.00	0.00	0.00	0.00	0.00	1.32	0.00	0.00	0.00	0.03	0.03	0.00	0.01
0.00	0.00	0.00	0.00	0.00	0.00	0.00	0.00	5.31	3.77	8.13	0.15	0.11	0.00	0.00
25.04	49.90	90.47	162.12	254.36	479.42	699.56	978.80	1 473.19	2 571.93	2 885.94	158.71	133.12	5.51	13.90
24.68	49.90	89.42	160.74	253.36	478.73	698.56	976.16	1 466.11	2 571.93	2 853.43	158.10	132.59	5.48	13.86

表 6-1-14 河南省城市肿瘤登记地区

部位		病例数	构成 (%)	年龄组 0–	1–	5–	10–	15–	20–	25–	30–
唇	C00	0	0.00	0.00	0.00	0.00	0.00	0.00	0.00	0.00	0.00
舌	C01–C02	4	0.12	0.00	0.00	0.00	0.00	0.00	0.00	0.00	0.00
口	C03–C06	11	0.32	0.00	0.00	0.00	0.00	0.00	0.00	0.00	0.00
唾液腺	C07–C08	4	0.12	0.00	0.00	0.00	0.00	0.00	0.00	0.66	0.00
扁桃体	C09	0	0.00	0.00	0.00	0.00	0.00	0.00	0.00	0.00	0.00
其他的口咽	C10	4	0.12	0.00	0.00	0.00	0.00	0.00	0.00	0.00	0.00
鼻咽	C11	14	0.41	0.00	0.00	0.00	0.00	0.00	0.00	0.00	0.82
喉咽	C12–C13	1	0.03	0.00	0.00	0.00	0.00	0.00	0.00	0.00	0.00
咽，部位不明	C14	5	0.15	0.00	0.00	0.00	0.00	0.00	0.00	0.00	0.00
食管	C15	478	13.97	0.00	0.00	0.00	0.00	0.00	0.62	0.00	0.00
胃	C16	536	15.67	0.00	0.00	0.00	0.00	0.00	0.00	0.66	0.82
小肠	C17	13	0.38	0.00	0.00	0.00	0.00	0.00	0.00	0.00	0.00
结肠	C18	109	3.19	0.00	0.00	0.00	0.00	0.00	0.62	1.33	0.00
直肠	C19–C20	128	3.74	0.00	0.00	0.00	0.00	0.00	0.00	0.00	0.00
肛门	C21	1	0.03	0.00	0.00	0.00	0.00	0.00	0.00	0.00	0.00
肝脏	C22	508	14.85	4.75	0.00	0.00	0.00	0.00	0.00	0.66	1.65
胆囊及其他	C23–C24	29	0.85	0.00	0.00	0.00	0.00	0.00	0.00	0.00	0.00
胰腺	C25	78	2.28	0.00	0.00	0.00	0.00	0.00	0.62	0.66	0.00
鼻、鼻窦及其他	C30–C31	1	0.03	0.00	0.00	0.00	0.00	0.00	0.00	0.00	0.00
喉	C32	23	0.67	0.00	0.00	0.00	0.00	0.00	0.00	0.00	0.00
气管、支气管、肺	C33–C34	1 029	30.08	0.00	0.00	0.00	0.00	0.00	1.23	1.99	2.47
其他的胸腔器官	C37–C38	13	0.38	0.00	0.00	0.00	0.00	0.00	0.00	0.00	0.00
骨	C40–C41	28	0.82	0.00	0.00	0.00	0.00	0.00	0.62	0.66	1.65
皮肤的黑色素瘤	C43	3	0.09	0.00	0.00	0.00	0.00	0.00	0.00	0.00	0.00
其他的皮肤	C44	10	0.29	0.00	0.00	0.00	0.00	0.00	0.00	0.00	0.00
间皮瘤	C45	1	0.03	0.00	0.00	0.00	0.00	0.00	0.00	0.00	0.00
卡波西肉瘤	C46	0	0.00	0.00	0.00	0.00	0.00	0.00	0.00	0.00	0.00
周围神经、其他结缔组织、软组织	C47;C49	4	0.12	0.00	0.00	0.00	0.00	0.00	0.00	0.00	0.82
乳房	C50	—	—	—	—	—	—	—	—	—	—
外阴	C51	—	—	—	—	—	—	—	—	—	—
阴道	C52	-	—	—	—	—	—	—	—	—	—
子宫颈	C53	—	—	—	—	—	—	—	—	—	—
子宫体	C54	—	—	—	—	—	—	—	—	—	—
子宫，部位不明	C55	—	—	—	—	—	—	—	—	—	—
卵巢	C56	—	—	—	—	—	—	—	—	—	—
其他的女性生殖器	C57	—	—	—	—	—	—	—	—	—	—
胎盘	C58	—	—	—	—	—	—	—	—	—	—
阴茎	C60	4	0.12	0.00	0.00	0.00	0.00	0.00	0.00	0.00	0.00
前列腺	C61	46	1.34	0.00	0.00	0.00	0.00	0.00	0.00	0.00	0.00
睾丸	C62	7	0.20	0.00	0.00	0.00	0.00	0.00	0.00	0.66	0.00
其他的男性生殖器	C63	0	0.00	0.00	0.00	0.00	0.00	0.00	0.00	0.00	0.00
肾	C64	35	1.02	0.00	1.04	0.00	0.00	0.00	0.00	0.00	0.00
肾盂	C65	4	0.12	0.00	0.00	0.00	0.00	0.00	0.00	0.00	0.00
输尿管	C66	8	0.23	0.00	0.00	0.00	0.00	0.00	0.00	0.00	0.00
膀胱	C67	41	1.20	0.00	0.00	0.00	0.00	0.00	0.00	0.00	0.00
其他的泌尿器官	C68	3	0.09	0.00	0.00	0.00	0.00	0.00	0.00	0.00	0.00
眼	C69	0	0.00	0.00	0.00	0.00	0.00	0.00	0.00	0.00	0.00
脑、神经系统	C70–C72	66	1.93	0.00	0.00	0.85	0.00	0.00	0.00	0.66	1.65
甲状腺	C73	8	0.23	0.00	0.00	0.00	0.00	0.00	0.00	0.00	0.82
肾上腺	C74	1	0.03	0.00	0.00	0.00	0.00	0.00	0.00	0.00	0.00
其他的内分泌腺	C75	1	0.03	0.00	0.00	0.00	0.00	0.00	0.00	0.00	0.00
霍奇金病	C81	11	0.32	0.00	0.00	0.00	0.00	0.00	0.00	0.00	0.00
非霍奇金淋巴瘤	C82–C85;C96	26	0.76	0.00	0.00	0.00	0.00	0.00	0.62	0.66	0.00
免疫增生性疾病	C88	0	0.00	0.00	0.00	0.00	0.00	0.00	0.00	0.00	0.00
多发性骨髓瘤	C90	4	0.12	0.00	0.00	0.00	0.00	0.00	0.00	0.00	0.00
淋巴样白血病	C91	17	0.50	0.00	1.04	0.00	0.00	0.85	0.62	0.00	0.00
髓样白血病	C92–C94	12	0.35	0.00	0.00	0.85	0.00	0.00	0.00	0.66	0.00
白血病，未特指	C95	37	1.08	0.00	0.00	1.71	0.95	0.00	1.23	0.00	1.65
其他的或未指明部位的	O&U	49	1.43	0.00	0.00	0.85	0.00	0.00	1.23	1.33	0.00
骨髓增殖性疾病	MPD	0	0.00	0.00	0.00	0.00	0.00	0.00	0.00	0.00	0.00
骨髓增生异常综合征	MDS	2	0.06	0.00	0.00	0.00	0.00	0.00	0.00	0.00	0.00
合计	ALL	3 421	100.00	4.75	2.07	4.27	0.95	0.85	7.40	10.60	12.36
所有部位除外 C44	ALL but C44	3 411	99.71	4.75	2.07	4.27	0.95	0.85	7.40	10.60	12.36

2014 年男性死亡主要指标 (1/10^5)

											粗率	世标率	累积率 (%)	
35–	40–	45–	50–	55–	60–	65–	70–	75–	80–	85–	(1/10^5 万)	(1/10^5 万)	0~64	0~74
0.00	0.00	0.00	0.00	0.00	0.00	0.00	0.00	0.00	0.00	0.00	0.00	0.00	0.00	0.00
0.00	0.00	0.68	0.00	0.00	1.37	4.05	0.00	0.00	0.00	0.00	0.23	0.22	0.01	0.03
0.00	0.00	0.68	0.90	0.00	1.37	6.07	2.71	7.54	8.59	21.72	0.63	0.60	0.01	0.06
0.00	0.00	0.00	0.00	0.00	0.00	0.00	0.00	7.54	0.00	21.72	0.23	0.24	0.00	0.00
0.00	0.00	0.00	0.00	0.00	0.00	0.00	0.00	0.00	0.00	0.00	0.00	0.00	0.00	0.00
0.00	0.00	0.68	0.00	0.00	0.00	0.00	0.00	7.54	0.00	21.72	0.23	0.23	0.00	0.00
0.68	0.00	0.68	1.81	0.00	0.00	12.14	0.00	3.77	8.59	21.72	0.80	0.78	0.02	0.08
0.00	0.00	0.00	0.00	0.00	0.00	0.00	0.00	0.00	8.59	0.00	0.06	0.04	0.00	0.00
0.00	0.00	0.00	0.00	2.01	0.00	0.00	0.00	3.77	8.59	21.72	0.28	0.27	0.01	0.01
0.68	2.50	8.90	16.28	49.16	89.04	153.83	192.45	271.55	730.12	499.57	27.20	24.44	0.84	2.57
2.72	7.51	7.53	28.04	42.13	95.89	176.10	214.14	339.44	669.99	651.61	30.50	27.66	0.93	2.88
0.00	0.63	0.68	0.90	1.00	0.00	4.05	8.13	3.77	8.59	43.44	0.74	0.75	0.02	0.08
0.68	0.63	2.05	5.43	11.03	9.59	28.34	24.40	98.06	180.38	152.04	6.20	5.43	0.16	0.42
0.00	2.50	2.74	9.04	8.03	21.92	46.55	40.66	67.89	163.20	238.92	7.28	6.86	0.22	0.66
0.00	0.00	0.00	0.00	0.00	0.00	0.00	2.71	0.00	0.00	0.00	0.06	0.05	0.00	0.01
7.47	17.53	25.32	45.22	66.21	95.89	151.81	154.51	169.72	343.58	543.01	28.91	25.79	1.30	2.84
0.00	0.00	0.00	1.81	1.00	8.22	8.10	8.13	18.86	51.54	43.44	1.65	1.53	0.06	0.14
0.68	0.63	2.74	3.62	4.01	12.33	28.34	32.53	45.26	60.13	173.76	4.44	4.30	0.13	0.43
0.00	0.00	0.00	0.00	0.00	0.00	0.00	2.71	0.00	0.00	0.00	0.06	0.05	0.00	0.01
0.00	0.00	0.68	0.90	4.01	1.37	4.05	8.13	26.40	34.36	0.00	1.31	1.02	0.03	0.10
5.43	8.77	29.43	49.75	98.31	197.26	255.04	441.83	656.26	1168.18	1303.21	58.56	52.74	1.97	5.46
0.00	0.63	0.68	0.90	2.01	0.00	0.00	2.71	7.54	8.59	86.88	0.74	0.81	0.02	0.03
0.00	0.00	2.74	0.90	4.01	1.37	8.10	10.84	11.31	8.59	43.44	1.59	1.46	0.06	0.15
0.00	0.00	0.00	0.00	0.00	1.37	2.02	0.00	0.00	0.00	21.72	0.17	0.22	0.01	0.02
0.00	0.00	0.68	0.90	2.01	0.00	0.00	5.42	11.31	0.00	21.72	0.57	0.50	0.02	0.05
0.00	0.00	0.68	0.00	0.00	0.00	0.00	0.00	0.00	0.00	0.00	0.06	0.04	0.00	0.00
0.00	0.00	0.00	0.00	0.00	0.00	0.00	0.00	0.00	0.00	0.00	0.00	0.00	0.00	0.00
0.00	0.00	0.68	0.00	0.00	0.00	0.00	0.00	7.54	0.00	0.00	0.23	0.17	0.01	0.01
—	—	—	—	—	—	—	—	—	—	—	—	—	—	—
—	—	—	—	—	—	—	—	—	—	—	—	—	—	—
—	—	—	—	—	—	—	—	—	—	—	—	—	—	—
—	—	—	—	—	—	—	—	—	—	—	—	—	—	—
—	—	—	—	—	—	—	—	—	—	—	—	—	—	—
—	—	—	—	—	—	—	—	—	—	—	—	—	—	—
—	—	—	—	—	—	—	—	—	—	—	—	—	—	—
—	—	—	—	—	—	—	—	—	—	—	—	—	—	—
—	—	—	—	—	—	—	—	—	—	—	—	—	—	—
0.00	0.00	0.00	0.00	0.00	0.00	0.00	2.71	11.31	0.00	0.00	0.23	0.17	0.00	0.01
0.00	0.00	0.00	0.90	1.00	4.11	4.05	8.13	30.17	163.20	195.48	2.62	2.63	0.03	0.09
0.00	0.00	0.00	0.90	0.00	0.00	0.00	0.00	7.54	25.77	0.00	0.40	0.30	0.01	0.01
0.00	0.00	0.00	0.00	0.00	0.00	0.00	0.00	0.00	0.00	0.00	0.00	0.00	0.00	0.00
0.68	0.00	0.68	1.81	5.02	8.22	10.12	21.68	7.54	34.36	0.00	1.99	1.79	0.09	0.25
0.00	0.63	0.00	0.00	0.00	0.00	0.00	5.42	0.00	8.59	0.00	0.23	0.19	0.00	0.03
0.00	0.00	0.68	0.90	0.00	1.37	0.00	2.71	3.77	8.59	43.44	0.46	0.49	0.01	0.03
0.00	0.00	0.00	0.00	2.01	8.22	8.10	18.97	22.63	94.49	108.60	2.33	2.27	0.05	0.19
0.00	0.00	0.00	0.00	1.00	1.37	0.00	0.00	0.00	8.59	0.00	0.17	0.14	0.01	0.01
0.00	0.00	0.00	0.00	0.00	0.00	0.00	0.00	0.00	0.00	0.00	0.00	0.00	0.00	0.00
0.68	1.88	2.05	5.43	7.02	16.44	10.12	13.55	22.63	85.90	86.88	3.76	3.39	0.18	0.30
0.00	0.63	1.37	0.00	1.00	2.74	0.00	2.71	0.00	0.00	0.00	0.46	0.37	0.03	0.05
0.00	0.00	0.00	0.00	0.00	1.37	0.00	0.00	0.00	0.00	0.00	0.06	0.05	0.01	0.01
0.00	0.00	0.00	0.00	0.00	0.00	2.02	0.00	0.00	0.00	0.00	0.06	0.06	0.00	0.01
0.00	0.00	0.68	0.90	1.00	0.00	6.07	5.42	7.54	0.00	21.72	0.63	0.60	0.01	0.07
0.00	0.63	0.68	2.71	2.01	0.00	8.10	8.13	22.63	25.77	21.72	1.48	1.27	0.04	0.12
0.00	0.00	0.00	0.00	0.00	0.00	0.00	0.00	0.00	0.00	0.00	0.00	0.00	0.00	0.00
0.00	0.00	0.00	0.00	0.00	1.37	0.00	2.71	3.77	0.00	21.72	0.23	0.26	0.01	0.02
0.00	0.00	0.00	0.90	2.01	4.11	8.10	5.42	7.54	0.00	0.00	0.97	0.94	0.05	0.11
0.68	0.00	0.00	0.90	1.00	1.37	2.02	8.13	3.77	8.59	0.00	0.68	0.62	0.03	0.08
0.00	2.50	0.68	1.81	3.01	6.85	2.02	13.55	15.09	34.36	21.72	2.11	1.89	0.10	0.18
1.36	1.88	0.00	0.90	3.01	9.59	6.07	18.97	30.17	51.54	86.88	2.79	2.59	0.10	0.23
0.00	0.00	0.00	0.00	0.00	0.00	0.00	0.00	0.00	0.00	0.00	0.00	0.00	0.00	0.00
0.00	0.00	0.00	0.00	0.00	0.00	0.00	0.00	3.77	8.59	0.00	0.11	0.08	0.00	0.00
21.73	49.46	95.81	184.51	324.02	604.12	955.39	1 292.96	1 965.00	4 028.52	4 561.25	194.69	176.57	6.59	17.83
21.73	49.46	95.12	183.61	322.02	604.12	955.39	1 287.54	1 953.68	4 028.52	4 539.53	194.12	176.07	6.58	17.79

表 6-1-15 河南省城市肿瘤登记地区

部位		病例数	构成 (%)	年龄组 0–	1–	5–	10–	15–	20–	25–	30–
唇	C00	0	0.00	0.00	0.00	0.00	0.00	0.00	0.00	0.00	0.00
舌	C01–C02	10	0.49	0.00	0.00	0.00	0.00	0.00	0.00	0.69	0.00
口	C03–C06	7	0.34	0.00	0.00	0.00	0.00	0.00	0.00	0.00	0.00
唾液腺	C07–C08	1	0.05	0.00	0.00	0.00	0.00	0.00	0.00	0.00	0.00
扁桃体	C09	0	0.00	0.00	0.00	0.00	0.00	0.00	0.00	0.00	0.00
其他的口咽	C10	1	0.05	0.00	0.00	0.00	0.00	0.00	0.00	0.00	0.00
鼻咽	C11	7	0.34	0.00	0.00	0.00	0.00	0.00	0.00	0.00	0.00
喉咽	C12–C13	2	0.10	0.00	0.00	0.00	0.00	0.00	0.00	0.00	0.00
咽，部位不明	C14	3	0.15	0.00	0.00	0.00	0.00	0.00	0.00	0.00	0.00
食管	C15	248	12.21	0.00	0.00	0.00	0.00	0.00	0.00	0.00	1.65
胃	C16	206	10.14	0.00	0.00	0.00	0.00	0.00	0.00	0.00	1.65
小肠	C17	11	0.54	0.00	0.00	0.00	0.00	0.00	0.00	0.00	0.00
结肠	C18	79	3.89	0.00	0.00	0.00	0.00	0.00	0.00	0.69	0.00
直肠	C19–C20	85	4.19	0.00	0.00	0.00	0.00	0.00	0.00	0.69	0.83
肛门	C21	5	0.25	0.00	0.00	0.00	0.00	0.00	0.00	0.00	0.00
肝脏	C22	189	9.31	0.00	0.00	0.00	1.12	0.00	0.00	0.00	1.65
胆囊及其他	C23–C24	36	1.77	0.00	0.00	0.00	0.00	0.00	0.00	0.00	0.00
胰腺	C25	53	2.61	0.00	0.00	0.00	0.00	0.00	0.00	0.69	0.00
鼻、鼻窦及其他	C30–C31	1	0.05	0.00	0.00	0.00	0.00	0.00	0.00	0.00	0.00
喉	C32	1	0.05	0.00	0.00	0.00	0.00	0.00	0.00	0.00	0.00
气管、支气管、肺	C33–C34	383	18.86	0.00	0.00	0.00	0.00	0.00	0.00	0.69	1.65
其他的胸腔器官	C37–C38	7	0.34	0.00	0.00	0.00	0.00	0.00	0.00	0.00	0.00
骨	C40–C41	21	1.03	0.00	0.00	0.00	0.00	0.00	0.00	0.00	0.00
皮肤的黑色素瘤	C43	2	0.10	0.00	0.00	0.00	0.00	0.00	0.00	0.00	0.00
其他的皮肤	C44	11	0.54	0.00	0.00	0.00	0.00	0.00	0.00	0.00	0.00
间皮瘤	C45	2	0.10	0.00	0.00	0.00	0.00	0.00	0.00	0.00	0.00
卡波西肉瘤	C46	0	0.00	0.00	0.00	0.00	0.00	0.00	0.00	0.00	0.00
周围神经、其他结缔组织、软组织	C47;C49	1	0.05	0.00	0.00	0.00	0.00	0.00	0.00	0.00	0.00
乳房	C50	233	11.47	0.00	0.00	0.00	0.00	0.00	0.00	1.38	1.65
外阴	C51	3	0.15	0.00	0.00	0.00	0.00	0.00	0.00	0.00	0.00
阴道	C52	1	0.05	0.00	0.00	0.00	0.00	0.00	0.00	0.00	0.00
子宫颈	C53	92	4.53	0.00	0.00	0.00	0.00	0.00	0.00	0.00	2.48
子宫体	C54	39	1.92	0.00	0.00	0.00	0.00	0.00	0.00	0.00	0.00
子宫，部位不明	C55	10	0.49	0.00	0.00	0.00	0.00	0.00	0.00	0.69	0.00
卵巢	C56	51	2.51	0.00	0.00	0.00	0.00	0.00	0.00	0.69	0.83
其他的女性生殖器	C57	2	0.10	0.00	0.00	0.00	0.00	0.00	0.00	0.00	0.00
胎盘	C58	0	0.00	0.00	0.00	0.00	0.00	0.00	0.00	0.00	0.00
阴茎	C60	—	—	—	—	—	—	—	—	—	—
前列腺	C61	—	—	—	—	—	—	—	—	—	—
睾丸	C62	—	—	—	—	—	—	—	—	—	—
其他的男性生殖器	C63	—	—	—	—	—	—	—	—	—	—
肾	C64	17	0.84	0.00	1.20	0.00	0.00	0.00	0.00	0.00	0.00
肾盂	C65	1	0.05	0.00	0.00	0.00	0.00	0.00	0.00	0.00	0.00
输尿管	C66	3	0.15	0.00	0.00	0.00	1.12	0.00	0.00	0.00	0.00
膀胱	C67	15	0.74	0.00	0.00	0.00	0.00	0.00	0.00	0.00	0.00
其他的泌尿器官	C68	2	0.10	0.00	0.00	0.00	0.00	0.00	0.00	0.00	0.00
眼	C69	1	0.05	0.00	0.00	0.00	1.12	0.00	0.00	0.00	0.00
脑、神经系统	C70–C72	44	2.17	0.00	0.00	0.00	1.12	0.00	0.00	0.00	0.83
甲状腺	C73	27	1.33	0.00	0.00	0.99	0.00	0.00	0.00	0.00	1.65
肾上腺	C74	2	0.10	0.00	0.00	0.99	0.00	0.00	0.00	0.00	0.00
其他的内分泌腺	C75	1	0.05	0.00	0.00	0.00	0.00	0.00	0.00	0.00	0.00
霍奇金病	C81	7	0.34	0.00	0.00	0.00	0.00	0.00	0.00	0.00	0.00
非霍奇金淋巴瘤	C82–C85;C96	14	0.69	0.00	0.00	0.00	0.00	0.87	0.00	0.00	0.00
免疫增生性疾病	C88	0	0.00	0.00	0.00	0.00	0.00	0.00	0.00	0.00	0.00
多发性骨髓瘤	C90	2	0.10	0.00	0.00	0.00	0.00	0.00	0.00	0.00	0.00
淋巴样白血病	C91	11	0.54	0.00	0.00	0.00	0.00	0.00	0.00	0.69	0.00
髓样白血病	C92–C94	9	0.44	0.00	1.20	0.99	0.00	0.00	0.00	0.69	0.00
白血病，未特指	C95	34	1.67	0.00	2.40	0.99	0.00	0.00	0.64	1.38	0.83
其他的或未指明部位的	O&U	34	1.67	0.00	0.00	0.00	1.12	0.00	0.64	0.69	0.00
骨髓增殖性疾病	MPD	1	0.05	0.00	0.00	0.00	0.00	0.00	0.00	0.00	0.00
骨髓增生异常综合征	MDS	3	0.15	0.00	0.00	0.00	0.00	0.00	0.00	0.00	0.00
合计	ALL	2 031	100.00	0.00	4.80	3.97	5.62	0.87	1.28	9.68	15.71
所有部位除外 C44	ALL but C44	2 020	99.46	0.00	4.80	3.97	5.62	0.87	1.28	9.68	15.71

2014 年女性死亡主要指标 (1/10^5)

											粗率	世标率	累积率 (%)	
35–	40–	45–	50–	55–	60–	65–	70–	75–	80–	85–	(1/10^5 万)	(1/10 万^5)	0~64	0~74
0.00	0.00	0.00	0.00	0.00	0.00	0.00	0.00	0.00	0.00	0.00	0.00	0.00	0.00	0.00
0.00	0.66	0.71	0.94	1.00	2.79	1.99	0.00	3.34	0.00	12.99	0.60	0.49	0.03	0.04
0.00	0.00	0.00	0.94	0.00	0.00	1.99	2.57	6.68	13.45	0.00	0.42	0.29	0.00	0.03
0.00	0.00	0.71	0.00	0.00	0.00	0.00	0.00	0.00	0.00	0.00	0.06	0.04	0.00	0.00
0.00	0.00	0.00	0.00	0.00	0.00	0.00	0.00	0.00	0.00	0.00	0.00	0.00	0.00	0.00
0.00	0.00	0.00	0.00	0.00	0.00	1.99	0.00	0.00	0.00	0.00	0.06	0.06	0.00	0.01
0.00	0.66	0.71	0.00	1.99	0.00	3.97	0.00	3.34	0.00	0.00	0.42	0.31	0.02	0.04
0.00	0.00	0.71	0.00	0.00	0.00	1.99	0.00	0.00	0.00	0.00	0.12	0.10	0.00	0.01
0.00	0.00	0.00	0.00	1.00	1.39	0.00	0.00	0.00	6.72	0.00	0.18	0.13	0.01	0.01
0.00	0.00	2.12	4.69	18.92	39.02	77.42	105.36	153.53	201.68	454.72	14.78	12.03	0.33	1.25
0.00	1.99	3.54	8.45	14.94	34.84	73.45	43.68	140.18	221.85	233.86	12.28	9.60	0.33	0.91
0.00	0.00	0.00	0.00	1.00	0.00	1.99	5.14	13.35	13.45	12.99	0.66	0.47	0.00	0.04
0.00	1.33	0.00	5.63	9.96	4.18	23.82	33.41	50.06	60.50	103.94	4.71	3.69	0.11	0.40
2.20	2.65	2.12	3.75	4.98	22.30	5.96	33.41	56.74	33.61	129.92	5.07	4.03	0.20	0.39
0.00	0.00	0.00	0.00	1.00	0.00	0.00	5.14	3.34	6.72	0.00	0.30	0.21	0.00	0.03
0.73	4.64	3.54	4.69	25.89	41.81	29.78	82.23	110.14	141.18	142.91	11.26	8.74	0.42	0.98
0.00	0.66	1.42	0.94	4.98	6.97	7.94	20.56	16.69	20.17	25.98	2.15	1.70	0.07	0.22
1.47	1.33	0.00	0.94	7.97	2.79	15.88	25.70	33.38	33.61	51.97	3.16	2.45	0.08	0.28
0.00	0.00	0.00	0.00	0.00	0.00	0.00	0.00	3.34	0.00	0.00	0.06	0.03	0.00	0.00
0.00	0.00	0.00	0.00	0.00	0.00	0.00	0.00	0.00	0.00	12.99	0.06	0.06	0.00	0.00
3.67	6.63	11.33	21.58	29.87	62.71	83.38	159.32	240.30	315.97	363.78	22.82	17.72	0.69	1.90
0.00	0.00	0.00	0.94	1.00	1.39	1.99	2.57	3.34	0.00	12.99	0.42	0.35	0.02	0.04
0.00	0.00	0.00	1.88	3.98	4.18	3.97	7.71	13.35	13.45	12.99	1.25	0.96	0.05	0.11
0.73	0.00	0.00	0.00	0.00	1.39	0.00	0.00	0.00	0.00	0.00	0.12	0.10	0.01	0.01
0.73	0.00	1.42	1.88	0.00	1.39	1.99	0.00	3.34	0.00	38.98	0.66	0.57	0.03	0.04
0.00	0.00	0.71	0.00	0.00	0.00	0.00	0.00	0.00	6.72	0.00	0.12	0.08	0.00	0.00
0.00	0.00	0.00	0.00	0.00	0.00	0.00	0.00	0.00	0.00	0.00	0.00	0.00	0.00	0.00
0.00	0.00	0.00	0.00	0.00	0.00	1.99	0.00	0.00	0.00	0.00	0.06	0.06	0.00	0.01
6.60	13.92	20.53	35.66	24.89	50.17	41.69	28.27	60.08	87.39	103.94	13.88	10.83	0.77	1.12
0.00	0.00	0.00	0.00	0.00	2.79	0.00	2.57	0.00	0.00	0.00	0.18	0.16	0.01	0.03
0.00	0.00	0.00	0.94	0.00	0.00	0.00	0.00	0.00	0.00	0.00	0.06	0.05	0.00	0.00
3.67	5.30	12.74	15.02	12.95	9.75	13.90	10.28	16.69	40.34	0.00	5.48	4.10	0.31	0.43
1.47	0.66	2.83	9.38	2.99	6.97	5.96	15.42	6.68	13.45	12.99	2.32	1.85	0.12	0.23
0.00	0.66	0.71	2.82	0.00	1.39	5.96	0.00	0.00	0.00	0.00	0.60	0.51	0.03	0.06
2.20	1.99	9.20	1.88	1.99	8.36	5.96	23.13	16.69	20.17	0.00	3.04	2.33	0.14	0.28
0.73	0.00	0.71	0.00	0.00	0.00	0.00	0.00	0.00	0.00	0.00	0.12	0.09	0.01	0.01
0.00	0.00	0.00	0.00	0.00	0.00	0.00	0.00	0.00	0.00	0.00	0.00	0.00	0.00	0.00
—	—	—	—	—	—	—	—	—	—	—	—	—	—	—
—	—	—	—	—	—	—	—	—	—	—	—	—	—	—
—	—	—	—	—	—	—	—	—	—	—	—	—	—	—
—	—	—	—	—	—	—	—	—	—	—	—	—	—	—
0.00	0.00	0.00	0.94	2.99	0.00	0.00	10.28	13.35	26.89	0.00	1.01	0.76	0.02	0.08
0.00	0.00	0.00	0.00	0.00	0.00	0.00	0.00	0.00	6.72	0.00	0.06	0.03	0.00	0.00
0.00	0.00	0.00	0.00	0.00	0.00	1.99	2.57	0.00	0.00	0.00	0.18	0.21	0.01	0.03
0.00	0.00	0.71	0.94	1.00	4.18	0.00	2.57	13.35	13.45	25.98	0.89	0.68	0.03	0.05
0.00	0.00	0.00	0.00	0.00	1.39	0.00	0.00	0.00	6.72	0.00	0.12	0.09	0.01	0.01
0.00	0.00	0.00	0.00	0.00	0.00	0.00	0.00	0.00	0.00	0.00	0.06	0.10	0.01	0.01
1.47	2.65	0.00	4.69	0.00	13.94	7.94	10.28	10.01	33.61	64.96	2.62	2.23	0.12	0.21
0.00	1.33	2.12	1.88	3.98	8.36	3.97	7.71	6.68	0.00	0.00	1.61	1.33	0.10	0.16
0.00	0.00	0.00	0.00	0.00	0.00	0.00	2.57	0.00	0.00	0.00	0.12	0.15	0.00	0.02
0.00	0.00	0.00	0.94	0.00	0.00	0.00	0.00	0.00	0.00	0.00	0.06	0.05	0.00	0.00
0.73	0.00	1.42	0.00	0.00	0.00	1.99	5.14	3.34	0.00	0.00	0.42	0.32	0.01	0.05
0.73	0.00	0.00	0.00	1.00	4.18	1.99	7.71	3.34	20.17	0.00	0.83	0.68	0.03	0.08
0.00	0.00	0.00	0.00	0.00	0.00	0.00	0.00	0.00	0.00	0.00	0.00	0.00	0.00	0.00
0.00	0.00	0.00	0.00	0.00	1.39	1.99	0.00	0.00	0.00	0.00	0.12	0.12	0.01	0.02
0.73	1.33	0.71	0.94	1.00	0.00	1.99	0.00	0.00	13.45	12.99	0.66	0.50	0.03	0.04
0.00	0.00	0.00	0.94	1.00	1.39	0.00	0.00	3.34	13.45	0.00	0.54	0.51	0.03	0.03
0.73	0.00	2.12	1.88	1.00	5.57	7.94	7.71	10.01	26.89	25.98	2.03	1.83	0.09	0.16
0.00	1.99	2.12	2.82	1.99	5.57	3.97	15.42	13.35	20.17	12.99	2.03	1.62	0.08	0.18
0.00	0.00	0.00	0.00	0.00	0.00	0.00	2.57	0.00	0.00	0.00	0.06	0.05	0.00	0.01
0.00	0.00	0.00	0.00	0.00	0.00	0.00	0.00	6.68	0.00	12.99	0.18	0.13	0.00	0.00
28.61	50.37	84.94	138.89	185.22	352.56	448.65	680.97	1 037.98	1 431.93	1 883.85	121.03	95.60	4.41	10.06
27.88	50.37	83.53	137.01	185.22	351.17	446.67	680.97	1 034.64	1 431.93	1 844.87	120.38	95.03	4.38	10.02

表 6-1-16 河南省农村肿瘤登记地区

部位		病例数	构成	年龄组							
			(%)	0–	1–	5–	10–	15–	20–	25–	30–
唇	C00	11	0.04	0.00	0.00	0.00	0.00	0.00	0.00	0.00	0.00
舌	C01–C02	27	0.10	0.00	0.00	0.00	0.00	0.00	0.00	0.00	0.00
口	C03–C06	48	0.17	0.00	0.00	0.00	0.00	0.00	0.00	0.00	0.00
唾液腺	C07–C08	21	0.08	0.00	0.00	0.00	0.00	0.00	0.00	0.07	0.08
扁桃体	C09	10	0.04	0.00	0.00	0.00	0.00	0.00	0.00	0.00	0.00
其他的口咽	C10	22	0.08	0.00	0.00	0.00	0.00	0.00	0.00	0.00	0.00
鼻咽	C11	105	0.38	0.00	0.00	0.08	0.00	0.00	0.13	0.07	0.23
喉咽	C12–C13	20	0.07	0.00	0.00	0.00	0.00	0.00	0.00	0.00	0.00
咽，部位不明	C14	28	0.10	0.00	0.00	0.00	0.00	0.00	0.00	0.00	0.00
食管	C15	4 776	17.37	0.00	0.00	0.00	0.00	0.00	0.07	0.20	0.54
胃	C16	5 204	18.92	0.00	0.00	0.00	0.00	0.00	0.39	1.18	1.78
小肠	C17	111	0.40	0.00	0.00	0.00	0.00	0.00	0.00	0.07	0.08
结肠	C18	512	1.86	0.00	0.00	0.00	0.00	0.00	0.07	0.26	0.46
直肠	C19–C20	750	2.73	0.00	0.00	0.00	0.00	0.00	0.00	0.20	0.54
肛门	C21	48	0.17	0.00	0.00	0.00	0.00	0.00	0.00	0.00	0.08
肝脏	C22	3 925	14.27	0.00	0.00	0.00	0.18	0.16	0.26	0.72	2.24
胆囊及其他	C23–C24	366	1.33	0.00	0.00	0.00	0.00	0.00	0.07	0.00	0.08
胰腺	C25	423	1.54	0.00	0.00	0.00	0.00	0.00	0.00	0.26	0.31
鼻、鼻窦及其他	C30–C31	30	0.11	0.00	0.00	0.00	0.09	0.00	0.00	0.07	0.31
喉	C32	135	0.49	0.00	0.00	0.00	0.00	0.00	0.00	0.00	0.08
气管、支气管、肺	C33–C34	6 228	22.65	0.00	0.00	0.00	0.00	0.00	0.00	0.59	1.70
其他的胸腔器官	C37–C38	53	0.19	0.46	0.00	0.00	0.18	0.00	0.07	0.13	0.15
骨	C40–C41	219	0.80	0.00	0.00	0.00	0.18	0.16	0.33	0.13	0.23
皮肤的黑色素瘤	C43	20	0.07	0.00	0.10	0.00	0.00	0.00	0.07	0.00	0.00
其他的皮肤	C44	95	0.35	0.00	0.00	0.00	0.00	0.16	0.00	0.00	0.08
间皮瘤	C45	4	0.01	0.00	0.00	0.00	0.00	0.00	0.00	0.00	0.00
卡波西肉瘤	C46	0	0.00	0.00	0.00	0.00	0.00	0.00	0.00	0.00	0.00
周围神经、其他结缔组织、软组织	C47;C49	21	0.08	0.00	0.10	0.00	0.00	0.00	0.00	0.00	0.08
乳房	C50	—	—	—	—	—	—	—	—	—	—
外阴	C51	—	—	—	—	—	—	—	—	—	—
阴道	C52	—	—	—	—	—	—	—	—	—	—
子宫颈	C53	—	—	—	—	—	—	—	—	—	—
子宫体	C54	—	—	—	—	—	—	—	—	—	—
子宫，部位不明	C55	—	—	—	—	—	—	—	—	—	—
卵巢	C56	—	—	—	—	—	—	—	—	—	—
其他的女性生殖器	C57	—	—	—	—	—	—	—	—	—	—
胎盘	C58	—	—	—	—	—	—	—	—	—	—
阴茎	C60	—	—	—	—	—	—	—	—	—	—
前列腺	C61	—	—	—	—	—	—	—	—	—	—
睾丸	C62	—	—	—	—	—	—	—	—	—	—
其他的男性生殖器	C63	—	—	—	—	—	—	—	—	—	—
肾	C64	120	0.44	0.00	0.00	0.08	0.09	0.08	0.07	0.13	0.00
肾盂	C65	23	0.08	0.00	0.00	0.00	0.00	0.00	0.00	0.00	0.00
输尿管	C66	18	0.07	0.00	0.00	0.00	0.00	0.00	0.00	0.00	0.00
膀胱	C67	199	0.72	0.00	0.00	0.00	0.09	0.00	0.00	0.07	0.00
其他的泌尿器官	C68	5	0.02	0.00	0.00	0.00	0.00	0.00	0.00	0.00	0.00
眼	C69	8	0.03	0.00	0.00	0.08	0.00	0.00	0.00	0.00	0.00
脑、神经系统	C70–C72	717	2.61	0.46	0.69	1.08	1.06	0.57	0.39	0.72	1.16
甲状腺	C73	96	0.35	0.00	0.00	0.08	0.00	0.00	0.00	0.00	0.00
肾上腺	C74	20	0.07	0.00	0.10	0.08	0.00	0.00	0.00	0.00	0.08
其他的内分泌腺	C75	13	0.05	0.00	0.00	0.00	0.00	0.00	0.00	0.00	0.00
霍奇金病	C81	32	0.12	0.00	0.00	0.00	0.09	0.00	0.00	0.00	0.08
非霍奇金淋巴瘤	C82–C85;C96	206	0.75	0.00	0.10	0.08	0.09	0.00	0.20	0.07	0.39
免疫增生性疾病	C88	2	0.01	0.00	0.00	0.00	0.00	0.00	0.00	0.00	0.00
多发性骨髓瘤	C90	57	0.21	0.00	0.00	0.00	0.00	0.00	0.07	0.00	0.08
淋巴样白血病	C91	93	0.34	0.46	0.20	0.25	0.44	0.40	0.79	0.39	0.31
髓样白血病	C92–C94	113	0.41	0.00	0.39	0.17	0.18	0.24	0.26	0.33	0.31
白血病，未特指	C95	299	1.09	0.00	1.18	1.50	1.15	1.05	0.85	1.24	0.46
其他的或未指明部位的	O&U	351	1.28	0.46	0.29	0.17	0.18	0.24	0.39	0.33	0.46
骨髓增殖性疾病	MPD	3	0.01	0.00	0.00	0.00	0.00	0.00	0.00	0.00	0.00
骨髓增生异常综合征	MDS	12	0.04	0.00	0.00	0.00	0.00	0.00	0.00	0.00	0.00
合计	ALL	27 500	100.00	1.85	3.14	3.75	3.98	3.23	4.98	7.59	13.85
所有部位除外 C44	ALL but C44	27 405	99.65	1.85	3.14	3.75	3.98	3.07	4.98	7.59	13.77

2014 年合计死亡主要指标 ($1/10^5$)

											粗率	世标率	累积率 (%)	
35–	40–	45–	50–	55–	60–	65–	70–	75–	80–	85–	($1/10^5$ 万)	($1/10^5$ 万)	0~64	0~74
0.00	0.07	0.07	0.00	0.10	0.25	0.18	0.00	0.98	0.56	0.94	0.06	0.05	0.00	0.00
0.08	0.07	0.14	0.09	0.31	0.51	0.72	0.99	1.30	1.67	0.00	0.15	0.12	0.01	0.01
0.15	0.21	0.07	0.00	0.42	1.01	1.27	1.23	2.61	3.34	3.76	0.27	0.21	0.01	0.02
0.08	0.00	0.14	0.28	0.21	0.63	0.54	0.25	0.65	0.00	0.00	0.12	0.10	0.01	0.01
0.00	0.00	0.00	0.00	0.00	0.38	0.36	0.00	0.65	1.11	0.94	0.06	0.04	0.00	0.00
0.00	0.14	0.14	0.00	0.31	0.51	0.36	0.49	0.65	1.67	1.88	0.12	0.10	0.01	0.01
0.00	0.50	0.58	1.31	1.26	2.03	2.90	2.22	1.96	3.89	2.82	0.60	0.48	0.03	0.06
0.00	0.00	0.14	0.09	0.31	0.51	0.36	0.49	0.98	1.11	0.94	0.11	0.09	0.01	0.01
0.08	0.00	0.14	0.47	0.52	0.38	0.72	0.99	0.65	0.56	0.94	0.16	0.13	0.01	0.02
0.98	2.43	7.24	20.32	42.63	92.59	157.53	184.31	232.16	335.35	310.96	27.12	21.08	0.84	2.54
1.97	7.37	12.09	23.04	49.66	103.48	147.03	192.69	254.66	352.59	296.87	29.55	22.85	1.00	2.70
0.15	0.36	0.43	0.56	1.05	2.03	2.72	3.45	4.56	6.67	8.46	0.63	0.49	0.02	0.05
0.23	1.14	2.68	3.18	4.93	10.64	13.58	15.52	16.63	36.15	24.43	2.91	2.27	0.12	0.26
0.68	1.14	3.91	4.68	8.61	13.05	17.02	25.87	32.28	43.93	46.03	4.26	3.29	0.16	0.38
0.15	0.29	0.29	0.84	0.52	0.76	1.27	0.74	0.65	1.11	2.82	0.27	0.22	0.01	0.02
5.00	12.45	19.84	35.69	51.13	85.37	104.84	102.01	120.97	167.40	146.56	22.29	17.69	1.07	2.10
0.23	0.07	1.23	1.50	3.25	6.08	7.79	15.03	21.19	22.25	36.64	2.08	1.59	0.06	0.18
0.23	0.50	2.03	3.00	4.41	7.35	12.67	17.74	14.67	16.68	26.31	2.40	1.92	0.09	0.24
0.00	0.07	0.07	0.19	0.42	0.38	1.09	0.25	0.33	1.67	1.88	0.17	0.14	0.01	0.01
0.08	0.07	0.29	1.03	1.78	2.66	3.80	6.90	4.56	6.67	3.76	0.77	0.61	0.03	0.08
3.26	8.59	17.16	35.03	56.07	118.43	185.59	227.68	289.55	391.52	388.00	35.37	27.54	1.20	3.27
0.00	0.29	0.14	0.37	0.52	1.01	0.72	1.72	1.30	2.78	1.88	0.30	0.25	0.01	0.03
0.23	0.57	0.87	1.97	3.57	4.43	6.34	4.19	6.20	8.90	4.70	1.24	1.00	0.06	0.12
0.00	0.00	0.22	0.00	0.00	0.38	0.36	1.48	0.33	0.56	1.88	0.11	0.10	0.00	0.01
0.08	0.07	0.22	0.28	0.84	1.14	1.27	2.71	3.59	8.34	21.61	0.54	0.41	0.01	0.03
0.00	0.00	0.00	0.09	0.00	0.13	0.18	0.00	0.00	0.56	0.00	0.02	0.02	0.00	0.00
0.00	0.00	0.00	0.00	0.00	0.00	0.00	0.00	0.00	0.00	0.00	0.00	0.00	0.00	0.00
0.00	0.14	0.14	0.19	0.10	0.51	0.18	0.74	0.33	1.11	0.94	0.12	0.10	0.01	0.01
—	—	—	—	—	—	—	—	—	—	—	—	—	—	—
—	—	—	—	—	—	—	—	—	—	—	—	—	—	—
—	—	—	—	—	—	—	—	—	—	—	—	—	—	—
—	—	—	—	—	—	—	—	—	—	—	—	—	—	—
—	—	—	—	—	—	—	—	—	—	—	—	—	—	—
—	—	—	—	—	—	—	—	—	—	—	—	—	—	—
—	—	—	—	—	—	—	—	—	—	—	—	—	—	—
—	—	—	—	—	—	—	—	—	—	—	—	—	—	—
—	—	—	—	—	—	—	—	—	—	—	—	—	—	—
—	—	—	—	—	—	—	—	—	—	—	—	—	—	—
—	—	—	—	—	—	—	—	—	—	—	—	—	—	—
—	—	—	—	—	—	—	—	—	—	—	—	—	—	—
—	—	—	—	—	—	—	—	—	—	—	—	—	—	—
0.00	0.21	0.51	1.03	1.36	1.52	3.44	3.70	4.56	7.79	5.64	0.68	0.54	0.03	0.06
0.08	0.14	0.14	0.09	0.31	0.25	0.54	0.49	0.65	1.67	1.88	0.13	0.10	0.01	0.01
0.00	0.00	0.00	0.00	0.31	0.25	0.54	1.23	0.98	0.00	1.88	0.10	0.08	0.00	0.01
0.08	0.14	0.43	0.94	1.15	2.66	7.42	7.88	10.76	14.46	13.15	1.13	0.88	0.03	0.10
0.00	0.00	0.00	0.00	0.00	0.25	0.00	0.00	0.33	0.00	1.88	0.03	0.02	0.00	0.00
0.00	0.00	0.00	0.00	0.10	0.38	0.18	0.25	0.00	0.00	0.94	0.05	0.04	0.00	0.00
2.73	2.50	4.34	4.87	7.14	12.92	15.75	16.02	16.63	31.70	30.06	4.07	3.38	0.20	0.36
0.08	0.29	0.58	0.75	0.73	1.52	2.53	3.20	4.89	3.89	5.64	0.55	0.43	0.02	0.05
0.00	0.00	0.07	0.28	0.21	0.00	0.36	0.49	0.98	1.11	1.88	0.11	0.09	0.00	0.01
0.08	0.00	0.07	0.09	0.10	0.13	0.00	0.49	0.98	1.67	0.00	0.07	0.05	0.00	0.00
0.15	0.07	0.07	0.09	0.31	0.89	0.36	1.48	0.33	2.22	1.88	0.18	0.15	0.01	0.02
0.23	0.64	0.58	2.44	2.73	3.93	3.44	7.39	5.54	8.90	8.46	1.17	0.94	0.06	0.11
0.00	0.00	0.00	0.00	0.00	0.00	0.18	0.00	0.00	0.00	0.94	0.01	0.01	0.00	0.00
0.00	0.21	0.43	0.28	0.73	1.39	1.45	1.72	2.28	1.11	0.94	0.32	0.26	0.02	0.03
0.38	0.50	0.65	0.28	0.42	0.63	0.54	1.72	2.28	1.67	1.88	0.53	0.48	0.03	0.04
0.53	0.72	0.80	0.47	1.57	1.52	1.63	0.74	3.26	3.34	0.94	0.64	0.55	0.04	0.05
0.68	1.22	1.30	1.40	2.62	4.43	5.43	5.17	5.22	7.23	5.64	1.70	1.59	0.09	0.15
0.76	0.86	1.67	2.06	3.99	5.95	7.79	8.87	14.02	19.46	13.15	1.99	1.59	0.09	0.17
0.00	0.00	0.00	0.09	0.00	0.00	0.00	0.25	0.33	0.00	0.00	0.02	0.01	0.00	0.00
0.00	0.00	0.00	0.19	0.10	0.38	0.36	0.00	0.00	1.11	1.88	0.07	0.05	0.00	0.01
23.40	51.73	97.52	169.53	280.24	531.46	762.65	919.58	1 134.07	1 601.12	1 510.67	156.17	122.68	5.97	14.38
23.33	51.66	97.31	169.25	279.40	530.32	761.39	916.87	1 130.49	1 592.77	1 489.06	155.63	122.27	5.96	14.35

表 6-1-17 河南省农村肿瘤登记地区

部位		病例数	构成	年龄组							
			(%)	0-	1-	5-	10-	15-	20-	25-	30-
唇	C00	6	0.04	0.00	0.00	0.00	0.00	0.00	0.00	0.00	0.00
舌	C01-C02	14	0.08	0.00	0.00	0.00	0.00	0.00	0.00	0.00	0.00
口	C03-C06	21	0.12	0.00	0.00	0.00	0.00	0.00	0.00	0.00	0.00
唾液腺	C07-C08	11	0.06	0.00	0.00	0.00	0.00	0.00	0.00	0.13	0.00
扁桃体	C09	7	0.04	0.00	0.00	0.00	0.00	0.00	0.00	0.00	0.00
其他的口咽	C10	13	0.08	0.00	0.00	0.00	0.00	0.00	0.00	0.00	0.00
鼻咽	C11	59	0.35	0.00	0.00	0.00	0.00	0.00	0.13	0.13	0.00
喉咽	C12-C13	18	0.11	0.00	0.00	0.00	0.00	0.00	0.00	0.00	0.00
咽，部位不明	C14	21	0.12	0.00	0.00	0.00	0.00	0.00	0.00	0.00	0.00
食管	C15	2 969	17.47	0.00	0.00	0.00	0.00	0.00	0.00	0.13	0.45
胃	C16	3 667	21.58	0.00	0.00	0.00	0.00	0.00	0.38	1.02	1.35
小肠	C17	65	0.38	0.00	0.00	0.00	0.00	0.00	0.00	0.00	0.00
结肠	C18	287	1.69	0.00	0.00	0.00	0.00	0.00	0.00	0.26	0.45
直肠	C19-C20	430	2.53	0.00	0.00	0.00	0.00	0.00	0.00	0.13	0.60
肛门	C21	27	0.16	0.00	0.00	0.00	0.00	0.00	0.00	0.00	0.15
肝脏	C22	2 693	15.85	0.00	0.00	0.00	0.00	0.31	0.25	0.89	3.30
胆囊及其他	C23-C24	148	0.87	0.00	0.00	0.00	0.00	0.00	0.13	0.00	0.00
胰腺	C25	236	1.39	0.00	0.00	0.00	0.00	0.00	0.00	0.51	0.45
鼻、鼻窦及其他	C30-C31	12	0.07	0.00	0.00	0.00	0.16	0.00	0.00	0.13	0.45
喉	C32	94	0.55	0.00	0.00	0.00	0.00	0.00	0.00	0.00	0.00
气管、支气管、肺	C33-C34	4 354	25.63	0.00	0.00	0.00	0.00	0.00	0.00	0.64	2.55
其他的胸腔器官	C37-C38	30	0.18	0.87	0.00	0.00	0.33	0.00	0.00	0.00	0.30
骨	C40-C41	130	0.77	0.00	0.00	0.00	0.16	0.31	0.51	0.13	0.30
皮肤的黑色素瘤	C43	9	0.05	0.00	0.18	0.00	0.00	0.00	0.00	0.00	0.00
其他的皮肤	C44	53	0.31	0.00	0.00	0.00	0.00	0.00	0.00	0.00	0.15
间皮瘤	C45	3	0.02	0.00	0.00	0.00	0.00	0.00	0.00	0.00	0.00
卡波西肉瘤	C46	0	0.00	0.00	0.00	0.00	0.00	0.00	0.00	0.00	0.00
周围神经、其他结缔组织、软组织	C47;C49	15	0.09	0.00	0.18	0.00	0.00	0.00	0.00	0.00	0.15
乳房	C50	—	—	—	—	—	—	—	—	—	—
外阴	C51	—	—	—	—	—	—	—	—	—	—
阴道	C52	—	—	—	—	—	—	—	—	—	—
子宫颈	C53	—	—	—	—	—	—	—	—	—	—
子宫体	C54	—	—	—	—	—	—	—	—	—	—
子宫，部位不明	C55	—	—	—	—	—	—	—	—	—	—
卵巢	C56	—	—	—	—	—	—	—	—	—	—
其他的女性生殖器	C57	—	—	—	—	—	—	—	—	—	—
胎盘	C58	—	—	—	—	—	—	—	—	—	—
阴茎	C60	11	0.06	0.00	0.00	0.00	0.00	0.00	0.00	0.00	0.00
前列腺	C61	146	0.86	0.00	0.00	0.15	0.00	0.15	0.00	0.00	0.00
睾丸	C62	13	0.08	0.00	0.00	0.00	0.00	0.00	0.00	0.00	0.00
其他的男性生殖器	C63	5	0.03	0.00	0.00	0.00	0.00	0.00	0.00	0.00	0.00
肾	C64	85	0.50	0.00	0.00	0.15	0.16	0.00	0.00	0.26	0.00
肾盂	C65	16	0.09	0.00	0.00	0.00	0.00	0.00	0.00	0.00	0.00
输尿管	C66	14	0.08	0.00	0.00	0.00	0.00	0.00	0.00	0.00	0.00
膀胱	C67	150	0.88	0.00	0.00	0.00	0.00	0.00	0.00	0.13	0.00
其他的泌尿器官	C68	2	0.01	0.00	0.00	0.00	0.00	0.00	0.00	0.00	0.00
眼	C69	5	0.03	0.00	0.00	0.15	0.00	0.00	0.00	0.00	0.00
脑、神经系统	C70-C72	390	2.30	0.87	0.72	1.39	1.14	0.62	0.38	0.89	1.65
甲状腺	C73	43	0.25	0.00	0.00	0.00	0.00	0.00	0.00	0.00	0.00
肾上腺	C74	14	0.08	0.00	0.18	0.00	0.00	0.00	0.00	0.00	0.15
其他的内分泌腺	C75	8	0.05	0.00	0.00	0.00	0.00	0.00	0.00	0.00	0.00
霍奇金病	C81	20	0.12	0.00	0.00	0.00	0.16	0.00	0.00	0.00	0.15
非霍奇金淋巴瘤	C82-C85;C96	129	0.76	0.00	0.18	0.00	0.16	0.00	0.13	0.13	0.30
免疫增生性疾病	C88	0	0.00	0.00	0.00	0.00	0.00	0.00	0.00	0.00	0.00
多发性骨髓瘤	C90	40	0.24	0.00	0.00	0.00	0.00	0.00	0.13	0.00	0.15
淋巴样白血病	C91	49	0.29	0.00	0.18	0.31	0.82	0.62	0.63	0.51	0.60
髓样白血病	C92-C94	66	0.39	0.00	0.36	0.15	0.33	0.31	0.25	0.26	0.30
白血病，未特指	C95	162	0.95	0.00	0.72	1.86	1.63	1.24	0.89	1.15	0.60
其他的或未指明部位的	O&U	210	1.24	0.87	0.36	0.15	0.16	0.15	0.51	0.38	0.60
骨髓增殖性疾病	MPD	2	0.01	0.00	0.00	0.00	0.00	0.00	0.00	0.00	0.00
骨髓增生异常综合征	MDS	10	0.06	0.00	0.00	0.00	0.00	0.00	0.00	0.00	0.00
合计	ALL	16 991	100.00	2.61	3.05	4.33	5.23	3.71	4.31	7.79	15.13
所有部位除外 C44	ALL but C44	16 938	99.69	2.61	3.05	4.33	5.23	3.71	4.31	7.79	14.98

2014 年男性死亡主要指标 (1/10^5)

											粗率	世标率	累积率 (%)	
35–	40–	45–	50–	55–	60–	65–	70–	75–	80–	85–	(1/10^5 万)	(1/10^5 万)	0~64	0~74
0.00	0.00	0.14	0.00	0.21	0.00	0.36	0.00	0.70	1.30	2.74	0.07	0.05	0.00	0.00
0.14	0.14	0.14	0.00	0.62	0.25	1.08	0.50	1.40	1.30	0.00	0.15	0.12	0.01	0.01
0.29	0.28	0.00	0.00	0.41	0.50	1.45	0.99	2.10	3.90	2.74	0.23	0.19	0.01	0.02
0.00	0.00	0.00	0.18	0.21	0.75	1.08	0.00	1.40	0.00	0.00	0.12	0.10	0.01	0.01
0.00	0.00	0.00	0.00	0.00	0.50	0.72	0.00	0.70	1.30	2.74	0.08	0.07	0.00	0.01
0.00	0.28	0.00	0.00	0.41	0.75	0.36	0.50	0.00	2.60	5.48	0.14	0.12	0.01	0.01
0.00	0.55	0.86	1.29	1.23	2.00	3.97	2.98	2.10	5.20	5.48	0.65	0.55	0.03	0.07
0.00	0.00	0.29	0.18	0.62	1.00	0.36	0.99	2.10	2.60	0.00	0.20	0.16	0.01	0.02
0.14	0.00	0.29	0.55	1.03	0.50	1.45	0.99	1.40	0.00	0.00	0.23	0.19	0.01	0.02
0.72	3.04	9.87	26.17	56.23	123.30	207.77	230.30	294.54	441.11	441.19	32.65	27.54	1.10	3.29
2.17	10.63	16.17	33.54	72.24	152.01	216.80	280.04	381.29	551.72	457.63	40.32	33.54	1.45	3.93
0.14	0.28	0.86	0.74	1.23	2.25	3.61	5.47	5.60	7.81	5.48	0.71	0.59	0.03	0.07
0.29	0.83	3.29	3.69	5.13	11.98	15.90	18.90	19.59	46.84	32.88	3.16	2.63	0.13	0.30
1.01	1.52	4.15	4.79	9.23	16.47	21.32	32.83	43.38	48.15	46.59	4.73	3.92	0.19	0.46
0.14	0.14	0.29	0.92	0.41	0.75	1.81	1.49	0.00	1.30	8.22	0.30	0.27	0.01	0.03
7.54	20.03	30.91	53.99	71.62	117.81	143.45	132.81	161.61	209.50	211.01	29.61	24.78	1.53	2.91
0.43	0.00	1.14	0.74	3.90	4.74	5.78	14.42	13.29	18.22	43.85	1.63	1.39	0.06	0.16
0.29	0.41	2.58	3.69	5.75	9.24	13.37	19.90	11.89	20.82	30.14	2.60	2.22	0.11	0.28
0.00	0.00	0.14	0.18	0.21	0.25	0.36	0.00	0.00	1.30	2.74	0.13	0.12	0.01	0.01
0.14	0.14	0.43	1.47	1.85	3.99	5.42	9.95	7.70	10.41	5.48	1.03	0.87	0.04	0.12
4.35	11.60	22.46	46.99	78.80	167.98	277.14	341.72	437.26	579.04	616.57	47.88	40.23	1.68	4.77
0.00	0.14	0.14	0.55	0.62	1.75	1.08	1.49	1.40	2.60	0.00	0.33	0.29	0.02	0.03
0.00	0.83	1.14	2.21	4.10	4.74	8.67	4.97	5.60	13.01	8.22	1.43	1.22	0.07	0.14
0.00	0.00	0.29	0.00	0.00	0.50	0.00	1.49	0.00	0.00	2.74	0.10	0.10	0.00	0.01
0.00	0.14	0.00	0.55	1.23	1.25	0.72	3.98	6.30	9.11	30.14	0.58	0.50	0.02	0.04
0.00	0.00	0.00	0.18	0.00	0.00	0.36	0.00	0.00	1.30	0.00	0.03	0.03	0.00	0.00
0.00	0.00	0.00	0.00	0.00	0.00	0.00	0.00	0.00	0.00	0.00	0.00	0.00	0.00	0.00
0.00	0.14	0.29	0.18	0.21	0.50	0.36	0.99	0.70	2.60	0.00	0.16	0.14	0.01	0.01
—	—	—	—	—	—	—	—	—	—	—	—	—	—	—
—	—	—	—	—	—	—	—	—	—	—	—	—	—	—
—	—	—	—	—	—	—	—	—	—	—	—	—	—	—
—	—	—	—	—	—	—	—	—	—	—	—	—	—	—
—	—	—	—	—	—	—	—	—	—	—	—	—	—	—
—	—	—	—	—	—	—	—	—	—	—	—	—	—	—
—	—	—	—	—	—	—	—	—	—	—	—	—	—	—
—	—	—	—	—	—	—	—	—	—	—	—	—	—	—
—	—	—	—	—	—	—	—	—	—	—	—	—	—	—
0.14	0.00	0.00	0.00	0.21	0.00	1.08	0.99	0.70	2.60	2.74	0.12	0.10	0.00	0.01
0.00	0.00	0.43	0.00	1.03	2.25	7.23	10.45	21.69	37.74	71.25	1.61	1.37	0.02	0.11
0.00	0.00	0.29	0.37	0.00	0.75	0.72	1.49	0.00	1.30	0.00	0.14	0.12	0.01	0.02
0.00	0.00	0.00	0.18	0.00	0.00	0.36	0.00	0.70	1.30	2.74	0.05	0.05	0.00	0.00
0.00	0.14	0.86	1.47	2.67	1.75	4.34	5.97	7.70	10.41	8.22	0.93	0.78	0.04	0.09
0.14	0.28	0.14	0.18	0.00	0.50	0.72	0.99	0.70	2.60	5.48	0.18	0.15	0.01	0.01
0.00	0.00	0.00	0.00	0.62	0.25	0.72	1.49	2.10	0.00	5.48	0.15	0.13	0.00	0.02
0.14	0.28	0.43	1.11	1.85	3.74	10.84	12.44	20.29	24.72	27.40	1.65	1.38	0.04	0.15
0.00	0.00	0.00	0.00	0.00	0.50	0.00	0.00	0.00	0.00	0.00	0.02	0.02	0.00	0.00
0.00	0.00	0.00	0.00	0.21	0.50	0.36	0.00	0.00	0.00	0.00	0.05	0.05	0.00	0.01
3.19	2.49	5.44	5.90	7.59	10.98	17.34	16.91	20.29	32.53	46.59	4.29	3.75	0.21	0.38
0.14	0.14	0.43	0.74	0.62	1.25	2.17	3.48	4.20	7.81	2.74	0.47	0.38	0.02	0.04
0.00	0.00	0.14	0.55	0.41	0.00	0.36	0.00	1.40	2.60	2.74	0.15	0.13	0.01	0.01
0.00	0.00	0.14	0.18	0.21	0.00	0.00	0.99	0.00	3.90	0.00	0.09	0.07	0.00	0.01
0.00	0.00	0.00	0.18	0.41	1.25	0.72	2.49	0.70	1.30	2.74	0.22	0.20	0.01	0.03
0.29	0.69	1.14	2.76	3.49	5.74	2.89	9.45	9.10	7.81	19.18	1.42	1.21	0.07	0.14
0.00	0.00	0.00	0.00	0.00	0.00	0.00	0.00	0.00	0.00	0.00	0.00	0.00	0.00	0.00
0.00	0.28	0.72	0.55	1.23	1.50	1.45	1.99	4.90	0.00	2.74	0.44	0.36	0.02	0.04
0.43	0.69	0.57	0.37	0.62	0.25	0.72	1.49	0.70	0.00	0.00	0.54	0.52	0.03	0.04
0.72	0.69	1.00	0.74	1.44	1.75	2.53	1.49	4.20	1.30	2.74	0.73	0.64	0.04	0.06
1.01	0.83	1.43	1.66	2.67	4.49	6.14	4.48	7.70	6.51	8.22	1.78	1.70	0.10	0.15
0.72	1.38	2.00	2.03	4.72	7.49	9.76	11.44	18.19	20.82	21.92	2.31	1.96	0.10	0.21
0.00	0.00	0.00	0.18	0.00	0.00	0.00	0.50	0.00	0.00	0.00	0.02	0.02	0.00	0.00
0.00	0.00	0.00	0.37	0.21	0.75	0.36	0.00	0.00	1.30	5.48	0.11	0.10	0.01	0.01
24.79	59.11	111.61	202.34	347.64	671.43	1 005.96	1 196.76	1 527.28	2 150.92	2 203.22	186.83	157.24	7.30	18.32
24.79	58.97	111.61	201.78	346.41	670.19	1 005.24	1 192.78	1 520.98	2 141.81	2 173.08	186.25	156.73	7.29	18.28

表 6-1-18　河南省农村肿瘤登记地区

部位		病例数	构成	年龄组							
			(%)	0–	1–	5–	10–	15–	20–	25–	30–
唇	C00	5	0.05	0.00	0.00	0.00	0.00	0.00	0.00	0.00	0.00
舌	C01–C02	13	0.12	0.00	0.00	0.00	0.00	0.00	0.00	0.00	0.00
口	C03–C06	27	0.26	0.00	0.00	0.00	0.00	0.00	0.00	0.00	0.00
唾液腺	C07–C08	10	0.10	0.00	0.00	0.00	0.00	0.00	0.00	0.00	0.16
扁桃体	C09	3	0.03	0.00	0.00	0.00	0.00	0.00	0.00	0.00	0.00
其他的口咽	C10	9	0.09	0.00	0.00	0.00	0.00	0.00	0.00	0.00	0.00
鼻咽	C11	46	0.44	0.00	0.00	0.18	0.00	0.00	0.14	0.00	0.48
喉咽	C12–C13	2	0.02	0.00	0.00	0.00	0.00	0.00	0.00	0.00	0.00
咽，部位不明	C14	7	0.07	0.00	0.00	0.00	0.00	0.00	0.00	0.00	0.00
食管	C15	1 807	17.19	0.00	0.00	0.00	0.00	0.00	0.14	0.27	0.64
胃	C16	1 537	14.63	0.00	0.00	0.00	0.00	0.00	0.41	1.34	2.24
小肠	C17	46	0.44	0.00	0.00	0.00	0.00	0.00	0.00	0.13	0.16
结肠	C18	225	2.14	0.00	0.00	0.00	0.00	0.00	0.14	0.27	0.48
直肠	C19–C20	320	3.05	0.00	0.00	0.00	0.00	0.00	0.00	0.27	0.48
肛门	C21	21	0.20	0.00	0.00	0.00	0.00	0.00	0.00	0.00	0.00
肝脏	C22	1 232	11.72	0.00	0.00	0.00	0.39	0.00	0.27	0.54	1.12
胆囊及其他	C23–C24	218	2.07	0.00	0.00	0.00	0.00	0.00	0.00	0.00	0.16
胰腺	C25	187	1.78	0.00	0.00	0.00	0.00	0.00	0.00	0.00	0.16
鼻、鼻窦及其他	C30–C31	18	0.17	0.00	0.00	0.00	0.00	0.00	0.00	0.00	0.16
喉	C32	41	0.39	0.00	0.00	0.00	0.00	0.00	0.00	0.00	0.16
气管、支气管、肺	C33–C34	1 874	17.83	0.00	0.00	0.00	0.00	0.00	0.00	0.54	0.80
其他的胸腔器官	C37–C38	23	0.22	0.00	0.00	0.00	0.00	0.00	0.14	0.27	0.00
骨	C40–C41	89	0.85	0.00	0.00	0.00	0.19	0.00	0.14	0.13	0.16
皮肤的黑色素瘤	C43	11	0.10	0.00	0.00	0.00	0.00	0.00	0.14	0.00	0.00
其他的皮肤	C44	42	0.40	0.00	0.00	0.00	0.00	0.34	0.00	0.00	0.00
间皮瘤	C45	1	0.01	0.00	0.00	0.00	0.00	0.00	0.00	0.00	0.00
卡波西肉瘤	C46	0	0.00	0.00	0.00	0.00	0.00	0.00	0.00	0.00	0.00
周围神经、其他结缔组织、软组织	C47;C49	6	0.06	0.00	0.00	0.00	0.00	0.00	0.00	0.00	0.00
乳房	C50	833	7.93	0.00	0.00	0.00	0.00	0.00	0.54	0.80	1.76
外阴	C51	5	0.05	0.00	0.00	0.00	0.00	0.00	0.00	0.00	0.00
阴道	C52	11	0.10	0.00	0.00	0.00	0.00	0.00	0.00	0.00	0.00
子宫颈	C53	433	4.12	0.00	0.00	0.00	0.00	0.00	0.00	0.00	0.96
子宫体	C54	127	1.21	0.00	0.00	0.00	0.00	0.00	0.00	0.00	0.16
子宫，部位不明	C55	75	0.71	0.00	0.00	0.00	0.00	0.00	0.00	0.00	0.00
卵巢	C56	222	2.11	0.00	0.00	0.00	0.00	0.17	0.54	0.00	0.00
其他的女性生殖器	C57	9	0.09	0.00	0.00	0.00	0.00	0.00	0.00	0.00	0.00
胎盘	C58	2	0.02	0.00	0.00	0.00	0.00	0.00	0.00	0.00	0.16
阴茎	C60	—	—	—	—	—	—	—	—	—	—
前列腺	C61	—	—	—	—	—	—	—	—	—	—
睾丸	C62	—	—	—	—	—	—	—	—	—	—
其他的男性生殖器	C63	—	—	—	—	—	—	—	—	—	—
肾	C64	35	0.33	0.00	0.00	0.00	0.00	0.17	0.14	0.00	0.00
肾盂	C65	7	0.07	0.00	0.00	0.00	0.00	0.00	0.00	0.00	0.00
输尿管	C66	4	0.04	0.00	0.00	0.00	0.00	0.00	0.00	0.00	0.00
膀胱	C67	49	0.47	0.00	0.00	0.00	0.19	0.00	0.00	0.00	0.00
其他的泌尿器官	C68	3	0.03	0.00	0.00	0.00	0.00	0.00	0.00	0.00	0.00
眼	C69	3	0.03	0.00	0.00	0.00	0.00	0.00	0.00	0.00	0.00
脑、神经系统	C70–C72	327	3.11	0.00	0.65	0.72	0.96	0.51	0.41	0.54	0.64
甲状腺	C73	53	0.50	0.00	0.00	0.18	0.00	0.00	0.00	0.00	0.00
肾上腺	C74	6	0.06	0.00	0.00	0.18	0.00	0.00	0.00	0.00	0.00
其他的内分泌腺	C75	5	0.05	0.00	0.00	0.00	0.00	0.00	0.00	0.00	0.00
霍奇金病	C81	12	0.11	0.00	0.00	0.00	0.00	0.00	0.00	0.00	0.00
非霍奇金淋巴瘤	C82–C85;C96	77	0.73	0.00	0.00	0.18	0.00	0.00	0.27	0.00	0.48
免疫增生性疾病	C88	2	0.02	0.00	0.00	0.00	0.00	0.00	0.00	0.00	0.00
多发性骨髓瘤	C90	17	0.16	0.00	0.00	0.00	0.00	0.00	0.00	0.00	0.00
淋巴样白血病	C91	44	0.42	0.99	0.22	0.18	0.00	0.17	0.95	0.27	0.00
髓样白血病	C92–C94	47	0.45	0.00	0.43	0.18	0.00	0.17	0.27	0.40	0.32
白血病，未特指	C95	137	1.30	0.00	1.73	1.08	0.58	0.85	0.81	1.34	0.32
其他的或未指明部位的	O&U	141	1.34	0.00	0.22	0.18	0.19	0.34	0.27	0.27	0.32
骨髓增殖性疾病	MPD	1	0.01	0.00	0.00	0.00	0.00	0.00	0.00	0.00	0.00
骨髓增生异常综合征	MDS	2	0.02	0.00	0.00	0.00	0.00	0.00	0.00	0.00	0.00
合计	ALL	10 509	100.00	0.99	3.25	3.07	2.51	2.71	5.70	7.38	12.48
所有部位除外 C44	ALL but C44	10 467	99.60	0.99	3.25	3.07	2.51	2.37	5.70	7.38	12.48

2014 年女性死亡主要指标 ($1/10^5$)

35–	40–	45–	50–	55–	60–	65–	70–	75–	80–	85–	粗率 ($1/10^5$万)	世标率 ($1/10^5$万)	累积率 (%) 0~64	累积率 (%) 0~74
0.00	0.15	0.00	0.00	0.00	0.51	0.00	0.00	1.22	0.00	0.00	0.06	0.04	0.00	0.00
0.00	0.00	0.15	0.19	0.00	0.77	0.36	1.46	1.22	1.94	0.00	0.15	0.11	0.01	0.01
0.00	0.15	0.15	0.00	0.43	1.54	1.09	1.46	3.05	2.91	4.29	0.32	0.23	0.01	0.02
0.16	0.00	0.29	0.38	0.21	0.51	0.00	0.49	0.00	0.00	0.00	0.12	0.09	0.01	0.01
0.00	0.00	0.00	0.00	0.00	0.26	0.00	0.00	0.61	0.97	0.00	0.04	0.02	0.00	0.00
0.00	0.00	0.29	0.00	0.21	0.26	0.36	0.49	1.22	0.97	0.00	0.11	0.07	0.00	0.01
0.00	0.45	0.29	1.33	1.29	2.06	1.81	1.46	1.83	2.91	1.43	0.54	0.43	0.03	0.05
0.00	0.00	0.00	0.00	0.00	0.00	0.36	0.00	0.00	0.00	1.43	0.02	0.02	0.00	0.00
0.00	0.00	0.00	0.38	0.00	0.26	0.00	0.98	0.00	0.97	1.43	0.08	0.06	0.00	0.01
1.27	1.78	4.54	14.29	28.38	60.94	107.07	139.16	177.71	256.41	243.03	21.22	15.08	0.56	1.79
1.74	3.86	7.91	12.19	26.01	53.49	76.94	106.94	144.12	203.96	213.01	18.05	12.85	0.55	1.47
0.16	0.45	0.00	0.38	0.86	1.80	1.81	1.46	3.66	5.83	10.01	0.54	0.38	0.02	0.04
0.16	1.48	2.05	2.67	4.73	9.26	11.25	12.21	14.05	28.17	20.01	2.64	1.94	0.11	0.22
0.32	0.74	3.66	4.57	7.95	9.51	12.70	19.04	22.60	40.79	45.75	3.76	2.68	0.14	0.30
0.16	0.45	0.29	0.76	0.64	0.77	0.73	0.00	1.22	0.97	0.00	0.25	0.19	0.02	0.02
2.22	4.31	8.50	16.76	29.67	51.94	66.05	71.78	85.50	135.97	112.94	14.47	10.69	0.58	1.27
0.00	0.15	1.32	2.29	2.58	7.46	9.80	15.63	28.09	25.25	32.88	2.56	1.79	0.07	0.20
0.16	0.59	1.47	2.29	3.01	5.40	11.98	15.63	17.10	13.60	24.30	2.20	1.63	0.07	0.20
0.00	0.15	0.00	0.19	0.64	0.51	1.81	0.49	0.61	1.94	1.43	0.21	0.16	0.01	0.02
0.00	0.00	0.15	0.57	1.72	1.29	2.18	3.91	1.83	3.88	2.86	0.48	0.36	0.02	0.05
2.06	5.34	11.72	22.67	32.25	67.37	93.64	115.73	160.61	251.55	268.76	22.01	15.69	0.71	1.76
0.00	0.45	0.15	0.19	0.43	0.26	0.36	1.95	1.22	2.91	2.86	0.27	0.20	0.01	0.02
0.48	0.30	0.59	1.71	3.01	4.11	3.99	3.42	6.72	5.83	2.86	1.05	0.80	0.05	0.09
0.00	0.00	0.15	0.00	0.00	0.26	0.73	1.46	0.61	0.97	1.43	0.13	0.10	0.00	0.01
0.16	0.00	0.44	0.00	0.43	1.03	1.81	1.46	1.22	7.77	17.15	0.49	0.35	0.01	0.03
0.00	0.00	0.00	0.00	0.00	0.26	0.00	0.00	0.00	0.00	0.00	0.01	0.01	0.00	0.00
0.00	0.00	0.00	0.00	0.00	0.00	0.00	0.00	0.00	0.00	0.00	0.00	0.00	0.00	0.00
0.00	0.15	0.00	0.19	0.00	0.51	0.00	0.49	0.00	0.00	1.43	0.07	0.06	0.00	0.01
4.12	9.35	18.03	23.05	24.94	32.66	28.67	31.25	22.60	37.88	24.30	9.78	7.58	0.58	0.88
0.00	0.00	0.29	0.00	0.00	0.26	0.00	0.00	1.22	0.00	0.00	0.06	0.04	0.00	0.00
0.00	0.00	0.00	0.19	0.21	0.26	0.73	1.95	0.00	1.94	0.00	0.13	0.10	0.00	0.02
1.90	3.41	4.98	8.95	11.82	19.03	20.32	24.90	17.71	29.14	22.87	5.08	3.90	0.26	0.48
0.48	0.89	2.05	2.67	3.65	4.63	4.72	6.84	7.33	10.68	5.72	1.49	1.11	0.07	0.13
0.48	0.59	1.76	0.76	1.72	3.09	3.99	2.93	3.05	4.86	7.15	0.88	0.67	0.04	0.08
1.11	1.48	2.93	3.81	4.08	9.51	10.16	14.65	12.82	14.57	14.30	2.61	2.00	0.12	0.24
0.16	0.00	0.15	0.38	0.00	0.26	0.36	0.98	0.61	0.00	0.00	0.11	0.08	0.00	0.01
0.00	0.00	0.00	0.19	0.00	0.00	0.00	0.00	0.00	0.00	0.00	0.02	0.02	0.00	0.00
—	—	—	—	—	—	—	—	—	—	—	—	—	—	—
—	—	—	—	—	—	—	—	—	—	—	—	—	—	—
—	—	—	—	—	—	—	—	—	—	—	—	—	—	—
—	—	—	—	—	—	—	—	—	—	—	—	—	—	—
0.00	0.30	0.15	0.57	0.00	1.29	2.54	1.46	1.83	5.83	4.29	0.41	0.31	0.01	0.03
0.00	0.00	0.15	0.00	0.64	0.00	0.36	0.00	0.61	0.97	0.00	0.08	0.06	0.00	0.01
0.00	0.00	0.00	0.00	0.00	0.26	0.36	0.98	0.00	0.00	0.00	0.05	0.04	0.00	0.01
0.00	0.00	0.44	0.76	0.43	1.54	3.99	3.42	2.44	6.80	5.72	0.58	0.44	0.02	0.05
0.00	0.00	0.00	0.00	0.00	0.00	0.00	0.00	0.61	0.00	2.86	0.04	0.02	0.00	0.00
0.00	0.00	0.00	0.00	0.00	0.26	0.00	0.49	0.00	0.00	1.43	0.04	0.03	0.00	0.00
2.22	2.52	3.22	3.81	6.66	14.91	14.15	15.14	13.44	31.08	21.44	3.84	3.04	0.19	0.33
0.00	0.45	0.73	0.76	0.86	1.80	2.90	2.93	5.50	0.97	7.15	0.62	0.47	0.02	0.05
0.00	0.00	0.00	0.00	0.00	0.00	0.36	0.98	0.61	0.00	1.43	0.07	0.06	0.00	0.01
0.16	0.00	0.00	0.00	0.00	0.26	0.00	0.00	1.83	0.00	0.00	0.06	0.04	0.00	0.00
0.32	0.15	0.15	0.00	0.21	0.51	0.00	0.49	0.00	2.91	1.43	0.14	0.10	0.01	0.01
0.16	0.59	0.00	2.10	1.93	2.06	3.99	5.37	2.44	9.71	2.86	0.90	0.69	0.04	0.09
0.00	0.00	0.00	0.00	0.00	0.00	0.36	0.00	0.00	0.00	1.43	0.02	0.02	0.00	0.00
0.00	0.15	0.15	0.00	0.21	1.29	1.45	1.46	0.00	1.94	0.00	0.20	0.16	0.01	0.02
0.32	0.30	0.73	0.19	0.21	1.03	0.36	1.95	3.66	2.91	2.86	0.52	0.43	0.02	0.04
0.32	0.74	0.59	0.19	1.72	1.29	0.73	0.00	2.44	4.86	0.00	0.55	0.45	0.03	0.04
0.32	1.63	1.17	1.14	2.58	4.37	4.72	5.86	3.05	7.77	4.29	1.61	1.47	0.09	0.14
0.79	0.30	1.32	2.10	3.22	4.37	5.81	6.35	10.38	18.45	8.58	1.66	1.24	0.07	0.13
0.00	0.00	0.00	0.00	0.00	0.00	0.00	0.00	0.61	0.00	0.00	0.01	0.01	0.00	0.00
0.00	0.00	0.00	0.00	0.00	0.00	0.36	0.00	0.00	0.97	0.00	0.02	0.02	0.00	0.00
21.89	43.80	83.10	135.62	209.62	387.26	518.27	647.48	790.85	1 190.74	1 149.38	123.41	90.60	4.59	10.42
21.73	43.80	82.66	135.62	209.19	386.23	516.46	646.02	789.63	1 182.97	1 132.22	122.92	90.26	4.58	10.39

二、河南省肿瘤登记地区发病和死亡主要结果

2. All Cancer Incidences and Mortalities in Each Cancer Registry in Henan Province

表 6-2-1a 2014 年河南省郸城县恶性肿瘤发病主要指标

部位		男性						女性					
		病例数	构成 (%)	粗率 (1/10⁵)	世标率 (1/10⁵)	累积率 (%) 0~64	累积率 (%) 0~74	病例数	构成 (%)	粗率 (1/10⁵)	世标率 (1/10⁵)	累积率 (%) 0~64	累积率 (%) 0~74
唇	C00	3	0.17	0.42	0.37	0.02	0.06	3	0.18	0.45	0.50	0.06	0.06
舌	C01–C02	6	0.34	0.85	1.01	0.06	0.16	9	0.54	1.35	1.43	0.12	0.18
口	C03–C06	5	0.29	0.71	0.49	0.03	0.07	8	0.48	1.20	1.26	0.13	0.17
唾液腺	C07–C08	5	0.29	0.71	0.65	0.05	0.08	5	0.30	0.75	0.69	0.06	0.06
扁桃体	C09	2	0.11	0.28	0.29	0.02	0.02	2	0.12	0.30	0.24	0.02	0.02
其他的口咽	C10	4	0.23	0.57	0.44	0.04	0.04	4	0.24	0.60	0.61	0.05	0.08
鼻咽	C11	12	0.69	1.70	1.25	0.09	0.12	9	0.54	1.35	1.59	0.16	0.22
喉咽	C12–C13	3	0.17	0.42	0.43	0.03	0.07	1	0.06	0.15	0.10	0.00	0.00
咽，部位不明	C14	6	0.34	0.85	0.86	0.08	0.11	2	0.12	0.30	0.29	0.01	0.04
食管	C15	252	14.43	35.68	38.75	2.17	5.36	193	11.56	28.95	29.03	1.57	4.18
胃	C16	246	14.09	34.83	36.00	2.48	4.87	186	11.14	27.90	26.43	2.25	3.18
小肠	C17	10	0.57	1.42	1.34	0.05	0.18	11	0.66	1.65	1.43	0.07	0.19
结肠	C18	32	1.83	4.53	5.02	0.24	0.75	40	2.40	6.00	5.70	0.49	0.75
直肠	C19–C20	49	2.81	6.94	6.31	0.50	0.73	54	3.23	8.10	7.43	0.44	0.94
肛门	C21	34	1.95	4.81	4.66	0.37	0.53	26	1.56	3.90	3.47	0.22	0.43
肝脏	C22	256	14.66	36.24	37.02	2.67	4.77	168	10.06	25.20	23.97	1.66	2.88
胆囊及其他	C23–C24	10	0.57	1.42	1.48	0.09	0.23	15	0.90	2.25	2.02	0.14	0.20
胰腺	C25	16	0.92	2.27	2.25	0.13	0.33	15	0.90	2.25	2.15	0.12	0.31
鼻、鼻窦及其他	C30–C31	3	0.17	0.42	0.46	0.03	0.06	9	0.54	1.35	1.23	0.06	0.15
喉	C32	20	1.15	2.83	3.04	0.16	0.42	14	0.84	2.10	2.08	0.16	0.24
气管、支气管、肺	C33–C34	535	30.64	75.74	76.40	5.05	10.25	199	11.92	29.85	29.25	2.08	4.03
其他的胸腔器官	C37–C38	5	0.29	0.71	0.87	0.09	0.12	7	0.42	1.05	1.10	0.12	0.12
骨	C40–C41	6	0.34	0.85	0.87	0.05	0.08	5	0.30	0.75	0.71	0.08	0.08
皮肤的黑色素瘤	C43	2	0.11	0.28	0.28	0.01	0.04	1	0.06	0.15	0.18	0.00	0.03
其他的皮肤	C44	15	0.86	2.12	2.09	0.09	0.26	14	0.84	2.10	1.97	0.08	0.23
间皮瘤	C45	1	0.06	0.14	0.12	0.00	0.00	0	0.00	0.00	0.00	0.00	0.00
卡波西肉瘤	C46	0	0.00	0.00	0.00	0.00	0.00	0	0.00	0.00	0.00	0.00	0.00
周围神经、其他结缔组织、软组织	C47;C49	2	0.11	0.28	0.25	0.01	0.05	2	0.12	0.30	0.22	0.02	0.02
乳房	C50	—	—	—	—	—	—	368	22.04	55.20	50.31	3.82	6.51
外阴	C51	—	—	—	—	—	—	1	0.06	0.15	0.14	0.01	0.01
阴道	C52	—	—	—	—	—	—	1	0.06	0.15	0.20	0.02	0.02
子宫颈	C53	—	—	—	—	—	—	74	4.43	11.10	9.19	0.76	1.04
子宫体	C54	—	—	—	—	—	—	16	0.96	2.40	2.24	0.23	0.26
子宫，部位不明	C55	—	—	—	—	—	—	24	1.44	3.60	3.70	0.32	0.47
卵巢	C56	—	—	—	—	—	—	43	2.57	6.45	5.95	0.56	0.69
其他的女性生殖器	C57	—	—	—	—	—	—	8	0.48	1.20	1.01	0.07	0.13
胎盘	C58	—	—	—	—	—	—	1	0.06	0.15	0.10	0.01	0.01
阴茎	C60	4	0.23	0.57	0.48	0.05	0.05	—	—	—	—	—	—
前列腺	C61	12	0.69	1.70	1.64	0.08	0.18	—	—	—	—	—	—
睾丸	C62	3	0.17	0.42	0.33	0.03	0.03	—	—	—	—	—	—
其他的男性生殖器	C63	3	0.17	0.42	0.44	0.03	0.03	—	—	—	—	—	—
肾	C64	9	0.52	1.27	1.46	0.12	0.15	6	0.36	0.90	0.71	0.06	0.06
肾盂	C65	2	0.11	0.28	0.18	0.02	0.02	1	0.06	0.15	0.12	0.01	0.01
输尿管	C66	5	0.29	0.71	0.70	0.06	0.06	1	0.06	0.15	0.10	0.01	0.01
膀胱	C67	11	0.63	1.56	1.87	0.05	0.24	8	0.48	1.20	1.21	0.07	0.10
其他的泌尿器官	C68	1	0.06	0.14	0.19	0.02	0.02	2	0.12	0.30	0.29	0.01	0.04
眼	C69	1	0.06	0.14	0.14	0.00	0.03	0	0.00	0.00	0.00	0.00	0.00
脑、神经系统	C70–C72	37	2.12	5.24	5.45	0.36	0.46	32	1.92	4.80	4.71	0.36	0.54
甲状腺	C73	11	0.63	1.56	1.30	0.10	0.14	14	0.84	2.10	1.94	0.12	0.24
肾上腺	C74	2	0.11	0.28	0.21	0.02	0.02	1	0.06	0.15	0.10	0.01	0.01
其他的内分泌腺	C75	0	0.00	0.00	0.00	0.00	0.00	0	0.00	0.00	0.00	0.00	0.00
霍奇金病	C81	3	0.17	0.42	0.61	0.05	0.05	2	0.12	0.30	0.27	0.00	0.03
非霍奇金淋巴瘤	C82–C85;C96	13	0.74	1.84	1.64	0.08	0.21	7	0.42	1.05	1.08	0.06	0.15
免疫增生性疾病	C88	0	0.00	0.00	0.00	0.00	0.00	0	0.00	0.00	0.00	0.00	0.00
多发性骨髓瘤	C90	7	0.40	0.99	1.05	0.09	0.09	4	0.24	0.60	0.66	0.00	0.12
淋巴样白血病	C91	10	0.57	1.42	1.32	0.09	0.12	8	0.48	1.20	1.04	0.07	0.10
髓样白血病	C92–C94	24	1.37	3.40	2.93	0.26	0.36	12	0.72	1.80	1.47	0.07	0.13
白血病，未特指	C95	30	1.72	4.25	6.28	0.31	0.38	23	1.38	3.45	6.10	0.28	0.34
其他的或未指明部位的	O&U	17	0.97	2.41	2.37	0.15	0.21	11	0.66	1.65	1.64	0.11	0.20
骨髓增殖性疾病	MPD	0	0.00	0.00	0.00	0.00	0.00	0	0.00	0.00	0.00	0.00	0.00
骨髓增生异常综合征	MDS	0	0.00	0.00	0.00	0.00	0.00	0	0.00	0.00	0.00	0.00	0.00
合计	ALL	1 746	100.00	247.19	253.74	16.61	32.62	1670	100.00	250.49	239.37	17.22	30.02
所有部位除外 C44	ALL but C44	1 731	99.14	245.06	251.64	16.51	32.37	1656	99.16	248.39	237.40	17.14	29.79

表 6-2-2a 2014 年河南省方城县恶性肿瘤发病主要指标

部位		男性						女性					
		病例数	构成 (%)	粗率 (1/10^5)	世标率 (1/10^5)	累积率 (%) 0~64	累积率 (%) 0~74	病例数	构成 (%)	粗率 (1/10^5)	世标率 (1/10^5)	累积率 (%) 0~64	累积率 (%) 0~74
唇	C00	1	0.06	0.17	0.15	0.01	0.01	0	0.00	0.00	0.00	0.00	0.00
舌	C01–C02	2	0.12	0.33	0.29	0.03	0.03	3	0.23	0.56	0.47	0.05	0.05
口	C03–C06	8	0.48	1.34	0.99	0.04	0.16	3	0.23	0.56	0.44	0.02	0.06
唾液腺	C07–C08	1	0.06	0.17	0.14	0.01	0.01	3	0.23	0.56	0.46	0.05	0.05
扁桃体	C09	0	0.00	0.00	0.00	0.00	0.00	0	0.00	0.00	0.00	0.00	0.00
其他的口咽	C10	0	0.00	0.00	0.00	0.00	0.00	0	0.00	0.00	0.00	0.00	0.00
鼻咽	C11	9	0.54	1.50	1.18	0.07	0.14	3	0.23	0.56	0.46	0.04	0.04
喉咽	C12–C13	0	0.00	0.00	0.00	0.00	0.00	1	0.08	0.19	0.14	0.01	0.01
咽，部位不明	C14	0	0.00	0.00	0.00	0.00	0.00	0	0.00	0.00	0.00	0.00	0.00
食管	C15	147	8.89	24.58	19.49	1.31	2.58	50	3.81	9.30	7.39	0.35	1.04
胃	C16	290	17.53	48.49	37.46	2.42	4.84	95	7.25	17.68	13.41	0.76	1.62
小肠	C17	10	0.60	1.67	1.27	0.04	0.18	5	0.38	0.93	0.81	0.03	0.12
结肠	C18	45	2.72	7.52	5.97	0.42	0.75	36	2.75	6.70	5.16	0.43	0.59
直肠	C19–C20	40	2.42	6.69	5.37	0.40	0.72	41	3.13	7.63	6.04	0.26	0.75
肛门	C21	0	0.00	0.00	0.00	0.00	0.00	0	0.00	0.00	0.00	0.00	0.00
肝脏	C22	171	10.34	28.59	23.05	1.63	2.59	70	5.34	13.02	9.60	0.53	1.17
胆囊及其他	C23–C24	9	0.54	1.50	1.20	0.09	0.16	7	0.53	1.30	1.09	0.08	0.14
胰腺	C25	15	0.91	2.51	1.89	0.14	0.17	11	0.84	2.05	1.41	0.06	0.11
鼻、鼻窦及其他	C30–C31	3	0.18	0.50	0.36	0.03	0.03	1	0.08	0.19	0.18	0.00	0.04
喉	C32	22	1.33	3.68	3.02	0.29	0.36	2	0.15	0.37	0.31	0.03	0.03
气管、支气管、肺	C33–C34	406	24.55	67.89	52.04	3.04	6.78	164	12.51	30.51	24.24	1.38	3.13
其他的胸腔器官	C37–C38	5	0.30	0.84	0.70	0.07	0.09	2	0.15	0.37	0.31	0.01	0.04
骨	C40–C41	22	1.33	3.68	3.21	0.20	0.35	15	1.14	2.79	2.45	0.19	0.19
皮肤的黑色素瘤	C43	1	0.06	0.17	0.14	0.02	0.02	0	0.00	0.00	0.00	0.00	0.00
其他的皮肤	C44	10	0.60	1.67	0.95	0.02	0.06	5	0.38	0.93	1.26	0.08	0.08
间皮瘤	C45	0	0.00	0.00	0.00	0.00	0.00	0	0.00	0.00	0.00	0.00	0.00
卡波西肉瘤	C46	0	0.00	0.00	0.00	0.00	0.00	0	0.00	0.00	0.00	0.00	0.00
周围神经、其他结缔组织、软组织	C47;C49	7	0.42	1.17	0.95	0.10	0.10	1	0.08	0.19	0.28	0.02	0.02
乳房	C50	—	—	—	—	—	—	295	22.50	54.89	44.00	3.77	4.51
外阴	C51	—	—	—	—	—	—	2	0.15	0.37	0.28	0.00	0.04
阴道	C52	—	—	—	—	—	—	2	0.15	0.37	0.29	0.03	0.03
子宫颈	C53	—	—	—	—	—	—	111	8.47	20.65	16.21	1.37	1.56
子宫体	C54	—	—	—	—	—	—	37	2.82	6.88	5.67	0.46	0.71
子宫，部位不明	C55	—	—	—	—	—	—	16	1.22	2.98	2.38	0.18	0.26
卵巢	C56	—	—	—	—	—	—	37	2.82	6.88	5.82	0.45	0.75
其他的女性生殖器	C57	—	—	—	—	—	—	0	0.00	0.00	0.00	0.00	0.00
胎盘	C58	—	—	—	—	—	—	1	0.08	0.19	0.14	0.01	0.01
阴茎	C60	4	0.24	0.67	0.48	0.00	0.07	—	—	—	—	—	—
前列腺	C61	26	1.57	4.35	3.22	0.12	0.40	—	—	—	—	—	—
睾丸	C62	1	0.06	0.17	0.23	0.01	0.01	—	—	—	—	—	—
其他的男性生殖器	C63	0	0.00	0.00	0.00	0.00	0.00	—	—	—	—	—	—
肾	C64	7	0.42	1.17	0.76	0.05	0.08	9	0.69	1.67	1.40	0.11	0.16
肾盂	C65	1	0.06	0.17	0.20	0.01	0.01	2	0.15	0.37	0.32	0.04	0.04
输尿管	C66	1	0.06	0.17	0.14	0.02	0.02	0	0.00	0.00	0.00	0.00	0.00
膀胱	C67	23	1.39	3.85	2.93	0.16	0.32	1	0.08	0.19	0.07	0.00	0.00
其他的泌尿器官	C68	1	0.06	0.17	0.13	0.00	0.02	0	0.00	0.00	0.00	0.00	0.00
眼	C69	3	0.18	0.50	0.40	0.04	0.04	2	0.15	0.37	0.29	0.03	0.03
脑、神经系统	C70–C72	20	1.21	3.34	2.84	0.23	0.23	21	1.60	3.91	3.27	0.24	0.24
甲状腺	C73	15	0.91	2.51	1.93	0.12	0.19	38	2.90	7.07	6.03	0.46	0.54
肾上腺	C74	5	0.30	0.84	0.61	0.06	0.06	1	0.08	0.19	0.14	0.01	0.01
其他的内分泌腺	C75	2	0.12	0.33	0.27	0.02	0.02	1	0.08	0.19	0.14	0.01	0.01
霍奇金病	C81	0	0.00	0.00	0.00	0.00	0.00	0	0.00	0.00	0.00	0.00	0.00
非霍奇金淋巴瘤	C82–C85;C96	1	0.06	0.17	0.14	0.02	0.02	5	0.38	0.93	0.76	0.06	0.09
免疫增生性疾病	C88	0	0.00	0.00	0.00	0.00	0.00	0	0.00	0.00	0.00	0.00	0.00
多发性骨髓瘤	C90	1	0.06	0.17	0.13	0.01	0.01	1	0.08	0.19	0.14	0.02	0.02
淋巴样白血病	C91	7	0.42	1.17	1.41	0.11	0.11	6	0.46	1.12	0.88	0.05	0.08
髓样白血病	C92–C94	3	0.18	0.50	0.33	0.01	0.03	3	0.23	0.56	0.56	0.04	0.04
白血病，未特指	C95	2	0.12	0.33	0.29	0.03	0.03	7	0.53	1.30	1.18	0.09	0.12
其他的或未指明部位的	O&U	306	18.50	51.17	40.11	2.53	4.77	194	14.80	36.09	27.26	1.80	2.95
骨髓增殖性疾病	MPD	0	0.00	0.00	0.00	0.00	0.00	1	0.08	0.19	0.14	0.01	0.01
骨髓增生异常综合征	MDS	0	0.00	0.00	0.00	0.00	0.00	0	0.00	0.00	0.00	0.00	0.00
合计	ALL	1 654	100.00	276.58	216.53	13.93	26.56	1 311	100.00	243.92	193.31	13.63	21.50
所有部位除外 C44	ALL but C44	1 644	99.40	274.91	215.58	13.91	26.50	1 306	99.62	242.99	192.04	13.56	21.43

表 6-2-3a 2014 年河南省鹤壁市恶性肿瘤发病主要指标

部位		男性						女性					
		病例数	构成(%)	粗率(1/10^5)	世标率(1/10^5)	累积率(%) 0~64	累积率(%) 0~74	病例数	构成(%)	粗率(1/10^5)	世标率(1/10^5)	累积率(%) 0~64	累积率(%) 0~74
唇	C00	1	0.11	0.31	0.32	0.00	0.05	0	0.00	0.00	0.00	0.00	0.00
舌	C01–C02	2	0.22	0.62	0.47	0.05	0.05	3	0.41	0.97	0.72	0.02	0.14
口	C03–C06	6	0.66	1.85	1.43	0.08	0.08	3	0.41	0.97	0.61	0.03	0.03
唾液腺	C07–C08	2	0.22	0.62	0.45	0.02	0.02	4	0.55	1.29	1.00	0.09	0.09
扁桃体	C09	0	0.00	0.00	0.00	0.00	0.00	0	0.00	0.00	0.00	0.00	0.00
其他的口咽	C10	3	0.33	0.92	0.82	0.06	0.12	0	0.00	0.00	0.00	0.00	0.00
鼻咽	C11	4	0.44	1.23	0.94	0.11	0.11	2	0.27	0.64	0.52	0.03	0.10
喉咽	C12–C13	1	0.11	0.31	0.23	0.00	0.00	3	0.41	0.97	0.81	0.02	0.12
咽，部位不明	C14	2	0.22	0.62	0.54	0.07	0.07	0	0.00	0.00	0.00	0.00	0.00
食管	C15	224	24.48	69.06	61.04	2.94	8.20	147	20.11	47.35	36.75	1.90	4.98
胃	C16	172	18.80	53.02	46.11	2.49	6.13	78	10.67	25.12	19.29	1.16	2.56
小肠	C17	4	0.44	1.23	1.01	0.12	0.12	2	0.27	0.64	0.53	0.07	0.07
结肠	C18	32	3.50	9.87	8.05	0.40	0.82	31	4.24	9.99	7.40	0.39	0.86
直肠	C19–C20	24	2.62	7.40	6.01	0.30	0.66	20	2.74	6.44	4.77	0.35	0.60
肛门	C21	3	0.33	0.92	0.75	0.00	0.05	4	0.55	1.29	0.95	0.04	0.17
肝脏	C22	86	9.40	26.51	21.67	1.46	2.51	36	4.92	11.60	8.40	0.51	0.99
胆囊及其他	C23–C24	7	0.77	2.16	1.82	0.10	0.21	15	2.05	4.83	3.80	0.12	0.55
胰腺	C25	11	1.20	3.39	2.94	0.22	0.43	13	1.78	4.19	3.15	0.13	0.42
鼻、鼻窦及其他	C30–C31	0	0.00	0.00	0.00	0.00	0.00	0	0.00	0.00	0.00	0.00	0.00
喉	C32	4	0.44	1.23	1.04	0.02	0.17	2	0.27	0.64	0.59	0.00	0.10
气管、支气管、肺	C33–C34	189	20.66	58.27	51.07	2.46	6.81	75	10.26	24.16	18.60	1.15	2.52
其他的胸腔器官	C37–C38	5	0.55	1.54	1.31	0.09	0.17	4	0.55	1.29	0.94	0.07	0.13
骨	C40–C41	5	0.55	1.54	1.18	0.11	0.11	4	0.55	1.29	1.12	0.02	0.07
皮肤的黑色素瘤	C43	2	0.22	0.62	0.45	0.03	0.03	0	0.00	0.00	0.00	0.00	0.00
其他的皮肤	C44	2	0.22	0.62	0.46	0.02	0.02	1	0.14	0.32	0.16	0.00	0.00
间皮瘤	C45	0	0.00	0.00	0.00	0.00	0.00	0	0.00	0.00	0.00	0.00	0.00
卡波西肉瘤	C46	0	0.00	0.00	0.00	0.00	0.00	0	0.00	0.00	0.00	0.00	0.00
周围神经、其他结缔组织、软组织	C47;C49	4	0.44	1.23	0.87	0.07	0.07	3	0.41	0.97	0.82	0.06	0.11
乳房	C50	—	—	—	—	—	—	116	15.87	37.36	27.57	2.26	2.93
外阴	C51	—	—	—	—	—	—	0	0.00	0.00	0.00	0.00	0.00
阴道	C52	—	—	—	—	—	—	0	0.00	0.00	0.00	0.00	0.00
子宫颈	C53	—	—	—	—	—	—	45	6.16	14.49	10.58	0.81	1.08
子宫体	C54	—	—	—	—	—	—	16	2.19	5.15	3.92	0.30	0.54
子宫，部位不明	C55	—	—	—	—	—	—	2	0.27	0.64	0.48	0.05	0.05
卵巢	C56	—	—	—	—	—	—	18	2.46	5.80	4.33	0.34	0.46
其他的女性生殖器	C57	—	—	—	—	—	—	0	0.00	0.00	0.00	0.00	0.00
胎盘	C58	—	—	—	—	—	—	0	0.00	0.00	0.00	0.00	0.00
阴茎	C60	2	0.22	0.62	0.53	0.00	0.05	—	—	—	—	—	—
前列腺	C61	14	1.53	4.32	3.81	0.13	0.34	—	—	—	—	—	—
睾丸	C62	3	0.33	0.92	0.66	0.05	0.05	—	—	—	—	—	—
其他的男性生殖器	C63	0	0.00	0.00	0.00	0.00	0.00	—	—	—	—	—	—
肾	C64	12	1.31	3.70	3.12	0.28	0.43	5	0.68	1.61	1.13	0.07	0.14
肾盂	C65	3	0.33	0.92	0.94	0.00	0.21	2	0.27	0.64	0.50	0.02	0.07
输尿管	C66	2	0.22	0.62	0.45	0.02	0.02	3	0.41	0.97	0.72	0.08	0.08
膀胱	C67	7	0.77	2.16	1.75	0.06	0.19	3	0.41	0.97	0.79	0.04	0.08
其他的泌尿器官	C68	0	0.00	0.00	0.00	0.00	0.00	0	0.00	0.00	0.00	0.00	0.00
眼	C69	1	0.11	0.31	0.23	0.02	0.02	1	0.14	0.32	0.30	0.00	0.05
脑、神经系统	C70–C72	24	2.62	7.40	5.81	0.43	0.54	11	1.50	3.54	2.92	0.26	0.32
甲状腺	C73	4	0.44	1.23	1.16	0.09	0.14	15	2.05	4.83	3.87	0.24	0.44
肾上腺	C74	2	0.22	0.62	0.44	0.00	0.00	2	0.27	0.64	0.57	0.03	0.08
其他的内分泌腺	C75	2	0.22	0.62	0.55	0.03	0.11	4	0.55	1.29	0.92	0.09	0.09
霍奇金病	C81	3	0.33	0.92	0.98	0.02	0.08	4	0.55	1.29	1.21	0.11	0.11
非霍奇金淋巴瘤	C82–C85;C96	2	0.22	0.62	0.53	0.00	0.08	4	0.55	1.29	0.99	0.08	0.08
免疫增生性疾病	C88	0	0.00	0.00	0.00	0.00	0.00	0	0.00	0.00	0.00	0.00	0.00
多发性骨髓瘤	C90	1	0.11	0.31	0.21	0.00	0.00	1	0.14	0.32	0.20	0.02	0.02
淋巴样白血病	C91	8	0.87	2.47	2.54	0.10	0.10	11	1.50	3.54	3.33	0.25	0.30
髓样白血病	C92–C94	5	0.55	1.54	1.38	0.11	0.11	2	0.27	0.64	0.39	0.02	0.02
白血病，未特指	C95	12	1.31	3.70	3.48	0.23	0.44	14	1.92	4.51	3.34	0.23	0.34
其他的或未指明部位的	O&U	12	1.31	3.70	3.50	0.13	0.55	2	0.27	0.64	0.45	0.03	0.03
骨髓增殖性疾病	MPD	0	0.00	0.00	0.00	0.00	0.00	0	0.00	0.00	0.00	0.00	0.00
骨髓增生异常综合征	MDS	0	0.00	0.00	0.00	0.00	0.00	0	0.00	0.00	0.00	0.00	0.00
合计	ALL	915	100.00	282.08	243.56	12.93	30.49	731	100.00	235.46	179.43	11.49	21.91
所有部位除外 C44	ALL but C44	913	99.78	281.46	243.10	12.91	30.46	730	99.86	235.14	179.27	11.49	21.91

表 6-2-4a 2014 年河南省辉县市恶性肿瘤发病主要指标

部位		男性						女性					
		病例数	构成 (%)	粗率 (1/10⁵)	世标率 (1/10⁵)	累积率 (%) 0~64	累积率 (%) 0~74	病例数	构成 (%)	粗率 (1/10⁵)	世标率 (1/10⁵)	累积率 (%) 0~64	累积率 (%) 0~74
唇	C00	1	0.08	0.23	0.26	0.02	0.02	1	0.10	0.23	0.17	0.02	0.02
舌	C01–C02	4	0.31	0.93	0.83	0.06	0.12	0	0.00	0.00	0.00	0.00	0.00
口	C03–C06	5	0.38	1.16	1.09	0.04	0.13	4	0.41	0.94	0.54	0.02	0.02
唾液腺	C07–C08	2	0.15	0.47	0.34	0.03	0.03	1	0.10	0.23	0.27	0.02	0.02
扁桃体	C09	0	0.00	0.00	0.00	0.00	0.00	0	0.00	0.00	0.00	0.00	0.00
其他的口咽	C10	1	0.08	0.23	0.15	0.00	0.00	0	0.00	0.00	0.00	0.00	0.00
鼻咽	C11	4	0.31	0.93	0.71	0.04	0.04	1	0.10	0.23	0.20	0.00	0.03
喉咽	C12–C13	1	0.08	0.23	0.15	0.00	0.00	0	0.00	0.00	0.00	0.00	0.00
咽，部位不明	C14	3	0.23	0.70	0.48	0.04	0.04	0	0.00	0.00	0.00	0.00	0.00
食管	C15	403	30.98	93.77	75.46	3.54	9.09	262	27.01	61.41	42.23	1.63	5.50
胃	C16	304	23.37	70.74	55.93	2.99	6.69	97	10.00	22.73	15.80	0.91	2.06
小肠	C17	4	0.31	0.93	0.69	0.03	0.07	3	0.31	0.70	0.51	0.03	0.06
结肠	C18	40	3.07	9.31	7.15	0.33	0.78	34	3.51	7.97	5.37	0.32	0.58
直肠	C19–C20	35	2.69	8.14	6.44	0.34	0.82	39	4.02	9.14	6.10	0.35	0.69
肛门	C21	0	0.00	0.00	0.00	0.00	0.00	1	0.10	0.23	0.10	0.00	0.00
肝脏	C22	148	11.38	34.44	26.65	1.93	3.06	63	6.49	14.77	9.87	0.59	0.95
胆囊及其他	C23–C24	12	0.92	2.79	2.23	0.21	0.33	10	1.03	2.34	1.44	0.09	0.14
胰腺	C25	16	1.23	3.72	2.71	0.18	0.18	9	0.93	2.11	1.61	0.02	0.28
鼻、鼻窦及其他	C30–C31	1	0.08	0.23	0.24	0.00	0.06	0	0.00	0.00	0.00	0.00	0.00
喉	C32	5	0.38	1.16	1.14	0.06	0.06	5	0.52	1.17	0.70	0.00	0.05
气管、支气管、肺	C33–C34	140	10.76	32.58	25.91	1.35	3.08	95	9.79	22.27	15.94	0.88	2.16
其他的胸腔器官	C37–C38	5	0.38	1.16	1.05	0.06	0.12	1	0.10	0.23	0.20	0.01	0.01
骨	C40–C41	6	0.46	1.40	1.66	0.07	0.15	6	0.62	1.41	1.02	0.08	0.11
皮肤的黑色素瘤	C43	1	0.08	0.23	0.22	0.00	0.04	4	0.41	0.94	0.96	0.03	0.12
其他的皮肤	C44	0	0.00	0.00	0.00	0.00	0.00	1	0.10	0.23	0.21	0.00	0.05
间皮瘤	C45	1	0.08	0.23	0.15	0.00	0.00	0	0.00	0.00	0.00	0.00	0.00
卡波西肉瘤	C46	0	0.00	0.00	0.00	0.00	0.00	0	0.00	0.00	0.00	0.00	0.00
周围神经、其他结缔组织、软组织	C47;C49	0	0.00	0.00	0.00	0.00	0.00	1	0.10	0.23	0.13	0.00	0.00
乳房	C50	—	—	—	—	—	—	122	12.58	28.59	20.86	1.82	2.23
外阴	C51	—	—	—	—	—	—	1	0.10	0.23	0.21	0.00	0.05
阴道	C52	—	—	—	—	—	—	1	0.10	0.23	0.15	0.01	0.01
子宫颈	C53	—	—	—	—	—	—	44	4.54	10.31	7.73	0.60	0.84
子宫体	C54	—	—	—	—	—	—	21	2.16	4.92	3.43	0.30	0.42
子宫，部位不明	C55	—	—	—	—	—	—	18	1.86	4.22	2.91	0.28	0.31
卵巢	C56	—	—	—	—	—	—	23	2.37	5.39	4.09	0.32	0.47
其他的女性生殖器	C57	—	—	—	—	—	—	0	0.00	0.00	0.00	0.00	0.00
胎盘	C58	—	—	—	—	—	—	1	0.10	0.23	0.15	0.01	0.01
阴茎	C60	5	0.38	1.16	0.91	0.08	0.12	—	—	—	—	—	—
前列腺	C61	13	1.00	3.02	2.32	0.06	0.19	—	—	—	—	—	—
睾丸	C62	2	0.15	0.47	0.35	0.04	0.04	—	—	—	—	—	—
其他的男性生殖器	C63	0	0.00	0.00	0.00	0.00	0.00	—	—	—	—	—	—
肾	C64	12	0.92	2.79	2.22	0.17	0.23	6	0.62	1.41	1.03	0.08	0.11
肾盂	C65	2	0.15	0.47	0.41	0.02	0.06	0	0.00	0.00	0.00	0.00	0.00
输尿管	C66	1	0.08	0.23	0.24	0.00	0.06	2	0.21	0.47	0.36	0.02	0.05
膀胱	C67	15	1.15	3.49	2.86	0.19	0.33	4	0.41	0.94	0.56	0.03	0.03
其他的泌尿器官	C68	0	0.00	0.00	0.00	0.00	0.00	1	0.10	0.23	0.17	0.02	0.02
眼	C69	0	0.00	0.00	0.00	0.00	0.00	0	0.00	0.00	0.00	0.00	0.00
脑、神经系统	C70–C72	35	2.69	8.14	6.65	0.45	0.73	25	2.58	5.86	5.05	0.30	0.53
甲状腺	C73	9	0.69	2.09	1.86	0.13	0.20	15	1.55	3.52	2.49	0.23	0.26
肾上腺	C74	1	0.08	0.23	0.22	0.00	0.04	0	0.00	0.00	0.00	0.00	0.00
其他的内分泌腺	C75	0	0.00	0.00	0.00	0.00	0.00	0	0.00	0.00	0.00	0.00	0.00
霍奇金病	C81	0	0.00	0.00	0.00	0.00	0.00	0	0.00	0.00	0.00	0.00	0.00
非霍奇金淋巴瘤	C82–C85;C96	16	1.23	3.72	3.22	0.17	0.41	14	1.44	3.28	2.91	0.21	0.27
免疫增生性疾病	C88	0	0.00	0.00	0.00	0.00	0.00	0	0.00	0.00	0.00	0.00	0.00
多发性骨髓瘤	C90	7	0.54	1.63	1.37	0.06	0.19	5	0.52	1.17	0.81	0.07	0.07
淋巴样白血病	C91	4	0.31	0.93	1.29	0.06	0.06	2	0.21	0.47	0.76	0.03	0.03
髓样白血病	C92–C94	10	0.77	2.33	1.98	0.10	0.20	6	0.62	1.41	1.24	0.09	0.12
白血病，未特指	C95	16	1.23	3.72	3.35	0.23	0.33	11	1.13	2.58	1.89	0.10	0.13
其他的或未指明部位的	O&U	9	0.69	2.09	1.69	0.10	0.26	6	0.62	1.41	1.04	0.08	0.11
骨髓增殖性疾病	MPD	1	0.08	0.23	0.14	0.02	0.02	4	0.41	0.94	0.93	0.07	0.07
骨髓增生异常综合征	MDS	0	0.00	0.00	0.00	0.00	0.00	0	0.00	0.00	0.00	0.00	0.00
合计	ALL	1 301	100.00	302.73	242.89	13.21	28.38	970	100.00	227.34	162.11	9.67	19.01
所有部位除外 C44	ALL but C44	1 301	100.00	302.73	242.89	13.21	28.38	969	99.90	227.11	161.90	9.67	18.96

表 6-2-5a 2014 年河南省济源市恶性肿瘤发病主要指标

部位		男性						女性					
		病例数	构成 (%)	粗率 ($1/10^5$)	世标率 ($1/10^5$)	累积率 (%) 0~64	累积率 (%) 0~74	病例数	构成 (%)	粗率 ($1/10^5$)	世标率 ($1/10^5$)	累积率 (%) 0~64	累积率 (%) 0~74
唇	C00	1	0.12	0.28	0.29	0.00	0.05	1	0.13	0.29	0.27	0.02	0.02
舌	C01–C02	0	0.00	0.00	0.00	0.00	0.00	3	0.39	0.88	0.85	0.05	0.10
口	C03–C06	3	0.35	0.83	0.67	0.04	0.04	2	0.26	0.59	0.50	0.04	0.04
唾液腺	C07–C08	1	0.12	0.28	0.29	0.04	0.04	2	0.26	0.59	0.60	0.00	0.10
扁桃体	C09	0	0.00	0.00	0.00	0.00	0.00	0	0.00	0.00	0.00	0.00	0.00
其他的口咽	C10	1	0.12	0.28	0.32	0.04	0.04	0	0.00	0.00	0.00	0.00	0.00
鼻咽	C11	3	0.35	0.83	0.77	0.05	0.05	1	0.13	0.29	0.30	0.00	0.05
喉咽	C12–C13	0	0.00	0.00	0.00	0.00	0.00	0	0.00	0.00	0.00	0.00	0.00
咽，部位不明	C14	1	0.12	0.28	0.27	0.03	0.03	0	0.00	0.00	0.00	0.00	0.00
食管	C15	112	13.13	31.14	31.41	2.05	3.98	98	12.83	28.73	26.33	1.61	2.78
胃	C16	289	33.88	80.36	82.12	5.73	10.27	104	13.61	30.49	27.31	1.43	2.95
小肠	C17	3	0.35	0.83	0.79	0.06	0.06	4	0.52	1.17	1.05	0.03	0.13
结肠	C18	19	2.23	5.28	5.57	0.55	0.71	19	2.49	5.57	5.37	0.54	0.54
直肠	C19–C20	24	2.81	6.67	6.80	0.36	0.89	28	3.66	8.21	8.08	0.66	1.01
肛门	C21	0	0.00	0.00	0.00	0.00	0.00	0	0.00	0.00	0.00	0.00	0.00
肝脏	C22	75	8.79	20.86	20.67	1.51	2.40	26	3.40	7.62	6.87	0.35	0.82
胆囊及其他	C23–C24	11	1.29	3.06	3.45	0.22	0.34	17	2.23	4.98	4.52	0.29	0.39
胰腺	C25	18	2.11	5.01	4.96	0.21	0.45	13	1.70	3.81	3.25	0.14	0.32
鼻、鼻窦及其他	C30–C31	2	0.23	0.56	0.73	0.04	0.04	0	0.00	0.00	0.00	0.00	0.00
喉	C32	7	0.82	1.95	1.94	0.11	0.22	1	0.13	0.29	0.17	0.01	0.01
气管、支气管、肺	C33–C34	115	13.48	31.98	32.47	1.83	3.99	65	8.51	19.06	18.00	1.17	2.24
其他的胸腔器官	C37–C38	3	0.35	0.83	0.86	0.10	0.10	0	0.00	0.00	0.00	0.00	0.00
骨	C40–C41	6	0.70	1.67	1.73	0.17	0.17	6	0.79	1.76	1.83	0.10	0.23
皮肤的黑色素瘤	C43	0	0.00	0.00	0.00	0.00	0.00	0	0.00	0.00	0.00	0.00	0.00
其他的皮肤	C44	1	0.12	0.28	0.24	0.00	0.00	3	0.39	0.88	0.76	0.02	0.07
间皮瘤	C45	0	0.00	0.00	0.00	0.00	0.00	0	0.00	0.00	0.00	0.00	0.00
卡波西肉瘤	C46	0	0.00	0.00	0.00	0.00	0.00	0	0.00	0.00	0.00	0.00	0.00
周围神经、其他结缔组织、软组织	C47;C49	0	0.00	0.00	0.00	0.00	0.00	0	0.00	0.00	0.00	0.00	0.00
乳房	C50	—	—	—	—	—	—	91	11.91	26.68	24.78	2.01	2.52
外阴	C51	—	—	—	—	—	—	1	0.13	0.29	0.30	0.00	0.05
阴道	C52	—	—	—	—	—	—	0	0.00	0.00	0.00	0.00	0.00
子宫颈	C53	—	—	—	—	—	—	73	9.55	21.40	21.39	2.07	2.46
子宫体	C54	—	—	—	—	—	—	19	2.49	5.57	5.89	0.64	0.69
子宫，部位不明	C55	—	—	—	—	—	—	15	1.96	4.40	3.90	0.28	0.38
卵巢	C56	—	—	—	—	—	—	35	4.58	10.26	9.79	0.77	1.12
其他的女性生殖器	C57	—	—	—	—	—	—	0	0.00	0.00	0.00	0.00	0.00
胎盘	C58	—	—	—	—	—	—	0	0.00	0.00	0.00	0.00	0.00
阴茎	C60	2	0.23	0.56	0.61	0.08	0.08	—	—	—	—	—	—
前列腺	C61	16	1.88	4.45	4.36	0.18	0.44	—	—	—	—	—	—
睾丸	C62	1	0.12	0.28	0.32	0.04	0.04	—	—	—	—	—	—
其他的男性生殖器	C63	0	0.00	0.00	0.00	0.00	0.00	—	—	—	—	—	—
肾	C64	15	1.76	4.17	4.12	0.32	0.49	9	1.18	2.64	2.35	0.07	0.33
肾盂	C65	1	0.12	0.28	0.29	0.00	0.05	0	0.00	0.00	0.00	0.00	0.00
输尿管	C66	0	0.00	0.00	0.00	0.00	0.00	1	0.13	0.29	0.35	0.04	0.04
膀胱	C67	18	2.11	5.01	5.19	0.38	0.66	8	1.05	2.35	2.14	0.17	0.22
其他的泌尿器官	C68	1	0.12	0.28	0.32	0.04	0.04	0	0.00	0.00	0.00	0.00	0.00
眼	C69	1	0.12	0.28	0.27	0.00	0.07	0	0.00	0.00	0.00	0.00	0.00
脑、神经系统	C70–C72	16	1.88	4.45	4.42	0.32	0.47	14	1.83	4.10	4.12	0.38	0.45
甲状腺	C73	8	0.94	2.22	2.21	0.24	0.24	25	3.27	7.33	6.97	0.58	0.74
肾上腺	C74	2	0.23	0.56	0.51	0.05	0.05	1	0.13	0.29	0.27	0.02	0.02
其他的内分泌腺	C75	3	0.35	0.83	0.70	0.04	0.10	2	0.26	0.59	0.47	0.04	0.04
霍奇金病	C81	0	0.00	0.00	0.00	0.00	0.00	1	0.13	0.29	0.17	0.00	0.00
非霍奇金淋巴瘤	C82–C85;C96	6	0.70	1.67	1.50	0.13	0.13	3	0.39	0.88	0.69	0.04	0.04
免疫增生性疾病	C88	0	0.00	0.00	0.00	0.00	0.00	0	0.00	0.00	0.00	0.00	0.00
多发性骨髓瘤	C90	0	0.00	0.00	0.00	0.00	0.00	0	0.00	0.00	0.00	0.00	0.00
淋巴样白血病	C91	1	0.12	0.28	0.16	0.01	0.01	3	0.39	0.88	1.19	0.07	0.07
髓样白血病	C92–C94	1	0.12	0.28	0.55	0.02	0.02	0	0.00	0.00	0.00	0.00	0.00
白血病，未特指	C95	15	1.76	4.17	4.55	0.31	0.38	14	1.83	4.10	4.05	0.29	0.34
其他的或未指明部位的	O&U	51	5.98	14.18	14.16	0.90	1.81	56	7.33	16.42	14.73	1.18	1.65
骨髓增殖性疾病	MPD	0	0.00	0.00	0.00	0.00	0.00	0	0.00	0.00	0.00	0.00	0.00
骨髓增生异常综合征	MDS	0	0.00	0.00	0.00	0.00	0.00	0	0.00	0.00	0.00	0.00	0.00
合计	ALL	853	100.00	237.20	240.59	16.18	28.96	764	100.00	224.00	209.60	15.14	22.99
所有部位除外 C44	ALL but C44	852	99.88	236.92	240.35	16.18	28.96	761	99.61	223.12	208.84	15.11	22.91

表 6-2-6a 2014 年河南省林州市恶性肿瘤发病主要指标

部位		男性						女性					
		病例数	构成(%)	粗率(1/10^5)	世标率(1/10^5)	累积率(%) 0~64	累积率(%) 0~74	病例数	构成(%)	粗率(1/10^5)	世标率(1/10^5)	累积率(%) 0~64	累积率(%) 0~74
唇	C00	1	0.06	0.18	0.13	0.00	0.02	1	0.07	0.19	0.12	0.00	0.00
舌	C01–C02	3	0.18	0.54	0.43	0.03	0.03	5	0.33	0.93	0.79	0.03	0.07
口	C03–C06	5	0.29	0.90	0.71	0.05	0.05	5	0.33	0.93	0.60	0.06	0.08
唾液腺	C07–C08	2	0.12	0.36	0.27	0.03	0.03	4	0.26	0.75	0.57	0.06	0.06
扁桃体	C09	0	0.00	0.00	0.00	0.00	0.00	1	0.07	0.19	0.11	0.01	0.01
其他的口咽	C10	2	0.12	0.36	0.32	0.01	0.06	0	0.00	0.00	0.00	0.00	0.00
鼻咽	C11	2	0.12	0.36	0.33	0.02	0.04	1	0.07	0.19	0.14	0.01	0.01
喉咽	C12–C13	3	0.18	0.54	0.44	0.00	0.07	0	0.00	0.00	0.00	0.00	0.00
咽，部位不明	C14	0	0.00	0.00	0.00	0.00	0.00	0	0.00	0.00	0.00	0.00	0.00
食管	C15	448	26.34	80.32	64.68	3.51	8.13	349	22.92	65.12	42.63	2.38	5.45
胃	C16	646	37.98	115.81	92.84	5.74	12.62	280	18.38	52.25	34.27	1.96	4.12
小肠	C17	2	0.12	0.36	0.26	0.02	0.02	6	0.39	1.12	0.78	0.01	0.11
结肠	C18	39	2.29	6.99	5.52	0.41	0.52	46	3.02	8.58	6.00	0.35	0.69
直肠	C19–C20	38	2.23	6.81	5.79	0.36	0.82	56	3.68	10.45	6.95	0.53	0.78
肛门	C21	0	0.00	0.00	0.00	0.00	0.00	0	0.00	0.00	0.00	0.00	0.00
肝脏	C22	122	7.17	21.87	17.63	1.12	2.24	58	3.81	10.82	7.15	0.45	0.90
胆囊及其他	C23–C24	17	1.00	3.05	2.59	0.10	0.37	25	1.64	4.66	2.99	0.20	0.32
胰腺	C25	10	0.59	1.79	1.48	0.06	0.24	20	1.31	3.73	2.44	0.14	0.26
鼻、鼻窦及其他	C30–C31	3	0.18	0.54	0.48	0.01	0.06	1	0.07	0.19	0.12	0.01	0.01
喉	C32	11	0.65	1.97	1.61	0.06	0.22	3	0.20	0.56	0.31	0.00	0.02
气管、支气管、肺	C33–C34	155	9.11	27.79	22.30	1.25	2.78	124	8.14	23.14	15.73	0.94	1.78
其他的胸腔器官	C37–C38	4	0.24	0.72	0.61	0.06	0.06	8	0.53	1.49	1.05	0.05	0.15
骨	C40–C41	12	0.71	2.15	1.81	0.12	0.16	13	0.85	2.43	1.83	0.13	0.17
皮肤的黑色素瘤	C43	7	0.41	1.25	1.26	0.08	0.12	5	0.33	0.93	1.16	0.07	0.07
其他的皮肤	C44	5	0.29	0.90	0.81	0.05	0.05	8	0.53	1.49	1.01	0.03	0.09
间皮瘤	C45	0	0.00	0.00	0.00	0.00	0.00	0	0.00	0.00	0.00	0.00	0.00
卡波西肉瘤	C46	0	0.00	0.00	0.00	0.00	0.00	1	0.07	0.19	0.18	0.01	0.01
周围神经、其他结缔组织、软组织	C47;C49	5	0.29	0.90	0.70	0.06	0.06	2	0.13	0.37	0.78	0.04	0.04
乳房	C50	—	—	—	—	—	—	169	11.10	31.53	23.56	2.03	2.33
外阴	C51	—	—	—	—	—	—	0	0.00	0.00	0.00	0.00	0.00
阴道	C52	—	—	—	—	—	—	0	0.00	0.00	0.00	0.00	0.00
子宫颈	C53	—	—	—	—	—	—	113	7.42	21.09	16.66	1.45	1.61
子宫体	C54	—	—	—	—	—	—	31	2.04	5.78	4.21	0.38	0.44
子宫，部位不明	C55	—	—	—	—	—	—	3	0.20	0.56	0.48	0.05	0.05
卵巢	C56	—	—	—	—	—	—	36	2.36	6.72	4.99	0.37	0.55
其他的女性生殖器	C57	—	—	—	—	—	—	2	0.13	0.37	0.28	0.03	0.03
胎盘	C58	—	—	—	—	—	—	0	0.00	0.00	0.00	0.00	0.00
阴茎	C60	2	0.12	0.36	0.27	0.00	0.04	—	—	—	—	—	—
前列腺	C61	6	0.35	1.08	0.80	0.05	0.07	—	—	—	—	—	—
睾丸	C62	0	0.00	0.00	0.00	0.00	0.00	—	—	—	—	—	—
其他的男性生殖器	C63	1	0.06	0.18	0.13	0.00	0.02	—	—	—	—	—	—
肾	C64	11	0.65	1.97	1.62	0.10	0.16	4	0.26	0.75	0.52	0.04	0.06
肾盂	C65	0	0.00	0.00	0.00	0.00	0.00	0	0.00	0.00	0.00	0.00	0.00
输尿管	C66	0	0.00	0.00	0.00	0.00	0.00	1	0.07	0.19	0.14	0.01	0.01
膀胱	C67	16	0.94	2.87	2.29	0.16	0.30	9	0.59	1.68	1.12	0.04	0.16
其他的泌尿器官	C68	0	0.00	0.00	0.00	0.00	0.00	1	0.07	0.19	0.12	0.00	0.00
眼	C69	4	0.24	0.72	0.75	0.05	0.05	1	0.07	0.19	0.08	0.00	0.00
脑、神经系统	C70–C72	32	1.88	5.74	5.03	0.37	0.53	43	2.82	8.02	6.26	0.42	0.69
甲状腺	C73	7	0.41	1.25	1.28	0.07	0.10	16	1.05	2.99	2.26	0.20	0.24
肾上腺	C74	1	0.06	0.18	0.15	0.01	0.01	0	0.00	0.00	0.00	0.00	0.00
其他的内分泌腺	C75	3	0.18	0.54	0.48	0.03	0.03	3	0.20	0.56	0.46	0.04	0.04
霍奇金病	C81	2	0.12	0.36	0.33	0.01	0.06	0	0.00	0.00	0.00	0.00	0.00
非霍奇金淋巴瘤	C82–C85;C96	23	1.35	4.12	3.54	0.27	0.38	14	0.92	2.61	1.98	0.17	0.21
免疫增生性疾病	C88	0	0.00	0.00	0.00	0.00	0.00	0	0.00	0.00	0.00	0.00	0.00
多发性骨髓瘤	C90	8	0.47	1.43	1.10	0.13	0.13	6	0.39	1.12	0.76	0.06	0.12
淋巴样白血病	C91	1	0.06	0.18	0.19	0.00	0.05	2	0.13	0.37	0.39	0.03	0.03
髓样白血病	C92–C94	3	0.18	0.54	0.48	0.05	0.05	6	0.39	1.12	0.87	0.09	0.09
白血病，未特指	C95	14	0.82	2.51	2.60	0.20	0.20	22	1.44	4.11	3.39	0.24	0.32
其他的或未指明部位的	O&U	22	1.29	3.94	3.66	0.23	0.32	17	1.12	3.17	2.37	0.13	0.23
骨髓增殖性疾病	MPD	0	0.00	0.00	0.00	0.00	0.00	2	0.13	0.37	0.25	0.03	0.03
骨髓增生异常综合征	MDS	0	0.00	0.00	0.00	0.00	0.00	0	0.00	0.00	0.00	0.00	0.00
合计	ALL	1 701	100.00	304.95	248.12	14.89	31.31	1523	100.00	284.18	198.85	13.31	22.43
所有部位除外 C44	ALL1 but C44	1 696	99.71	304.05	247.30	14.84	31.27	1515	99.47	282.69	197.84	13.28	22.33

表 6-2-7a　2014 年河南省鲁山县恶性肿瘤发病主要指标

部位		男性						女性					
		病例数	构成 (%)	粗率 (1/10^5)	世标率 (1/10^5)	累积率 (%) 0~64	累积率 (%) 0~74	病例数	构成 (%)	粗率 (1/10^5)	世标率 (1/10^5)	累积率 (%) 0~64	累积率 (%) 0~74
唇	C00	0	0.00	0.00	0.00	0.00	0.00	0	0.00	0.00	0.00	0.00	0.00
舌	C01–C02	1	0.07	0.22	0.21	0.02	0.02	1	0.11	0.23	0.19	0.02	0.02
口	C03–C06	3	0.22	0.65	0.53	0.04	0.04	1	0.11	0.23	0.19	0.02	0.02
唾液腺	C07–C08	1	0.07	0.22	0.25	0.01	0.01	1	0.11	0.23	0.19	0.02	0.02
扁桃体	C09	0	0.00	0.00	0.00	0.00	0.00	0	0.00	0.00	0.00	0.00	0.00
其他的口咽	C10	0	0.00	0.00	0.00	0.00	0.00	3	0.34	0.69	0.40	0.01	0.01
鼻咽	C11	7	0.51	1.51	1.23	0.07	0.11	0	0.00	0.00	0.00	0.00	0.00
喉咽	C12–C13	3	0.22	0.65	0.60	0.04	0.08	0	0.00	0.00	0.00	0.00	0.00
咽，部位不明	C14	0	0.00	0.00	0.00	0.00	0.00	0	0.00	0.00	0.00	0.00	0.00
食管	C15	258	18.64	55.71	57.06	1.87	5.86	113	12.99	26.03	22.80	0.81	2.24
胃	C16	281	20.30	60.67	59.45	2.51	6.62	91	10.46	20.96	17.39	0.61	1.53
小肠	C17	4	0.29	0.86	0.86	0.08	0.12	1	0.11	0.23	0.25	0.00	0.04
结肠	C18	22	1.59	4.75	4.17	0.19	0.53	14	1.61	3.22	2.70	0.20	0.28
直肠	C19–C20	35	2.53	7.56	7.98	0.40	0.83	21	2.41	4.84	5.11	0.16	0.66
肛门	C21	0	0.00	0.00	0.00	0.00	0.00	0	0.00	0.00	0.00	0.00	0.00
肝脏	C22	190	13.73	41.03	41.00	2.48	4.03	77	8.85	17.73	16.11	0.69	1.48
胆囊及其他	C23–C24	11	0.79	2.38	1.90	0.09	0.13	14	1.61	3.22	2.89	0.02	0.19
胰腺	C25	21	1.52	4.53	3.99	0.23	0.45	13	1.49	2.99	2.89	0.13	0.34
鼻、鼻窦及其他	C30–C31	0	0.00	0.00	0.00	0.00	0.00	1	0.11	0.23	0.11	0.00	0.00
喉	C32	2	0.14	0.43	0.32	0.02	0.02	0	0.00	0.00	0.00	0.00	0.00
气管、支气管、肺	C33–C34	399	28.83	86.15	81.57	3.75	9.12	142	16.32	32.71	28.90	1.19	2.48
其他的胸腔器官	C37–C38	2	0.14	0.43	0.35	0.00	0.04	0	0.00	0.00	0.00	0.00	0.00
骨	C40–C41	16	1.16	3.45	3.31	0.17	0.46	12	1.38	2.76	2.34	0.23	0.23
皮肤的黑色素瘤	C43	0	0.00	0.00	0.00	0.00	0.00	0	0.00	0.00	0.00	0.00	0.00
其他的皮肤	C44	2	0.14	0.43	0.89	0.02	0.02	2	0.23	0.46	0.47	0.05	0.05
间皮瘤	C45	0	0.00	0.00	0.00	0.00	0.00	0	0.00	0.00	0.00	0.00	0.00
卡波西肉瘤	C46	0	0.00	0.00	0.00	0.00	0.00	0	0.00	0.00	0.00	0.00	0.00
周围神经、其他结缔组织、软组织	C47;C49	1	0.07	0.22	0.18	0.02	0.02	0	0.00	0.00	0.00	0.00	0.00
乳房	C50	—	—	—	—	—	—	89	10.23	20.50	18.82	1.42	1.90
外阴	C51	—	—	—	—	—	—	0	0.00	0.00	0.00	0.00	0.00
阴道	C52	—	—	—	—	—	—	0	0.00	0.00	0.00	0.00	0.00
子宫颈	C53	—	—	—	—	—	—	69	7.93	15.89	15.22	1.25	1.72
子宫体	C54	—	—	—	—	—	—	123	14.14	28.33	25.80	2.18	2.64
子宫，部位不明	C55	—	—	—	—	—	—	1	0.11	0.23	0.25	0.00	0.04
卵巢	C56	—	—	—	—	—	—	9	1.03	2.07	1.83	0.12	0.21
其他的女性生殖器	C57	—	—	—	—	—	—	0	0.00	0.00	0.00	0.00	0.00
胎盘	C58	—	—	—	—	—	—	0	0.00	0.00	0.00	0.00	0.00
阴茎	C60	5	0.36	1.08	0.88	0.04	0.08	—	—	—	—	—	—
前列腺	C61	10	0.72	2.16	2.50	0.08	0.17	—	—	—	—	—	—
睾丸	C62	3	0.22	0.65	0.56	0.04	0.04	—	—	—	—	—	—
其他的男性生殖器	C63	0	0.00	0.00	0.00	0.00	0.00	—	—	—	—	—	—
肾	C64	13	0.94	2.81	2.66	0.16	0.32	4	0.46	0.92	0.97	0.09	0.09
肾盂	C65	1	0.07	0.22	0.71	0.00	0.00	0	0.00	0.00	0.00	0.00	0.00
输尿管	C66	0	0.00	0.00	0.00	0.00	0.00	0	0.00	0.00	0.00	0.00	0.00
膀胱	C67	18	1.30	3.89	3.80	0.12	0.38	1	0.11	0.23	0.25	0.00	0.04
其他的泌尿器官	C68	0	0.00	0.00	0.00	0.00	0.00	0	0.00	0.00	0.00	0.00	0.00
眼	C69	0	0.00	0.00	0.00	0.00	0.00	0	0.00	0.00	0.00	0.00	0.00
脑、神经系统	C70–C72	44	3.18	9.50	8.69	0.44	1.12	27	3.10	6.22	6.77	0.33	0.63
甲状腺	C73	2	0.14	0.43	0.38	0.03	0.03	22	2.53	5.07	4.01	0.30	0.34
肾上腺	C74	1	0.07	0.22	0.17	0.00	0.00	0	0.00	0.00	0.00	0.00	0.00
其他的内分泌腺	C75	0	0.00	0.00	0.00	0.00	0.00	0	0.00	0.00	0.00	0.00	0.00
霍奇金病	C81	7	0.51	1.51	1.31	0.07	0.19	3	0.34	0.69	0.61	0.05	0.05
非霍奇金淋巴瘤	C82–C85;C96	1	0.07	0.22	0.18	0.00	0.04	0	0.00	0.00	0.00	0.00	0.00
免疫增生性疾病	C88	0	0.00	0.00	0.00	0.00	0.00	0	0.00	0.00	0.00	0.00	0.00
多发性骨髓瘤	C90	2	0.14	0.43	0.43	0.02	0.06	0	0.00	0.00	0.00	0.00	0.00
淋巴样白血病	C91	3	0.22	0.65	0.60	0.03	0.03	3	0.34	0.69	0.83	0.04	0.04
髓样白血病	C92–C94	2	0.14	0.43	0.46	0.03	0.03	2	0.23	0.46	0.58	0.03	0.03
白血病，未特指	C95	3	0.22	0.65	0.47	0.03	0.03	1	0.11	0.23	0.19	0.02	0.02
其他的或未指明部位的	O&U	8	0.58	1.73	1.42	0.04	0.16	9	1.03	2.07	1.86	0.17	0.21
骨髓增殖性疾病	MPD	0	0.00	0.00	0.00	0.00	0.00	0	0.00	0.00	0.00	0.00	0.00
骨髓增生异常综合征	MDS	0	0.00	0.00	0.00	0.00	0.00	0	0.00	0.00	0.00	0.00	0.00
合计	ALL	1 384	100.00	298.84	292.01	13.13	31.24	870	100.00	200.38	180.92	10.17	17.57
所有部位除外 C44	ALL but C44	1 382	99.86	298.41	291.12	13.11	31.22	868	99.77	199.92	180.45	10.11	17.51

表 6-2-8a　2014 年河南省罗山县恶性肿瘤发病主要指标

部位		男性						女性					
		病例数	构成 (%)	粗率 ($1/10^5$)	世标率 ($1/10^5$)	累积率 (%) 0~64	累积率 (%) 0~74	病例数	构成 (%)	粗率 ($1/10^5$)	世标率 ($1/10^5$)	累积率 (%) 0~64	累积率 (%) 0~74
唇	C00	0	0.00	0.00	0.00	0.00	0.00	0	0.00	0.00	0.00	0.00	0.00
舌	C01–C02	0	0.00	0.00	0.00	0.00	0.00	0	0.00	0.00	0.00	0.00	0.00
口	C03–C06	3	0.27	0.77	0.69	0.08	0.08	0	0.00	0.00	0.00	0.00	0.00
唾液腺	C07–C08	1	0.09	0.26	0.32	0.00	0.05	0	0.00	0.00	0.00	0.00	0.00
扁桃体	C09	0	0.00	0.00	0.00	0.00	0.00	0	0.00	0.00	0.00	0.00	0.00
其他的口咽	C10	3	0.27	0.77	0.93	0.04	0.09	0	0.00	0.00	0.00	0.00	0.00
鼻咽	C11	32	2.88	8.18	7.64	0.49	0.98	9	1.35	2.54	2.04	0.18	0.24
喉咽	C12–C13	0	0.00	0.00	0.00	0.00	0.00	0	0.00	0.00	0.00	0.00	0.00
咽，部位不明	C14	1	0.09	0.26	0.21	0.02	0.02	0	0.00	0.00	0.00	0.00	0.00
食管	C15	94	8.47	24.03	26.46	1.23	3.02	23	3.45	6.49	6.01	0.18	0.50
胃	C16	272	24.50	69.54	77.19	3.64	8.81	86	12.89	24.27	22.16	1.38	2.27
小肠	C17	0	0.00	0.00	0.00	0.00	0.00	0	0.00	0.00	0.00	0.00	0.00
结肠	C18	89	8.02	22.75	23.90	1.26	2.63	68	10.19	19.19	17.73	0.88	2.10
直肠	C19–C20	10	0.90	2.56	3.56	0.18	0.30	11	1.65	3.10	2.61	0.20	0.30
肛门	C21	0	0.00	0.00	0.00	0.00	0.00	1	0.15	0.28	0.27	0.00	0.07
肝脏	C22	173	15.59	44.23	43.09	2.46	4.74	70	10.49	19.75	17.99	0.75	2.30
胆囊及其他	C23–C24	3	0.27	0.77	0.77	0.05	0.05	6	0.90	1.69	1.45	0.07	0.19
胰腺	C25	19	1.71	4.86	4.50	0.32	0.55	11	1.65	3.10	3.03	0.18	0.48
鼻、鼻窦及其他	C30–C31	5	0.45	1.28	1.32	0.03	0.14	0	0.00	0.00	0.00	0.00	0.00
喉	C32	3	0.27	0.77	0.83	0.06	0.12	2	0.30	0.56	0.40	0.05	0.05
气管、支气管、肺	C33–C34	264	23.78	67.49	72.27	3.56	8.81	93	13.94	26.24	25.63	1.01	2.31
其他的胸腔器官	C37–C38	3	0.27	0.77	0.78	0.09	0.09	1	0.15	0.28	0.23	0.01	0.01
骨	C40–C41	15	1.35	3.83	3.44	0.18	0.37	5	0.75	1.41	1.29	0.07	0.12
皮肤的黑色素瘤	C43	0	0.00	0.00	0.00	0.00	0.00	0	0.00	0.00	0.00	0.00	0.00
其他的皮肤	C44	5	0.45	1.28	1.26	0.07	0.07	3	0.45	0.85	0.65	0.02	0.02
间皮瘤	C45	0	0.00	0.00	0.00	0.00	0.00	0	0.00	0.00	0.00	0.00	0.00
卡波西肉瘤	C46	0	0.00	0.00	0.00	0.00	0.00	0	0.00	0.00	0.00	0.00	0.00
周围神经、其他结缔组织、软组织	C47;C49	1	0.09	0.26	0.21	0.02	0.02	0	0.00	0.00	0.00	0.00	0.00
乳房	C50	—	—	—	—	—	—	74	11.09	20.88	16.72	1.57	1.77
外阴	C51	—	—	—	—	—	—	1	0.15	0.28	0.20	0.02	0.02
阴道	C52	—	—	—	—	—	—	0	0.00	0.00	0.00	0.00	0.00
子宫颈	C53	—	—	—	—	—	—	74	11.09	20.88	16.95	1.36	1.79
子宫体	C54	—	—	—	—	—	—	5	0.75	1.41	1.17	0.11	0.11
子宫，部位不明	C55	—	—	—	—	—	—	0	0.00	0.00	0.00	0.00	0.00
卵巢	C56	—	—	—	—	—	—	8	1.20	2.26	1.65	0.16	0.16
其他的女性生殖器	C57	—	—	—	—	—	—	0	0.00	0.00	0.00	0.00	0.00
胎盘	C58	—	—	—	—	—	—	0	0.00	0.00	0.00	0.00	0.00
阴茎	C60	0	0.00	0.00	0.00	0.00	0.00	—	—	—	—	—	—
前列腺	C61	14	1.26	3.58	4.97	0.23	0.39	—	—	—	—	—	—
睾丸	C62	0	0.00	0.00	0.00	0.00	0.00	—	—	—	—	—	—
其他的男性生殖器	C63	1	0.09	0.26	0.19	0.02	0.02	—	—	—	—	—	—
肾	C64	7	0.63	1.79	2.91	0.11	0.16	6	0.90	1.69	1.45	0.10	0.15
肾盂	C65	0	0.00	0.00	0.00	0.00	0.00	0	0.00	0.00	0.00	0.00	0.00
输尿管	C66	0	0.00	0.00	0.00	0.00	0.00	0	0.00	0.00	0.00	0.00	0.00
膀胱	C67	12	1.08	3.07	3.29	0.10	0.50	2	0.30	0.56	0.51	0.06	0.06
其他的泌尿器官	C68	0	0.00	0.00	0.00	0.00	0.00	0	0.00	0.00	0.00	0.00	0.00
眼	C69	2	0.18	0.51	0.75	0.05	0.05	0	0.00	0.00	0.00	0.00	0.00
脑、神经系统	C70–C72	28	2.52	7.16	6.09	0.61	0.67	29	4.35	8.18	7.13	0.39	0.99
甲状腺	C73	4	0.36	1.02	0.88	0.08	0.08	52	7.80	14.67	11.13	0.96	1.08
肾上腺	C74	0	0.00	0.00	0.00	0.00	0.00	0	0.00	0.00	0.00	0.00	0.00
其他的内分泌腺	C75	0	0.00	0.00	0.00	0.00	0.00	0	0.00	0.00	0.00	0.00	0.00
霍奇金病	C81	0	0.00	0.00	0.00	0.00	0.00	0	0.00	0.00	0.00	0.00	0.00
非霍奇金淋巴瘤	C82–C85;C96	14	1.26	3.58	3.37	0.23	0.40	13	1.95	3.67	3.31	0.25	0.45
免疫增生性疾病	C88	0	0.00	0.00	0.00	0.00	0.00	0	0.00	0.00	0.00	0.00	0.00
多发性骨髓瘤	C90	0	0.00	0.00	0.00	0.00	0.00	0	0.00	0.00	0.00	0.00	0.00
淋巴样白血病	C91	2	0.18	0.51	0.35	0.04	0.04	0	0.00	0.00	0.00	0.00	0.00
髓样白血病	C92–C94	0	0.00	0.00	0.00	0.00	0.00	0	0.00	0.00	0.00	0.00	0.00
白血病，未特指	C95	17	1.53	4.35	4.42	0.30	0.47	4	0.60	1.13	1.29	0.11	0.11
其他的或未指明部位的	O&U	9	0.81	2.30	2.93	0.11	0.18	10	1.50	2.82	2.39	0.16	0.29
骨髓增殖性疾病	MPD	0	0.00	0.00	0.00	0.00	0.00	0	0.00	0.00	0.00	0.00	0.00
骨髓增生异常综合征	MDS	0	0.00	0.00	0.00	0.00	0.00	0	0.00	0.00	0.00	0.00	0.00
合计	ALL	1 110	100.00	283.79	300.38	15.73	34.01	667	100.00	188.20	165.38	10.22	17.94
所有部位除外 C44	ALL but C44	1 105	99.55	282.51	299.12	15.66	33.94	664	99.55	187.35	164.74	10.20	17.92

表 6-2-9a 2014 年河南省洛阳市恶性肿瘤发病主要指标

部位		男性						女性					
		病例数	构成	粗率	世标率	累积率 (%)		病例数	构成	粗率	世标率	累积率 (%)	
			(%)	(1/10^5)	(1/10^5)	0~64	0~74		(%)	(1/10^5)	(1/10^5)	0~64	0~74
唇	C00	0	0.00	0.00	0.00	0.00	0.00	0	0.00	0.00	0.00	0.00	0.00
舌	C01–C02	1	0.06	0.17	0.12	0.01	0.01	2	0.16	0.37	0.35	0.03	0.03
口	C03–C06	5	0.31	0.87	0.84	0.03	0.10	2	0.16	0.37	0.28	0.02	0.02
唾液腺	C07–C08	8	0.50	1.39	1.68	0.07	0.07	1	0.08	0.18	0.15	0.01	0.01
扁桃体	C09	0	0.00	0.00	0.00	0.00	0.00	0	0.00	0.00	0.00	0.00	0.00
其他的口咽	C10	0	0.00	0.00	0.00	0.00	0.00	0	0.00	0.00	0.00	0.00	0.00
鼻咽	C11	10	0.62	1.74	1.96	0.05	0.22	5	0.39	0.92	0.73	0.08	0.08
喉咽	C12–C13	2	0.12	0.35	0.33	0.01	0.05	1	0.08	0.18	0.15	0.00	0.00
咽，部位不明	C14	0	0.00	0.00	0.00	0.00	0.00	3	0.24	0.55	0.72	0.00	0.00
食管	C15	121	7.54	21.09	23.89	0.96	2.27	71	5.56	13.02	14.15	0.25	1.27
胃	C16	213	13.28	37.13	43.20	1.21	3.86	85	6.66	15.58	14.68	0.54	1.56
小肠	C17	7	0.44	1.22	1.42	0.05	0.13	8	0.63	1.47	1.31	0.03	0.10
结肠	C18	80	4.99	13.95	14.90	0.49	1.50	63	4.94	11.55	10.44	0.39	0.95
直肠	C19–C20	70	4.36	12.20	13.41	0.52	1.17	60	4.70	11.00	9.54	0.31	0.81
肛门	C21	0	0.00	0.00	0.00	0.00	0.00	2	0.16	0.37	0.38	0.03	0.07
肝脏	C22	198	12.34	34.52	38.71	1.76	3.38	86	6.74	15.77	15.93	0.49	1.54
胆囊及其他	C23–C24	22	1.37	3.84	5.14	0.21	0.29	33	2.59	6.05	6.40	0.20	0.39
胰腺	C25	45	2.81	7.84	9.26	0.21	0.81	25	1.96	4.58	4.35	0.04	0.55
鼻、鼻窦及其他	C30–C31	5	0.31	0.87	0.75	0.02	0.11	2	0.16	0.37	0.32	0.00	0.04
喉	C32	13	0.81	2.27	2.16	0.09	0.18	1	0.08	0.18	0.43	0.00	0.00
气管、支气管、肺	C33–C34	465	28.99	81.06	87.81	3.09	8.19	180	14.11	33.00	32.33	1.12	3.22
其他的胸腔器官	C37–C38	8	0.50	1.39	2.69	0.06	0.10	1	0.08	0.18	0.13	0.01	0.01
骨	C40–C41	5	0.31	0.87	0.81	0.09	0.09	13	1.02	2.38	1.96	0.08	0.24
皮肤的黑色素瘤	C43	0	0.00	0.00	0.00	0.00	0.00	0	0.00	0.00	0.00	0.00	0.00
其他的皮肤	C44	4	0.25	0.70	0.70	0.01	0.08	9	0.71	1.65	1.82	0.07	0.07
间皮瘤	C45	1	0.06	0.17	0.12	0.01	0.01	1	0.08	0.18	0.15	0.01	0.01
卡波西肉瘤	C46	0	0.00	0.00	0.00	0.00	0.00	0	0.00	0.00	0.00	0.00	0.00
周围神经、其他结缔组织、软组织	C47;C49	4	0.25	0.70	0.56	0.03	0.08	2	0.16	0.37	0.34	0.01	0.04
乳房	C50	—	—	—	—	—	—	245	19.20	44.91	36.74	2.77	4.07
外阴	C51	—	—	—	—	—	—	0	0.00	0.00	0.00	0.00	0.00
阴道	C52	—	—	—	—	—	—	2	0.16	0.37	0.54	0.02	0.05
子宫颈	C53	—	—	—	—	—	—	71	5.56	13.02	10.75	0.90	1.12
子宫体	C54	—	—	—	—	—	—	33	2.59	6.05	5.45	0.40	0.62
子宫，部位不明	C55	—	—	—	—	—	—	11	0.86	2.02	1.56	0.11	0.24
卵巢	C56	—	—	—	—	—	—	37	2.90	6.78	6.18	0.32	0.65
其他的女性生殖器	C57	—	—	—	—	—	—	2	0.16	0.37	0.35	0.04	0.04
胎盘	C58	—	—	—	—	—	—	0	0.00	0.00	0.00	0.00	0.00
阴茎	C60	1	0.06	0.17	0.14	0.01	0.01	—	—	—	—	—	—
前列腺	C61	45	2.81	7.84	9.34	0.07	0.67	—	—	—	—	—	—
睾丸	C62	3	0.19	0.52	0.45	0.02	0.06	—	—	—	—	—	—
其他的男性生殖器	C63	1	0.06	0.17	0.15	0.00	0.00	—	—	—	—	—	—
肾	C64	40	2.49	6.97	7.86	0.39	0.97	21	1.65	3.85	3.62	0.20	0.41
肾盂	C65	5	0.31	0.87	0.78	0.06	0.06	3	0.24	0.55	0.49	0.01	0.09
输尿管	C66	5	0.31	0.87	1.39	0.08	0.13	2	0.16	0.37	0.35	0.00	0.09
膀胱	C67	51	3.18	8.89	9.59	0.38	0.86	22	1.72	4.03	3.94	0.12	0.24
其他的泌尿器官	C68	1	0.06	0.17	0.20	0.00	0.00	0	0.00	0.00	0.00	0.00	0.00
眼	C69	2	0.12	0.35	0.77	0.00	0.00	2	0.16	0.37	0.56	0.03	0.03
脑、神经系统	C70–C72	33	2.06	5.75	6.22	0.30	0.38	45	3.53	8.25	7.98	0.53	0.79
甲状腺	C73	17	1.06	2.96	2.24	0.20	0.20	47	3.68	8.62	6.77	0.53	0.71
肾上腺	C74	2	0.12	0.35	0.31	0.02	0.06	1	0.08	0.18	0.21	0.03	0.03
其他的内分泌腺	C75	1	0.06	0.17	0.18	0.00	0.05	1	0.08	0.18	0.12	0.01	0.01
霍奇金病	C81	1	0.06	0.17	0.20	0.01	0.01	1	0.08	0.18	0.17	0.00	0.04
非霍奇金淋巴瘤	C82–C85;C96	16	1.00	2.79	3.36	0.09	0.22	19	1.49	3.48	3.20	0.15	0.47
免疫增生性疾病	C88	1	0.06	0.17	0.15	0.00	0.00	0	0.00	0.00	0.00	0.00	0.00
多发性骨髓瘤	C90	6	0.37	1.05	1.50	0.04	0.07	4	0.31	0.73	0.65	0.02	0.09
淋巴样白血病	C91	7	0.44	1.22	1.29	0.05	0.21	3	0.24	0.55	0.98	0.03	0.03
髓样白血病	C92–C94	10	0.62	1.74	1.61	0.06	0.24	4	0.31	0.73	0.56	0.05	0.05
白血病，未特指	C95	33	2.06	5.75	5.66	0.26	0.47	18	1.41	3.30	3.61	0.15	0.34
其他的或未指明部位的	O&U	24	1.50	4.18	4.94	0.16	0.35	23	1.80	4.22	4.28	0.12	0.44
骨髓增殖性疾病	MPD	2	0.12	0.35	0.23	0.02	0.02	2	0.16	0.37	0.60	0.00	0.04
骨髓增生异常综合征	MDS	3	0.19	0.52	0.50	0.01	0.10	1	0.08	0.18	0.14	0.02	0.02
合计	ALL	1 604	100.00	279.62	310.68	11.26	27.92	1 276	100.00	233.92	216.86	10.35	21.74
所有部位除外 C44	ALL but C44	1 600	99.75	278.92	309.97	11.25	27.84	1 267	99.29	232.27	215.05	10.28	21.67

表 6-2-10a　2014 年河南省孟津县恶性肿瘤发病主要指标

部位		男性						女性					
		病例数	构成 (%)	粗率 $(1/10^5)$	世标率 $(1/10^5)$	累积率 (%) 0~64	累积率 (%) 0~74	病例数	构成 (%)	粗率 $(1/10^5)$	世标率 $(1/10^5)$	累积率 (%) 0~64	累积率 (%) 0~74
唇	C00	0	0.00	0.00	0.00	0.00	0.00	0	0.00	0.00	0.00	0.00	0.00
舌	C01–C02	2	0.33	0.87	0.68	0.07	0.07	0	0.00	0.00	0.00	0.00	0.00
口	C03–C06	1	0.16	0.43	0.34	0.04	0.04	3	0.59	1.31	1.08	0.07	0.14
唾液腺	C07–C08	1	0.16	0.43	0.29	0.00	0.00	1	0.20	0.44	0.30	0.02	0.02
扁桃体	C09	0	0.00	0.00	0.00	0.00	0.00	0	0.00	0.00	0.00	0.00	0.00
其他的口咽	C10	0	0.00	0.00	0.00	0.00	0.00	0	0.00	0.00	0.00	0.00	0.00
鼻咽	C11	1	0.16	0.43	0.39	0.00	0.06	0	0.00	0.00	0.00	0.00	0.00
喉咽	C12–C13	1	0.16	0.43	0.34	0.03	0.03	0	0.00	0.00	0.00	0.00	0.00
咽，部位不明	C14	0	0.00	0.00	0.00	0.00	0.00	1	0.20	0.44	0.22	0.00	0.00
食管	C15	110	18.00	47.58	39.23	1.60	4.80	68	13.33	29.77	20.10	0.48	2.75
胃	C16	124	20.29	53.63	43.66	1.73	6.16	52	10.20	22.77	16.18	0.74	2.08
小肠	C17	4	0.65	1.73	1.46	0.07	0.23	4	0.78	1.75	0.99	0.04	0.04
结肠	C18	15	2.45	6.49	5.36	0.28	0.60	10	1.96	4.38	3.17	0.24	0.48
直肠	C19–C20	17	2.78	7.35	6.20	0.29	0.74	12	2.35	5.25	3.60	0.24	0.44
肛门	C21	0	0.00	0.00	0.00	0.00	0.00	0	0.00	0.00	0.00	0.00	0.00
肝脏	C22	53	8.67	22.92	18.37	1.10	1.91	32	6.27	14.01	10.32	0.25	1.58
胆囊及其他	C23–C24	15	2.45	6.49	5.64	0.21	0.57	13	2.55	5.69	4.28	0.22	0.62
胰腺	C25	10	1.64	4.33	3.69	0.08	0.69	7	1.37	3.06	1.99	0.14	0.20
鼻、鼻窦及其他	C30–C31	0	0.00	0.00	0.00	0.00	0.00	0	0.00	0.00	0.00	0.00	0.00
喉	C32	4	0.65	1.73	1.23	0.03	0.10	0	0.00	0.00	0.00	0.00	0.00
气管、支气管、肺	C33–C34	144	23.57	62.28	50.28	2.13	5.79	83	16.27	36.34	24.55	1.30	3.05
其他的胸腔器官	C37–C38	2	0.33	0.87	0.68	0.08	0.08	3	0.59	1.31	0.88	0.07	0.07
骨	C40–C41	4	0.65	1.73	1.27	0.10	0.10	2	0.39	0.88	0.55	0.00	0.06
皮肤的黑色素瘤	C43	2	0.33	0.87	0.54	0.03	0.03	2	0.39	0.88	0.60	0.00	0.06
其他的皮肤	C44	3	0.49	1.30	0.94	0.03	0.10	2	0.39	0.88	0.51	0.03	0.03
间皮瘤	C45	0	0.00	0.00	0.00	0.00	0.00	0	0.00	0.00	0.00	0.00	0.00
卡波西肉瘤	C46	0	0.00	0.00	0.00	0.00	0.00	0	0.00	0.00	0.00	0.00	0.00
周围神经、其他结缔组织、软组织	C47;C49	0	0.00	0.00	0.00	0.00	0.00	1	0.20	0.44	0.33	0.03	0.03
乳房	C50	—	—	—	—	—	—	94	18.43	41.16	30.09	2.54	3.52
外阴	C51	—	—	—	—	—	—	0	0.00	0.00	0.00	0.00	0.00
阴道	C52	—	—	—	—	—	—	0	0.00	0.00	0.00	0.00	0.00
子宫颈	C53	—	—	—	—	—	—	24	4.71	10.51	7.83	0.41	1.08
子宫体	C54	—	—	—	—	—	—	15	2.94	6.57	4.84	0.37	0.53
子宫，部位不明	C55	—	—	—	—	—	—	2	0.39	0.88	0.51	0.03	0.03
卵巢	C56	—	—	—	—	—	—	9	1.76	3.94	2.83	0.28	0.28
其他的女性生殖器	C57	—	—	—	—	—	—	1	0.20	0.44	0.33	0.03	0.03
胎盘	C58	—	—	—	—	—	—	0	0.00	0.00	0.00	0.00	0.00
阴茎	C60	1	0.16	0.43	0.29	0.00	0.00	—	—	—	—	—	—
前列腺	C61	7	1.15	3.03	2.74	0.07	0.40	—	—	—	—	—	—
睾丸	C62	0	0.00	0.00	0.00	0.00	0.00	—	—	—	—	—	—
其他的男性生殖器	C63	0	0.00	0.00	0.00	0.00	0.00	—	—	—	—	—	—
肾	C64	7	1.15	3.03	2.49	0.21	0.40	5	0.98	2.19	1.68	0.14	0.20
肾盂	C65	0	0.00	0.00	0.00	0.00	0.00	1	0.20	0.44	0.25	0.03	0.03
输尿管	C66	1	0.16	0.43	0.25	0.03	0.03	0	0.00	0.00	0.00	0.00	0.00
膀胱	C67	13	2.13	5.62	4.58	0.14	0.69	2	0.39	0.88	0.60	0.00	0.06
其他的泌尿器官	C68	0	0.00	0.00	0.00	0.00	0.00	0	0.00	0.00	0.00	0.00	0.00
眼	C69	0	0.00	0.00	0.00	0.00	0.00	0	0.00	0.00	0.00	0.00	0.00
脑、神经系统	C70–C72	17	2.78	7.35	5.87	0.37	0.49	25	4.90	10.95	9.84	0.55	1.06
甲状腺	C73	4	0.65	1.73	1.23	0.11	0.11	8	1.57	3.50	2.45	0.15	0.21
肾上腺	C74	0	0.00	0.00	0.00	0.00	0.00	0	0.00	0.00	0.00	0.00	0.00
其他的内分泌腺	C75	2	0.33	0.87	0.68	0.06	0.06	1	0.20	0.44	0.35	0.03	0.03
霍奇金病	C81	2	0.33	0.87	0.85	0.05	0.05	0	0.00	0.00	0.00	0.00	0.00
非霍奇金淋巴瘤	C82–C85;C96	13	2.13	5.62	5.30	0.24	0.47	8	1.57	3.50	2.75	0.20	0.26
免疫增生性疾病	C88	0	0.00	0.00	0.00	0.00	0.00	0	0.00	0.00	0.00	0.00	0.00
多发性骨髓瘤	C90	1	0.16	0.43	0.39	0.00	0.06	0	0.00	0.00	0.00	0.00	0.00
淋巴样白血病	C91	1	0.16	0.43	0.34	0.03	0.03	1	0.20	0.44	0.89	0.04	0.04
髓样白血病	C92–C94	3	0.49	1.30	1.03	0.11	0.11	1	0.20	0.44	0.45	0.02	0.02
白血病，未特指	C95	13	2.13	5.62	4.84	0.22	0.44	8	1.57	3.50	2.53	0.17	0.17
其他的或未指明部位的	O&U	12	1.96	5.19	4.14	0.19	0.58	9	1.76	3.94	2.45	0.16	0.23
骨髓增殖性疾病	MPD	0	0.00	0.00	0.00	0.00	0.00	0	0.00	0.00	0.00	0.00	0.00
骨髓增生异常综合征	MDS	1	0.16	0.43	0.34	0.04	0.04	0	0.00	0.00	0.00	0.00	0.00
合计	ALL	611	100.00	264.27	215.93	9.77	26.06	510	100.00	223.29	160.29	9.02	19.46
所有部位除外 C44	ALL but C44	608	99.51	262.98	215.00	9.73	25.97	508	99.61	222.42	159.78	8.99	19.43

表 6-2-11a 2014 年河南省南阳市恶性肿瘤发病主要指标

部位		男性						女性					
		病例数	构成 (%)	粗率 ($1/10^5$)	世标率 ($1/10^5$)	累积率 (%) 0~64	累积率 (%) 0~74	病例数	构成 (%)	粗率 ($1/10^5$)	世标率 ($1/10^5$)	累积率 (%) 0~64	累积率 (%) 0~74
唇	C00	0	0.00	0.00	0.00	0.00	0.00	0	0.00	0.00	0.00	0.00	0.00
舌	C01–C02	1	0.07	0.21	0.15	0.02	0.02	2	0.21	0.45	0.39	0.03	0.03
口	C03–C06	7	0.46	1.50	1.40	0.07	0.14	5	0.53	1.13	0.93	0.00	0.09
唾液腺	C07–C08	2	0.13	0.43	0.42	0.03	0.03	3	0.32	0.68	0.53	0.04	0.04
扁桃体	C09	0	0.00	0.00	0.00	0.00	0.00	0	0.00	0.00	0.00	0.00	0.00
其他的口咽	C10	2	0.13	0.43	0.31	0.02	0.02	0	0.00	0.00	0.00	0.00	0.00
鼻咽	C11	6	0.39	1.28	0.98	0.06	0.09	3	0.32	0.68	0.60	0.00	0.08
喉咽	C12–C13	1	0.07	0.21	0.19	0.02	0.02	0	0.00	0.00	0.00	0.00	0.00
咽，部位不明	C14	2	0.13	0.43	0.36	0.02	0.02	1	0.11	0.23	0.20	0.03	0.03
食管	C15	299	19.59	63.91	55.52	2.39	6.50	119	12.61	26.79	22.06	0.80	2.47
胃	C16	338	22.15	72.24	63.12	3.12	7.49	120	12.71	27.02	22.53	0.94	2.35
小肠	C17	7	0.46	1.50	1.22	0.04	0.16	8	0.85	1.80	1.49	0.09	0.18
结肠	C18	37	2.42	7.91	7.34	0.24	0.66	20	2.12	4.50	3.87	0.11	0.50
直肠	C19–C20	53	3.47	11.33	10.28	0.56	1.26	37	3.92	8.33	6.32	0.41	0.64
肛门	C21	2	0.13	0.43	0.37	0.00	0.05	1	0.11	0.23	0.21	0.00	0.05
肝脏	C22	194	12.71	41.47	36.22	1.90	4.46	64	6.78	14.41	11.73	0.74	1.52
胆囊及其他	C23–C24	5	0.33	1.07	0.77	0.07	0.07	0	0.00	0.00	0.00	0.00	0.00
胰腺	C25	5	0.33	1.07	0.88	0.02	0.17	7	0.74	1.58	1.32	0.10	0.15
鼻、鼻窦及其他	C30–C31	2	0.13	0.43	0.31	0.03	0.03	2	0.21	0.45	0.25	0.00	0.00
喉	C32	4	0.26	0.85	0.70	0.02	0.09	1	0.11	0.23	0.13	0.02	0.02
气管、支气管、肺	C33–C34	382	25.03	81.65	70.25	3.12	8.32	142	15.04	31.97	27.26	1.38	3.23
其他的胸腔器官	C37–C38	5	0.33	1.07	0.77	0.05	0.10	6	0.64	1.35	1.10	0.03	0.11
骨	C40–C41	14	0.92	2.99	2.60	0.14	0.34	14	1.48	3.15	2.47	0.18	0.28
皮肤的黑色素瘤	C43	2	0.13	0.43	0.45	0.02	0.06	2	0.21	0.45	0.43	0.04	0.04
其他的皮肤	C44	3	0.20	0.64	0.63	0.04	0.04	5	0.53	1.13	0.90	0.05	0.05
间皮瘤	C45	0	0.00	0.00	0.00	0.00	0.00	1	0.11	0.23	0.25	0.02	0.02
卡波西肉瘤	C46	0	0.00	0.00	0.00	0.00	0.00	0	0.00	0.00	0.00	0.00	0.00
周围神经、其他结缔组织、软组织	C47;C49	1	0.07	0.21	0.13	0.00	0.00	2	0.21	0.45	0.38	0.03	0.03
乳房	C50	—	—	—	—	—	—	155	16.42	34.89	28.87	2.42	3.04
外阴	C51	—	—	—	—	—	—	1	0.11	0.23	0.25	0.02	0.02
阴道	C52	—	—	—	—	—	—	0	0.00	0.00	0.00	0.00	0.00
子宫颈	C53	—	—	—	—	—	—	75	7.94	16.88	14.52	1.10	1.67
子宫体	C54	—	—	—	—	—	—	26	2.75	5.85	4.81	0.41	0.51
子宫，部位不明	C55	—	—	—	—	—	—	5	0.53	1.13	1.11	0.04	0.16
卵巢	C56	—	—	—	—	—	—	24	2.54	5.40	4.46	0.34	0.47
其他的女性生殖器	C57	—	—	—	—	—	—	1	0.11	0.23	0.18	0.01	0.01
胎盘	C58	—	—	—	—	—	—	0	0.00	0.00	0.00	0.00	0.00
阴茎	C60	3	0.20	0.64	0.40	0.02	0.02	—	—	—	—	—	—
前列腺	C61	12	0.79	2.56	2.21	0.00	0.19	—	—	—	—	—	—
睾丸	C62	3	0.20	0.64	0.47	0.01	0.01	—	—	—	—	—	—
其他的男性生殖器	C63	0	0.00	0.00	0.00	0.00	0.00	—	—	—	—	—	—
肾	C64	3	0.20	0.64	0.60	0.05	0.05	2	0.21	0.45	0.31	0.00	0.00
肾盂	C65	0	0.00	0.00	0.00	0.00	0.00	0	0.00	0.00	0.00	0.00	0.00
输尿管	C66	1	0.07	0.21	0.24	0.02	0.02	0	0.00	0.00	0.00	0.00	0.00
膀胱	C67	13	0.85	2.78	2.72	0.09	0.34	2	0.21	0.45	0.33	0.00	0.05
其他的泌尿器官	C68	7	0.46	1.50	1.08	0.09	0.09	2	0.21	0.45	0.36	0.04	0.04
眼	C69	0	0.00	0.00	0.00	0.00	0.00	0	0.00	0.00	0.00	0.00	0.00
脑、神经系统	C70–C72	39	2.56	8.34	7.54	0.36	0.76	29	3.07	6.53	5.56	0.35	0.57
甲状腺	C73	3	0.20	0.64	0.54	0.03	0.08	19	2.01	4.28	3.53	0.33	0.33
肾上腺	C74	0	0.00	0.00	0.00	0.00	0.00	1	0.11	0.23	0.15	0.01	0.01
其他的内分泌腺	C75	2	0.13	0.43	0.40	0.02	0.06	0	0.00	0.00	0.00	0.00	0.00
霍奇金病	C81	5	0.33	1.07	1.15	0.03	0.03	4	0.42	0.90	0.88	0.05	0.09
非霍奇金淋巴瘤	C82–C85;C96	12	0.79	2.56	2.01	0.10	0.22	8	0.85	1.80	1.76	0.14	0.24
免疫增生性疾病	C88	0	0.00	0.00	0.00	0.00	0.00	0	0.00	0.00	0.00	0.00	0.00
多发性骨髓瘤	C90	1	0.07	0.21	0.24	0.02	0.02	2	0.21	0.45	0.44	0.03	0.06
淋巴样白血病	C91	3	0.20	0.64	0.55	0.04	0.08	2	0.21	0.45	0.31	0.03	0.03
髓样白血病	C92–C94	1	0.07	0.21	0.26	0.02	0.02	1	0.11	0.23	0.30	0.01	0.01
白血病，未特指	C95	11	0.72	2.35	1.82	0.16	0.16	6	0.64	1.35	1.33	0.05	0.14
其他的或未指明部位的	O&U	29	1.90	6.20	5.35	0.37	0.55	14	1.48	3.15	2.43	0.20	0.25
骨髓增殖性疾病	MPD	0	0.00	0.00	0.00	0.00	0.00	0	0.00	0.00	0.00	0.00	0.00
骨髓增生异常综合征	MDS	0	0.00	0.00	0.00	0.00	0.00	0	0.00	0.00	0.00	0.00	0.00
合计	ALL	1 526	100.00	326.17	283.84	13.49	32.86	944	100.00	212.52	177.22	10.61	19.63
所有部位除外 C44	ALL but C44	1 523	99.80	325.53	283.21	13.45	32.82	939	99.47	211.40	176.32	10.56	19.58

表 6-2-12a 2014 年河南省内乡县恶性肿瘤发病主要指标

部位		男性						女性					
		病例数	构成 (%)	粗率 ($1/10^5$)	世标率 ($1/10^5$)	累积率 (%) 0~64	累积率 (%) 0~74	病例数	构成 (%)	粗率 ($1/10^5$)	世标率 ($1/10^5$)	累积率 (%) 0~64	累积率 (%) 0~74
唇	C00	1	0.09	0.27	0.25	0.03	0.03	1	0.13	0.29	0.22	0.00	0.06
舌	C01–C02	2	0.17	0.54	0.41	0.02	0.08	0	0.00	0.00	0.00	0.00	0.00
口	C03–C06	1	0.09	0.27	0.25	0.03	0.03	2	0.27	0.57	0.50	0.06	0.06
唾液腺	C07–C08	1	0.09	0.27	0.27	0.00	0.04	1	0.13	0.29	0.15	0.00	0.00
扁桃体	C09	1	0.09	0.27	0.25	0.03	0.03	0	0.00	0.00	0.00	0.00	0.00
其他的口咽	C10	2	0.17	0.54	0.44	0.04	0.04	0	0.00	0.00	0.00	0.00	0.00
鼻咽	C11	2	0.17	0.54	0.47	0.04	0.04	2	0.27	0.57	0.48	0.05	0.05
喉咽	C12–C13	3	0.26	0.81	0.57	0.06	0.06	0	0.00	0.00	0.00	0.00	0.00
咽，部位不明	C14	0	0.00	0.00	0.00	0.00	0.00	0	0.00	0.00	0.00	0.00	0.00
食管	C15	357	30.75	96.98	79.22	4.73	10.47	166	22.40	47.33	35.70	1.99	4.61
胃	C16	354	30.49	96.17	78.73	4.25	10.66	107	14.44	30.51	23.27	1.14	3.16
小肠	C17	0	0.00	0.00	0.00	0.00	0.00	1	0.13	0.29	0.19	0.02	0.02
结肠	C18	16	1.38	4.35	3.81	0.31	0.41	6	0.81	1.71	1.26	0.11	0.16
直肠	C19–C20	32	2.76	8.69	7.00	0.47	0.76	39	5.26	11.12	8.21	0.58	0.96
肛门	C21	0	0.00	0.00	0.00	0.00	0.00	0	0.00	0.00	0.00	0.00	0.00
肝脏	C22	86	7.41	23.36	19.22	1.54	2.52	41	5.53	11.69	9.49	0.60	1.30
胆囊及其他	C23–C24	4	0.34	1.09	0.91	0.07	0.13	5	0.67	1.43	1.09	0.07	0.12
胰腺	C25	12	1.03	3.26	2.78	0.24	0.38	6	0.81	1.71	1.12	0.08	0.08
鼻、鼻窦及其他	C30–C31	0	0.00	0.00	0.00	0.00	0.00	0	0.00	0.00	0.00	0.00	0.00
喉	C32	4	0.34	1.09	0.82	0.07	0.12	1	0.13	0.29	0.22	0.00	0.06
气管、支气管、肺	C33–C34	177	15.25	48.08	39.33	2.75	5.35	67	9.04	19.10	14.43	0.93	1.85
其他的胸腔器官	C37–C38	3	0.26	0.81	0.64	0.02	0.06	1	0.13	0.29	0.21	0.02	0.02
骨	C40–C41	12	1.03	3.26	3.04	0.23	0.34	12	1.62	3.42	2.69	0.20	0.26
皮肤的黑色素瘤	C43	0	0.00	0.00	0.00	0.00	0.00	0	0.00	0.00	0.00	0.00	0.00
其他的皮肤	C44	5	0.43	1.36	1.04	0.04	0.21	5	0.67	1.43	1.00	0.04	0.15
间皮瘤	C45	2	0.17	0.54	0.50	0.02	0.07	1	0.13	0.29	0.30	0.02	0.02
卡波西肉瘤	C46	0	0.00	0.00	0.00	0.00	0.00	0	0.00	0.00	0.00	0.00	0.00
周围神经、其他结缔组织、软组织	C47;C49	0	0.00	0.00	0.00	0.00	0.00	1	0.13	0.29	0.18	0.02	0.02
乳房	C50	—	—	—	—	—	—	125	16.87	35.64	26.83	2.34	2.85
外阴	C51	—	—	—	—	—	—	0	0.00	0.00	0.00	0.00	0.00
阴道	C52	—	—	—	—	—	—	3	0.40	0.86	0.62	0.04	0.10
子宫颈	C53	—	—	—	—	—	—	31	4.18	8.84	6.95	0.57	0.71
子宫体	C54	—	—	—	—	—	—	34	4.59	9.69	7.37	0.62	0.86
子宫，部位不明	C55	—	—	—	—	—	—	0	0.00	0.00	0.00	0.00	0.00
卵巢	C56	—	—	—	—	—	—	22	2.97	6.27	5.41	0.42	0.51
其他的女性生殖器	C57	—	—	—	—	—	—	0	0.00	0.00	0.00	0.00	0.00
胎盘	C58	—	—	—	—	—	—	0	0.00	0.00	0.00	0.00	0.00
阴茎	C60	1	0.09	0.27	0.16	0.00	0.00	—	—	—	—	—	—
前列腺	C61	7	0.60	1.90	1.28	0.06	0.06	—	—	—	—	—	—
睾丸	C62	1	0.09	0.27	0.27	0.00	0.04	—	—	—	—	—	—
其他的男性生殖器	C63	0	0.00	0.00	0.00	0.00	0.00	—	—	—	—	—	—
肾	C64	5	0.43	1.36	1.18	0.06	0.15	3	0.40	0.86	1.03	0.05	0.10
肾盂	C65	2	0.17	0.54	0.50	0.06	0.06	6	0.81	1.71	1.31	0.11	0.11
输尿管	C66	0	0.00	0.00	0.00	0.00	0.00	0	0.00	0.00	0.00	0.00	0.00
膀胱	C67	10	0.86	2.72	2.26	0.20	0.31	3	0.40	0.86	0.64	0.02	0.06
其他的泌尿器官	C68	0	0.00	0.00	0.00	0.00	0.00	0	0.00	0.00	0.00	0.00	0.00
眼	C69	0	0.00	0.00	0.00	0.00	0.00	1	0.13	0.29	0.30	0.02	0.02
脑、神经系统	C70–C72	10	0.86	2.72	2.77	0.21	0.27	10	1.35	2.85	2.36	0.16	0.21
甲状腺	C73	2	0.17	0.54	0.48	0.05	0.05	16	2.16	4.56	3.75	0.23	0.33
肾上腺	C74	0	0.00	0.00	0.00	0.00	0.00	2	0.27	0.57	0.40	0.04	0.04
其他的内分泌腺	C75	1	0.09	0.27	0.18	0.02	0.02	0	0.00	0.00	0.00	0.00	0.00
霍奇金病	C81	3	0.26	0.81	0.68	0.03	0.08	0	0.00	0.00	0.00	0.00	0.00
非霍奇金淋巴瘤	C82–C85;C96	13	1.12	3.53	2.65	0.14	0.25	4	0.54	1.14	0.88	0.11	0.11
免疫增生性疾病	C88	0	0.00	0.00	0.00	0.00	0.00	1	0.13	0.29	0.19	0.00	0.00
多发性骨髓瘤	C90	2	0.17	0.54	0.47	0.03	0.09	2	0.27	0.57	0.81	0.05	0.05
淋巴样白血病	C91	0	0.00	0.00	0.00	0.00	0.00	1	0.13	0.29	0.19	0.02	0.02
髓样白血病	C92–C94	7	0.60	1.90	1.61	0.11	0.15	3	0.40	0.86	0.58	0.05	0.05
白血病，未特指	C95	10	0.86	2.72	2.45	0.11	0.27	7	0.94	2.00	1.45	0.10	0.10
其他的或未指明部位的	O&U	8	0.69	2.17	1.84	0.13	0.23	2	0.27	0.57	0.45	0.03	0.03
骨髓增殖性疾病	MPD	0	0.00	0.00	0.00	0.00	0.00	0	0.00	0.00	0.00	0.00	0.00
骨髓增生异常综合征	MDS	1	0.09	0.27	0.18	0.02	0.02	0	0.00	0.00	0.00	0.00	0.00
合计	ALL	1 161	100.00	315.39	259.05	16.23	33.91	741	100.00	211.26	162.26	10.91	19.20
所有部位除外 C44	ALL but C44	1 156	99.57	314.03	258.02	16.20	33.70	736	99.33	209.84	161.26	10.87	19.04

表 6-2-13a 2014 年河南省汝阳县恶性肿瘤发病主要指标

部位		男性						女性					
		病例数	构成 (%)	粗率 (1/10^5)	世标率 (1/10^5)	累积率 (%) 0~64	累积率 (%) 0~74	病例数	构成 (%)	粗率 (1/10^5)	世标率 (1/10^5)	累积率 (%) 0~64	累积率 (%) 0~74
唇	C00	1	0.14	0.38	0.29	0.02	0.02	0	0.00	0.00	0.00	0.00	0.00
舌	C01–C02	1	0.14	0.38	0.51	0.02	0.02	0	0.00	0.00	0.00	0.00	0.00
口	C03–C06	2	0.28	0.76	0.87	0.02	0.10	3	0.52	1.22	1.18	0.06	0.14
唾液腺	C07–C08	5	0.71	1.89	1.49	0.14	0.14	2	0.35	0.81	0.67	0.06	0.06
扁桃体	C09	0	0.00	0.00	0.00	0.00	0.00	0	0.00	0.00	0.00	0.00	0.00
其他的口咽	C10	1	0.14	0.38	0.23	0.00	0.00	0	0.00	0.00	0.00	0.00	0.00
鼻咽	C11	0	0.00	0.00	0.00	0.00	0.00	2	0.35	0.81	0.68	0.00	0.08
喉咽	C12–C13	1	0.14	0.38	0.28	0.03	0.03	1	0.17	0.41	0.51	0.00	0.08
咽，部位不明	C14	0	0.00	0.00	0.00	0.00	0.00	0	0.00	0.00	0.00	0.00	0.00
食管	C15	149	21.23	56.37	51.20	1.74	6.83	89	15.45	36.24	27.16	0.58	2.94
胃	C16	186	26.50	70.37	63.21	3.05	7.01	72	12.50	29.32	23.40	0.82	3.07
小肠	C17	1	0.14	0.38	0.37	0.05	0.05	1	0.17	0.41	0.39	0.05	0.05
结肠	C18	13	1.85	4.92	4.14	0.14	0.39	16	2.78	6.51	5.60	0.32	0.83
直肠	C19–C20	17	2.42	6.43	5.25	0.29	0.29	20	3.47	8.14	6.28	0.30	0.66
肛门	C21	0	0.00	0.00	0.00	0.00	0.00	1	0.17	0.41	0.31	0.04	0.04
肝脏	C22	44	6.27	16.65	15.18	0.87	2.14	21	3.65	8.55	6.36	0.20	0.66
胆囊及其他	C23–C24	8	1.14	3.03	2.51	0.07	0.35	10	1.74	4.07	2.90	0.13	0.34
胰腺	C25	8	1.14	3.03	2.95	0.11	0.36	11	1.91	4.48	4.10	0.23	0.49
鼻、鼻窦及其他	C30–C31	1	0.14	0.38	0.46	0.00	0.08	0	0.00	0.00	0.00	0.00	0.00
喉	C32	4	0.57	1.51	1.14	0.03	0.13	2	0.35	0.81	0.57	0.05	0.05
气管、支气管、肺	C33–C34	165	23.50	62.43	57.16	2.43	7.00	68	11.81	27.69	22.71	1.07	2.88
其他的胸腔器官	C37–C38	1	0.14	0.38	0.28	0.03	0.03	1	0.17	0.41	0.21	0.00	0.00
骨	C40–C41	4	0.57	1.51	1.64	0.07	0.25	4	0.69	1.63	1.43	0.12	0.12
皮肤的黑色素瘤	C43	1	0.14	0.38	0.46	0.00	0.08	2	0.35	0.81	0.74	0.07	0.07
其他的皮肤	C44	1	0.14	0.38	0.37	0.05	0.05	8	1.39	3.26	2.25	0.10	0.18
间皮瘤	C45	1	0.14	0.38	0.28	0.03	0.03	0	0.00	0.00	0.00	0.00	0.00
卡波西肉瘤	C46	0	0.00	0.00	0.00	0.00	0.00	0	0.00	0.00	0.00	0.00	0.00
周围神经、其他结缔组织、软组织	C47;C49	1	0.14	0.38	0.30	0.02	0.02	1	0.17	0.41	0.42	0.04	0.04
乳房	C50	—	—	—	—	—	—	67	11.63	27.28	22.82	1.70	2.44
外阴	C51	—	—	—	—	—	—	1	0.17	0.41	0.31	0.04	0.04
阴道	C52	—	—	—	—	—	—	0	0.00	0.00	0.00	0.00	0.00
子宫颈	C53	—	—	—	—	—	—	58	10.07	23.61	20.80	1.46	2.37
子宫体	C54	—	—	—	—	—	—	17	2.95	6.92	6.09	0.52	0.71
子宫，部位不明	C55	—	—	—	—	—	—	0	0.00	0.00	0.00	0.00	0.00
卵巢	C56	—	—	—	—	—	—	13	2.26	5.29	4.71	0.28	0.58
其他的女性生殖器	C57	—	—	—	—	—	—	2	0.35	0.81	0.62	0.07	0.07
胎盘	C58	—	—	—	—	—	—	0	0.00	0.00	0.00	0.00	0.00
阴茎	C60	3	0.43	1.14	1.07	0.05	0.12	—	—	—	—	—	—
前列腺	C61	9	1.28	3.41	3.20	0.06	0.41	—	—	—	—	—	—
睾丸	C62	1	0.14	0.38	0.31	0.03	0.03	—	—	—	—	—	—
其他的男性生殖器	C63	0	0.00	0.00	0.00	0.00	0.00	—	—	—	—	—	—
肾	C64	1	0.14	0.38	0.33	0.03	0.03	4	0.69	1.63	1.23	0.12	0.12
肾盂	C65	1	0.14	0.38	0.31	0.03	0.03	0	0.00	0.00	0.00	0.00	0.00
输尿管	C66	1	0.14	0.38	0.40	0.03	0.03	1	0.17	0.41	0.51	0.00	0.08
膀胱	C67	8	1.14	3.03	2.52	0.17	0.27	2	0.35	0.81	0.86	0.04	0.12
其他的泌尿器官	C68	0	0.00	0.00	0.00	0.00	0.00	0	0.00	0.00	0.00	0.00	0.00
眼	C69	1	0.14	0.38	0.29	0.02	0.02	1	0.17	0.41	0.57	0.02	0.02
脑、神经系统	C70–C72	15	2.14	5.68	5.30	0.28	0.54	24	4.17	9.77	8.71	0.72	0.89
甲状腺	C73	4	0.57	1.51	1.30	0.16	0.16	18	3.13	7.33	6.21	0.59	0.59
肾上腺	C74	0	0.00	0.00	0.00	0.00	0.00	0	0.00	0.00	0.00	0.00	0.00
其他的内分泌腺	C75	2	0.28	0.76	0.61	0.06	0.06	0	0.00	0.00	0.00	0.00	0.00
霍奇金病	C81	1	0.14	0.38	0.40	0.03	0.03	0	0.00	0.00	0.00	0.00	0.00
非霍奇金淋巴瘤	C82–C85;C96	6	0.85	2.27	2.09	0.10	0.30	7	1.22	2.85	2.26	0.17	0.28
免疫增生性疾病	C88	0	0.00	0.00	0.00	0.00	0.00	0	0.00	0.00	0.00	0.00	0.00
多发性骨髓瘤	C90	1	0.14	0.38	0.41	0.00	0.00	2	0.35	0.81	0.74	0.04	0.15
淋巴样白血病	C91	5	0.71	1.89	1.82	0.09	0.09	2	0.35	0.81	0.77	0.07	0.07
髓样白血病	C92–C94	5	0.71	1.89	1.71	0.12	0.12	4	0.69	1.63	1.37	0.02	0.11
白血病，未特指	C95	13	1.85	4.92	4.53	0.26	0.51	8	1.39	3.26	3.07	0.20	0.37
其他的或未指明部位的	O&U	8	1.14	3.03	2.61	0.09	0.37	8	1.39	3.26	2.11	0.17	0.17
骨髓增殖性疾病	MPD	1	0.14	0.38	0.31	0.03	0.03	2	0.35	0.81	0.71	0.08	0.08
骨髓增生异常综合征	MDS	0	0.00	0.00	0.00	0.00	0.00	0	0.00	0.00	0.00	0.00	0.00
合计	ALL	702	100.00	265.60	240.11	10.89	28.58	576	100.00	234.52	192.35	10.51	22.03
所有部位除外 C44	ALL but C44	701	99.86	265.22	239.74	10.85	28.53	568	98.61	231.26	190.10	10.41	21.85

表 6-2-14a 2014 年河南省三门峡市恶性肿瘤发病主要指标

部位		男性						女性					
		病例数	构成 (%)	粗率 ($1/10^5$)	世标率 ($1/10^5$)	累积率 (%) 0~64	累积率 (%) 0~74	病例数	构成 (%)	粗率 ($1/10^5$)	世标率 ($1/10^5$)	累积率 (%) 0~64	累积率 (%) 0~74
唇	C00	0	0.00	0.00	0.00	0.00	0.00	0	0.00	0.00	0.00	0.00	0.00
舌	C01–C02	1	0.23	0.68	0.53	0.04	0.04	1	0.26	0.68	0.23	0.00	0.00
口	C03–C06	2	0.46	1.37	1.11	0.00	0.23	3	0.79	2.05	1.10	0.09	0.09
唾液腺	C07–C08	1	0.23	0.68	0.40	0.04	0.04	1	0.26	0.68	0.42	0.04	0.04
扁桃体	C09	0	0.00	0.00	0.00	0.00	0.00	0	0.00	0.00	0.00	0.00	0.00
其他的口咽	C10	1	0.23	0.68	0.58	0.00	0.00	0	0.00	0.00	0.00	0.00	0.00
鼻咽	C11	3	0.68	2.05	1.51	0.10	0.19	1	0.26	0.68	0.25	0.00	0.00
喉咽	C12–C13	2	0.46	1.37	0.88	0.00	0.14	0	0.00	0.00	0.00	0.00	0.00
咽，部位不明	C14	0	0.00	0.00	0.00	0.00	0.00	0	0.00	0.00	0.00	0.00	0.00
食管	C15	26	5.94	17.78	11.31	0.60	1.20	15	3.95	10.24	6.79	0.26	0.93
胃	C16	53	12.10	36.25	24.65	0.89	2.93	16	4.21	10.92	6.06	0.26	0.56
小肠	C17	1	0.23	0.68	0.40	0.04	0.04	1	0.26	0.68	0.37	0.03	0.03
结肠	C18	13	2.97	8.89	5.25	0.22	0.63	9	2.37	6.14	3.45	0.19	0.28
直肠	C19–C20	28	6.39	19.15	12.27	0.56	1.35	22	5.79	15.02	9.69	0.46	1.27
肛门	C21	0	0.00	0.00	0.00	0.00	0.00	1	0.26	0.68	0.25	0.00	0.00
肝脏	C22	57	13.01	38.99	24.71	1.42	2.57	28	7.37	19.11	11.23	0.54	1.42
胆囊及其他	C23–C24	3	0.68	2.05	1.28	0.04	0.18	7	1.84	4.78	2.54	0.11	0.20
胰腺	C25	12	2.74	8.21	5.29	0.27	0.64	12	3.16	8.19	5.26	0.15	0.72
鼻、鼻窦及其他	C30–C31	0	0.00	0.00	0.00	0.00	0.00	0	0.00	0.00	0.00	0.00	0.00
喉	C32	6	1.37	4.10	3.03	0.09	0.55	1	0.26	0.68	0.56	0.07	0.07
气管、支气管、肺	C33–C34	120	27.40	82.08	52.40	2.09	5.79	57	15.00	38.91	22.85	1.30	2.54
其他的胸腔器官	C37–C38	1	0.23	0.68	0.58	0.00	0.00	2	0.53	1.37	0.79	0.07	0.07
骨	C40–C41	5	1.14	3.42	2.59	0.00	0.33	3	0.79	2.05	1.39	0.15	0.15
皮肤的黑色素瘤	C43	0	0.00	0.00	0.00	0.00	0.00	0	0.00	0.00	0.00	0.00	0.00
其他的皮肤	C44	8	1.83	5.47	3.68	0.15	0.38	4	1.05	2.73	1.46	0.11	0.11
间皮瘤	C45	0	0.00	0.00	0.00	0.00	0.00	0	0.00	0.00	0.00	0.00	0.00
卡波西肉瘤	C46	0	0.00	0.00	0.00	0.00	0.00	0	0.00	0.00	0.00	0.00	0.00
周围神经、其他结缔组织、软组织	C47;C49	1	0.23	0.68	0.55	0.07	0.07	1	0.26	0.68	0.42	0.04	0.04
乳房	C50	—	—	—	—	—	—	68	17.89	46.42	29.38	2.30	3.01
外阴	C51	—	—	—	—	—	—	1	0.26	0.68	0.42	0.03	0.03
阴道	C52	—	—	—	—	—	—	0	0.00	0.00	0.00	0.00	0.00
子宫颈	C53	—	—	—	—	—	—	29	7.63	19.80	13.19	1.11	1.32
子宫体	C54	—	—	—	—	—	—	14	3.68	9.56	6.19	0.46	0.79
子宫，部位不明	C55	—	—	—	—	—	—	6	1.58	4.10	2.69	0.32	0.32
卵巢	C56	—	—	—	—	—	—	10	2.63	6.83	4.57	0.39	0.48
其他的女性生殖器	C57	—	—	—	—	—	—	1	0.26	0.68	0.42	0.04	0.04
胎盘	C58	—	—	—	—	—	—	0	0.00	0.00	0.00	0.00	0.00
阴茎	C60	0	0.00	0.00	0.00	0.00	0.00	—	—	—	—	—	—
前列腺	C61	22	5.02	15.05	9.43	0.14	0.65	—	—	—	—	—	—
睾丸	C62	1	0.23	0.68	0.62	0.04	0.04	—	—	—	—	—	—
其他的男性生殖器	C63	0	0.00	0.00	0.00	0.00	0.00	—	—	—	—	—	—
肾	C64	9	2.05	6.16	4.89	0.21	0.44	2	0.53	1.37	0.99	0.05	0.15
肾盂	C65	0	0.00	0.00	0.00	0.00	0.00	0	0.00	0.00	0.00	0.00	0.00
输尿管	C66	0	0.00	0.00	0.00	0.00	0.00	0	0.00	0.00	0.00	0.00	0.00
膀胱	C67	10	2.28	6.84	4.48	0.26	0.36	4	1.05	2.73	1.62	0.04	0.16
其他的泌尿器官	C68	2	0.46	1.37	0.97	0.04	0.13	1	0.26	0.68	0.56	0.07	0.07
眼	C69	0	0.00	0.00	0.00	0.00	0.00	0	0.00	0.00	0.00	0.00	0.00
脑、神经系统	C70–C72	4	0.91	2.74	1.75	0.17	0.17	9	2.37	6.14	4.17	0.16	0.58
甲状腺	C73	14	3.20	9.58	5.97	0.54	0.68	28	7.37	19.11	13.83	1.09	1.40
肾上腺	C74	0	0.00	0.00	0.00	0.00	0.00	0	0.00	0.00	0.00	0.00	0.00
其他的内分泌腺	C75	0	0.00	0.00	0.00	0.00	0.00	0	0.00	0.00	0.00	0.00	0.00
霍奇金病	C81	0	0.00	0.00	0.00	0.00	0.00	0	0.00	0.00	0.00	0.00	0.00
非霍奇金淋巴瘤	C82–C85;C96	6	1.37	4.10	2.45	0.16	0.30	4	1.05	2.73	1.92	0.12	0.24
免疫增生性疾病	C88	0	0.00	0.00	0.00	0.00	0.00	0	0.00	0.00	0.00	0.00	0.00
多发性骨髓瘤	C90	3	0.68	2.05	1.28	0.03	0.17	1	0.26	0.68	0.56	0.07	0.07
淋巴样白血病	C91	2	0.46	1.37	2.83	0.13	0.13	1	0.26	0.68	0.56	0.00	0.09
髓样白血病	C92–C94	10	2.28	6.84	4.76	0.33	0.52	5	1.32	3.41	2.21	0.15	0.15
白血病，未特指	C95	3	0.68	2.05	1.81	0.06	0.19	4	1.05	2.73	3.80	0.21	0.21
其他的或未指明部位的	O&U	6	1.37	4.10	2.65	0.07	0.30	7	1.84	4.78	3.03	0.27	0.27
骨髓增殖性疾病	MPD	0	0.00	0.00	0.00	0.00	0.00	0	0.00	0.00	0.00	0.00	0.00
骨髓增生异常综合征	MDS	1	0.23	0.68	0.41	0.05	0.05	0	0.00	0.00	0.00	0.00	0.00
合计	ALL	438	100.00	299.59	197.67	8.89	21.47	380	100.00	259.41	165.21	10.78	17.93
所有部位除外 C44	ALL but C44	430	98.17	294.12	193.99	8.74	21.08	376	98.95	256.68	163.75	10.67	17.82

表 6-2-15a 2014 年河南省沈丘县恶性肿瘤发病主要指标

部位		男性						女性					
		病例数	构成 (%)	粗率 (1/10⁵)	世标率 (1/10⁵)	累积率 (%) 0~64	累积率 (%) 0~74	病例数	构成 (%)	粗率 (1/10⁵)	世标率 (1/10⁵)	累积率 (%) 0~64	累积率 (%) 0~74
唇	C00	1	0.06	0.17	0.19	0.02	0.02	1	0.07	0.17	0.19	0.02	0.02
舌	C01-C02	1	0.06	0.17	0.08	0.00	0.00	2	0.14	0.34	0.33	0.03	0.03
口	C03-C06	2	0.11	0.34	0.32	0.02	0.05	1	0.07	0.17	0.07	0.00	0.00
唾液腺	C07-C08	0	0.00	0.00	0.00	0.00	0.00	2	0.14	0.34	0.39	0.05	0.05
扁桃体	C09	0	0.00	0.00	0.00	0.00	0.00	1	0.07	0.17	0.12	0.00	0.03
其他的口咽	C10	3	0.17	0.50	0.38	0.01	0.06	1	0.07	0.17	0.19	0.02	0.02
鼻咽	C11	13	0.74	2.18	1.83	0.17	0.20	3	0.21	0.52	0.40	0.04	0.04
喉咽	C12-C13	2	0.11	0.34	0.35	0.03	0.03	0	0.00	0.00	0.00	0.00	0.00
咽，部位不明	C14	2	0.11	0.34	0.31	0.02	0.05	0	0.00	0.00	0.00	0.00	0.00
食管	C15	181	10.30	30.33	25.85	1.62	3.25	136	9.45	23.41	17.78	0.90	2.16
胃	C16	211	12.00	35.36	30.07	1.74	3.71	111	7.71	19.11	14.34	0.78	1.66
小肠	C17	8	0.46	1.34	1.08	0.08	0.11	1	0.07	0.17	0.12	0.00	0.03
结肠	C18	25	1.42	4.19	3.35	0.24	0.29	33	2.29	5.68	4.36	0.24	0.52
直肠	C19-C20	78	4.44	13.07	11.45	0.83	1.35	71	4.93	12.22	9.36	0.68	0.98
肛门	C21	0	0.00	0.00	0.00	0.00	0.00	0	0.00	0.00	0.00	0.00	0.00
肝脏	C22	357	20.31	59.82	52.70	3.69	6.37	143	9.94	24.62	19.46	1.27	2.22
胆囊及其他	C23-C24	12	0.68	2.01	2.07	0.16	0.26	22	1.53	3.79	2.62	0.07	0.33
胰腺	C25	26	1.48	4.36	3.84	0.22	0.54	16	1.11	2.75	2.26	0.15	0.31
鼻、鼻窦及其他	C30-C31	1	0.06	0.17	0.15	0.00	0.02	2	0.14	0.34	0.31	0.01	0.01
喉	C32	18	1.02	3.02	2.52	0.18	0.28	5	0.35	0.86	0.61	0.03	0.08
气管、支气管、肺	C33-C34	561	31.91	94.00	79.52	4.48	9.69	286	19.87	49.23	38.22	2.42	4.53
其他的胸腔器官	C37-C38	1	0.06	0.17	0.12	0.01	0.01	4	0.28	0.69	0.65	0.07	0.07
骨	C40-C41	29	1.65	4.86	4.76	0.37	0.50	19	1.32	3.27	3.03	0.23	0.26
皮肤的黑色素瘤	C43	2	0.11	0.34	0.28	0.01	0.01	2	0.14	0.34	0.20	0.00	0.03
其他的皮肤	C44	8	0.46	1.34	0.99	0.06	0.12	8	0.56	1.38	1.08	0.07	0.10
间皮瘤	C45	0	0.00	0.00	0.00	0.00	0.00	0	0.00	0.00	0.00	0.00	0.00
卡波西肉瘤	C46	0	0.00	0.00	0.00	0.00	0.00	0	0.00	0.00	0.00	0.00	0.00
周围神经、其他结缔组织、软组织	C47;C49	2	0.11	0.34	0.29	0.02	0.02	0	0.00	0.00	0.00	0.00	0.00
乳房	C50	—	—	—	—	—	—	197	13.69	33.91	30.26	2.59	3.25
外阴	C51	—	—	—	—	—	—	1	0.07	0.17	0.15	0.00	0.02
阴道	C52	—	—	—	—	—	—	0	0.00	0.00	0.00	0.00	0.00
子宫颈	C53	—	—	—	—	—	—	105	7.30	18.07	15.47	1.25	1.78
子宫体	C54	—	—	—	—	—	—	16	1.11	2.75	2.55	0.20	0.30
子宫，部位不明	C55	—	—	—	—	—	—	0	0.00	0.00	0.00	0.00	0.00
卵巢	C56	—	—	—	—	—	—	35	2.43	6.02	5.58	0.49	0.61
其他的女性生殖器	C57	—	—	—	—	—	—	0	0.00	0.00	0.00	0.00	0.00
胎盘	C58	—	—	—	—	—	—	0	0.00	0.00	0.00	0.00	0.00
阴茎	C60	4	0.23	0.67	0.54	0.05	0.05	—	—	—	—	—	—
前列腺	C61	11	0.63	1.84	1.31	0.02	0.14	—	—	—	—	—	—
睾丸	C62	3	0.17	0.50	0.56	0.04	0.04	—	—	—	—	—	—
其他的男性生殖器	C63	1	0.06	0.17	0.15	0.02	0.02	—	—	—	—	—	—
肾	C64	13	0.74	2.18	2.10	0.19	0.27	7	0.49	1.20	1.08	0.10	0.13
肾盂	C65	0	0.00	0.00	0.00	0.00	0.00	0	0.00	0.00	0.00	0.00	0.00
输尿管	C66	1	0.06	0.17	0.19	0.02	0.02	0	0.00	0.00	0.00	0.00	0.00
膀胱	C67	36	2.05	6.03	5.27	0.19	0.65	12	0.83	2.07	1.41	0.04	0.17
其他的泌尿器官	C68	0	0.00	0.00	0.00	0.00	0.00	0	0.00	0.00	0.00	0.00	0.00
眼	C69	4	0.23	0.67	0.72	0.05	0.05	0	0.00	0.00	0.00	0.00	0.00
脑、神经系统	C70-C72	71	4.04	11.90	10.84	0.78	1.19	87	6.05	14.98	13.74	1.08	1.51
甲状腺	C73	7	0.40	1.17	1.06	0.09	0.12	30	2.08	5.16	4.30	0.35	0.43
肾上腺	C74	1	0.06	0.17	0.19	0.02	0.02	0	0.00	0.00	0.00	0.00	0.00
其他的内分泌腺	C75	1	0.06	0.17	0.19	0.02	0.02	2	0.14	0.34	0.27	0.02	0.02
霍奇金病	C81	7	0.40	1.17	0.90	0.05	0.08	15	1.04	2.58	2.56	0.22	0.27
非霍奇金淋巴瘤	C82-C85;C96	15	0.85	2.51	2.22	0.14	0.28	19	1.32	3.27	2.75	0.17	0.30
免疫增生性疾病	C88	0	0.00	0.00	0.00	0.00	0.00	0	0.00	0.00	0.00	0.00	0.00
多发性骨髓瘤	C90	0	0.00	0.00	0.00	0.00	0.00	1	0.07	0.17	0.13	0.01	0.01
淋巴样白血病	C91	1	0.06	0.17	0.25	0.01	0.01	3	0.21	0.52	0.79	0.04	0.04
髓样白血病	C92-C94	1	0.06	0.17	0.19	0.02	0.02	0	0.00	0.00	0.00	0.00	0.00
白血病，未特指	C95	37	2.10	6.20	6.04	0.36	0.47	39	2.71	6.71	7.06	0.43	0.60
其他的或未指明部位的	O&U	0	0.00	0.00	0.00	0.00	0.00	0	0.00	0.00	0.00	0.00	0.00
骨髓增殖性疾病	MPD	0	0.00	0.00	0.00	0.00	0.00	0	0.00	0.00	0.00	0.00	0.00
骨髓增生异常综合征	MDS	0	0.00	0.00	0.00	0.00	0.00	0	0.00	0.00	0.00	0.00	0.00
合计	ALL	1 758	100.00	294.57	255.23	16.07	30.42	1439	100.00	247.71	204.18	14.06	22.94
所有部位除外 C44	ALL but C44	1 750	99.54	293.23	254.24	16.01	30.30	1431	99.44	246.33	203.10	13.99	22.85

表 6-2-16a　2014 年河南省西平县恶性肿瘤发病主要指标

部位		男性						女性					
		病例数	构成 (%)	粗率 ($1/10^5$)	世标率 ($1/10^5$)	累积率 (%) 0~64	累积率 (%) 0~74	病例数	构成 (%)	粗率 ($1/10^5$)	世标率 ($1/10^5$)	累积率 (%) 0~64	累积率 (%) 0~74
唇	C00	0	0.00	0.00	0.00	0.00	0.00	0	0.00	0.00	0.00	0.00	0.00
舌	C01–C02	2	0.19	0.44	0.29	0.00	0.04	1	0.11	0.24	0.18	0.01	0.01
口	C03–C06	4	0.38	0.89	0.57	0.03	0.03	1	0.11	0.24	0.16	0.01	0.01
唾液腺	C07–C08	3	0.29	0.67	0.53	0.03	0.06	4	0.43	0.94	0.75	0.06	0.09
扁桃体	C09	1	0.10	0.22	0.13	0.00	0.00	0	0.00	0.00	0.00	0.00	0.00
其他的口咽	C10	0	0.00	0.00	0.00	0.00	0.00	0	0.00	0.00	0.00	0.00	0.00
鼻咽	C11	8	0.77	1.78	1.29	0.09	0.13	4	0.43	0.94	0.66	0.05	0.09
喉咽	C12–C13	2	0.19	0.44	0.29	0.02	0.02	0	0.00	0.00	0.00	0.00	0.00
咽，部位不明	C14	0	0.00	0.00	0.00	0.00	0.00	0	0.00	0.00	0.00	0.00	0.00
食管	C15	141	13.52	31.34	25.63	1.05	2.54	87	9.38	20.48	13.20	0.38	1.67
胃	C16	112	10.74	24.89	19.66	0.87	2.02	55	5.93	12.94	8.23	0.38	0.80
小肠	C17	4	0.38	0.89	0.73	0.04	0.12	6	0.65	1.41	0.92	0.05	0.09
结肠	C18	37	3.55	8.22	6.15	0.46	0.64	26	2.80	6.12	4.39	0.33	0.54
直肠	C19–C20	35	3.36	7.78	5.94	0.33	0.81	36	3.88	8.47	5.66	0.28	0.66
肛门	C21	0	0.00	0.00	0.00	0.00	0.00	0	0.00	0.00	0.00	0.00	0.00
肝脏	C22	159	15.24	35.34	27.16	1.84	2.91	76	8.19	17.89	11.57	0.64	1.26
胆囊及其他	C23–C24	19	1.82	4.22	3.21	0.14	0.33	31	3.34	7.30	5.08	0.25	0.52
胰腺	C25	19	1.82	4.22	3.42	0.12	0.37	14	1.51	3.30	2.37	0.16	0.27
鼻、鼻窦及其他	C30–C31	4	0.38	0.89	0.65	0.04	0.08	2	0.22	0.47	0.27	0.02	0.02
喉	C32	13	1.25	2.89	2.40	0.20	0.20	0	0.00	0.00	0.00	0.00	0.00
气管、支气管、肺	C33–C34	289	27.71	64.23	50.77	2.15	5.66	125	13.47	29.42	18.83	1.05	1.86
其他的胸腔器官	C37–C38	5	0.48	1.11	0.90	0.05	0.13	4	0.43	0.94	1.15	0.06	0.09
骨	C40–C41	9	0.86	2.00	1.72	0.07	0.16	11	1.19	2.59	1.86	0.12	0.23
皮肤的黑色素瘤	C43	2	0.19	0.44	0.50	0.04	0.04	1	0.11	0.24	0.16	0.00	0.04
其他的皮肤	C44	7	0.67	1.56	1.43	0.06	0.19	6	0.65	1.41	0.76	0.03	0.07
间皮瘤	C45	0	0.00	0.00	0.00	0.00	0.00	0	0.00	0.00	0.00	0.00	0.00
卡波西肉瘤	C46	0	0.00	0.00	0.00	0.00	0.00	0	0.00	0.00	0.00	0.00	0.00
周围神经、其他结缔组织、软组织	C47;C49	4	0.38	0.89	0.88	0.03	0.06	4	0.43	0.94	0.77	0.06	0.10
乳房	C50	—	—	—	—	—	—	164	17.67	38.60	28.16	2.56	2.90
外阴	C51	—	—	—	—	—	—	3	0.32	0.71	0.53	0.04	0.07
阴道	C52	—	—	—	—	—	—	1	0.11	0.24	0.17	0.02	0.02
子宫颈	C53	—	—	—	—	—	—	65	7.00	15.30	11.38	0.95	1.22
子宫体	C54	—	—	—	—	—	—	23	2.48	5.41	4.01	0.37	0.47
子宫，部位不明	C55	—	—	—	—	—	—	8	0.86	1.88	1.46	0.13	0.16
卵巢	C56	—	—	—	—	—	—	32	3.45	7.53	6.22	0.47	0.63
其他的女性生殖器	C57	—	—	—	—	—	—	1	0.11	0.24	0.17	0.02	0.02
胎盘	C58	—	—	—	—	—	—	5	0.54	1.18	1.00	0.07	0.07
阴茎	C60	1	0.10	0.22	0.20	0.03	0.03	—	—	—	—	—	—
前列腺	C61	18	1.73	4.00	3.33	0.12	0.32	—	—	—	—	—	—
睾丸	C62	0	0.00	0.00	0.00	0.00	0.00	—	—	—	—	—	—
其他的男性生殖器	C63	1	0.10	0.22	0.22	0.01	0.01	—	—	—	—	—	—
肾	C64	6	0.58	1.33	1.40	0.06	0.14	4	0.43	0.94	0.60	0.03	0.07
肾盂	C65	1	0.10	0.22	0.17	0.02	0.02	2	0.22	0.47	0.37	0.05	0.05
输尿管	C66	2	0.19	0.44	0.36	0.04	0.04	0	0.00	0.00	0.00	0.00	0.00
膀胱	C67	17	1.63	3.78	2.68	0.09	0.33	7	0.75	1.65	0.84	0.05	0.05
其他的泌尿器官	C68	0	0.00	0.00	0.00	0.00	0.00	1	0.11	0.24	0.08	0.00	0.00
眼	C69	0	0.00	0.00	0.00	0.00	0.00	1	0.11	0.24	0.10	0.00	0.00
脑、神经系统	C70–C72	32	3.07	7.11	7.41	0.42	0.56	28	3.02	6.59	5.17	0.39	0.53
甲状腺	C73	2	0.19	0.44	0.37	0.03	0.03	25	2.69	5.88	4.57	0.32	0.38
肾上腺	C74	1	0.10	0.22	0.20	0.03	0.03	0	0.00	0.00	0.00	0.00	0.00
其他的内分泌腺	C75	0	0.00	0.00	0.00	0.00	0.00	3	0.32	0.71	0.66	0.07	0.07
霍奇金病	C81	2	0.19	0.44	0.31	0.03	0.03	3	0.32	0.71	0.49	0.04	0.08
非霍奇金淋巴瘤	C82–C85;C96	29	2.78	6.45	5.42	0.37	0.60	14	1.51	3.30	2.46	0.22	0.29
免疫增生性疾病	C88	0	0.00	0.00	0.00	0.00	0.00	0	0.00	0.00	0.00	0.00	0.00
多发性骨髓瘤	C90	12	1.15	2.67	1.98	0.19	0.19	3	0.32	0.71	0.43	0.02	0.06
淋巴样白血病	C91	6	0.58	1.33	1.37	0.11	0.11	7	0.75	1.65	1.91	0.11	0.14
髓样白血病	C92–C94	17	1.63	3.78	3.35	0.22	0.26	9	0.97	2.12	1.34	0.03	0.12
白血病，未特指	C95	5	0.48	1.11	0.99	0.05	0.14	9	0.97	2.12	1.71	0.10	0.13
其他的或未指明部位的	O&U	12	1.15	2.67	2.57	0.17	0.21	13	1.40	3.06	2.66	0.21	0.25
骨髓增殖性疾病	MPD	0	0.00	0.00	0.00	0.00	0.00	1	0.11	0.24	0.19	0.00	0.03
骨髓增生异常综合征	MDS	0	0.00	0.00	0.00	0.00	0.00	2	0.22	0.47	0.42	0.03	0.03
合计	ALL	1 043	100.00	231.81	186.58	9.65	19.57	928	100.00	218.42	154.05	10.22	16.28
所有部位除外 C44	ALL but C44	1 036	99.33	230.25	185.16	9.59	19.38	922	99.35	217.00	153.29	10.20	16.21

表 6-2-17a　2014 年河南省开封市祥符区恶性肿瘤发病主要指标

部位		男性						女性					
		病例数	构成 (%)	粗率 ($1/10^5$)	世标率 ($1/10^5$)	累积率 (%) 0~64	累积率 (%) 0~74	病例数	构成 (%)	粗率 ($1/10^5$)	世标率 ($1/10^5$)	累积率 (%) 0~64	累积率 (%) 0~74
唇	C00	2	0.23	0.56	0.61	0.00	0.13	1	0.13	0.29	0.15	0.00	0.00
舌	C01–C02	2	0.23	0.56	0.41	0.03	0.03	1	0.13	0.29	0.25	0.03	0.03
口	C03–C06	5	0.58	1.40	1.18	0.10	0.10	7	0.91	2.02	1.48	0.10	0.10
唾液腺	C07–C08	2	0.23	0.56	0.54	0.06	0.06	3	0.39	0.87	0.68	0.07	0.07
扁桃体	C09	0	0.00	0.00	0.00	0.00	0.00	0	0.00	0.00	0.00	0.00	0.00
其他的口咽	C10	4	0.47	1.12	1.02	0.10	0.10	1	0.13	0.29	0.31	0.02	0.02
鼻咽	C11	9	1.05	2.52	2.14	0.18	0.18	4	0.52	1.15	0.97	0.08	0.08
喉咽	C12–C13	3	0.35	0.84	0.85	0.06	0.11	0	0.00	0.00	0.00	0.00	0.00
咽，部位不明	C14	0	0.00	0.00	0.00	0.00	0.00	0	0.00	0.00	0.00	0.00	0.00
食管	C15	84	9.78	23.50	21.05	0.66	2.49	31	4.01	8.95	6.83	0.14	1.04
胃	C16	95	11.06	26.58	23.00	1.60	2.75	46	5.95	13.28	10.09	0.44	1.46
小肠	C17	56	6.52	15.67	14.31	0.70	1.79	26	3.36	7.50	6.26	0.39	0.87
结肠	C18	27	3.14	7.55	6.88	0.50	0.76	17	2.20	4.91	3.75	0.25	0.44
直肠	C19–C20	38	4.42	10.63	9.28	0.40	1.14	20	2.59	5.77	4.23	0.23	0.48
肛门	C21	5	0.58	1.40	1.11	0.05	0.10	7	0.91	2.02	1.75	0.12	0.17
肝脏	C22	113	13.15	31.61	28.76	2.15	3.53	44	5.69	12.70	10.10	0.65	1.32
胆囊及其他	C23–C24	16	1.86	4.48	4.14	0.18	0.53	15	1.94	4.33	3.36	0.23	0.42
胰腺	C25	17	1.98	4.76	4.47	0.21	0.61	14	1.81	4.04	3.05	0.26	0.26
鼻、鼻窦及其他	C30–C31	2	0.23	0.56	0.59	0.05	0.05	3	0.39	0.87	0.64	0.02	0.07
喉	C32	14	1.63	3.92	3.17	0.26	0.31	1	0.13	0.29	0.17	0.02	0.02
气管、支气管、肺	C33–C34	218	25.38	60.98	55.15	2.34	6.74	110	14.23	31.75	24.21	1.25	3.13
其他的胸腔器官	C37–C38	4	0.47	1.12	1.11	0.10	0.10	0	0.00	0.00	0.00	0.00	0.00
骨	C40–C41	15	1.75	4.20	4.08	0.26	0.39	11	1.42	3.18	2.65	0.14	0.31
皮肤的黑色素瘤	C43	3	0.35	0.84	0.94	0.01	0.17	7	0.91	2.02	1.80	0.06	0.11
其他的皮肤	C44	8	0.93	2.24	2.14	0.09	0.21	10	1.29	2.89	2.47	0.08	0.20
间皮瘤	C45	0	0.00	0.00	0.00	0.00	0.00	0	0.00	0.00	0.00	0.00	0.00
卡波西肉瘤	C46	0	0.00	0.00	0.00	0.00	0.00	0	0.00	0.00	0.00	0.00	0.00
周围神经、其他结缔组织、软组织	C47;C49	3	0.35	0.84	0.71	0.05	0.05	6	0.78	1.73	1.70	0.11	0.18
乳房	C50	—	—	—	—	—	—	158	20.44	45.61	37.80	3.30	3.57
外阴	C51	—	—	—	—	—	—	1	0.13	0.29	0.25	0.02	0.02
阴道	C52	—	—	—	—	—	—	0	0.00	0.00	0.00	0.00	0.00
子宫颈	C53	—	—	—	—	—	—	47	6.08	13.57	10.72	0.79	1.13
子宫体	C54	—	—	—	—	—	—	25	3.23	7.22	5.91	0.51	0.56
子宫，部位不明	C55	—	—	—	—	—	—	2	0.26	0.58	0.56	0.02	0.07
卵巢	C56	—	—	—	—	—	—	34	4.40	9.81	9.02	0.54	0.98
其他的女性生殖器	C57	—	—	—	—	—	—	4	0.52	1.15	0.92	0.07	0.07
胎盘	C58	—	—	—	—	—	—	0	0.00	0.00	0.00	0.00	0.00
阴茎	C60	0	0.00	0.00	0.00	0.00	0.00	—	—	—	—	—	—
前列腺	C61	2	0.23	0.56	0.46	0.02	0.02	—	—	—	—	—	—
睾丸	C62	2	0.23	0.56	0.68	0.05	0.05	—	—	—	—	—	—
其他的男性生殖器	C63	0	0.00	0.00	0.00	0.00	0.00	—	—	—	—	—	—
肾	C64	2	0.23	0.56	0.60	0.04	0.04	2	0.26	0.58	0.72	0.02	0.07
肾盂	C65	3	0.35	0.84	0.70	0.06	0.06	4	0.52	1.15	0.82	0.07	0.07
输尿管	C66	0	0.00	0.00	0.00	0.00	0.00	0	0.00	0.00	0.00	0.00	0.00
膀胱	C67	25	2.91	6.99	6.10	0.20	0.68	5	0.65	1.44	1.22	0.05	0.19
其他的泌尿器官	C68	1	0.12	0.28	0.25	0.03	0.03	1	0.13	0.29	0.21	0.01	0.01
眼	C69	1	0.12	0.28	0.25	0.02	0.02	0	0.00	0.00	0.00	0.00	0.00
脑、神经系统	C70–C72	20	2.33	5.59	5.24	0.24	0.47	14	1.81	4.04	3.64	0.31	0.38
甲状腺	C73	10	1.16	2.80	2.74	0.17	0.38	47	6.08	13.57	11.55	0.92	1.23
肾上腺	C74	2	0.23	0.56	0.51	0.06	0.06	0	0.00	0.00	0.00	0.00	0.00
其他的内分泌腺	C75	3	0.35	0.84	0.51	0.02	0.02	5	0.65	1.44	1.32	0.12	0.12
霍奇金病	C81	0	0.00	0.00	0.00	0.00	0.00	0	0.00	0.00	0.00	0.00	0.00
非霍奇金淋巴瘤	C82–C85;C96	9	1.05	2.52	2.20	0.12	0.20	6	0.78	1.73	1.71	0.10	0.22
免疫增生性疾病	C88	0	0.00	0.00	0.00	0.00	0.00	0	0.00	0.00	0.00	0.00	0.00
多发性骨髓瘤	C90	5	0.58	1.40	1.10	0.07	0.15	2	0.26	0.58	0.38	0.00	0.07
淋巴样白血病	C91	9	1.05	2.52	2.78	0.15	0.23	16	2.07	4.62	4.00	0.29	0.39
髓样白血病	C92–C94	6	0.70	1.68	1.82	0.11	0.16	7	0.91	2.02	1.71	0.11	0.18
白血病，未特指	C95	9	1.05	2.52	2.44	0.12	0.27	3	0.39	0.87	0.89	0.02	0.14
其他的或未指明部位的	O&U	1	0.12	0.28	0.31	0.00	0.08	3	0.39	0.87	0.72	0.02	0.16
骨髓增殖性疾病	MPD	1	0.12	0.28	0.29	0.02	0.02	0	0.00	0.00	0.00	0.00	0.00
骨髓增生异常综合征	MDS	0	0.00	0.00	0.00	0.00	0.00	2	0.26	0.58	0.52	0.04	0.04
合计	ALL	859	100.00	240.30	217.49	11.67	25.49	773	100.00	223.13	181.48	12.04	20.57
所有部位除外 C44	ALLL but C44	851	99.07	238.06	215.36	11.58	25.28	763	98.71	220.24	179.01	11.96	20.36

表 6-2-18a　2014 年河南省新安县恶性肿瘤发病主要指标

部位		男性						女性					
		病例数	构成 (%)	粗率 (1/10^5)	世标率 (1/10^5)	累积率 (%) 0~64	累积率 (%) 0~74	病例数	构成 (%)	粗率 (1/10^5)	世标率 (1/10^5)	累积率 (%) 0~64	累积率 (%) 0~74
唇	C00	0	0.00	0.00	0.00	0.00	0.00	0	0.00	0.00	0.00	0.00	0.00
舌	C01–C02	0	0.00	0.00	0.00	0.00	0.00	2	0.40	0.77	0.54	0.00	0.06
口	C03–C06	0	0.00	0.00	0.00	0.00	0.00	0	0.00	0.00	0.00	0.00	0.00
唾液腺	C07–C08	0	0.00	0.00	0.00	0.00	0.00	0	0.00	0.00	0.00	0.00	0.00
扁桃体	C09	0	0.00	0.00	0.00	0.00	0.00	0	0.00	0.00	0.00	0.00	0.00
其他的口咽	C10	1	0.14	0.36	0.33	0.00	0.05	0	0.00	0.00	0.00	0.00	0.00
鼻咽	C11	4	0.57	1.45	1.12	0.09	0.09	2	0.40	0.77	0.27	0.00	0.00
喉咽	C12–C13	0	0.00	0.00	0.00	0.00	0.00	0	0.00	0.00	0.00	0.00	0.00
咽，部位不明	C14	1	0.14	0.36	0.33	0.03	0.03	0	0.00	0.00	0.00	0.00	0.00
食管	C15	108	15.47	39.20	28.48	1.14	3.67	54	10.76	20.87	14.91	0.64	1.87
胃	C16	158	22.64	57.35	43.18	2.06	5.70	78	15.54	30.14	21.40	0.92	2.73
小肠	C17	2	0.29	0.73	0.59	0.03	0.09	1	0.20	0.39	0.14	0.00	0.00
结肠	C18	12	1.72	4.36	3.16	0.25	0.39	9	1.79	3.48	2.51	0.14	0.28
直肠	C19–C20	32	4.58	11.62	8.88	0.49	1.15	25	4.98	9.66	7.24	0.43	0.92
肛门	C21	1	0.14	0.36	0.26	0.03	0.03	0	0.00	0.00	0.00	0.00	0.00
肝脏	C22	102	14.61	37.02	27.64	1.65	3.35	67	13.35	25.89	19.07	0.90	2.33
胆囊及其他	C23–C24	4	0.57	1.45	1.16	0.03	0.16	18	3.59	6.96	4.47	0.16	0.59
胰腺	C25	11	1.58	3.99	2.65	0.17	0.30	9	1.79	3.48	2.43	0.18	0.26
鼻、鼻窦及其他	C30–C31	1	0.14	0.36	0.33	0.03	0.03	0	0.00	0.00	0.00	0.00	0.00
喉	C32	7	1.00	2.54	2.11	0.07	0.29	0	0.00	0.00	0.00	0.00	0.00
气管、支气管、肺	C33–C34	167	23.93	60.62	44.02	2.18	4.86	79	15.74	30.53	20.26	1.12	2.31
其他的胸腔器官	C37–C38	0	0.00	0.00	0.00	0.00	0.00	1	0.20	0.39	0.33	0.03	0.03
骨	C40–C41	7	1.00	2.54	2.16	0.15	0.27	3	0.60	1.16	0.95	0.08	0.16
皮肤的黑色素瘤	C43	0	0.00	0.00	0.00	0.00	0.00	0	0.00	0.00	0.00	0.00	0.00
其他的皮肤	C44	2	0.29	0.73	0.41	0.00	0.07	2	0.40	0.77	0.54	0.05	0.05
间皮瘤	C45	0	0.00	0.00	0.00	0.00	0.00	0	0.00	0.00	0.00	0.00	0.00
卡波西肉瘤	C46	0	0.00	0.00	0.00	0.00	0.00	0	0.00	0.00	0.00	0.00	0.00
周围神经、其他结缔组织、软组织	C47;C49	0	0.00	0.00	0.00	0.00	0.00	0	0.00	0.00	0.00	0.00	0.00
乳房	C50	—	—	—	—	—	—	43	8.57	16.62	13.39	1.09	1.43
外阴	C51	—	—	—	—	—	—	1	0.20	0.39	0.37	0.05	0.05
阴道	C52	—	—	—	—	—	—	1	0.20	0.39	0.28	0.03	0.03
子宫颈	C53	—	—	—	—	—	—	31	6.18	11.98	9.71	0.69	1.09
子宫体	C54	—	—	—	—	—	—	11	2.19	4.25	3.47	0.38	0.38
子宫，部位不明	C55	—	—	—	—	—	—	18	3.59	6.96	4.49	0.27	0.41
卵巢	C56	—	—	—	—	—	—	7	1.39	2.70	2.05	0.20	0.27
其他的女性生殖器	C57	—	—	—	—	—	—	0	0.00	0.00	0.00	0.00	0.00
胎盘	C58	—	—	—	—	—	—	0	0.00	0.00	0.00	0.00	0.00
阴茎	C60	2	0.29	0.73	0.63	0.04	0.09	—	—	—	—	—	—
前列腺	C61	14	2.01	5.08	3.34	0.07	0.32	—	—	—	—	—	—
睾丸	C62	1	0.14	0.36	0.27	0.00	0.07	—	—	—	—	—	—
其他的男性生殖器	C63	0	0.00	0.00	0.00	0.00	0.00	—	—	—	—	—	—
肾	C64	9	1.29	3.27	2.45	0.11	0.37	8	1.59	3.09	1.93	0.13	0.13
肾盂	C65	1	0.14	0.36	0.17	0.00	0.00	2	0.40	0.77	0.54	0.05	0.05
输尿管	C66	0	0.00	0.00	0.00	0.00	0.00	0	0.00	0.00	0.00	0.00	0.00
膀胱	C67	6	0.86	2.18	1.80	0.13	0.27	2	0.40	0.77	0.59	0.03	0.11
其他的泌尿器官	C68	0	0.00	0.00	0.00	0.00	0.00	0	0.00	0.00	0.00	0.00	0.00
眼	C69	0	0.00	0.00	0.00	0.00	0.00	0	0.00	0.00	0.00	0.00	0.00
脑、神经系统	C70–C72	15	2.15	5.44	4.10	0.23	0.42	15	2.99	5.80	4.43	0.23	0.50
甲状腺	C73	6	0.86	2.18	1.65	0.15	0.15	1	0.20	0.39	0.17	0.00	0.00
肾上腺	C74	0	0.00	0.00	0.00	0.00	0.00	0	0.00	0.00	0.00	0.00	0.00
其他的内分泌腺	C75	0	0.00	0.00	0.00	0.00	0.00	0	0.00	0.00	0.00	0.00	0.00
霍奇金病	C81	1	0.14	0.36	0.14	0.00	0.00	0	0.00	0.00	0.00	0.00	0.00
非霍奇金淋巴瘤	C82–C85;C96	4	0.57	1.45	1.24	0.05	0.12	2	0.40	0.77	0.65	0.02	0.10
免疫增生性疾病	C88	0	0.00	0.00	0.00	0.00	0.00	0	0.00	0.00	0.00	0.00	0.00
多发性骨髓瘤	C90	0	0.00	0.00	0.00	0.00	0.00	0	0.00	0.00	0.00	0.00	0.00
淋巴样白血病	C91	0	0.00	0.00	0.00	0.00	0.00	0	0.00	0.00	0.00	0.00	0.00
髓样白血病	C92–C94	0	0.00	0.00	0.00	0.00	0.00	0	0.00	0.00	0.00	0.00	0.00
白血病，未特指	C95	7	1.00	2.54	2.09	0.13	0.18	2	0.40	0.77	0.71	0.02	0.08
其他的或未指明部位的	O&U	11	1.58	3.99	3.38	0.17	0.36	8	1.59	3.09	2.92	0.19	0.27
骨髓增殖性疾病	MPD	0	0.00	0.00	0.00	0.00	0.00	0	0.00	0.00	0.00	0.00	0.00
骨髓增生异常综合征	MDS	1	0.14	0.36	0.14	0.00	0.00	0	0.00	0.00	0.00	0.00	0.00
合计	ALL	698	100.00	253.35	188.21	9.49	22.89	502	100.00	193.98	140.74	8.03	16.49
所有部位除外 C44	ALL but C44	696	99.71	252.63	187.80	9.49	22.82	500	99.60	193.21	140.20	7.98	16.44

表 6-2-19a 2014 年河南省宜阳县恶性肿瘤发病主要指标

部位		男性						女性					
		病例数	构成 (%)	粗率 $(1/10^5)$	世标率 $(1/10^5)$	累积率 (%) 0~64	累积率 (%) 0~74	病例数	构成 (%)	粗率 $(1/10^5)$	世标率 $(1/10^5)$	累积率 (%) 0~64	累积率 (%) 0~74
唇	C00	0	0.00	0.00	0.00	0.00	0.00	0	0.00	0.00	0.00	0.00	0.00
舌	C01–C02	0	0.00	0.00	0.00	0.00	0.00	1	0.12	0.30	0.33	0.03	0.03
口	C03–C06	1	0.09	0.28	0.17	0.00	0.00	0	0.00	0.00	0.00	0.00	0.00
唾液腺	C07–C08	0	0.00	0.00	0.00	0.00	0.00	2	0.23	0.59	0.59	0.05	0.05
扁桃体	C09	0	0.00	0.00	0.00	0.00	0.00	0	0.00	0.00	0.00	0.00	0.00
其他的口咽	C10	0	0.00	0.00	0.00	0.00	0.00	0	0.00	0.00	0.00	0.00	0.00
鼻咽	C11	7	0.60	1.96	1.80	0.16	0.16	0	0.00	0.00	0.00	0.00	0.00
喉咽	C12–C13	0	0.00	0.00	0.00	0.00	0.00	0	0.00	0.00	0.00	0.00	0.00
咽，部位不明	C14	0	0.00	0.00	0.00	0.00	0.00	0	0.00	0.00	0.00	0.00	0.00
食管	C15	359	30.97	100.34	88.77	3.73	10.78	211	24.65	62.48	47.71	2.14	6.18
胃	C16	278	23.99	77.70	66.26	2.89	7.72	107	12.50	31.68	24.77	1.13	3.08
小肠	C17	4	0.35	1.12	1.04	0.00	0.26	3	0.35	0.89	0.71	0.00	0.12
结肠	C18	25	2.16	6.99	6.34	0.30	0.91	20	2.34	5.92	4.70	0.27	0.56
直肠	C19–C20	24	2.07	6.71	6.41	0.36	0.78	26	3.04	7.70	6.38	0.38	0.77
肛门	C21	1	0.09	0.28	0.26	0.00	0.07	1	0.12	0.30	0.33	0.03	0.03
肝脏	C22	88	7.59	24.60	22.39	0.98	2.29	51	5.96	15.10	10.55	0.42	0.88
胆囊及其他	C23–C24	10	0.86	2.79	2.61	0.03	0.31	14	1.64	4.15	3.36	0.27	0.38
胰腺	C25	13	1.12	3.63	3.20	0.21	0.39	11	1.29	3.26	2.35	0.18	0.24
鼻、鼻窦及其他	C30–C31	2	0.17	0.56	0.45	0.05	0.05	0	0.00	0.00	0.00	0.00	0.00
喉	C32	10	0.86	2.79	2.42	0.13	0.38	3	0.35	0.89	0.59	0.02	0.08
气管、支气管、肺	C33–C34	181	15.62	50.59	44.08	1.79	5.68	92	10.75	27.24	20.68	1.29	2.32
其他的胸腔器官	C37–C38	1	0.09	0.28	0.32	0.02	0.02	4	0.47	1.18	1.04	0.05	0.16
骨	C40–C41	24	2.07	6.71	5.88	0.40	0.57	14	1.64	4.15	3.46	0.24	0.36
皮肤的黑色素瘤	C43	0	0.00	0.00	0.00	0.00	0.00	0	0.00	0.00	0.00	0.00	0.00
其他的皮肤	C44	2	0.17	0.56	0.46	0.00	0.05	1	0.12	0.30	0.25	0.00	0.06
间皮瘤	C45	0	0.00	0.00	0.00	0.00	0.00	0	0.00	0.00	0.00	0.00	0.00
卡波西肉瘤	C46	1	0.09	0.28	0.20	0.02	0.02	0	0.00	0.00	0.00	0.00	0.00
周围神经、其他结缔组织、软组织	C47;C49	0	0.00	0.00	0.00	0.00	0.00	0	0.00	0.00	0.00	0.00	0.00
乳房	C50	—	—	—	—	—	—	119	13.90	35.24	28.11	2.43	2.94
外阴	C51	—	—	—	—	—	—	0	0.00	0.00	0.00	0.00	0.00
阴道	C52	—	—	—	—	—	—	0	0.00	0.00	0.00	0.00	0.00
子宫颈	C53	—	—	—	—	—	—	41	4.79	12.14	9.81	0.66	1.22
子宫体	C54	—	—	—	—	—	—	19	2.22	5.63	4.78	0.44	0.50
子宫，部位不明	C55	—	—	—	—	—	—	6	0.70	1.78	1.44	0.09	0.14
卵巢	C56	—	—	—	—	—	—	21	2.45	6.22	5.35	0.34	0.56
其他的女性生殖器	C57	—	—	—	—	—	—	0	0.00	0.00	0.00	0.00	0.00
胎盘	C58	—	—	—	—	—	—	0	0.00	0.00	0.00	0.00	0.00
阴茎	C60	3	0.26	0.84	0.63	0.06	0.06	—	—	—	—	—	—
前列腺	C61	6	0.52	1.68	1.37	0.06	0.11	—	—	—	—	—	—
睾丸	C62	2	0.17	0.56	0.55	0.06	0.06	—	—	—	—	—	—
其他的男性生殖器	C63	0	0.00	0.00	0.00	0.00	0.00	—	—	—	—	—	—
肾	C64	9	0.78	2.52	1.94	0.16	0.27	5	0.58	1.48	1.29	0.11	0.16
肾盂	C65	0	0.00	0.00	0.00	0.00	0.00	0	0.00	0.00	0.00	0.00	0.00
输尿管	C66	0	0.00	0.00	0.00	0.00	0.00	0	0.00	0.00	0.00	0.00	0.00
膀胱	C67	22	1.90	6.15	5.75	0.25	0.57	6	0.70	1.78	1.53	0.12	0.12
其他的泌尿器官	C68	0	0.00	0.00	0.00	0.00	0.00	0	0.00	0.00	0.00	0.00	0.00
眼	C69	1	0.09	0.28	0.46	0.02	0.02	1	0.12	0.30	0.31	0.00	0.05
脑、神经系统	C70–C72	20	1.73	5.59	5.00	0.39	0.44	29	3.39	8.59	7.36	0.53	0.77
甲状腺	C73	10	0.86	2.79	2.33	0.13	0.24	14	1.64	4.15	3.13	0.30	0.30
肾上腺	C74	3	0.26	0.84	0.77	0.06	0.11	0	0.00	0.00	0.00	0.00	0.00
其他的内分泌腺	C75	0	0.00	0.00	0.00	0.00	0.00	0	0.00	0.00	0.00	0.00	0.00
霍奇金病	C81	0	0.00	0.00	0.00	0.00	0.00	0	0.00	0.00	0.00	0.00	0.00
非霍奇金淋巴瘤	C82–C85;C96	3	0.26	0.84	0.77	0.02	0.13	5	0.58	1.48	1.24	0.06	0.18
免疫增生性疾病	C88	0	0.00	0.00	0.00	0.00	0.00	0	0.00	0.00	0.00	0.00	0.00
多发性骨髓瘤	C90	0	0.00	0.00	0.00	0.00	0.00	0	0.00	0.00	0.00	0.00	0.00
淋巴样白血病	C91	2	0.17	0.56	0.81	0.04	0.04	2	0.23	0.59	0.76	0.04	0.04
髓样白血病	C92–C94	2	0.17	0.56	0.47	0.06	0.06	1	0.12	0.30	0.20	0.02	0.02
白血病，未特指	C95	28	2.42	7.83	8.99	0.44	0.61	15	1.75	4.44	3.98	0.29	0.35
其他的或未指明部位的	O&U	15	1.29	4.19	4.23	0.14	0.32	11	1.29	3.26	2.79	0.17	0.30
骨髓增殖性疾病	MPD	1	0.09	0.28	0.23	0.03	0.03	0	0.00	0.00	0.00	0.00	0.00
骨髓增生异常综合征	MDS	0	0.00	0.00	0.00	0.00	0.00	0	0.00	0.00	0.00	0.00	0.00
合计	ALL	1 159	100.00	323.94	287.60	12.98	33.59	856	100.00	253.46	199.87	12.09	22.95
所有部位除外 C44	ALL but C44	1 157	99.83	323.38	287.14	12.98	33.54	855	99.88	253.16	199.62	12.09	22.88

表 6-2-20a 2014 年河南省虞城县恶性肿瘤发病主要指标

部位		男性						女性					
		病例数	构成 (%)	粗率 (1/10⁵)	世标率 (1/10⁵)	累积率 (%) 0~64	累积率 (%) 0~74	病例数	构成 (%)	粗率 (1/10⁵)	世标率 (1/10⁵)	累积率 (%) 0~64	累积率 (%) 0~74
唇	C00	3	0.22	0.52	0.60	0.03	0.03	0	0.00	0.00	0.00	0.00	0.00
舌	C01–C02	2	0.14	0.35	0.31	0.01	0.05	2	0.16	0.38	0.33	0.04	0.04
口	C03–C06	2	0.14	0.35	0.33	0.04	0.04	1	0.08	0.19	0.08	0.00	0.00
唾液腺	C07–C08	1	0.07	0.17	0.14	0.01	0.01	3	0.25	0.56	0.46	0.03	0.07
扁桃体	C09	2	0.14	0.35	0.34	0.02	0.05	1	0.08	0.19	0.12	0.00	0.00
其他的口咽	C10	3	0.22	0.52	0.44	0.02	0.02	0	0.00	0.00	0.00	0.00	0.00
鼻咽	C11	7	0.51	1.22	1.19	0.07	0.13	16	1.31	3.00	2.54	0.23	0.30
喉咽	C12–C13	4	0.29	0.70	0.51	0.03	0.03	1	0.08	0.19	0.06	0.00	0.00
咽，部位不明	C14	10	0.72	1.75	1.62	0.12	0.21	2	0.16	0.38	0.34	0.02	0.05
食管	C15	213	15.41	37.18	34.15	2.03	4.99	223	18.25	41.86	36.48	3.14	4.46
胃	C16	306	22.14	53.41	47.18	2.33	6.04	117	9.57	21.96	17.84	1.36	2.16
小肠	C17	37	2.68	6.46	5.73	0.42	0.64	13	1.06	2.44	1.91	0.16	0.20
结肠	C18	41	2.97	7.16	6.37	0.44	0.90	28	2.29	5.26	4.12	0.25	0.56
直肠	C19–C20	65	4.70	11.35	10.19	0.49	1.39	21	1.72	3.94	3.39	0.18	0.47
肛门	C21	5	0.36	0.87	0.74	0.02	0.12	3	0.25	0.56	0.40	0.03	0.03
肝脏	C22	203	14.69	35.43	31.69	1.75	4.17	136	11.13	25.53	21.69	1.75	2.89
胆囊及其他	C23–C24	11	0.80	1.92	1.56	0.08	0.22	13	1.06	2.44	1.94	0.19	0.19
胰腺	C25	14	1.01	2.44	2.28	0.20	0.32	11	0.90	2.06	1.68	0.13	0.24
鼻、鼻窦及其他	C30–C31	1	0.07	0.17	0.15	0.02	0.02	4	0.33	0.75	0.60	0.07	0.07
喉	C32	15	1.09	2.62	2.27	0.09	0.37	28	2.29	5.26	4.60	0.29	0.66
气管、支气管、肺	C33–C34	298	21.56	52.01	46.55	2.84	5.91	176	14.40	33.04	27.86	2.21	3.34
其他的胸腔器官	C37–C38	1	0.07	0.17	0.18	0.01	0.01	1	0.08	0.19	0.15	0.02	0.02
骨	C40–C41	6	0.43	1.05	1.08	0.03	0.13	10	0.82	1.88	1.76	0.12	0.22
皮肤的黑色素瘤	C43	0	0.00	0.00	0.00	0.00	0.00	0	0.00	0.00	0.00	0.00	0.00
其他的皮肤	C44	1	0.07	0.17	0.20	0.00	0.00	1	0.08	0.19	0.19	0.00	0.03
间皮瘤	C45	0	0.00	0.00	0.00	0.00	0.00	0	0.00	0.00	0.00	0.00	0.00
卡波西肉瘤	C46	0	0.00	0.00	0.00	0.00	0.00	0	0.00	0.00	0.00	0.00	0.00
周围神经、其他结缔组织、软组织	C47;C49	1	0.07	0.17	0.18	0.02	0.02	4	0.33	0.75	0.66	0.08	0.08
乳房	C50	—	—	—	—	—	—	130	10.64	24.40	20.73	1.47	2.54
外阴	C51	—	—	—	—	—	—	4	0.33	0.75	0.66	0.05	0.08
阴道	C52	—	—	—	—	—	—	6	0.49	1.13	0.98	0.04	0.18
子宫颈	C53	—	—	—	—	—	—	68	5.56	12.76	10.40	0.82	1.22
子宫体	C54	—	—	—	—	—	—	28	2.29	5.26	4.15	0.33	0.43
子宫，部位不明	C55	—	—	—	—	—	—	7	0.57	1.31	1.10	0.08	0.15
卵巢	C56	—	—	—	—	—	—	54	4.42	10.14	7.80	0.48	0.84
其他的女性生殖器	C57	—	—	—	—	—	—	0	0.00	0.00	0.00	0.00	0.00
胎盘	C58	—	—	—	—	—	—	0	0.00	0.00	0.00	0.00	0.00
阴茎	C60	3	0.22	0.52	0.47	0.02	0.02	—	—	—	—	—	—
前列腺	C61	18	1.30	3.14	2.55	0.04	0.28	—	—	—	—	—	—
睾丸	C62	3	0.22	0.52	0.38	0.00	0.04	—	—	—	—	—	—
其他的男性生殖器	C63	0	0.00	0.00	0.00	0.00	0.00	—	—	—	—	—	—
肾	C64	5	0.36	0.87	0.76	0.02	0.06	4	0.33	0.75	0.58	0.04	0.04
肾盂	C65	5	0.36	0.87	0.75	0.07	0.07	1	0.08	0.19	0.12	0.00	0.00
输尿管	C66	3	0.22	0.52	0.46	0.02	0.02	0	0.00	0.00	0.00	0.00	0.00
膀胱	C67	6	0.43	1.05	0.83	0.06	0.09	10	0.82	1.88	1.61	0.14	0.24
其他的泌尿器官	C68	0	0.00	0.00	0.00	0.00	0.00	0	0.00	0.00	0.00	0.00	0.00
眼	C69	1	0.07	0.17	0.29	0.01	0.01	0	0.00	0.00	0.00	0.00	0.00
脑、神经系统	C70–C72	19	1.37	3.32	3.16	0.22	0.38	18	1.47	3.38	2.66	0.21	0.28
甲状腺	C73	12	0.87	2.09	1.84	0.10	0.23	13	1.06	2.44	2.02	0.15	0.22
肾上腺	C74	3	0.22	0.52	0.45	0.05	0.05	0	0.00	0.00	0.00	0.00	0.00
其他的内分泌腺	C75	0	0.00	0.00	0.00	0.00	0.00	0	0.00	0.00	0.00	0.00	0.00
霍奇金病	C81	0	0.00	0.00	0.00	0.00	0.00	0	0.00	0.00	0.00	0.00	0.00
非霍奇金淋巴瘤	C82–C85;C96	5	0.36	0.87	0.83	0.09	0.09	5	0.41	0.94	0.51	0.01	0.04
免疫增生性疾病	C88	0	0.00	0.00	0.00	0.00	0.00	0	0.00	0.00	0.00	0.00	0.00
多发性骨髓瘤	C90	0	0.00	0.00	0.00	0.00	0.00	1	0.08	0.19	0.20	0.02	0.02
淋巴样白血病	C91	2	0.14	0.35	0.36	0.01	0.04	3	0.25	0.56	0.49	0.00	0.06
髓样白血病	C92–C94	4	0.29	0.70	0.65	0.04	0.07	0	0.00	0.00	0.00	0.00	0.00
白血病，未特指	C95	24	1.74	4.19	3.94	0.32	0.35	26	2.13	4.88	4.71	0.34	0.57
其他的或未指明部位的	O&U	15	1.09	2.62	2.58	0.15	0.31	29	2.37	5.44	5.09	0.36	0.61
骨髓增殖性疾病	MPD	0	0.00	0.00	0.00	0.00	0.00	0	0.00	0.00	0.00	0.00	0.00
骨髓增生异常综合征	MDS	0	0.00	0.00	0.00	0.00	0.00	0	0.00	0.00	0.00	0.00	0.00
合计	ALL	1 382	100.00	241.22	216.66	12.35	27.99	1 222	100.00	229.38	193.01	14.85	23.59
所有部位除外 C44	ALL but C44	1 381	99.93	241.04	216.45	12.35	27.99	1 221	99.92	229.20	192.82	14.85	23.55

表 6-2-21a　2014 年河南省禹州市恶性肿瘤发病主要指标

部位		男性						女性					
		病例数	构成 (%)	粗率 (1/10^5)	世标率 (1/10^5)	累积率 (%) 0~64	累积率 (%) 0~74	病例数	构成 (%)	粗率 (1/10^5)	世标率 (1/10^5)	累积率 (%) 0~64	累积率 (%) 0~74
唇	C00	0	0.00	0.00	0.00	0.00	0.00	0	0.00	0.00	0.00	0.00	0.00
舌	C01–C02	0	0.00	0.00	0.00	0.00	0.00	0	0.00	0.00	0.00	0.00	0.00
口	C03–C06	1	0.06	0.17	0.11	0.01	0.01	0	0.00	0.00	0.00	0.00	0.00
唾液腺	C07–C08	1	0.06	0.17	0.12	0.01	0.01	2	0.17	0.37	0.38	0.02	0.06
扁桃体	C09	0	0.00	0.00	0.00	0.00	0.00	0	0.00	0.00	0.00	0.00	0.00
其他的口咽	C10	1	0.06	0.17	0.09	0.00	0.00	0	0.00	0.00	0.00	0.00	0.00
鼻咽	C11	7	0.42	1.17	1.23	0.03	0.14	12	1.04	2.24	1.74	0.14	0.14
喉咽	C12–C13	0	0.00	0.00	0.00	0.00	0.00	1	0.09	0.19	0.13	0.01	0.01
咽，部位不明	C14	2	0.12	0.33	0.27	0.01	0.04	0	0.00	0.00	0.00	0.00	0.00
食管	C15	159	9.46	26.57	20.62	0.77	2.85	74	6.38	13.81	9.22	0.39	1.21
胃	C16	194	11.54	32.42	24.64	1.08	3.37	58	5.00	10.82	6.82	0.31	0.77
小肠	C17	13	0.77	2.17	1.86	0.07	0.33	10	0.86	1.87	1.41	0.06	0.21
结肠	C18	35	2.08	5.85	4.43	0.20	0.63	27	2.33	5.04	3.68	0.18	0.50
直肠	C19–C20	71	4.22	11.87	9.07	0.44	1.23	50	4.31	9.33	6.39	0.28	0.83
肛门	C21	0	0.00	0.00	0.00	0.00	0.00	0	0.00	0.00	0.00	0.00	0.00
肝脏	C22	243	14.46	40.61	31.39	1.82	3.86	94	8.11	17.54	11.83	0.66	1.55
胆囊及其他	C23–C24	7	0.42	1.17	1.07	0.03	0.17	15	1.29	2.80	1.75	0.12	0.19
胰腺	C25	22	1.31	3.68	2.57	0.16	0.30	14	1.21	2.61	1.97	0.07	0.27
鼻、鼻窦及其他	C30–C31	1	0.06	0.17	0.11	0.01	0.01	2	0.17	0.37	0.27	0.01	0.04
喉	C32	7	0.42	1.17	0.90	0.01	0.14	4	0.35	0.75	0.56	0.03	0.06
气管、支气管、肺	C33–C34	766	45.57	128.03	97.78	4.45	12.36	256	22.09	47.76	32.18	1.48	3.94
其他的胸腔器官	C37–C38	2	0.12	0.33	0.27	0.01	0.04	4	0.35	0.75	0.55	0.06	0.06
骨	C40–C41	18	1.07	3.01	2.45	0.17	0.25	17	1.47	3.17	2.56	0.16	0.39
皮肤的黑色素瘤	C43	0	0.00	0.00	0.00	0.00	0.00	0	0.00	0.00	0.00	0.00	0.00
其他的皮肤	C44	10	0.59	1.67	1.06	0.04	0.10	6	0.52	1.12	0.68	0.04	0.07
间皮瘤	C45	0	0.00	0.00	0.00	0.00	0.00	0	0.00	0.00	0.00	0.00	0.00
卡波西肉瘤	C46	0	0.00	0.00	0.00	0.00	0.00	0	0.00	0.00	0.00	0.00	0.00
周围神经、其他结缔组织、软组织	C47;C49	0	0.00	0.00	0.00	0.00	0.00	0	0.00	0.00	0.00	0.00	0.00
乳房	C50	—	—	—	—	—	—	207	17.86	38.62	28.01	2.20	2.96
外阴	C51	—	—	—	—	—	—	1	0.09	0.19	0.07	0.00	0.00
阴道	C52	—	—	—	—	—	—	0	0.00	0.00	0.00	0.00	0.00
子宫颈	C53	—	—	—	—	—	—	200	17.26	37.31	26.65	2.15	2.85
子宫体	C54	—	—	—	—	—	—	1	0.09	0.19	0.10	0.00	0.00
子宫，部位不明	C55	—	—	—	—	—	—	0	0.00	0.00	0.00	0.00	0.00
卵巢	C56	—	—	—	—	—	—	25	2.16	4.66	3.32	0.22	0.44
其他的女性生殖器	C57	—	—	—	—	—	—	0	0.00	0.00	0.00	0.00	0.00
胎盘	C58	—	—	—	—	—	—	0	0.00	0.00	0.00	0.00	0.00
阴茎	C60	5	0.30	0.84	0.76	0.03	0.14	—	—	—	—	—	—
前列腺	C61	6	0.36	1.00	0.70	0.01	0.05	—	—	—	—	—	—
睾丸	C62	0	0.00	0.00	0.00	0.00	0.00	—	—	—	—	—	—
其他的男性生殖器	C63	0	0.00	0.00	0.00	0.00	0.00	—	—	—	—	—	—
肾	C64	9	0.54	1.50	1.19	0.04	0.17	5	0.43	0.93	0.84	0.03	0.13
肾盂	C65	0	0.00	0.00	0.00	0.00	0.00	0	0.00	0.00	0.00	0.00	0.00
输尿管	C66	1	0.06	0.17	0.16	0.00	0.03	0	0.00	0.00	0.00	0.00	0.00
膀胱	C67	19	1.13	3.18	2.26	0.11	0.25	2	0.17	0.37	0.25	0.00	0.03
其他的泌尿器官	C68	0	0.00	0.00	0.00	0.00	0.00	0	0.00	0.00	0.00	0.00	0.00
眼	C69	0	0.00	0.00	0.00	0.00	0.00	0	0.00	0.00	0.00	0.00	0.00
脑、神经系统	C70–C72	35	2.08	5.85	4.72	0.32	0.49	30	2.59	5.60	4.25	0.16	0.54
甲状腺	C73	8	0.48	1.34	1.09	0.09	0.15	19	1.64	3.54	2.61	0.22	0.30
肾上腺	C74	0	0.00	0.00	0.00	0.00	0.00	0	0.00	0.00	0.00	0.00	0.00
其他的内分泌腺	C75	0	0.00	0.00	0.00	0.00	0.00	0	0.00	0.00	0.00	0.00	0.00
霍奇金病	C81	0	0.00	0.00	0.00	0.00	0.00	0	0.00	0.00	0.00	0.00	0.00
非霍奇金淋巴瘤	C82–C85;C96	0	0.00	0.00	0.00	0.00	0.00	0	0.00	0.00	0.00	0.00	0.00
免疫增生性疾病	C88	0	0.00	0.00	0.00	0.00	0.00	0	0.00	0.00	0.00	0.00	0.00
多发性骨髓瘤	C90	0	0.00	0.00	0.00	0.00	0.00	0	0.00	0.00	0.00	0.00	0.00
淋巴样白血病	C91	0	0.00	0.00	0.00	0.00	0.00	0	0.00	0.00	0.00	0.00	0.00
髓样白血病	C92–C94	0	0.00	0.00	0.00	0.00	0.00	0	0.00	0.00	0.00	0.00	0.00
白血病，未特指	C95	0	0.00	0.00	0.00	0.00	0.00	0	0.00	0.00	0.00	0.00	0.00
其他的或未指明部位的	O&U	38	2.26	6.35	5.21	0.29	0.51	23	1.98	4.29	4.02	0.19	0.42
骨髓增殖性疾病	MPD	0	0.00	0.00	0.00	0.00	0.00	0	0.00	0.00	0.00	0.00	0.00
骨髓增生异常综合征	MDS	0	0.00	0.00	0.00	0.00	0.00	0	0.00	0.00	0.00	0.00	0.00
合计	ALL	1 681	100.00	280.96	216.14	10.20	27.65	1159	100.00	216.24	152.24	9.21	17.95
所有部位除外 C44	ALL but C44	1 671	99.41	279.28	215.09	10.17	27.55	1153	99.48	215.12	151.56	9.16	17.88

表 6-2-22a 2014 年河南省漯河市召陵区恶性肿瘤发病主要指标

部位		男性						女性					
		病例数	构成 (%)	粗率 ($1/10^5$)	世标率 ($1/10^5$)	累积率 (%) 0~64	累积率 (%) 0~74	病例数	构成 (%)	粗率 ($1/10^5$)	世标率 ($1/10^5$)	累积率 (%) 0~64	累积率 (%) 0~74
唇	C00	0	0.00	0.00	0.00	0.00	0.00	0	0.00	0.00	0.00	0.00	0.00
舌	C01–C02	3	0.48	1.22	1.21	0.08	0.15	7	1.31	3.02	2.13	0.17	0.17
口	C03–C06	0	0.00	0.00	0.00	0.00	0.00	4	0.75	1.73	1.33	0.08	0.15
唾液腺	C07–C08	2	0.32	0.82	0.76	0.09	0.09	2	0.37	0.86	0.85	0.07	0.07
扁桃体	C09	0	0.00	0.00	0.00	0.00	0.00	0	0.00	0.00	0.00	0.00	0.00
其他的口咽	C10	0	0.00	0.00	0.00	0.00	0.00	0	0.00	0.00	0.00	0.00	0.00
鼻咽	C11	5	0.81	2.04	1.80	0.19	0.19	3	0.56	1.30	1.06	0.12	0.12
喉咽	C12–C13	0	0.00	0.00	0.00	0.00	0.00	0	0.00	0.00	0.00	0.00	0.00
咽，部位不明	C14	0	0.00	0.00	0.00	0.00	0.00	0	0.00	0.00	0.00	0.00	0.00
食管	C15	62	9.98	25.29	22.57	1.01	3.18	37	6.93	15.99	11.48	0.45	1.13
胃	C16	38	6.12	15.50	12.98	0.84	1.64	21	3.93	9.07	7.21	0.38	0.97
小肠	C17	1	0.16	0.41	0.25	0.03	0.03	2	0.37	0.86	0.81	0.03	0.10
结肠	C18	15	2.42	6.12	5.00	0.43	0.52	18	3.37	7.78	6.07	0.35	0.69
直肠	C19–C20	32	5.15	13.05	11.74	0.61	1.32	25	4.68	10.80	9.25	0.47	0.88
肛门	C21	1	0.16	0.41	0.37	0.03	0.03	0	0.00	0.00	0.00	0.00	0.00
肝脏	C22	109	17.55	44.47	38.67	2.26	4.90	36	6.74	15.55	11.18	0.95	1.28
胆囊及其他	C23–C24	7	1.13	2.86	2.33	0.16	0.33	5	0.94	2.16	1.35	0.05	0.12
胰腺	C25	15	2.42	6.12	5.69	0.23	0.78	4	0.75	1.73	1.34	0.06	0.13
鼻、鼻窦及其他	C30–C31	0	0.00	0.00	0.00	0.00	0.00	0	0.00	0.00	0.00	0.00	0.00
喉	C32	0	0.00	0.00	0.00	0.00	0.00	0	0.00	0.00	0.00	0.00	0.00
气管、支气管、肺	C33–C34	208	33.49	84.86	72.25	3.38	9.42	86	16.10	37.16	26.90	1.22	2.96
其他的胸腔器官	C37–C38	5	0.81	2.04	1.87	0.11	0.19	0	0.00	0.00	0.00	0.00	0.00
骨	C40–C41	9	1.45	3.67	3.17	0.13	0.37	3	0.56	1.30	1.10	0.08	0.17
皮肤的黑色素瘤	C43	1	0.16	0.41	0.45	0.00	0.07	0	0.00	0.00	0.00	0.00	0.00
其他的皮肤	C44	4	0.64	1.63	1.16	0.10	0.10	4	0.75	1.73	1.10	0.07	0.07
间皮瘤	C45	0	0.00	0.00	0.00	0.00	0.00	0	0.00	0.00	0.00	0.00	0.00
卡波西肉瘤	C46	0	0.00	0.00	0.00	0.00	0.00	0	0.00	0.00	0.00	0.00	0.00
周围神经、其他结缔组织、软组织	C47;C49	3	0.48	1.22	1.04	0.06	0.06	0	0.00	0.00	0.00	0.00	0.00
乳房	C50	—	—	—	—	—	—	125	23.41	54.01	42.20	3.63	4.58
外阴	C51	—	—	—	—	—	—	0	0.00	0.00	0.00	0.00	0.00
阴道	C52	—	—	—	—	—	—	0	0.00	0.00	0.00	0.00	0.00
子宫颈	C53	—	—	—	—	—	—	47	8.80	20.31	16.32	1.44	1.51
子宫体	C54	—	—	—	—	—	—	19	3.56	8.21	6.64	0.40	0.89
子宫，部位不明	C55	—	—	—	—	—	—	3	0.56	1.30	1.09	0.11	0.11
卵巢	C56	—	—	—	—	—	—	23	4.31	9.94	8.18	0.70	1.13
其他的女性生殖器	C57	—	—	—	—	—	—	1	0.19	0.43	0.38	0.05	0.05
胎盘	C58	—	—	—	—	—	—	0	0.00	0.00	0.00	0.00	0.00
阴茎	C60	1	0.16	0.41	0.45	0.00	0.07	—	—	—	—	—	—
前列腺	C61	11	1.77	4.49	4.16	0.11	0.38	—	—	—	—	—	—
睾丸	C62	0	0.00	0.00	0.00	0.00	0.00	—	—	—	—	—	—
其他的男性生殖器	C63	0	0.00	0.00	0.00	0.00	0.00	—	—	—	—	—	—
肾	C64	7	1.13	2.86	2.67	0.20	0.35	4	0.75	1.73	1.48	0.11	0.11
肾盂	C65	1	0.16	0.41	0.37	0.04	0.04	0	0.00	0.00	0.00	0.00	0.00
输尿管	C66	1	0.16	0.41	0.31	0.03	0.03	2	0.37	0.86	0.53	0.00	0.09
膀胱	C67	14	2.25	5.71	4.88	0.20	0.39	6	1.12	2.59	1.82	0.10	0.19
其他的泌尿器官	C68	0	0.00	0.00	0.00	0.00	0.00	0	0.00	0.00	0.00	0.00	0.00
眼	C69	1	0.16	0.41	0.25	0.03	0.03	1	0.19	0.43	0.15	0.00	0.00
脑、神经系统	C70–C72	15	2.42	6.12	5.43	0.44	0.61	8	1.50	3.46	2.39	0.21	0.21
甲状腺	C73	6	0.97	2.45	2.11	0.20	0.20	12	2.25	5.18	4.43	0.34	0.41
肾上腺	C74	0	0.00	0.00	0.00	0.00	0.00	1	0.19	0.43	0.24	0.03	0.03
其他的内分泌腺	C75	0	0.00	0.00	0.00	0.00	0.00	1	0.19	0.43	0.45	0.00	0.07
霍奇金病	C81	8	1.29	3.26	2.51	0.07	0.33	1	0.19	0.43	0.30	0.02	0.02
非霍奇金淋巴瘤	C82–C85;C96	0	0.00	0.00	0.00	0.00	0.00	1	0.19	0.43	0.24	0.03	0.03
免疫增生性疾病	C88	0	0.00	0.00	0.00	0.00	0.00	0	0.00	0.00	0.00	0.00	0.00
多发性骨髓瘤	C90	0	0.00	0.00	0.00	0.00	0.00	0	0.00	0.00	0.00	0.00	0.00
淋巴样白血病	C91	9	1.45	3.67	3.35	0.24	0.41	5	0.94	2.16	1.72	0.06	0.13
髓样白血病	C92–C94	13	2.09	5.30	5.25	0.34	0.50	7	1.31	3.02	2.03	0.11	0.18
白血病，未特指	C95	0	0.00	0.00	0.00	0.00	0.00	0	0.00	0.00	0.00	0.00	0.00
其他的或未指明部位的	O&U	14	2.25	5.71	5.06	0.33	0.74	9	1.69	3.89	3.31	0.26	0.34
骨髓增殖性疾病	MPD	0	0.00	0.00	0.00	0.00	0.00	1	0.19	0.43	0.37	0.04	0.04
骨髓增生异常综合征	MDS	0	0.00	0.00	0.00	0.00	0.00	0	0.00	0.00	0.00	0.00	0.00
合计	ALL	621	100.00	253.34	220.12	11.97	27.45	534	100.00	230.71	177.42	12.16	19.14
所有部位除外 C44	ALL but C44	617	99.36	251.71	218.96	11.87	27.34	530	99.25	228.98	176.32	12.09	19.07

表 6-2-23a　2014 年河南省偃师市恶性肿瘤发病主要指标

部位		男性						女性					
		病例数	构成 (%)	粗率 $(1/10^5)$	世标率 $(1/10^5)$	累积率 (%) 0~64	累积率 (%) 0~74	病例数	构成 (%)	粗率 $(1/10^5)$	世标率 $(1/10^5)$	累积率 (%) 0~64	累积率 (%) 0~74
唇	C00	0	0.00	0.00	0.00	0.00	0.00	1	0.14	0.33	0.15	0.00	0.00
舌	C01–C02	1	0.14	0.32	0.26	0.03	0.03	0	0.00	0.00	0.00	0.00	0.00
口	C03–C06	3	0.41	0.96	0.74	0.05	0.05	2	0.29	0.65	0.29	0.02	0.02
唾液腺	C07–C08	5	0.69	1.60	1.18	0.10	0.15	2	0.29	0.65	0.64	0.03	0.03
扁桃体	C09	0	0.00	0.00	0.00	0.00	0.00	0	0.00	0.00	0.00	0.00	0.00
其他的口咽	C10	1	0.14	0.32	0.28	0.00	0.07	1	0.14	0.33	0.26	0.00	0.06
鼻咽	C11	1	0.14	0.32	0.27	0.02	0.02	4	0.58	1.30	0.64	0.02	0.02
喉咽	C12–C13	0	0.00	0.00	0.00	0.00	0.00	0	0.00	0.00	0.00	0.00	0.00
咽，部位不明	C14	1	0.14	0.32	0.19	0.02	0.02	0	0.00	0.00	0.00	0.00	0.00
食管	C15	120	16.53	38.31	29.84	0.88	3.23	81	11.74	26.37	17.10	0.47	2.09
胃	C16	145	19.97	46.29	37.00	1.50	4.50	45	6.67	14.97	9.91	0.47	1.08
小肠	C17	5	0.69	1.60	1.33	0.08	0.22	2	0.29	0.65	0.50	0.03	0.10
结肠	C18	22	3.03	7.02	5.37	0.33	0.55	25	3.62	8.14	5.53	0.23	0.68
直肠	C19–C20	22	3.03	7.02	5.39	0.35	0.73	19	2.75	6.19	4.35	0.16	0.53
肛门	C21	0	0.00	0.00	0.00	0.00	0.00	1	0.14	0.33	0.16	0.00	0.00
肝脏	C22	86	11.85	27.45	21.67	1.47	2.58	46	6.67	14.97	9.98	0.64	1.16
胆囊及其他	C23–C24	14	1.93	4.47	3.27	0.13	0.30	12	1.74	3.91	2.44	0.10	0.25
胰腺	C25	13	1.79	4.15	3.55	0.07	0.41	6	0.87	1.95	1.26	0.10	0.16
鼻、鼻窦及其他	C30–C31	1	0.14	0.32	0.23	0.02	0.02	1	0.14	0.33	0.26	0.00	0.06
喉	C32	6	0.83	1.92	1.39	0.10	0.15	2	0.29	0.65	0.51	0.00	0.13
气管、支气管、肺	C33–C34	112	15.43	35.75	28.15	1.38	3.53	71	10.29	23.11	14.86	0.55	1.62
其他的胸腔器官	C37–C38	2	0.28	0.64	0.50	0.04	0.04	4	0.58	1.30	0.80	0.05	0.05
骨	C40–C41	10	1.38	3.19	2.55	0.23	0.30	5	0.72	1.63	1.14	0.09	0.16
皮肤的黑色素瘤	C43	0	0.00	0.00	0.00	0.00	0.00	2	0.29	0.65	0.37	0.02	0.02
其他的皮肤	C44	3	0.41	0.96	0.84	0.03	0.03	8	1.16	2.60	1.66	0.09	0.14
间皮瘤	C45	0	0.00	0.00	0.00	0.00	0.00	0	0.00	0.00	0.00	0.00	0.00
卡波西肉瘤	C46	0	0.00	0.00	0.00	0.00	0.00	0	0.00	0.00	0.00	0.00	0.00
周围神经、其他结缔组织、软组织	C47;C49	4	0.55	1.28	0.94	0.05	0.12	4	0.58	1.30	1.10	0.09	0.09
乳房	C50	—	—	—	—	—	—	116	16.81	37.76	27.84	2.30	2.90
外阴	C51	—	—	—	—	—	—	0	0.00	0.00	0.00	0.00	0.00
阴道	C52	—	—	—	—	—	—	1	0.14	0.33	0.11	0.00	0.00
子宫颈	C53	—	—	—	—	—	—	49	7.10	15.95	11.58	0.94	1.22
子宫体	C54	—	—	—	—	—	—	29	4.20	9.44	6.74	0.54	0.64
子宫，部位不明	C55	—	—	—	—	—	—	4	0.58	1.30	0.91	0.07	0.07
卵巢	C56	—	—	—	—	—	—	23	3.33	7.49	5.63	0.39	0.62
其他的女性生殖器	C57	—	—	—	—	—	—	4	0.58	1.30	0.91	0.07	0.07
胎盘	C58	—	—	—	—	—	—	0	0.00	0.00	0.00	0.00	0.00
阴茎	C60	0	0.00	0.00	0.00	0.00	0.00	—	—	—	—	—	—
前列腺	C61	21	2.89	6.70	5.65	0.02	0.83	—	—	—	—	—	—
睾丸	C62	0	0.00	0.00	0.00	0.00	0.00	—	—	—	—	—	—
其他的男性生殖器	C63	1	0.14	0.32	0.30	0.00	0.05	—	—	—	—	—	—
肾	C64	13	1.79	4.15	3.17	0.22	0.41	5	0.72	1.63	1.33	0.07	0.19
肾盂	C65	1	0.14	0.32	0.30	0.00	0.05	0	0.00	0.00	0.00	0.00	0.00
输尿管	C66	2	0.28	0.64	0.44	0.06	0.06	0	0.00	0.00	0.00	0.00	0.00
膀胱	C67	12	1.65	3.83	3.13	0.13	0.44	4	0.58	1.30	0.82	0.05	0.05
其他的泌尿器官	C68	0	0.00	0.00	0.00	0.00	0.00	0	0.00	0.00	0.00	0.00	0.00
眼	C69	1	0.14	0.32	0.26	0.03	0.03	1	0.14	0.33	0.25	0.03	0.03
脑、神经系统	C70–C72	34	4.68	10.85	9.03	0.57	1.08	32	4.64	10.42	8.12	0.55	0.90
甲状腺	C73	11	1.52	3.51	2.71	0.21	0.28	31	4.49	10.09	7.55	0.60	0.77
肾上腺	C74	1	0.14	0.32	0.19	0.00	0.00	0	0.00	0.00	0.00	0.00	0.00
其他的内分泌腺	C75	3	0.41	0.96	0.70	0.08	0.08	10	1.45	3.26	2.32	0.15	0.27
霍奇金病	C81	0	0.00	0.00	0.00	0.00	0.00	0	0.00	0.00	0.00	0.00	0.00
非霍奇金淋巴瘤	C82–C85;C96	14	1.93	4.47	4.35	0.17	0.43	12	1.74	3.91	2.66	0.17	0.35
免疫增生性疾病	C88	0	0.00	0.00	0.00	0.00	0.00	0	0.00	0.00	0.00	0.00	0.00
多发性骨髓瘤	C90	6	0.83	1.92	1.25	0.05	0.05	4	0.58	1.30	0.89	0.09	0.09
淋巴样白血病	C91	2	0.28	0.64	1.08	0.05	0.05	2	0.29	0.65	0.94	0.05	0.05
髓样白血病	C92–C94	2	0.28	0.64	0.44	0.03	0.03	2	0.29	0.65	0.61	0.05	0.05
白血病，未特指	C95	10	1.38	3.19	3.05	0.15	0.30	9	1.30	2.93	2.97	0.21	0.21
其他的或未指明部位的	O&U	10	1.38	3.19	2.92	0.11	0.23	7	1.01	2.28	1.50	0.13	0.13
骨髓增殖性疾病	MPD	0	0.00	0.00	0.00	0.00	0.00	0	0.00	0.00	0.00	0.00	0.00
骨髓增生异常综合征	MDS	0	0.00	0.00	0.00	0.00	0.00	0	0.00	0.00	0.00	0.00	0.00
合计	ALL	726	100.00	231.76	184.98	8.83	21.58	690	100.00	224.62	157.62	9.63	17.08
所有部位除外 C44	ALL but C44	723	99.59	230.80	184.14	8.80	21.54	682	98.84	222.02	155.96	9.54	16.93

表 6-2-24a 2014 年河南省嵩县恶性肿瘤发病主要指标

部位		男性						女性					
		病例数	构成 (%)	粗率 ($1/10^5$)	世标率 ($1/10^5$)	累积率 (%) 0~64	累积率 (%) 0~74	病例数	构成 (%)	粗率 ($1/10^5$)	世标率 ($1/10^5$)	累积率 (%) 0~64	累积率 (%) 0~74
唇	C00	1	0.13	0.32	0.23	0.02	0.02	0	0.00	0.00	0.00	0.00	0.00
舌	C01-C02	0	0.00	0.00	0.00	0.00	0.00	1	0.18	0.35	0.19	0.00	0.00
口	C03-C06	0	0.00	0.00	0.00	0.00	0.00	2	0.35	0.70	0.53	0.07	0.07
唾液腺	C07-C08	2	0.26	0.64	0.47	0.04	0.04	2	0.35	0.70	0.66	0.07	0.07
扁桃体	C09	0	0.00	0.00	0.00	0.00	0.00	0	0.00	0.00	0.00	0.00	0.00
其他的口咽	C10	0	0.00	0.00	0.00	0.00	0.00	0	0.00	0.00	0.00	0.00	0.00
鼻咽	C11	1	0.13	0.32	0.23	0.02	0.02	3	0.53	1.05	0.64	0.06	0.06
喉咽	C12-C13	0	0.00	0.00	0.00	0.00	0.00	0	0.00	0.00	0.00	0.00	0.00
咽，部位不明	C14	1	0.13	0.32	0.33	0.00	0.06	0	0.00	0.00	0.00	0.00	0.00
食管	C15	278	36.53	88.61	70.46	4.10	8.81	162	28.47	56.80	45.32	2.11	6.41
胃	C16	240	31.54	76.50	62.24	3.76	8.40	85	14.94	29.80	22.76	1.22	2.73
小肠	C17	1	0.13	0.32	0.24	0.02	0.02	0	0.00	0.00	0.00	0.00	0.00
结肠	C18	20	2.63	6.37	5.09	0.31	0.62	15	2.64	5.26	4.33	0.21	0.59
直肠	C19-C20	17	2.23	5.42	4.24	0.22	0.46	17	2.99	5.96	4.93	0.26	0.74
肛门	C21	0	0.00	0.00	0.00	0.00	0.00	0	0.00	0.00	0.00	0.00	0.00
肝脏	C22	59	7.75	18.81	15.39	1.04	2.11	37	6.50	12.97	9.45	0.54	1.23
胆囊及其他	C23-C24	3	0.39	0.96	0.91	0.03	0.17	8	1.41	2.80	2.24	0.06	0.28
胰腺	C25	10	1.31	3.19	2.87	0.16	0.40	7	1.23	2.45	1.86	0.08	0.24
鼻、鼻窦及其他	C30-C31	1	0.13	0.32	0.33	0.00	0.06	1	0.18	0.35	0.25	0.03	0.03
喉	C32	1	0.13	0.32	0.22	0.03	0.03	0	0.00	0.00	0.00	0.00	0.00
气管、支气管、肺	C33-C34	45	5.91	14.34	11.59	0.69	1.45	32	5.62	11.22	8.19	0.48	0.95
其他的胸腔器官	C37-C38	2	0.26	0.64	0.55	0.03	0.08	2	0.35	0.70	0.40	0.03	0.03
骨	C40-C41	7	0.92	2.23	1.87	0.17	0.17	4	0.70	1.40	1.16	0.05	0.11
皮肤的黑色素瘤	C43	0	0.00	0.00	0.00	0.00	0.00	1	0.18	0.35	0.37	0.00	0.06
其他的皮肤	C44	0	0.00	0.00	0.00	0.00	0.00	1	0.18	0.35	0.38	0.00	0.10
间皮瘤	C45	0	0.00	0.00	0.00	0.00	0.00	0	0.00	0.00	0.00	0.00	0.00
卡波西肉瘤	C46	0	0.00	0.00	0.00	0.00	0.00	0	0.00	0.00	0.00	0.00	0.00
周围神经、其他结缔组织、软组织	C47;C49	1	0.13	0.32	0.22	0.03	0.03	0	0.00	0.00	0.00	0.00	0.00
乳房	C50	—	—	—	—	—	—	50	8.79	17.53	14.09	1.26	1.61
外阴	C51	—	—	—	—	—	—	3	0.53	1.05	0.72	0.05	0.05
阴道	C52	—	—	—	—	—	—	3	0.53	1.05	0.77	0.08	0.08
子宫颈	C53	—	—	—	—	—	—	53	9.31	18.58	14.90	1.06	1.81
子宫体	C54	—	—	—	—	—	—	15	2.64	5.26	3.87	0.34	0.44
子宫，部位不明	C55	—	—	—	—	—	—	9	1.58	3.16	2.53	0.27	0.27
卵巢	C56	—	—	—	—	—	—	8	1.41	2.80	2.36	0.15	0.24
其他的女性生殖器	C57	—	—	—	—	—	—	0	0.00	0.00	0.00	0.00	0.00
胎盘	C58	—	—	—	—	—	—	0	0.00	0.00	0.00	0.00	0.00
阴茎	C60	1	0.13	0.32	0.34	0.03	0.03	—	—	—	—	—	—
前列腺	C61	7	0.92	2.23	1.85	0.02	0.25	—	—	—	—	—	—
睾丸	C62	3	0.39	0.96	0.74	0.03	0.03	—	—	—	—	—	—
其他的男性生殖器	C63	0	0.00	0.00	0.00	0.00	0.00	—	—	—	—	—	—
肾	C64	7	0.92	2.23	2.02	0.16	0.22	4	0.70	1.40	1.02	0.09	0.09
肾盂	C65	1	0.13	0.32	0.25	0.03	0.03	0	0.00	0.00	0.00	0.00	0.00
输尿管	C66	0	0.00	0.00	0.00	0.00	0.00	1	0.18	0.35	0.38	0.00	0.10
膀胱	C67	13	1.71	4.14	3.37	0.15	0.50	3	0.53	1.05	0.85	0.03	0.13
其他的泌尿器官	C68	0	0.00	0.00	0.00	0.00	0.00	0	0.00	0.00	0.00	0.00	0.00
眼	C69	0	0.00	0.00	0.00	0.00	0.00	0	0.00	0.00	0.00	0.00	0.00
脑、神经系统	C70-C72	11	1.45	3.51	3.00	0.23	0.32	12	2.11	4.21	3.56	0.30	0.36
甲状腺	C73	4	0.53	1.27	1.26	0.04	0.22	16	2.81	5.61	4.21	0.38	0.38
肾上腺	C74	3	0.39	0.96	1.06	0.06	0.15	0	0.00	0.00	0.00	0.00	0.00
其他的内分泌腺	C75	0	0.00	0.00	0.00	0.00	0.00	1	0.18	0.35	0.13	0.00	0.00
霍奇金病	C81	0	0.00	0.00	0.00	0.00	0.00	0	0.00	0.00	0.00	0.00	0.00
非霍奇金淋巴瘤	C82-C85;C96	1	0.13	0.32	0.23	0.02	0.02	0	0.00	0.00	0.00	0.00	0.00
免疫增生性疾病	C88	0	0.00	0.00	0.00	0.00	0.00	0	0.00	0.00	0.00	0.00	0.00
多发性骨髓瘤	C90	1	0.13	0.32	0.25	0.03	0.03	0	0.00	0.00	0.00	0.00	0.00
淋巴样白血病	C91	2	0.26	0.64	0.32	0.00	0.00	0	0.00	0.00	0.00	0.00	0.00
髓样白血病	C92-C94	0	0.00	0.00	0.00	0.00	0.00	0	0.00	0.00	0.00	0.00	0.00
白血病，未特指	C95	5	0.66	1.59	1.12	0.07	0.07	4	0.70	1.40	1.43	0.10	0.10
其他的或未指明部位的	O&U	12	1.58	3.82	3.30	0.26	0.26	7	1.23	2.45	2.29	0.13	0.23
骨髓增殖性疾病	MPD	0	0.00	0.00	0.00	0.00	0.00	0	0.00	0.00	0.00	0.00	0.00
骨髓增生异常综合征	MDS	0	0.00	0.00	0.00	0.00	0.00	0	0.00	0.00	0.00	0.00	0.00
合计	ALL	761	100.00	242.55	196.59	11.79	25.07	569	100.00	199.48	156.77	9.54	19.58
所有部位除外 C44	ALL but C44	761	100.00	242.55	196.59	11.79	25.07	568	99.82	199.13	156.39	9.54	19.48

表 6-2-25a　2014 年河南省漯河市恶性肿瘤发病主要指标

部位		男性						女性					
		病例数	构成 (%)	粗率 ($1/10^5$)	世标率 ($1/10^5$)	累积率 (%) 0~64	累积率 (%) 0~74	病例数	构成 (%)	粗率 ($1/10^5$)	世标率 ($1/10^5$)	累积率 (%) 0~64	累积率 (%) 0~74
唇	C00	0	0.00	0.00	0.00	0.00	0.00	0	0.00	0.00	0.00	0.00	0.00
舌	C01–C02	3	0.48	1.22	1.21	0.08	0.15	7	1.31	3.02	2.13	0.17	0.17
口	C03–C06	0	0.00	0.00	0.00	0.00	0.00	4	0.75	1.73	1.33	0.08	0.15
唾液腺	C07–C08	2	0.32	0.82	0.76	0.09	0.09	2	0.37	0.86	0.85	0.07	0.07
扁桃体	C09	0	0.00	0.00	0.00	0.00	0.00	0	0.00	0.00	0.00	0.00	0.00
其他的口咽	C10	0	0.00	0.00	0.00	0.00	0.00	0	0.00	0.00	0.00	0.00	0.00
鼻咽	C11	5	0.81	2.04	1.80	0.19	0.19	3	0.56	1.30	1.06	0.12	0.12
喉咽	C12–C13	0	0.00	0.00	0.00	0.00	0.00	0	0.00	0.00	0.00	0.00	0.00
咽，部位不明	C14	0	0.00	0.00	0.00	0.00	0.00	0	0.00	0.00	0.00	0.00	0.00
食管	C15	62	9.98	25.29	22.57	1.01	3.18	37	6.93	15.99	11.48	0.45	1.13
胃	C16	38	6.12	15.50	12.98	0.84	1.64	21	3.93	9.07	7.21	0.38	0.97
小肠	C17	1	0.16	0.41	0.25	0.03	0.03	2	0.37	0.86	0.81	0.03	0.10
结肠	C18	15	2.42	6.12	5.00	0.43	0.52	18	3.37	7.78	6.07	0.35	0.69
直肠	C19–C20	32	5.15	13.05	11.74	0.61	1.32	25	4.68	10.80	9.25	0.47	0.88
肛门	C21	1	0.16	0.41	0.37	0.03	0.03	0	0.00	0.00	0.00	0.00	0.00
肝脏	C22	109	17.55	44.47	38.67	2.26	4.90	36	6.74	15.55	11.18	0.95	1.28
胆囊及其他	C23–C24	7	1.13	2.86	2.33	0.16	0.33	5	0.94	2.16	1.35	0.05	0.12
胰腺	C25	15	2.42	6.12	5.69	0.23	0.78	4	0.75	1.73	1.34	0.06	0.13
鼻、鼻窦及其他	C30–C31	0	0.00	0.00	0.00	0.00	0.00	0	0.00	0.00	0.00	0.00	0.00
喉	C32	0	0.00	0.00	0.00	0.00	0.00	0	0.00	0.00	0.00	0.00	0.00
气管、支气管、肺	C33–C34	208	33.49	84.86	72.25	3.38	9.42	86	16.10	37.16	26.90	1.22	2.96
其他的胸腔器官	C37–C38	5	0.81	2.04	1.87	0.11	0.19	0	0.00	0.00	0.00	0.00	0.00
骨	C40–C41	9	1.45	3.67	3.17	0.13	0.37	3	0.56	1.30	1.10	0.08	0.17
皮肤的黑色素瘤	C43	1	0.16	0.41	0.45	0.00	0.07	0	0.00	0.00	0.00	0.00	0.00
其他的皮肤	C44	4	0.64	1.63	1.16	0.10	0.10	4	0.75	1.73	1.10	0.07	0.07
间皮瘤	C45	0	0.00	0.00	0.00	0.00	0.00	0	0.00	0.00	0.00	0.00	0.00
卡波西肉瘤	C46	0	0.00	0.00	0.00	0.00	0.00	0	0.00	0.00	0.00	0.00	0.00
周围神经、其他结缔组织、软组织	C47;C49	3	0.48	1.22	1.04	0.06	0.06	0	0.00	0.00	0.00	0.00	0.00
乳房	C50	—	—	—	—	—	—	125	23.41	54.01	42.20	3.63	4.58
外阴	C51	—	—	—	—	—	—	0	0.00	0.00	0.00	0.00	0.00
阴道	C52	—	—	—	—	—	—	0	0.00	0.00	0.00	0.00	0.00
子宫颈	C53	—	—	—	—	—	—	47	8.80	20.31	16.32	1.44	1.51
子宫体	C54	—	—	—	—	—	—	19	3.56	8.21	6.64	0.40	0.89
子宫，部位不明	C55	—	—	—	—	—	—	3	0.56	1.30	1.09	0.11	0.11
卵巢	C56	—	—	—	—	—	—	23	4.31	9.94	8.18	0.70	1.13
其他的女性生殖器	C57	—	—	—	—	—	—	1	0.19	0.43	0.38	0.05	0.05
胎盘	C58	—	—	—	—	—	—	0	0.00	0.00	0.00	0.00	0.00
阴茎	C60	1	0.16	0.41	0.45	0.00	0.07	—	—	—	—	—	—
前列腺	C61	11	1.77	4.49	4.16	0.11	0.38	—	—	—	—	—	—
睾丸	C62	0	0.00	0.00	0.00	0.00	0.00	—	—	—	—	—	—
其他的男性生殖器	C63	0	0.00	0.00	0.00	0.00	0.00	—	—	—	—	—	—
肾	C64	7	1.13	2.86	2.67	0.20	0.35	4	0.75	1.73	1.48	0.11	0.11
肾盂	C65	1	0.16	0.41	0.37	0.04	0.04	0	0.00	0.00	0.00	0.00	0.00
输尿管	C66	1	0.16	0.41	0.31	0.03	0.03	2	0.37	0.86	0.53	0.00	0.09
膀胱	C67	14	2.25	5.71	4.88	0.20	0.39	6	1.12	2.59	1.82	0.10	0.19
其他的泌尿器官	C68	0	0.00	0.00	0.00	0.00	0.00	0	0.00	0.00	0.00	0.00	0.00
眼	C69	1	0.16	0.41	0.25	0.03	0.03	1	0.19	0.43	0.15	0.00	0.00
脑、神经系统	C70–C72	15	2.42	6.12	5.43	0.44	0.61	8	1.50	3.46	2.39	0.21	0.21
甲状腺	C73	6	0.97	2.45	2.11	0.20	0.20	12	2.25	5.18	4.43	0.34	0.41
肾上腺	C74	0	0.00	0.00	0.00	0.00	0.00	1	0.19	0.43	0.24	0.03	0.03
其他的内分泌腺	C75	0	0.00	0.00	0.00	0.00	0.00	1	0.19	0.43	0.45	0.00	0.07
霍奇金病	C81	8	1.29	3.26	2.51	0.07	0.33	1	0.19	0.43	0.30	0.02	0.02
非霍奇金淋巴瘤	C82–C85;C96	0	0.00	0.00	0.00	0.00	0.00	1	0.19	0.43	0.24	0.03	0.03
免疫增生性疾病	C88	0	0.00	0.00	0.00	0.00	0.00	0	0.00	0.00	0.00	0.00	0.00
多发性骨髓瘤	C90	0	0.00	0.00	0.00	0.00	0.00	0	0.00	0.00	0.00	0.00	0.00
淋巴样白血病	C91	9	1.45	3.67	3.35	0.24	0.41	5	0.94	2.16	1.72	0.06	0.13
髓样白血病	C92–C94	13	2.09	5.30	5.25	0.34	0.50	7	1.31	3.02	2.03	0.11	0.18
白血病，未特指	C95	0	0.00	0.00	0.00	0.00	0.00	0	0.00	0.00	0.00	0.00	0.00
其他的或未指明部位的	O&U	14	2.25	5.71	5.06	0.33	0.74	9	1.69	3.89	3.31	0.26	0.34
骨髓增殖性疾病	MPD	0	0.00	0.00	0.00	0.00	0.00	1	0.19	0.43	0.37	0.04	0.04
骨髓增生异常综合征	MDS	0	0.00	0.00	0.00	0.00	0.00	0	0.00	0.00	0.00	0.00	0.00
合计	ALL	621	100.00	253.34	220.12	11.97	27.45	534	100.00	230.71	177.42	12.16	19.14
所有部位除外 C44	ALL but C44	617	99.36	251.71	218.96	11.87	27.34	530	99.25	228.98	176.32	12.09	19.07

表 6-2-26a 2014 年河南省栾川县恶性肿瘤发病主要指标

部位		男性						女性					
		病例数	构成 (%)	粗率 (1/10^5)	世标率 (1/10^5)	累积率 (%) 0~64	累积率 (%) 0~74	病例数	构成 (%)	粗率 (1/10^5)	世标率 (1/10^5)	累积率 (%) 0~64	累积率 (%) 0~74
唇	C00	0	0.00	0.00	0.00	0.00	0.00	0	0.00	0.00	0.00	0.00	0.00
舌	C01-C02	0	0.00	0.00	0.00	0.00	0.00	0	0.00	0.00	0.00	0.00	0.00
口	C03-C06	1	0.21	0.54	0.38	0.05	0.05	0	0.00	0.00	0.00	0.00	0.00
唾液腺	C07-C08	0	0.00	0.00	0.00	0.00	0.00	0	0.00	0.00	0.00	0.00	0.00
扁桃体	C09	0	0.00	0.00	0.00	0.00	0.00	0	0.00	0.00	0.00	0.00	0.00
其他的口咽	C10	0	0.00	0.00	0.00	0.00	0.00	1	0.30	0.62	0.49	0.04	0.04
鼻咽	C11	5	1.03	2.69	2.04	0.15	0.15	1	0.30	0.62	0.34	0.00	0.00
喉咽	C12-C13	0	0.00	0.00	0.00	0.00	0.00	0	0.00	0.00	0.00	0.00	0.00
咽，部位不明	C14	0	0.00	0.00	0.00	0.00	0.00	1	0.30	0.62	0.42	0.03	0.03
食管	C15	97	19.96	52.15	36.02	1.86	4.69	50	14.84	31.06	20.72	0.96	2.29
胃	C16	139	28.60	74.73	50.78	3.54	6.12	36	10.68	22.36	15.58	1.10	1.40
小肠	C17	0	0.00	0.00	0.00	0.00	0.00	0	0.00	0.00	0.00	0.00	0.00
结肠	C18	11	2.26	5.91	3.84	0.23	0.37	7	2.08	4.35	3.04	0.21	0.38
直肠	C19-C20	10	2.06	5.38	3.97	0.26	0.44	14	4.15	8.70	5.92	0.44	0.79
肛门	C21	0	0.00	0.00	0.00	0.00	0.00	0	0.00	0.00	0.00	0.00	0.00
肝脏	C22	59	12.14	31.72	22.74	1.63	2.48	25	7.42	15.53	11.40	0.59	1.53
胆囊及其他	C23-C24	1	0.21	0.54	0.43	0.00	0.07	8	2.37	4.97	3.82	0.34	0.43
胰腺	C25	9	1.85	4.84	3.67	0.27	0.57	6	1.78	3.73	2.80	0.05	0.30
鼻、鼻窦及其他	C30-C31	0	0.00	0.00	0.00	0.00	0.00	0	0.00	0.00	0.00	0.00	0.00
喉	C32	5	1.03	2.69	1.92	0.08	0.30	1	0.30	0.62	0.37	0.04	0.04
气管、支气管、肺	C33-C34	78	16.05	41.93	28.78	1.52	3.25	36	10.68	22.36	15.19	0.81	1.88
其他的胸腔器官	C37-C38	0	0.00	0.00	0.00	0.00	0.00	1	0.30	0.62	0.42	0.03	0.03
骨	C40-C41	11	2.26	5.91	4.94	0.30	0.55	6	1.78	3.73	3.19	0.26	0.26
皮肤的黑色素瘤	C43	0	0.00	0.00	0.00	0.00	0.00	0	0.00	0.00	0.00	0.00	0.00
其他的皮肤	C44	2	0.41	1.08	0.67	0.00	0.11	1	0.30	0.62	0.22	0.00	0.00
间皮瘤	C45	0	0.00	0.00	0.00	0.00	0.00	0	0.00	0.00	0.00	0.00	0.00
卡波西肉瘤	C46	0	0.00	0.00	0.00	0.00	0.00	0	0.00	0.00	0.00	0.00	0.00
周围神经、其他结缔组织、软组织	C47;C49	2	0.41	1.08	0.90	0.07	0.07	1	0.30	0.62	0.44	0.06	0.06
乳房	C50	—	—	—	—	—	—	35	10.39	21.74	16.95	1.38	1.60
外阴	C51	—	—	—	—	—	—	1	0.30	0.62	0.63	0.05	0.05
阴道	C52	—	—	—	—	—	—	0	0.00	0.00	0.00	0.00	0.00
子宫颈	C53	—	—	—	—	—	—	44	13.06	27.33	19.40	1.46	2.22
子宫体	C54	—	—	—	—	—	—	9	2.67	5.59	3.89	0.37	0.37
子宫，部位不明	C55	—	—	—	—	—	—	2	0.59	1.24	1.00	0.00	0.17
卵巢	C56	—	—	—	—	—	—	5	1.48	3.11	2.43	0.24	0.24
其他的女性生殖器	C57	—	—	—	—	—	—	0	0.00	0.00	0.00	0.00	0.00
胎盘	C58	—	—	—	—	—	—	0	0.00	0.00	0.00	0.00	0.00
阴茎	C60	0	0.00	0.00	0.00	0.00	0.00	—	—	—	—	—	—
前列腺	C61	1	0.21	0.54	0.32	0.00	0.00	—	—	—	—	—	—
睾丸	C62	2	0.41	1.08	0.89	0.09	0.09	—	—	—	—	—	—
其他的男性生殖器	C63	0	0.00	0.00	0.00	0.00	0.00	—	—	—	—	—	—
肾	C64	4	0.82	2.15	1.45	0.05	0.19	0	0.00	0.00	0.00	0.00	0.00
肾盂	C65	0	0.00	0.00	0.00	0.00	0.00	0	0.00	0.00	0.00	0.00	0.00
输尿管	C66	0	0.00	0.00	0.00	0.00	0.00	0	0.00	0.00	0.00	0.00	0.00
膀胱	C67	3	0.62	1.61	1.06	0.00	0.11	3	0.89	1.86	1.37	0.00	0.22
其他的泌尿器官	C68	0	0.00	0.00	0.00	0.00	0.00	1	0.30	0.62	0.37	0.04	0.04
眼	C69	0	0.00	0.00	0.00	0.00	0.00	0	0.00	0.00	0.00	0.00	0.00
脑、神经系统	C70-C72	8	1.65	4.30	3.85	0.26	0.41	23	6.82	14.29	11.09	1.05	1.21
甲状腺	C73	7	1.44	3.76	2.74	0.07	0.37	6	1.78	3.73	2.61	0.23	0.23
肾上腺	C74	1	0.21	0.54	0.22	0.00	0.00	0	0.00	0.00	0.00	0.00	0.00
其他的内分泌腺	C75	0	0.00	0.00	0.00	0.00	0.00	0	0.00	0.00	0.00	0.00	0.00
霍奇金病	C81	3	0.62	1.61	1.36	0.10	0.10	2	0.59	1.24	1.14	0.08	0.08
非霍奇金淋巴瘤	C82-C85;C96	0	0.00	0.00	0.00	0.00	0.00	2	0.59	1.24	1.13	0.05	0.14
免疫增生性疾病	C88	0	0.00	0.00	0.00	0.00	0.00	0	0.00	0.00	0.00	0.00	0.00
多发性骨髓瘤	C90	0	0.00	0.00	0.00	0.00	0.00	1	0.30	0.62	0.41	0.05	0.05
淋巴样白血病	C91	0	0.00	0.00	0.00	0.00	0.00	0	0.00	0.00	0.00	0.00	0.00
髓样白血病	C92-C94	3	0.62	1.61	1.66	0.11	0.11	1	0.30	0.62	0.44	0.06	0.06
白血病，未特指	C95	0	0.00	0.00	0.00	0.00	0.00	0	0.00	0.00	0.00	0.00	0.00
其他的或未指明部位的	O&U	18	3.70	9.68	7.34	0.55	0.98	7	2.08	4.35	4.16	0.32	0.32
骨髓增殖性疾病	MPD	0	0.00	0.00	0.00	0.00	0.00	0	0.00	0.00	0.00	0.00	0.00
骨髓增生异常综合征	MDS	0	0.00	0.00	0.00	0.00	0.00	0	0.00	0.00	0.00	0.00	0.00
合计	ALL	486	100.00	261.27	184.21	11.26	21.92	337	100.00	209.34	151.40	10.36	16.45
所有部位除外 C44	ALL but C44	484	99.59	260.20	183.53	11.26	21.81	336	99.70	208.72	151.18	10.36	16.45

表 6-2-27a　2014 年河南省睢县恶性肿瘤发病主要指标

部位		男性						女性					
		病例数	构成 (%)	粗率 (1/10⁵)	世标率 (1/10⁵)	累积率 (%) 0~64	累积率 (%) 0~74	病例数	构成 (%)	粗率 (1/10⁵)	世标率 (1/10⁵)	累积率 (%) 0~64	累积率 (%) 0~74
唇	C00	1	0.09	0.23	0.22	0.00	0.05	2	0.19	0.49	0.34	0.02	0.02
舌	C01−C02	2	0.18	0.45	0.37	0.05	0.05	1	0.10	0.24	0.22	0.02	0.02
口	C03−C06	2	0.18	0.45	0.50	0.00	0.10	4	0.38	0.98	0.75	0.02	0.09
唾液腺	C07−C08	2	0.18	0.45	0.41	0.03	0.03	1	0.10	0.24	0.23	0.02	0.02
扁桃体	C09	1	0.09	0.23	0.29	0.00	0.00	1	0.10	0.24	0.17	0.02	0.02
其他的口咽	C10	2	0.18	0.45	0.43	0.05	0.05	0	0.00	0.00	0.00	0.00	0.00
鼻咽	C11	11	0.97	2.49	2.28	0.19	0.24	6	0.58	1.47	1.13	0.13	0.13
喉咽	C12−C13	0	0.00	0.00	0.00	0.00	0.00	0	0.00	0.00	0.00	0.00	0.00
咽，部位不明	C14	0	0.00	0.00	0.00	0.00	0.00	0	0.00	0.00	0.00	0.00	0.00
食管	C15	61	5.36	13.82	12.60	0.69	1.85	65	6.26	15.91	11.28	0.62	1.44
胃	C16	110	9.67	24.92	22.57	1.18	2.74	66	6.35	16.16	11.69	0.76	1.28
小肠	C17	4	0.35	0.91	0.79	0.08	0.08	5	0.48	1.22	0.90	0.07	0.11
结肠	C18	36	3.17	8.15	7.50	0.38	0.97	25	2.41	6.12	4.65	0.33	0.44
直肠	C19−C20	37	3.25	8.38	7.88	0.48	1.03	53	5.10	12.97	9.13	0.50	1.00
肛门	C21	0	0.00	0.00	0.00	0.00	0.00	0	0.00	0.00	0.00	0.00	0.00
肝脏	C22	265	23.31	60.03	52.73	3.97	6.27	90	8.66	22.03	15.48	0.92	1.87
胆囊及其他	C23−C24	23	2.02	5.21	5.05	0.24	0.70	33	3.18	8.08	6.14	0.44	0.71
胰腺	C25	28	2.46	6.34	5.66	0.34	0.63	17	1.64	4.16	2.55	0.09	0.33
鼻、鼻窦及其他	C30−C31	5	0.44	1.13	0.92	0.09	0.09	0	0.00	0.00	0.00	0.00	0.00
喉	C32	17	1.50	3.85	3.62	0.16	0.50	0	0.00	0.00	0.00	0.00	0.00
气管、支气管、肺	C33−C34	310	27.26	70.22	64.50	3.35	9.07	144	13.86	35.25	25.65	1.62	3.00
其他的胸腔器官	C37−C38	1	0.09	0.23	0.16	0.02	0.02	1	0.10	0.24	0.17	0.02	0.02
骨	C40−C41	18	1.58	4.08	3.74	0.20	0.34	9	0.87	2.20	1.52	0.09	0.16
皮肤的黑色素瘤	C43	0	0.00	0.00	0.00	0.00	0.00	0	0.00	0.00	0.00	0.00	0.00
其他的皮肤	C44	8	0.70	1.81	1.80	0.07	0.18	3	0.29	0.73	0.37	0.00	0.04
间皮瘤	C45	0	0.00	0.00	0.00	0.00	0.00	0	0.00	0.00	0.00	0.00	0.00
卡波西肉瘤	C46	0	0.00	0.00	0.00	0.00	0.00	0	0.00	0.00	0.00	0.00	0.00
周围神经、其他结缔组织、软组织	C47;C49	1	0.09	0.23	0.19	0.02	0.02	2	0.19	0.49	0.33	0.02	0.06
乳房	C50	—	—	—	—	—	—	204	19.63	49.94	41.23	3.58	4.22
外阴	C51	—	—	—	—	—	—	1	0.10	0.24	0.11	0.00	0.00
阴道	C52	—	—	—	—	—	—	0	0.00	0.00	0.00	0.00	0.00
子宫颈	C53	—	—	—	—	—	—	62	5.97	15.18	12.45	1.10	1.28
子宫体	C54	—	—	—	—	—	—	51	4.91	12.48	10.32	0.95	1.05
子宫，部位不明	C55	—	—	—	—	—	—	4	0.38	0.98	0.82	0.09	0.09
卵巢	C56	—	—	—	—	—	—	28	2.69	6.85	6.06	0.52	0.55
其他的女性生殖器	C57	—	—	—	—	—	—	0	0.00	0.00	0.00	0.00	0.00
胎盘	C58	—	—	—	—	—	—	0	0.00	0.00	0.00	0.00	0.00
阴茎	C60	2	0.18	0.45	0.29	0.00	0.00	—	—	—	—	—	—
前列腺	C61	5	0.44	1.13	1.06	0.00	0.15	—	—	—	—	—	—
睾丸	C62	4	0.35	0.91	0.77	0.05	0.10	—	—	—	—	—	—
其他的男性生殖器	C63	0	0.00	0.00	0.00	0.00	0.00	—	—	—	—	—	—
肾	C64	16	1.41	3.62	3.68	0.14	0.53	11	1.06	2.69	2.25	0.19	0.23
肾盂	C65	0	0.00	0.00	0.00	0.00	0.00	0	0.00	0.00	0.00	0.00	0.00
输尿管	C66	0	0.00	0.00	0.00	0.00	0.00	1	0.10	0.24	0.23	0.02	0.02
膀胱	C67	22	1.93	4.98	4.14	0.25	0.40	7	0.67	1.71	1.03	0.04	0.04
其他的泌尿器官	C68	0	0.00	0.00	0.00	0.00	0.00	0	0.00	0.00	0.00	0.00	0.00
眼	C69	2	0.18	0.45	0.50	0.03	0.07	0	0.00	0.00	0.00	0.00	0.00
脑、神经系统	C70−C72	56	4.93	12.68	12.66	0.79	1.24	49	4.72	11.99	9.53	0.70	0.97
甲状腺	C73	15	1.32	3.40	2.82	0.22	0.27	39	3.75	9.55	7.75	0.59	0.77
肾上腺	C74	1	0.09	0.23	0.37	0.02	0.02	1	0.10	0.24	0.22	0.02	0.02
其他的内分泌腺	C75	0	0.00	0.00	0.00	0.00	0.00	0	0.00	0.00	0.00	0.00	0.00
霍奇金病	C81	7	0.62	1.59	1.50	0.11	0.22	8	0.77	1.96	1.44	0.07	0.19
非霍奇金淋巴瘤	C82−C85;C96	1	0.09	0.23	0.22	0.03	0.03	0	0.00	0.00	0.00	0.00	0.00
免疫增生性疾病	C88	0	0.00	0.00	0.00	0.00	0.00	0	0.00	0.00	0.00	0.00	0.00
多发性骨髓瘤	C90	1	0.09	0.23	0.22	0.03	0.03	0	0.00	0.00	0.00	0.00	0.00
淋巴样白血病	C91	1	0.09	0.23	0.19	0.02	0.02	3	0.29	0.73	0.51	0.04	0.04
髓样白血病	C92−C94	21	1.85	4.76	5.19	0.27	0.42	8	0.77	1.96	1.40	0.10	0.10
白血病，未特指	C95	36	3.17	8.15	9.16	0.59	0.78	28	2.69	6.85	6.10	0.38	0.57
其他的或未指明部位的	O&U	2	0.18	0.45	0.32	0.02	0.02	6	0.58	1.47	1.21	0.11	0.15
骨髓增殖性疾病	MPD	0	0.00	0.00	0.00	0.00	0.00	0	0.00	0.00	0.00	0.00	0.00
骨髓增生异常综合征	MDS	0	0.00	0.00	0.00	0.00	0.00	0	0.00	0.00	0.00	0.00	0.00
合计	ALL	1 137	100.00	257.55	237.30	14.13	29.32	1039	100.00	254.33	195.36	14.19	21.06
所有部位除外 C44	ALL but C44	1 129	99.30	255.73	235.49	14.06	29.14	1036	99.71	253.60	194.99	14.19	21.02

表 6-2-1b　2014 年河南省郸城县恶性肿瘤死亡主要指标

部位		男性						女性					
		病例数	构成 (%)	粗率 (1/10^5)	世标率 (1/10^5)	累积率 (%) 0~64	0~74	病例数	构成 (%)	粗率 (1/10^5)	世标率 (1/10^5)	累积率 (%) 0~64	0~74
唇	C00	2	0.14	0.28	0.22	0.01	0.01	2	0.17	0.30	0.30	0.03	0.03
舌	C01–C02	4	0.27	0.57	0.61	0.05	0.08	5	0.43	0.75	0.75	0.06	0.09
口	C03–C06	3	0.20	0.42	0.38	0.03	0.03	7	0.60	1.05	1.08	0.07	0.11
唾液腺	C07–C08	3	0.20	0.42	0.41	0.03	0.03	3	0.26	0.45	0.39	0.04	0.04
扁桃体	C09	1	0.07	0.14	0.10	0.00	0.00	1	0.09	0.15	0.20	0.02	0.02
其他的口咽	C10	3	0.20	0.42	0.40	0.01	0.01	3	0.26	0.45	0.49	0.03	0.06
鼻咽	C11	8	0.55	1.13	0.91	0.06	0.12	6	0.52	0.90	1.14	0.10	0.16
喉咽	C12–C13	2	0.14	0.28	0.29	0.02	0.02	0	0.00	0.00	0.00	0.00	0.00
咽，部位不明	C14	4	0.27	0.57	0.48	0.05	0.05	1	0.09	0.15	0.10	0.01	0.01
食管	C15	209	14.25	29.59	33.23	2.06	4.77	158	13.60	23.70	23.34	1.12	3.34
胃	C16	209	14.25	29.59	27.41	1.67	3.20	146	12.56	21.90	20.39	1.31	2.55
小肠	C17	6	0.41	0.85	0.77	0.02	0.12	7	0.60	1.05	1.00	0.06	0.15
结肠	C18	19	1.30	2.69	2.57	0.11	0.21	25	2.15	3.75	3.27	0.22	0.44
直肠	C19–C20	33	2.25	4.67	4.79	0.37	0.53	31	2.67	4.65	4.36	0.28	0.50
肛门	C21	20	1.36	2.83	2.93	0.14	0.34	15	1.29	2.25	1.82	0.16	0.19
肝脏	C22	244	16.63	34.54	34.80	2.90	4.37	154	13.25	23.10	22.33	1.60	2.67
胆囊及其他	C23–C24	8	0.55	1.13	1.01	0.04	0.14	12	1.03	1.80	1.73	0.10	0.19
胰腺	C25	15	1.02	2.12	2.33	0.14	0.33	14	1.20	2.10	2.06	0.07	0.36
鼻、鼻窦及其他	C30–C31	2	0.14	0.28	0.28	0.01	0.04	7	0.60	1.05	1.05	0.05	0.14
喉	C32	19	1.30	2.69	2.64	0.13	0.33	11	0.95	1.65	1.57	0.10	0.22
气管、支气管、肺	C33–C34	475	32.38	67.25	70.77	3.88	9.49	177	15.23	26.55	26.23	1.69	3.34
其他的胸腔器官	C37–C38	4	0.27	0.57	0.62	0.03	0.10	7	0.60	1.05	0.91	0.06	0.13
骨	C40–C41	5	0.34	0.71	0.61	0.03	0.07	5	0.43	0.75	0.69	0.08	0.08
皮肤的黑色素瘤	C43	1	0.07	0.14	0.14	0.00	0.03	1	0.09	0.15	0.13	0.00	0.03
其他的皮肤	C44	8	0.55	1.13	0.90	0.03	0.10	7	0.60	1.05	0.97	0.03	0.13
间皮瘤	C45	1	0.07	0.14	0.12	0.00	0.00	0	0.00	0.00	0.00	0.00	0.00
卡波西肉瘤	C46	0	0.00	0.00	0.00	0.00	0.00	0	0.00	0.00	0.00	0.00	0.00
周围神经、其他结缔组织、软组织	C47;C49	2	0.14	0.28	0.26	0.00	0.03	1	0.09	0.15	0.10	0.01	0.01
乳房	C50	—	—	—	—	—	—	150	12.91	22.50	18.10	1.47	2.14
外阴	C51	—	—	—	—	—	—	1	0.09	0.15	0.12	0.01	0.01
阴道	C52	—	—	—	—	—	—	1	0.09	0.15	0.18	0.00	0.03
子宫颈	C53	—	—	—	—	—	—	38	3.27	5.70	4.71	0.35	0.50
子宫体	C54	—	—	—	—	—	—	13	1.12	1.95	1.95	0.22	0.22
子宫，部位不明	C55	—	—	—	—	—	—	15	1.29	2.25	2.21	0.19	0.25
卵巢	C56	—	—	—	—	—	—	30	2.58	4.50	4.07	0.23	0.49
其他的女性生殖器	C57	—	—	—	—	—	—	7	0.60	1.05	0.94	0.05	0.15
胎盘	C58	—	—	—	—	—	—	1	0.09	0.15	0.10	0.01	0.01
阴茎	C60	3	0.20	0.42	0.44	0.01	0.08	—	—	—	—	—	—
前列腺	C61	8	0.55	1.13	1.12	0.06	0.06	—	—	—	—	—	—
睾丸	C62	3	0.20	0.42	0.49	0.03	0.06	—	—	—	—	—	—
其他的男性生殖器	C63	2	0.14	0.28	0.20	0.01	0.01	—	—	—	—	—	—
肾	C64	7	0.48	0.99	1.03	0.10	0.10	4	0.34	0.60	0.46	0.04	0.04
肾盂	C65	2	0.14	0.28	0.19	0.01	0.01	1	0.09	0.15	0.12	0.01	0.01
输尿管	C66	4	0.27	0.57	0.67	0.02	0.09	1	0.09	0.15	0.13	0.00	0.03
膀胱	C67	9	0.61	1.27	1.39	0.03	0.18	7	0.60	1.05	1.11	0.07	0.10
其他的泌尿器官	C68	1	0.07	0.14	0.19	0.02	0.02	1	0.09	0.15	0.17	0.00	0.00
眼	C69	1	0.07	0.14	0.19	0.00	0.03	1	0.09	0.15	0.13	0.00	0.03
脑、神经系统	C70–C72	33	2.25	4.67	4.43	0.30	0.46	26	2.24	3.90	3.81	0.27	0.49
甲状腺	C73	7	0.48	0.99	0.87	0.08	0.08	9	0.77	1.35	1.27	0.05	0.17
肾上腺	C74	2	0.14	0.28	0.22	0.01	0.01	1	0.09	0.15	0.18	0.00	0.03
其他的内分泌腺	C75	1	0.07	0.14	0.12	0.00	0.00	0	0.00	0.00	0.00	0.00	0.00
霍奇金病	C81	2	0.14	0.28	0.38	0.05	0.05	1	0.09	0.15	0.10	0.00	0.00
非霍奇金淋巴瘤	C82–C85;C96	10	0.68	1.42	1.15	0.05	0.15	4	0.34	0.60	0.53	0.03	0.07
免疫增生性疾病	C88	0	0.00	0.00	0.00	0.00	0.00	0	0.00	0.00	0.00	0.00	0.00
多发性骨髓瘤	C90	5	0.34	0.71	0.71	0.06	0.09	3	0.26	0.45	0.49	0.00	0.09
淋巴样白血病	C91	6	0.41	0.85	0.76	0.05	0.05	5	0.43	0.75	0.64	0.02	0.02
髓样白血病	C92–C94	19	1.30	2.69	2.25	0.19	0.25	10	0.86	1.50	1.24	0.07	0.10
白血病，未特指	C95	18	1.23	2.55	3.82	0.20	0.23	15	1.29	2.25	3.93	0.21	0.21
其他的或未指明部位的	O&U	13	0.89	1.84	1.88	0.13	0.16	11	0.95	1.65	1.57	0.06	0.21
骨髓增殖性疾病	MPD	0	0.00	0.00	0.00	0.00	0.00	0	0.00	0.00	0.00	0.00	0.00
骨髓增生异常综合征	MDS	0	0.00	0.00	0.00	0.00	0.00	0	0.00	0.00	0.00	0.00	0.00
合计	ALL	1 467	100.00	207.69	212.62	13.25	26.75	1162	100.00	174.29	164.66	10.68	20.40
所有部位除外 C44	ALL but C44	1 459	99.45	206.55	211.72	13.22	26.65	1155	99.40	173.24	163.70	10.65	20.27

表 6-2-2b 2014 年河南省方城县恶性肿瘤死亡主要指标

部位		男性						女性					
		病例数	构成 (%)	粗率 (1/10^5)	世标率 (1/10^5)	累积率 (%) 0~64	累积率 (%) 0~74	病例数	构成 (%)	粗率 (1/10^5)	世标率 (1/10^5)	累积率 (%) 0~64	累积率 (%) 0~74
唇	C00	0	0.00	0.00	0.00	0.00	0.00	1	0.25	0.19	0.10	0.00	0.00
舌	C01–C02	0	0.00	0.00	0.00	0.00	0.00	1	0.25	0.19	0.18	0.00	0.04
口	C03–C06	2	0.24	0.33	0.22	0.00	0.02	1	0.25	0.19	0.17	0.00	0.03
唾液腺	C07–C08	0	0.00	0.00	0.00	0.00	0.00	0	0.00	0.00	0.00	0.00	0.00
扁桃体	C09	0	0.00	0.00	0.00	0.00	0.00	0	0.00	0.00	0.00	0.00	0.00
其他的口咽	C10	0	0.00	0.00	0.00	0.00	0.00	0	0.00	0.00	0.00	0.00	0.00
鼻咽	C11	6	0.71	1.00	0.82	0.03	0.09	0	0.00	0.00	0.00	0.00	0.00
喉咽	C12–C13	0	0.00	0.00	0.00	0.00	0.00	1	0.25	0.19	0.10	0.00	0.00
咽，部位不明	C14	1	0.12	0.17	0.13	0.00	0.02	1	0.25	0.19	0.18	0.00	0.04
食管	C15	84	9.91	14.05	9.72	0.31	1.01	26	6.53	4.84	3.09	0.04	0.31
胃	C16	174	20.52	29.10	20.85	0.99	2.29	59	14.82	10.98	7.65	0.32	0.79
小肠	C17	4	0.47	0.67	0.49	0.00	0.07	0	0.00	0.00	0.00	0.00	0.00
结肠	C18	11	1.30	1.84	1.37	0.07	0.19	9	2.26	1.67	1.20	0.07	0.13
直肠	C19–C20	20	2.36	3.34	2.32	0.14	0.24	17	4.27	3.16	2.29	0.07	0.25
肛门	C21	0	0.00	0.00	0.00	0.00	0.00	0	0.00	0.00	0.00	0.00	0.00
肝脏	C22	154	18.16	25.75	20.00	1.40	2.18	53	13.32	9.86	7.29	0.36	0.86
胆囊及其他	C23–C24	4	0.47	0.67	0.51	0.05	0.05	5	1.26	0.93	0.75	0.03	0.09
胰腺	C25	10	1.18	1.67	1.29	0.06	0.14	8	2.01	1.49	1.06	0.02	0.14
鼻、鼻窦及其他	C30–C31	2	0.24	0.33	0.28	0.03	0.03	0	0.00	0.00	0.00	0.00	0.00
喉	C32	0	0.00	0.00	0.00	0.00	0.00	0	0.00	0.00	0.00	0.00	0.00
气管、支气管、肺	C33–C34	242	28.54	40.47	28.96	1.22	3.17	90	22.61	16.74	12.33	0.48	1.60
其他的胸腔器官	C37–C38	1	0.12	0.17	0.14	0.00	0.03	4	1.01	0.74	0.39	0.00	0.04
骨	C40–C41	11	1.30	1.84	1.45	0.08	0.20	8	2.01	1.49	1.20	0.10	0.17
皮肤的黑色素瘤	C43	0	0.00	0.00	0.00	0.00	0.00	0	0.00	0.00	0.00	0.00	0.00
其他的皮肤	C44	2	0.24	0.33	0.21	0.00	0.03	3	0.75	0.56	0.28	0.00	0.00
间皮瘤	C45	0	0.00	0.00	0.00	0.00	0.00	0	0.00	0.00	0.00	0.00	0.00
卡波西肉瘤	C46	0	0.00	0.00	0.00	0.00	0.00	0	0.00	0.00	0.00	0.00	0.00
周围神经、其他结缔组织、软组织	C47;C49	1	0.12	0.17	0.14	0.02	0.02	0	0.00	0.00	0.00	0.00	0.00
乳房	C50	—	—	—	—	—	—	26	6.53	4.84	4.09	0.31	0.59
外阴	C51	—	—	—	—	—	—	1	0.25	0.19	0.10	0.00	0.00
阴道	C52	—	—	—	—	—	—	0	0.00	0.00	0.00	0.00	0.00
子宫颈	C53	—	—	—	—	—	—	11	2.76	2.05	1.55	0.10	0.19
子宫体	C54	—	—	—	—	—	—	1	0.25	0.19	0.14	0.01	0.01
子宫，部位不明	C55	—	—	—	—	—	—	9	2.26	1.67	1.36	0.07	0.21
卵巢	C56	—	—	—	—	—	—	4	1.01	0.74	0.55	0.03	0.08
其他的女性生殖器	C57	—	—	—	—	—	—	0	0.00	0.00	0.00	0.00	0.00
胎盘	C58	—	—	—	—	—	—	0	0.00	0.00	0.00	0.00	0.00
阴茎	C60	1	0.12	0.17	0.14	0.00	0.03	—	—	—	—	—	—
前列腺	C61	8	0.94	1.34	0.83	0.00	0.06	—	—	—	—	—	—
睾丸	C62	0	0.00	0.00	0.00	0.00	0.00	—	—	—	—	—	—
其他的男性生殖器	C63	0	0.00	0.00	0.00	0.00	0.00	—	—	—	—	—	—
肾	C64	0	0.00	0.00	0.00	0.00	0.00	1	0.25	0.19	0.18	0.00	0.04
肾盂	C65	2	0.24	0.33	0.27	0.00	0.06	0	0.00	0.00	0.00	0.00	0.00
输尿管	C66	0	0.00	0.00	0.00	0.00	0.00	0	0.00	0.00	0.00	0.00	0.00
膀胱	C67	6	0.71	1.00	0.79	0.03	0.08	2	0.50	0.37	0.21	0.02	0.02
其他的泌尿器官	C68	0	0.00	0.00	0.00	0.00	0.00	0	0.00	0.00	0.00	0.00	0.00
眼	C69	0	0.00	0.00	0.00	0.00	0.00	0	0.00	0.00	0.00	0.00	0.00
脑、神经系统	C70–C72	19	2.24	3.18	2.41	0.08	0.30	16	4.02	2.98	2.24	0.15	0.24
甲状腺	C73	1	0.12	0.17	0.09	0.00	0.00	3	0.75	0.56	0.39	0.00	0.04
肾上腺	C74	0	0.00	0.00	0.00	0.00	0.00	0	0.00	0.00	0.00	0.00	0.00
其他的内分泌腺	C75	0	0.00	0.00	0.00	0.00	0.00	0	0.00	0.00	0.00	0.00	0.00
霍奇金病	C81	0	0.00	0.00	0.00	0.00	0.00	0	0.00	0.00	0.00	0.00	0.00
非霍奇金淋巴瘤	C82–C85;C96	7	0.83	1.17	0.94	0.05	0.08	0	0.00	0.00	0.00	0.00	0.00
免疫增生性疾病	C88	0	0.00	0.00	0.00	0.00	0.00	0	0.00	0.00	0.00	0.00	0.00
多发性骨髓瘤	C90	6	0.71	1.00	0.85	0.03	0.07	2	0.50	0.37	0.29	0.03	0.03
淋巴样白血病	C91	8	0.94	1.34	1.23	0.07	0.13	4	1.01	0.74	0.72	0.04	0.04
髓样白血病	C92–C94	0	0.00	0.00	0.00	0.00	0.00	1	0.25	0.19	0.14	0.01	0.01
白血病，未特指	C95	2	0.24	0.33	0.28	0.03	0.03	2	0.50	0.37	0.29	0.03	0.03
其他的或未指明部位的	O&U	59	6.96	9.87	7.39	0.50	0.75	28	7.04	5.21	3.76	0.24	0.41
骨髓增殖性疾病	MPD	0	0.00	0.00	0.00	0.00	0.00	0	0.00	0.00	0.00	0.00	0.00
骨髓增生异常综合征	MDS	0	0.00	0.00	0.00	0.00	0.00	0	0.00	0.00	0.00	0.00	0.00
合计	ALL	848	100.00	141.80	104.12	5.18	11.38	398	100.00	74.05	54.28	2.53	6.45
所有部位除外 C44	ALL but C44	846	99.76	141.47	103.91	5.18	11.35	395	99.25	73.49	54.00	2.53	6.45

表 6-2-3b　2014 年河南省鹤壁市恶性肿瘤死亡主要指标

部位		男性						女性					
		病例数	构成	粗率	世标率	累积率 (%)		病例数	构成	粗率	世标率	累积率 (%)	
			(%)	(1/10⁵)	(1/10⁵)	0~64	0~74		(%)	(1/10⁵)	(1/10⁵)	0~64	0~74
唇	C00	0	0.00	0.00	0.00	0.00	0.00	0	0.00	0.00	0.00	0.00	0.00
舌	C01–C02	1	0.16	0.31	0.32	0.00	0.05	2	0.49	0.64	0.54	0.02	0.07
口	C03–C06	3	0.47	0.92	0.79	0.03	0.11	1	0.24	0.32	0.30	0.00	0.05
唾液腺	C07–C08	1	0.16	0.31	0.21	0.00	0.00	0	0.00	0.00	0.00	0.00	0.00
扁桃体	C09	0	0.00	0.00	0.00	0.00	0.00	0	0.00	0.00	0.00	0.00	0.00
其他的口咽	C10	1	0.16	0.31	0.20	0.02	0.02	0	0.00	0.00	0.00	0.00	0.00
鼻咽	C11	1	0.16	0.31	0.32	0.00	0.05	1	0.24	0.32	0.26	0.03	0.03
喉咽	C12–C13	0	0.00	0.00	0.00	0.00	0.00	2	0.49	0.64	0.51	0.02	0.07
咽，部位不明	C14	1	0.16	0.31	0.21	0.00	0.00	0	0.00	0.00	0.00	0.00	0.00
食管	C15	157	24.84	48.40	41.50	1.88	4.89	98	23.90	31.57	24.03	1.06	2.85
胃	C16	108	17.09	33.29	28.17	1.07	3.60	53	12.93	17.07	12.60	0.40	1.39
小肠	C17	3	0.47	0.92	0.95	0.04	0.04	0	0.00	0.00	0.00	0.00	0.00
结肠	C18	22	3.48	6.78	5.34	0.34	0.45	23	5.61	7.41	5.57	0.21	0.66
直肠	C19–C20	15	2.37	4.62	4.08	0.18	0.50	4	0.98	1.29	0.97	0.10	0.10
肛门	C21	0	0.00	0.00	0.00	0.00	0.00	3	0.73	0.97	0.67	0.03	0.09
肝脏	C22	72	11.39	22.20	18.39	1.16	2.07	31	7.56	9.99	7.37	0.42	0.90
胆囊及其他	C23–C24	5	0.79	1.54	1.48	0.07	0.28	7	1.71	2.25	1.83	0.08	0.31
胰腺	C25	10	1.58	3.08	2.89	0.11	0.40	9	2.20	2.90	2.24	0.16	0.26
鼻、鼻窦及其他	C30–C31	0	0.00	0.00	0.00	0.00	0.00	0	0.00	0.00	0.00	0.00	0.00
喉	C32	3	0.47	0.92	0.63	0.02	0.02	0	0.00	0.00	0.00	0.00	0.00
气管、支气管、肺	C33–C34	159	25.16	49.02	42.09	1.88	5.16	63	15.37	20.29	14.92	0.71	1.76
其他的胸腔器官	C37–C38	1	0.16	0.31	0.23	0.02	0.02	0	0.00	0.00	0.00	0.00	0.00
骨	C40–C41	4	0.63	1.23	1.05	0.10	0.10	2	0.49	0.64	0.44	0.00	0.00
皮肤的黑色素瘤	C43	1	0.16	0.31	0.53	0.00	0.00	0	0.00	0.00	0.00	0.00	0.00
其他的皮肤	C44	1	0.16	0.31	0.24	0.03	0.03	0	0.00	0.00	0.00	0.00	0.00
间皮瘤	C45	0	0.00	0.00	0.00	0.00	0.00	2	0.49	0.64	0.38	0.02	0.02
卡波西肉瘤	C46	0	0.00	0.00	0.00	0.00	0.00	0	0.00	0.00	0.00	0.00	0.00
周围神经、其他结缔组织、软组织	C47;C49	0	0.00	0.00	0.00	0.00	0.00	0	0.00	0.00	0.00	0.00	0.00
乳房	C50	—	—	—	—	—	—	31	7.56	9.99	7.27	0.61	0.71
外阴	C51	—	—	—	—	—	—	2	0.49	0.64	0.52	0.03	0.10
阴道	C52	—	—	—	—	—	—	0	0.00	0.00	0.00	0.00	0.00
子宫颈	C53	—	—	—	—	—	—	16	3.90	5.15	3.74	0.37	0.37
子宫体	C54	—	—	—	—	—	—	7	1.71	2.25	1.73	0.16	0.16
子宫，部位不明	C55	—	—	—	—	—	—	1	0.24	0.32	0.22	0.02	0.02
卵巢	C56	—	—	—	—	—	—	9	2.20	2.90	2.01	0.12	0.25
其他的女性生殖器	C57	—	—	—	—	—	—	0	0.00	0.00	0.00	0.00	0.00
胎盘	C58	—	—	—	—	—	—	0	0.00	0.00	0.00	0.00	0.00
阴茎	C60	1	0.16	0.31	0.21	0.00	0.00	—	—	—	—	—	—
前列腺	C61	7	1.11	2.16	1.87	0.03	0.03	—	—	—	—	—	—
睾丸	C62	0	0.00	0.00	0.00	0.00	0.00	—	—	—	—	—	—
其他的男性生殖器	C63	0	0.00	0.00	0.00	0.00	0.00	—	—	—	—	—	—
肾	C64	4	0.63	1.23	1.14	0.05	0.18	3	0.73	0.97	0.75	0.02	0.15
肾盂	C65	2	0.32	0.62	0.62	0.00	0.16	0	0.00	0.00	0.00	0.00	0.00
输尿管	C66	1	0.16	0.31	0.27	0.03	0.03	2	0.49	0.64	0.68	0.02	0.09
膀胱	C67	3	0.47	0.92	0.82	0.06	0.12	1	0.24	0.32	0.22	0.02	0.02
其他的泌尿器官	C68	0	0.00	0.00	0.00	0.00	0.00	0	0.00	0.00	0.00	0.00	0.00
眼	C69	0	0.00	0.00	0.00	0.00	0.00	1	0.24	0.32	0.42	0.02	0.02
脑、神经系统	C70–C72	18	2.85	5.55	4.68	0.21	0.44	9	2.20	2.90	2.33	0.24	0.24
甲状腺	C73	0	0.00	0.00	0.00	0.00	0.00	6	1.46	1.93	1.84	0.06	0.28
肾上腺	C74	1	0.16	0.31	0.27	0.03	0.03	1	0.24	0.32	0.25	0.00	0.06
其他的内分泌腺	C75	0	0.00	0.00	0.00	0.00	0.00	0	0.00	0.00	0.00	0.00	0.00
霍奇金病	C81	0	0.00	0.00	0.00	0.00	0.00	3	0.73	0.97	0.64	0.02	0.08
非霍奇金淋巴瘤	C82–C85;C96	1	0.16	0.31	0.31	0.00	0.08	0	0.00	0.00	0.00	0.00	0.00
免疫增生性疾病	C88	0	0.00	0.00	0.00	0.00	0.00	0	0.00	0.00	0.00	0.00	0.00
多发性骨髓瘤	C90	0	0.00	0.00	0.00	0.00	0.00	0	0.00	0.00	0.00	0.00	0.00
淋巴样白血病	C91	4	0.63	1.23	1.33	0.08	0.08	4	0.98	1.29	0.98	0.09	0.09
髓样白血病	C92–C94	2	0.32	0.62	0.64	0.05	0.05	2	0.49	0.64	0.87	0.06	0.06
白血病，未特指	C95	8	1.27	2.47	2.72	0.11	0.32	10	2.44	3.22	2.53	0.12	0.17
其他的或未指明部位的	O&U	11	1.74	3.39	2.93	0.13	0.28	1	0.24	0.32	0.18	0.00	0.00
骨髓增殖性疾病	MPD	0	0.00	0.00	0.00	0.00	0.00	0	0.00	0.00	0.00	0.00	0.00
骨髓增生异常综合征	MDS	0	0.00	0.00	0.00	0.00	0.00	0	0.00	0.00	0.00	0.00	0.00
合计	ALL	632	100.00	194.84	167.44	7.73	19.58	410	100.00	132.06	99.81	5.27	11.44
所有部位除外 C44	ALL but C44	631	99.84	194.53	167.20	7.70	19.55	410	100.00	132.06	99.81	5.27	11.44

表 6-2-4b　2014 年河南省辉县市恶性肿瘤死亡主要指标

部位		男性						女性					
		病例数	构成 (%)	粗率 ($1/10^5$)	世标率 ($1/10^5$)	累积率 (%) 0~64	累积率 (%) 0~74	病例数	构成 (%)	粗率 ($1/10^5$)	世标率 ($1/10^5$)	累积率 (%) 0~64	累积率 (%) 0~74
唇	C00	0	0.00	0.00	0.00	0.00	0.00	0	0.00	0.00	0.00	0.00	0.00
舌	C01–C02	1	0.11	0.23	0.26	0.02	0.02	0	0.00	0.00	0.00	0.00	0.00
口	C03–C06	3	0.33	0.70	0.56	0.02	0.08	3	0.58	0.70	0.50	0.00	0.08
唾液腺	C07–C08	0	0.00	0.00	0.00	0.00	0.00	0	0.00	0.00	0.00	0.00	0.00
扁桃体	C09	0	0.00	0.00	0.00	0.00	0.00	0	0.00	0.00	0.00	0.00	0.00
其他的口咽	C10	0	0.00	0.00	0.00	0.00	0.00	0	0.00	0.00	0.00	0.00	0.00
鼻咽	C11	4	0.44	0.93	0.70	0.04	0.07	0	0.00	0.00	0.00	0.00	0.00
喉咽	C12–C13	1	0.11	0.23	0.14	0.02	0.02	0	0.00	0.00	0.00	0.00	0.00
咽，部位不明	C14	2	0.22	0.47	0.38	0.02	0.08	1	0.19	0.23	0.10	0.00	0.00
食管	C15	311	34.25	72.37	58.86	2.21	6.68	182	35.14	42.66	28.26	0.79	3.19
胃	C16	193	21.26	44.91	35.77	1.21	4.20	77	14.86	18.05	12.08	0.31	1.58
小肠	C17	3	0.33	0.70	0.47	0.03	0.03	2	0.39	0.47	0.33	0.02	0.05
结肠	C18	17	1.87	3.96	2.97	0.16	0.30	15	2.90	3.52	2.30	0.14	0.21
直肠	C19–C20	19	2.09	4.42	3.62	0.17	0.51	13	2.51	3.05	1.93	0.11	0.16
肛门	C21	0	0.00	0.00	0.00	0.00	0.00	0	0.00	0.00	0.00	0.00	0.00
肝脏	C22	112	12.33	26.06	20.04	1.29	2.34	42	8.11	9.84	6.24	0.29	0.64
胆囊及其他	C23–C24	6	0.66	1.40	1.24	0.06	0.22	7	1.35	1.64	0.93	0.02	0.07
胰腺	C25	14	1.54	3.26	2.51	0.15	0.19	9	1.74	2.11	1.53	0.03	0.24
鼻、鼻窦及其他	C30–C31	1	0.11	0.23	0.38	0.02	0.02	1	0.19	0.23	0.14	0.02	0.02
喉	C32	2	0.22	0.47	0.38	0.02	0.08	0	0.00	0.00	0.00	0.00	0.00
气管、支气管、肺	C33–C34	122	13.44	28.39	22.37	1.13	2.74	63	12.16	14.77	9.66	0.41	0.92
其他的胸腔器官	C37–C38	4	0.44	0.93	1.10	0.07	0.07	0	0.00	0.00	0.00	0.00	0.00
骨	C40–C41	5	0.55	1.16	0.83	0.04	0.07	6	1.16	1.41	0.87	0.09	0.09
皮肤的黑色素瘤	C43	1	0.11	0.23	0.18	0.02	0.02	1	0.19	0.23	0.20	0.01	0.01
其他的皮肤	C44	1	0.11	0.23	0.13	0.00	0.00	1	0.19	0.23	0.14	0.02	0.02
间皮瘤	C45	0	0.00	0.00	0.00	0.00	0.00	0	0.00	0.00	0.00	0.00	0.00
卡波西肉瘤	C46	0	0.00	0.00	0.00	0.00	0.00	0	0.00	0.00	0.00	0.00	0.00
周围神经、其他结缔组织、软组织	C47;C49	0	0.00	0.00	0.00	0.00	0.00	1	0.19	0.23	0.17	0.02	0.02
乳房	C50	—	—	—	—	—	—	25	4.83	5.86	4.34	0.37	0.55
外阴	C51	—	—	—	—	—	—	0	0.00	0.00	0.00	0.00	0.00
阴道	C52	—	—	—	—	—	—	0	0.00	0.00	0.00	0.00	0.00
子宫颈	C53	—	—	—	—	—	—	11	2.12	2.58	2.00	0.12	0.24
子宫体	C54	—	—	—	—	—	—	3	0.58	0.70	0.56	0.02	0.12
子宫，部位不明	C55	—	—	—	—	—	—	13	2.51	3.05	2.34	0.14	0.34
卵巢	C56	—	—	—	—	—	—	3	0.58	0.70	0.48	0.06	0.06
其他的女性生殖器	C57	—	—	—	—	—	—	0	0.00	0.00	0.00	0.00	0.00
胎盘	C58	—	—	—	—	—	—	0	0.00	0.00	0.00	0.00	0.00
阴茎	C60	3	0.33	0.70	0.58	0.00	0.07	—	—	—	—	—	—
前列腺	C61	5	0.55	1.16	0.72	0.02	0.02	—	—	—	—	—	—
睾丸	C62	1	0.11	0.23	0.18	0.02	0.02	—	—	—	—	—	—
其他的男性生殖器	C63	0	0.00	0.00	0.00	0.00	0.00	—	—	—	—	—	—
肾	C64	11	1.21	2.56	1.81	0.13	0.19	0	0.00	0.00	0.00	0.00	0.00
肾盂	C65	0	0.00	0.00	0.00	0.00	0.00	0	0.00	0.00	0.00	0.00	0.00
输尿管	C66	1	0.11	0.23	0.14	0.02	0.02	1	0.19	0.23	0.20	0.00	0.03
膀胱	C67	5	0.55	1.16	1.00	0.06	0.16	0	0.00	0.00	0.00	0.00	0.00
其他的泌尿器官	C68	0	0.00	0.00	0.00	0.00	0.00	0	0.00	0.00	0.00	0.00	0.00
眼	C69	0	0.00	0.00	0.00	0.00	0.00	0	0.00	0.00	0.00	0.00	0.00
脑、神经系统	C70–C72	19	2.09	4.42	4.07	0.17	0.48	13	2.51	3.05	2.91	0.15	0.35
甲状腺	C73	2	0.22	0.47	0.46	0.00	0.10	0	0.00	0.00	0.00	0.00	0.00
肾上腺	C74	0	0.00	0.00	0.00	0.00	0.00	0	0.00	0.00	0.00	0.00	0.00
其他的内分泌腺	C75	0	0.00	0.00	0.00	0.00	0.00	0	0.00	0.00	0.00	0.00	0.00
霍奇金病	C81	0	0.00	0.00	0.00	0.00	0.00	0	0.00	0.00	0.00	0.00	0.00
非霍奇金淋巴瘤	C82–C85;C96	10	1.10	2.33	2.02	0.10	0.38	6	1.16	1.41	1.01	0.05	0.15
免疫增生性疾病	C88	0	0.00	0.00	0.00	0.00	0.00	0	0.00	0.00	0.00	0.00	0.00
多发性骨髓瘤	C90	5	0.55	1.16	0.87	0.08	0.08	4	0.77	0.94	0.63	0.04	0.08
淋巴样白血病	C91	1	0.11	0.23	0.22	0.00	0.04	0	0.00	0.00	0.00	0.00	0.00
髓样白血病	C92–C94	7	0.77	1.63	1.18	0.05	0.08	5	0.97	1.17	1.05	0.09	0.09
白血病，未特指	C95	9	0.99	2.09	2.38	0.15	0.22	7	1.35	1.64	1.29	0.05	0.13
其他的或未指明部位的	O&U	5	0.55	1.16	1.12	0.04	0.11	2	0.39	0.47	0.23	0.00	0.00
骨髓增殖性疾病	MPD	0	0.00	0.00	0.00	0.00	0.00	0	0.00	0.00	0.00	0.00	0.00
骨髓增生异常综合征	MDS	2	0.22	0.47	0.44	0.02	0.02	1	0.19	0.23	0.10	0.00	0.00
合计	ALL	908	100.00	211.28	170.10	7.56	19.74	518	100.00	121.40	82.52	3.36	9.45
所有部位除外 C44	ALL but C44	907	99.89	211.05	169.97	7.56	19.74	517	99.81	121.17	82.39	3.34	9.44

表 6-2-5b　2014 年河南省济源市恶性肿瘤死亡主要指标

部位		男性						女性					
		病例数	构成 (%)	粗率 (1/10⁵)	世标率 (1/10⁵)	累积率 (%) 0~64	累积率 (%) 0~74	病例数	构成 (%)	粗率 (1/10⁵)	世标率 (1/10⁵)	累积率 (%) 0~64	累积率 (%) 0~74
唇	C00	1	0.15	0.28	0.41	0.00	0.00	0	0.00	0.00	0.00	0.00	0.00
舌	C01–C02	0	0.00	0.00	0.00	0.00	0.00	0	0.00	0.00	0.00	0.00	0.00
口	C03–C06	1	0.15	0.28	0.19	0.02	0.02	2	0.52	0.59	0.38	0.00	0.00
唾液腺	C07–C08	1	0.15	0.28	0.29	0.00	0.05	0	0.00	0.00	0.00	0.00	0.00
扁桃体	C09	0	0.00	0.00	0.00	0.00	0.00	0	0.00	0.00	0.00	0.00	0.00
其他的口咽	C10	0	0.00	0.00	0.00	0.00	0.00	0	0.00	0.00	0.00	0.00	0.00
鼻咽	C11	2	0.30	0.56	0.67	0.03	0.03	0	0.00	0.00	0.00	0.00	0.00
喉咽	C12–C13	0	0.00	0.00	0.00	0.00	0.00	0	0.00	0.00	0.00	0.00	0.00
咽，部位不明	C14	0	0.00	0.00	0.00	0.00	0.00	1	0.26	0.29	0.29	0.03	0.03
食管	C15	100	14.84	27.81	27.84	1.50	2.79	66	17.23	19.35	16.65	0.68	1.34
胃	C16	239	35.46	66.46	66.20	3.16	6.77	85	22.19	24.92	21.35	1.00	1.91
小肠	C17	1	0.15	0.28	0.23	0.00	0.00	1	0.26	0.29	0.17	0.00	0.00
结肠	C18	17	2.52	4.73	4.67	0.14	0.40	9	2.35	2.64	2.39	0.10	0.27
直肠	C19–C20	21	3.12	5.84	5.48	0.43	0.47	8	2.09	2.35	1.91	0.16	0.16
肛门	C21	0	0.00	0.00	0.00	0.00	0.00	0	0.00	0.00	0.00	0.00	0.00
肝脏	C22	74	10.98	20.58	20.96	1.17	2.32	27	7.05	7.92	6.33	0.30	0.48
胆囊及其他	C23–C24	8	1.19	2.22	2.46	0.16	0.27	8	2.09	2.35	2.06	0.07	0.12
胰腺	C25	17	2.52	4.73	4.65	0.22	0.41	11	2.87	3.23	2.94	0.15	0.25
鼻、鼻窦及其他	C30–C31	0	0.00	0.00	0.00	0.00	0.00	0	0.00	0.00	0.00	0.00	0.00
喉	C32	4	0.59	1.11	1.13	0.08	0.13	1	0.26	0.29	0.17	0.01	0.01
气管、支气管、肺	C33–C34	101	14.99	28.09	28.35	1.23	3.25	48	12.53	14.07	12.23	0.65	1.16
其他的胸腔器官	C37–C38	1	0.15	0.28	0.27	0.03	0.03	0	0.00	0.00	0.00	0.00	0.00
骨	C40–C41	12	1.78	3.34	3.57	0.28	0.38	5	1.31	1.47	1.43	0.11	0.18
皮肤的黑色素瘤	C43	0	0.00	0.00	0.00	0.00	0.00	1	0.26	0.29	0.19	0.00	0.00
其他的皮肤	C44	1	0.15	0.28	0.32	0.04	0.04	1	0.26	0.29	0.35	0.04	0.04
间皮瘤	C45	0	0.00	0.00	0.00	0.00	0.00	0	0.00	0.00	0.00	0.00	0.00
卡波西肉瘤	C46	0	0.00	0.00	0.00	0.00	0.00	0	0.00	0.00	0.00	0.00	0.00
周围神经、其他结缔组织、软组织	C47;C49	0	0.00	0.00	0.00	0.00	0.00	0	0.00	0.00	0.00	0.00	0.00
乳房	C50	—	—	—	—	—	—	18	4.70	5.28	4.85	0.41	0.47
外阴	C51	—	—	—	—	—	—	0	0.00	0.00	0.00	0.00	0.00
阴道	C52	—	—	—	—	—	—	0	0.00	0.00	0.00	0.00	0.00
子宫颈	C53	—	—	—	—	—	—	14	3.66	4.10	3.90	0.29	0.34
子宫体	C54	—	—	—	—	—	—	3	0.78	0.88	0.87	0.06	0.11
子宫，部位不明	C55	—	—	—	—	—	—	9	2.35	2.64	2.44	0.18	0.25
卵巢	C56	—	—	—	—	—	—	10	2.61	2.93	2.71	0.20	0.33
其他的女性生殖器	C57	—	—	—	—	—	—	0	0.00	0.00	0.00	0.00	0.00
胎盘	C58	—	—	—	—	—	—	0	0.00	0.00	0.00	0.00	0.00
阴茎	C60	0	0.00	0.00	0.00	0.00	0.00	—	—	—	—	—	—
前列腺	C61	10	1.48	2.78	2.88	0.08	0.40	—	—	—	—	—	—
睾丸	C62	1	0.15	0.28	0.29	0.00	0.05	—	—	—	—	—	—
其他的男性生殖器	C63	0	0.00	0.00	0.00	0.00	0.00	—	—	—	—	—	—
肾	C64	4	0.59	1.11	0.94	0.00	0.00	3	0.78	0.88	0.79	0.00	0.10
肾盂	C65	1	0.15	0.28	0.24	0.00	0.00	2	0.52	0.59	0.56	0.06	0.06
输尿管	C66	0	0.00	0.00	0.00	0.00	0.00	1	0.26	0.29	0.35	0.04	0.04
膀胱	C67	6	0.89	1.67	1.55	0.05	0.10	1	0.26	0.29	0.17	0.00	0.00
其他的泌尿器官	C68	1	0.15	0.28	0.32	0.04	0.04	0	0.00	0.00	0.00	0.00	0.00
眼	C69	0	0.00	0.00	0.00	0.00	0.00	1	0.26	0.29	0.28	0.00	0.00
脑、神经系统	C70–C72	18	2.67	5.01	4.84	0.38	0.50	14	3.66	4.10	3.91	0.29	0.34
甲状腺	C73	0	0.00	0.00	0.00	0.00	0.00	2	0.52	0.59	0.58	0.00	0.05
肾上腺	C74	1	0.15	0.28	0.27	0.03	0.03	1	0.26	0.29	0.26	0.00	0.06
其他的内分泌腺	C75	0	0.00	0.00	0.00	0.00	0.00	1	0.26	0.29	0.20	0.02	0.02
霍奇金病	C81	0	0.00	0.00	0.00	0.00	0.00	1	0.26	0.29	0.17	0.00	0.00
非霍奇金淋巴瘤	C82–C85;C96	3	0.45	0.83	0.64	0.03	0.03	7	1.83	2.05	1.88	0.10	0.20
免疫增生性疾病	C88	0	0.00	0.00	0.00	0.00	0.00	0	0.00	0.00	0.00	0.00	0.00
多发性骨髓瘤	C90	1	0.15	0.28	0.29	0.04	0.04	1	0.26	0.29	0.25	0.02	0.02
淋巴样白血病	C91	4	0.59	1.11	0.89	0.06	0.13	8	2.09	2.35	2.52	0.16	0.23
髓样白血病	C92–C94	5	0.74	1.39	1.89	0.13	0.13	0	0.00	0.00	0.00	0.00	0.00
白血病，未特指	C95	11	1.63	3.06	3.31	0.32	0.37	3	0.78	0.88	0.80	0.06	0.06
其他的或未指明部位的	O&U	7	1.04	1.95	1.97	0.10	0.33	9	2.35	2.64	2.23	0.13	0.19
骨髓增殖性疾病	MPD	0	0.00	0.00	0.00	0.00	0.00	0	0.00	0.00	0.00	0.00	0.00
骨髓增生异常综合征	MDS	0	0.00	0.00	0.00	0.00	0.00	0	0.00	0.00	0.00	0.00	0.00
合计	ALL	674	100.00	187.42	187.99	9.71	19.51	383	100.00	112.29	98.51	5.32	8.82
所有部位除外 C44	ALL but C44	673	99.85	187.15	187.67	9.67	19.47	382	99.74	112.00	98.16	5.28	8.77

表 6-2-6b 2014 年河南省林州市恶性肿瘤死亡主要指标

部位		男性						女性					
		病例数	构成 (%)	粗率 ($1/10^5$)	世标率 ($1/10^5$)	累积率 (%)		病例数	构成 (%)	粗率 ($1/10^5$)	世标率 ($1/10^5$)	累积率 (%)	
						0~64	0~74					0~64	0~74
唇	C00	0	0.00	0.00	0.00	0.00	0.00	2	0.23	0.37	0.23	0.01	0.01
舌	C01–C02	2	0.15	0.36	0.28	0.01	0.03	0	0.00	0.00	0.00	0.00	0.00
口	C03–C06	3	0.23	0.54	0.51	0.01	0.01	2	0.23	0.37	0.25	0.03	0.03
唾液腺	C07–C08	0	0.00	0.00	0.00	0.00	0.00	1	0.11	0.19	0.12	0.01	0.01
扁桃体	C09	0	0.00	0.00	0.00	0.00	0.00	0	0.00	0.00	0.00	0.00	0.00
其他的口咽	C10	0	0.00	0.00	0.00	0.00	0.00	1	0.11	0.19	0.13	0.02	0.02
鼻咽	C11	1	0.08	0.18	0.15	0.01	0.01	0	0.00	0.00	0.00	0.00	0.00
喉咽	C12–C13	4	0.31	0.72	0.58	0.03	0.07	0	0.00	0.00	0.00	0.00	0.00
咽，部位不明	C14	1	0.08	0.18	0.13	0.00	0.02	0	0.00	0.00	0.00	0.00	0.00
食管	C15	376	28.79	67.41	55.03	2.12	6.52	256	29.36	47.77	30.10	1.26	3.44
胃	C16	475	36.37	85.16	68.63	3.41	8.93	204	23.39	38.06	24.50	1.16	2.89
小肠	C17	2	0.15	0.36	0.27	0.03	0.03	4	0.46	0.75	0.47	0.04	0.04
结肠	C18	14	1.07	2.51	2.05	0.12	0.14	22	2.52	4.11	2.78	0.15	0.26
直肠	C19–C20	30	2.30	5.38	4.46	0.21	0.44	28	3.21	5.22	3.56	0.21	0.41
肛门	C21	0	0.00	0.00	0.00	0.00	0.00	0	0.00	0.00	0.00	0.00	0.00
肝脏	C22	115	8.81	20.62	16.25	0.87	1.98	52	5.96	9.70	6.03	0.41	0.52
胆囊及其他	C23–C24	17	1.30	3.05	2.63	0.12	0.35	20	2.29	3.73	2.41	0.17	0.28
胰腺	C25	11	0.84	1.97	1.72	0.06	0.29	17	1.95	3.17	2.03	0.06	0.25
鼻、鼻窦及其他	C30–C31	2	0.15	0.36	0.29	0.01	0.01	0	0.00	0.00	0.00	0.00	0.00
喉	C32	10	0.77	1.79	1.55	0.02	0.27	3	0.34	0.56	0.31	0.00	0.02
气管、支气管、肺	C33–C34	145	11.10	25.99	21.23	1.03	2.54	92	10.55	17.17	11.28	0.59	1.25
其他的胸腔器官	C37–C38	2	0.15	0.36	0.27	0.02	0.04	3	0.34	0.56	0.54	0.02	0.06
骨	C40–C41	4	0.31	0.72	0.59	0.00	0.07	7	0.80	1.31	0.89	0.01	0.15
皮肤的黑色素瘤	C43	1	0.08	0.18	0.19	0.00	0.05	0	0.00	0.00	0.00	0.00	0.00
其他的皮肤	C44	1	0.08	0.18	0.24	0.00	0.00	2	0.23	0.37	0.19	0.00	0.00
间皮瘤	C45	0	0.00	0.00	0.00	0.00	0.00	0	0.00	0.00	0.00	0.00	0.00
卡波西肉瘤	C46	0	0.00	0.00	0.00	0.00	0.00	0	0.00	0.00	0.00	0.00	0.00
周围神经、其他结缔组织、软组织	C47;C49	0	0.00	0.00	0.00	0.00	0.00	0	0.00	0.00	0.00	0.00	0.00
乳房	C50	—	—	—	—	—	—	45	5.16	8.40	5.65	0.39	0.66
外阴	C51	—	—	—	—	—	—	1	0.11	0.19	0.12	0.00	0.00
阴道	C52	—	—	—	—	—	—	0	0.00	0.00	0.00	0.00	0.00
子宫颈	C53	—	—	—	—	—	—	17	1.95	3.17	2.09	0.20	0.20
子宫体	C54	—	—	—	—	—	—	5	0.57	0.93	0.61	0.03	0.08
子宫，部位不明	C55	—	—	—	—	—	—	0	0.00	0.00	0.00	0.00	0.00
卵巢	C56	—	—	—	—	—	—	23	2.64	4.29	2.82	0.19	0.32
其他的女性生殖器	C57	—	—	—	—	—	—	0	0.00	0.00	0.00	0.00	0.00
胎盘	C58	—	—	—	—	—	—	0	0.00	0.00	0.00	0.00	0.00
阴茎	C60	0	0.00	0.00	0.00	0.00	0.00	—	—	—	—	—	—
前列腺	C61	7	0.54	1.25	1.13	0.00	0.09	—	—	—	—	—	—
睾丸	C62	0	0.00	0.00	0.00	0.00	0.00	—	—	—	—	—	—
其他的男性生殖器	C63	0	0.00	0.00	0.00	0.00	0.00	—	—	—	—	—	—
肾	C64	6	0.46	1.08	0.87	0.03	0.14	1	0.11	0.19	0.12	0.01	0.01
肾盂	C65	0	0.00	0.00	0.00	0.00	0.00	0	0.00	0.00	0.00	0.00	0.00
输尿管	C66	0	0.00	0.00	0.00	0.00	0.00	0	0.00	0.00	0.00	0.00	0.00
膀胱	C67	9	0.69	1.61	1.32	0.07	0.18	4	0.46	0.75	0.46	0.00	0.08
其他的泌尿器官	C68	0	0.00	0.00	0.00	0.00	0.00	1	0.11	0.19	0.12	0.00	0.00
眼	C69	2	0.15	0.36	0.27	0.03	0.03	0	0.00	0.00	0.00	0.00	0.00
脑、神经系统	C70–C72	25	1.91	4.48	3.70	0.17	0.45	19	2.18	3.55	2.53	0.16	0.20
甲状腺	C73	2	0.15	0.36	0.27	0.00	0.04	2	0.23	0.37	0.23	0.01	0.03
肾上腺	C74	1	0.08	0.18	0.15	0.00	0.00	0	0.00	0.00	0.00	0.00	0.00
其他的内分泌腺	C75	0	0.00	0.00	0.00	0.00	0.00	0	0.00	0.00	0.00	0.00	0.00
霍奇金病	C81	0	0.00	0.00	0.00	0.00	0.00	2	0.23	0.37	0.33	0.03	0.03
非霍奇金淋巴瘤	C82–C85;C96	9	0.69	1.61	1.40	0.10	0.15	5	0.57	0.93	0.66	0.04	0.06
免疫增生性疾病	C88	0	0.00	0.00	0.00	0.00	0.00	0	0.00	0.00	0.00	0.00	0.00
多发性骨髓瘤	C90	7	0.54	1.25	0.96	0.09	0.11	1	0.11	0.19	0.11	0.00	0.02
淋巴样白血病	C91	0	0.00	0.00	0.00	0.00	0.00	2	0.23	0.37	0.19	0.01	0.01
髓样白血病	C92–C94	5	0.38	0.90	0.95	0.04	0.06	4	0.46	0.75	0.69	0.05	0.05
白血病，未特指	C95	11	0.84	1.97	1.77	0.09	0.09	14	1.61	2.61	2.02	0.14	0.18
其他的或未指明部位的	O&U	6	0.46	1.08	1.02	0.02	0.14	10	1.15	1.87	1.23	0.06	0.12
骨髓增殖性疾病	MPD	0	0.00	0.00	0.00	0.00	0.00	0	0.00	0.00	0.00	0.00	0.00
骨髓增生异常综合征	MDS	0	0.00	0.00	0.00	0.00	0.00	0	0.00	0.00	0.00	0.00	0.00
合计	ALL	1 306	100.00	234.13	190.83	8.73	23.29	872	100.00	162.71	105.82	5.47	11.71
所有部位除外 C44	ALL but C44	1 305	99.92	233.95	190.59	8.73	23.29	870	99.77	162.34	105.63	5.47	11.71

表 6-2-7b　2014 年河南省鲁山县恶性肿瘤死亡主要指标

部位		男性						女性					
		病例数	构成 (%)	粗率 (1/10^5)	世标率 (1/10^5)	累积率 (%) 0~64	累积率 (%) 0~74	病例数	构成 (%)	粗率 (1/10^5)	世标率 (1/10^5)	累积率 (%) 0~64	累积率 (%) 0~74
唇	C00	0	0.00	0.00	0.00	0.00	0.00	0	0.00	0.00	0.00	0.00	0.00
舌	C01–C02	0	0.00	0.00	0.00	0.00	0.00	0	0.00	0.00	0.00	0.00	0.00
口	C03–C06	0	0.00	0.00	0.00	0.00	0.00	1	0.30	0.23	0.28	0.03	0.03
唾液腺	C07–C08	0	0.00	0.00	0.00	0.00	0.00	0	0.00	0.00	0.00	0.00	0.00
扁桃体	C09	0	0.00	0.00	0.00	0.00	0.00	0	0.00	0.00	0.00	0.00	0.00
其他的口咽	C10	0	0.00	0.00	0.00	0.00	0.00	1	0.30	0.23	0.11	0.00	0.00
鼻咽	C11	1	0.14	0.22	0.14	0.00	0.00	0	0.00	0.00	0.00	0.00	0.00
喉咽	C12–C13	0	0.00	0.00	0.00	0.00	0.00	0	0.00	0.00	0.00	0.00	0.00
咽，部位不明	C14	1	0.14	0.22	0.18	0.02	0.02	0	0.00	0.00	0.00	0.00	0.00
食管	C15	148	20.03	31.96	32.75	0.72	3.20	56	16.92	12.90	10.54	0.28	1.06
胃	C16	140	18.94	30.23	28.18	1.00	2.66	37	11.18	8.52	6.92	0.15	0.64
小肠	C17	0	0.00	0.00	0.00	0.00	0.00	0	0.00	0.00	0.00	0.00	0.00
结肠	C18	6	0.81	1.30	1.18	0.03	0.20	5	1.51	1.15	0.85	0.04	0.08
直肠	C19–C20	14	1.89	3.02	2.97	0.05	0.18	3	0.91	0.69	0.57	0.02	0.07
肛门	C21	0	0.00	0.00	0.00	0.00	0.00	0	0.00	0.00	0.00	0.00	0.00
肝脏	C22	114	15.43	24.62	26.01	1.28	2.44	54	16.31	12.44	10.96	0.57	1.00
胆囊及其他	C23–C24	1	0.14	0.22	0.17	0.00	0.00	5	1.51	1.15	1.21	0.00	0.04
胰腺	C25	5	0.68	1.08	0.91	0.04	0.12	7	2.11	1.61	1.50	0.09	0.23
鼻、鼻窦及其他	C30–C31	0	0.00	0.00	0.00	0.00	0.00	0	0.00	0.00	0.00	0.00	0.00
喉	C32	1	0.14	0.22	0.14	0.00	0.00	0	0.00	0.00	0.00	0.00	0.00
气管、支气管、肺	C33–C34	247	33.42	53.33	51.27	1.86	5.04	87	26.28	20.04	18.97	0.69	1.48
其他的胸腔器官	C37–C38	1	0.14	0.22	0.18	0.02	0.02	0	0.00	0.00	0.00	0.00	0.00
骨	C40–C41	7	0.95	1.51	1.52	0.11	0.19	3	0.91	0.69	0.65	0.07	0.07
皮肤的黑色素瘤	C43	0	0.00	0.00	0.00	0.00	0.00	0	0.00	0.00	0.00	0.00	0.00
其他的皮肤	C44	0	0.00	0.00	0.00	0.00	0.00	0	0.00	0.00	0.00	0.00	0.00
间皮瘤	C45	0	0.00	0.00	0.00	0.00	0.00	0	0.00	0.00	0.00	0.00	0.00
卡波西肉瘤	C46	0	0.00	0.00	0.00	0.00	0.00	0	0.00	0.00	0.00	0.00	0.00
周围神经、其他结缔组织、软组织	C47;C49	0	0.00	0.00	0.00	0.00	0.00	0	0.00	0.00	0.00	0.00	0.00
乳房	C50	—	—	—	—	—	—	16	4.83	3.69	3.19	0.25	0.25
外阴	C51	—	—	—	—	—	—	0	0.00	0.00	0.00	0.00	0.00
阴道	C52	—	—	—	—	—	—	0	0.00	0.00	0.00	0.00	0.00
子宫颈	C53	—	—	—	—	—	—	18	5.44	4.15	3.71	0.21	0.39
子宫体	C54	—	—	—	—	—	—	12	3.63	2.76	2.26	0.14	0.23
子宫，部位不明	C55	—	—	—	—	—	—	0	0.00	0.00	0.00	0.00	0.00
卵巢	C56	—	—	—	—	—	—	5	1.51	1.15	1.08	0.04	0.17
其他的女性生殖器	C57	—	—	—	—	—	—	0	0.00	0.00	0.00	0.00	0.00
胎盘	C58	—	—	—	—	—	—	0	0.00	0.00	0.00	0.00	0.00
阴茎	C60	1	0.14	0.22	0.14	0.00	0.00	—	—	—	—	—	—
前列腺	C61	5	0.68	1.08	2.10	0.03	0.08	—	—	—	—	—	—
睾丸	C62	1	0.14	0.22	0.21	0.02	0.02	—	—	—	—	—	—
其他的男性生殖器	C63	0	0.00	0.00	0.00	0.00	0.00	—	—	—	—	—	—
肾	C64	3	0.41	0.65	0.59	0.02	0.06	0	0.00	0.00	0.00	0.00	0.00
肾盂	C65	1	0.14	0.22	0.71	0.00	0.00	0	0.00	0.00	0.00	0.00	0.00
输尿管	C66	0	0.00	0.00	0.00	0.00	0.00	0	0.00	0.00	0.00	0.00	0.00
膀胱	C67	10	1.35	2.16	1.66	0.03	0.17	2	0.60	0.46	0.46	0.02	0.06
其他的泌尿器官	C68	0	0.00	0.00	0.00	0.00	0.00	0	0.00	0.00	0.00	0.00	0.00
眼	C69	0	0.00	0.00	0.00	0.00	0.00	0	0.00	0.00	0.00	0.00	0.00
脑、神经系统	C70–C72	20	2.71	4.32	4.45	0.21	0.38	12	3.63	2.76	2.54	0.16	0.21
甲状腺	C73	1	0.14	0.22	0.17	0.00	0.00	2	0.60	0.46	0.31	0.02	0.02
肾上腺	C74	1	0.14	0.22	0.17	0.00	0.00	0	0.00	0.00	0.00	0.00	0.00
其他的内分泌腺	C75	0	0.00	0.00	0.00	0.00	0.00	1	0.30	0.23	0.11	0.00	0.00
霍奇金病	C81	3	0.41	0.65	0.59	0.00	0.13	2	0.60	0.46	0.46	0.05	0.05
非霍奇金淋巴瘤	C82–C85;C96	0	0.00	0.00	0.00	0.00	0.00	0	0.00	0.00	0.00	0.00	0.00
免疫增生性疾病	C88	0	0.00	0.00	0.00	0.00	0.00	0	0.00	0.00	0.00	0.00	0.00
多发性骨髓瘤	C90	2	0.27	0.43	0.42	0.04	0.04	0	0.00	0.00	0.00	0.00	0.00
淋巴样白血病	C91	0	0.00	0.00	0.00	0.00	0.00	1	0.30	0.23	0.21	0.02	0.02
髓样白血病	C92–C94	2	0.27	0.43	0.42	0.03	0.03	1	0.30	0.23	0.31	0.01	0.01
白血病，未特指	C95	0	0.00	0.00	0.00	0.00	0.00	0	0.00	0.00	0.00	0.00	0.00
其他的或未指明部位的	O&U	2	0.27	0.43	0.48	0.00	0.08	0	0.00	0.00	0.00	0.00	0.00
骨髓增殖性疾病	MPD	0	0.00	0.00	0.00	0.00	0.00	0	0.00	0.00	0.00	0.00	0.00
骨髓增生异常综合征	MDS	0	0.00	0.00	0.00	0.00	0.00	0	0.00	0.00	0.00	0.00	0.00
合计	ALL	739	100.00	159.57	158.45	5.50	15.06	331	100.00	76.24	67.21	2.87	6.10
所有部位除外 C44	ALL but C44	739	100.00	159.57	158.45	5.50	15.06	331	100.00	76.24	67.21	2.87	6.10

表 6-2-8b 2014 年河南省罗山县恶性肿瘤死亡主要指标

部位		男性						女性					
		病例数	构成 (%)	粗率 $(1/10^5)$	世标率 $(1/10^5)$	累积率 (%) 0~64	累积率 (%) 0~74	病例数	构成 (%)	粗率 $(1/10^5)$	世标率 $(1/10^5)$	累积率 (%) 0~64	累积率 (%) 0~74
唇	C00	1	0.14	0.26	0.21	0.02	0.02	0	0.00	0.00	0.00	0.00	0.00
舌	C01–C02	1	0.14	0.26	0.19	0.02	0.02	0	0.00	0.00	0.00	0.00	0.00
口	C03–C06	1	0.14	0.26	0.19	0.02	0.02	0	0.00	0.00	0.00	0.00	0.00
唾液腺	C07–C08	0	0.00	0.00	0.00	0.00	0.00	0	0.00	0.00	0.00	0.00	0.00
扁桃体	C09	0	0.00	0.00	0.00	0.00	0.00	0	0.00	0.00	0.00	0.00	0.00
其他的口咽	C10	0	0.00	0.00	0.00	0.00	0.00	0	0.00	0.00	0.00	0.00	0.00
鼻咽	C11	8	1.10	2.05	1.99	0.09	0.34	2	0.51	0.56	0.40	0.05	0.05
喉咽	C12–C13	1	0.14	0.26	0.23	0.00	0.00	0	0.00	0.00	0.00	0.00	0.00
咽，部位不明	C14	1	0.14	0.26	0.21	0.02	0.02	0	0.00	0.00	0.00	0.00	0.00
食管	C15	52	7.13	13.29	15.10	0.52	1.42	19	4.85	5.36	5.09	0.09	0.53
胃	C16	169	23.18	43.21	49.85	1.78	5.05	69	17.60	19.47	17.75	0.77	1.62
小肠	C17	2	0.27	0.51	0.48	0.02	0.08	1	0.26	0.28	0.20	0.02	0.02
结肠	C18	40	5.49	10.23	11.70	0.61	1.10	33	8.42	9.31	8.92	0.57	0.90
直肠	C19–C20	6	0.82	1.53	2.58	0.09	0.15	13	3.32	3.67	3.31	0.26	0.43
肛门	C21	0	0.00	0.00	0.00	0.00	0.00	0	0.00	0.00	0.00	0.00	0.00
肝脏	C22	133	18.24	34.00	33.14	1.87	3.70	49	12.50	13.83	13.07	0.53	1.75
胆囊及其他	C23–C24	1	0.14	0.26	0.16	0.01	0.01	5	1.28	1.41	1.28	0.06	0.13
胰腺	C25	16	2.19	4.09	4.79	0.20	0.45	5	1.28	1.41	1.18	0.05	0.11
鼻、鼻窦及其他	C30–C31	1	0.14	0.26	0.21	0.02	0.02	1	0.26	0.28	0.23	0.00	0.00
喉	C32	3	0.41	0.77	0.76	0.06	0.12	2	0.51	0.56	0.45	0.03	0.03
气管、支气管、肺	C33–C34	206	28.26	52.67	59.68	2.72	6.68	81	20.66	22.85	23.39	0.85	2.23
其他的胸腔器官	C37–C38	1	0.14	0.26	0.31	0.04	0.04	1	0.26	0.28	0.23	0.01	0.01
骨	C40–C41	8	1.10	2.05	1.99	0.14	0.26	2	0.51	0.56	0.53	0.00	0.05
皮肤的黑色素瘤	C43	0	0.00	0.00	0.00	0.00	0.00	0	0.00	0.00	0.00	0.00	0.00
其他的皮肤	C44	1	0.14	0.26	1.23	0.00	0.00	1	0.26	0.28	0.28	0.02	0.02
间皮瘤	C45	0	0.00	0.00	0.00	0.00	0.00	0	0.00	0.00	0.00	0.00	0.00
卡波西肉瘤	C46	0	0.00	0.00	0.00	0.00	0.00	0	0.00	0.00	0.00	0.00	0.00
周围神经、其他结缔组织、软组织	C47;C49	1	0.14	0.26	0.32	0.00	0.05	0	0.00	0.00	0.00	0.00	0.00
乳房	C50	—	—	—	—	—	—	28	7.14	7.90	6.69	0.57	0.67
外阴	C51	—	—	—	—	—	—	0	0.00	0.00	0.00	0.00	0.00
阴道	C52	—	—	—	—	—	—	0	0.00	0.00	0.00	0.00	0.00
子宫颈	C53	—	—	—	—	—	—	26	6.63	7.34	6.26	0.42	0.74
子宫体	C54	—	—	—	—	—	—	2	0.51	0.56	0.46	0.02	0.09
子宫，部位不明	C55	—	—	—	—	—	—	0	0.00	0.00	0.00	0.00	0.00
卵巢	C56	—	—	—	—	—	—	7	1.79	1.98	1.85	0.19	0.26
其他的女性生殖器	C57	—	—	—	—	—	—	0	0.00	0.00	0.00	0.00	0.00
胎盘	C58	—	—	—	—	—	—	0	0.00	0.00	0.00	0.00	0.00
阴茎	C60	1	0.14	0.26	0.16	0.01	0.01	—	—	—	—	—	—
前列腺	C61	12	1.65	3.07	4.30	0.10	0.34	—	—	—	—	—	—
睾丸	C62	0	0.00	0.00	0.00	0.00	0.00	—	—	—	—	—	—
其他的男性生殖器	C63	0	0.00	0.00	0.00	0.00	0.00	—	—	—	—	—	—
肾	C64	4	0.55	1.02	1.92	0.04	0.04	2	0.51	0.56	0.54	0.04	0.04
肾盂	C65	0	0.00	0.00	0.00	0.00	0.00	0	0.00	0.00	0.00	0.00	0.00
输尿管	C66	0	0.00	0.00	0.00	0.00	0.00	0	0.00	0.00	0.00	0.00	0.00
膀胱	C67	5	0.69	1.28	1.13	0.04	0.11	1	0.26	0.28	0.19	0.02	0.02
其他的泌尿器官	C68	0	0.00	0.00	0.00	0.00	0.00	0	0.00	0.00	0.00	0.00	0.00
眼	C69	1	0.14	0.26	0.55	0.03	0.03	0	0.00	0.00	0.00	0.00	0.00
脑、神经系统	C70–C72	19	2.61	4.86	4.47	0.38	0.48	20	5.10	5.64	4.84	0.28	0.58
甲状腺	C73	0	0.00	0.00	0.00	0.00	0.00	3	0.77	0.85	0.81	0.06	0.13
肾上腺	C74	0	0.00	0.00	0.00	0.00	0.00	0	0.00	0.00	0.00	0.00	0.00
其他的内分泌腺	C75	0	0.00	0.00	0.00	0.00	0.00	0	0.00	0.00	0.00	0.00	0.00
霍奇金病	C81	1	0.14	0.26	0.31	0.04	0.04	0	0.00	0.00	0.00	0.00	0.00
非霍奇金淋巴瘤	C82–C85;C96	7	0.96	1.79	1.77	0.13	0.25	8	2.04	2.26	2.08	0.14	0.30
免疫增生性疾病	C88	0	0.00	0.00	0.00	0.00	0.00	0	0.00	0.00	0.00	0.00	0.00
多发性骨髓瘤	C90	0	0.00	0.00	0.00	0.00	0.00	0	0.00	0.00	0.00	0.00	0.00
淋巴样白血病	C91	2	0.27	0.51	0.40	0.04	0.04	0	0.00	0.00	0.00	0.00	0.00
髓样白血病	C92–C94	2	0.27	0.51	0.49	0.02	0.07	1	0.26	0.28	0.21	0.03	0.03
白血病，未特指	C95	13	1.78	3.32	3.10	0.27	0.27	5	1.28	1.41	1.41	0.11	0.18
其他的或未指明部位的	O&U	8	1.10	2.05	2.79	0.08	0.22	5	1.28	1.41	1.15	0.04	0.17
骨髓增殖性疾病	MPD	0	0.00	0.00	0.00	0.00	0.00	0	0.00	0.00	0.00	0.00	0.00
骨髓增生异常综合征	MDS	0	0.00	0.00	0.00	0.00	0.00	0	0.00	0.00	0.00	0.00	0.00
合计	ALL	729	100.00	186.38	207.04	9.41	21.50	392	100.00	110.61	102.81	5.21	11.08
所有部位除外 C44	ALL but C44	728	99.86	186.12	205.81	9.41	21.50	391	99.74	110.32	102.53	5.19	11.06

表 6-2-9b 2014 年河南省洛阳市恶性肿瘤死亡主要指标

部位		男性						女性					
		病例数	构成(%)	粗率($1/10^5$)	世标率($1/10^5$)	累积率(%)		病例数	构成(%)	粗率($1/10^5$)	世标率($1/10^5$)	累积率(%)	
						0~64	0~74					0~64	0~74
唇	C00	0	0.00	0.00	0.00	0.00	0.00	0	0.00	0.00	0.00	0.00	0.00
舌	C01–C02	1	0.09	0.17	0.22	0.00	0.04	0	0.00	0.00	0.00	0.00	0.00
口	C03–C06	4	0.35	0.70	1.08	0.01	0.05	1	0.13	0.18	0.12	0.01	0.01
唾液腺	C07–C08	2	0.18	0.35	0.72	0.00	0.00	0	0.00	0.00	0.00	0.00	0.00
扁桃体	C09	0	0.00	0.00	0.00	0.00	0.00	0	0.00	0.00	0.00	0.00	0.00
其他的口咽	C10	0	0.00	0.00	0.00	0.00	0.00	1	0.13	0.18	0.19	0.00	0.03
鼻咽	C11	8	0.70	1.39	1.74	0.03	0.14	1	0.13	0.18	0.14	0.02	0.02
喉咽	C12–C13	1	0.09	0.17	0.20	0.00	0.00	0	0.00	0.00	0.00	0.00	0.00
咽，部位不明	C14	2	0.18	0.35	0.70	0.02	0.02	2	0.27	0.37	0.35	0.03	0.03
食管	C15	87	7.63	15.17	18.91	0.41	1.15	63	8.43	11.55	14.49	0.15	0.92
胃	C16	153	13.42	26.67	32.02	0.58	2.36	52	6.96	9.53	9.23	0.32	0.72
小肠	C17	3	0.26	0.52	0.91	0.00	0.05	6	0.80	1.10	1.24	0.00	0.08
结肠	C18	45	3.95	7.84	9.33	0.18	0.46	36	4.82	6.60	6.54	0.14	0.51
直肠	C19–C20	42	3.68	7.32	9.11	0.23	0.67	32	4.28	5.87	5.46	0.23	0.45
肛门	C21	0	0.00	0.00	0.00	0.00	0.00	1	0.13	0.18	0.17	0.00	0.04
肝脏	C22	165	14.47	28.76	32.35	1.39	2.74	75	10.04	13.75	13.63	0.39	1.19
胆囊及其他	C23–C24	16	1.40	2.79	3.61	0.05	0.13	23	3.08	4.22	4.07	0.20	0.47
胰腺	C25	44	3.86	7.67	10.86	0.20	0.64	24	3.21	4.40	4.07	0.04	0.40
鼻、鼻窦及其他	C30–C31	1	0.09	0.17	0.18	0.00	0.05	0	0.00	0.00	0.00	0.00	0.00
喉	C32	14	1.23	2.44	2.46	0.08	0.20	1	0.13	0.18	0.43	0.00	0.00
气管、支气管、肺	C33–C34	369	32.37	64.33	75.39	2.31	5.95	157	21.02	28.78	28.67	0.84	2.58
其他的胸腔器官	C37–C38	6	0.53	1.05	2.18	0.03	0.03	2	0.27	0.37	0.32	0.01	0.04
骨	C40–C41	3	0.26	0.52	0.91	0.01	0.05	8	1.07	1.47	1.29	0.03	0.18
皮肤的黑色素瘤	C43	1	0.09	0.17	0.21	0.03	0.03	1	0.13	0.18	0.21	0.03	0.03
其他的皮肤	C44	6	0.53	1.05	0.92	0.03	0.07	7	0.94	1.28	1.85	0.04	0.04
间皮瘤	C45	0	0.00	0.00	0.00	0.00	0.00	0	0.00	0.00	0.00	0.00	0.00
卡波西肉瘤	C46	0	0.00	0.00	0.00	0.00	0.00	0	0.00	0.00	0.00	0.00	0.00
周围神经、其他结缔组织、软组织	C47;C49	2	0.18	0.35	0.30	0.01	0.01	1	0.13	0.18	0.19	0.00	0.03
乳房	C50	—	—	—	—	—	—	81	10.84	14.85	12.92	0.80	1.26
外阴	C51	—	—	—	—	—	—	1	0.13	0.18	0.21	0.03	0.03
阴道	C52	—	—	—	—	—	—	1	0.13	0.18	0.12	0.01	0.01
子宫颈	C53	—	—	—	—	—	—	27	3.61	4.95	3.82	0.29	0.33
子宫体	C54	—	—	—	—	—	—	15	2.01	2.75	2.64	0.12	0.28
子宫，部位不明	C55	—	—	—	—	—	—	0	0.00	0.00	0.00	0.00	0.00
卵巢	C56	—	—	—	—	—	—	23	3.08	4.22	3.66	0.14	0.47
其他的女性生殖器	C57	—	—	—	—	—	—	1	0.13	0.18	0.15	0.01	0.01
胎盘	C58	—	—	—	—	—	—	0	0.00	0.00	0.00	0.00	0.00
阴茎	C60	1	0.09	0.17	0.18	0.00	0.05	—	—	—	—	—	—
前列腺	C61	25	2.19	4.36	6.68	0.05	0.23	—	—	—	—	—	—
睾丸	C62	4	0.35	0.70	0.68	0.01	0.01	—	—	—	—	—	—
其他的男性生殖器	C63	0	0.00	0.00	0.00	0.00	0.00	—	—	—	—	—	—
肾	C64	18	1.58	3.14	3.16	0.14	0.45	11	1.47	2.02	1.91	0.07	0.16
肾盂	C65	1	0.09	0.17	0.20	0.00	0.00	1	0.13	0.18	0.14	0.00	0.00
输尿管	C66	2	0.18	0.35	0.75	0.00	0.05	1	0.13	0.18	0.19	0.00	0.03
膀胱	C67	20	1.75	3.49	4.49	0.10	0.23	12	1.61	2.20	2.20	0.11	0.11
其他的泌尿器官	C68	1	0.09	0.17	0.20	0.00	0.00	0	0.00	0.00	0.00	0.00	0.00
眼	C69	0	0.00	0.00	0.00	0.00	0.00	0	0.00	0.00	0.00	0.00	0.00
脑、神经系统	C70–C72	19	1.67	3.31	3.83	0.19	0.34	18	2.41	3.30	4.01	0.12	0.26
甲状腺	C73	3	0.26	0.52	0.46	0.03	0.07	6	0.80	1.10	0.90	0.06	0.06
肾上腺	C74	0	0.00	0.00	0.00	0.00	0.00	1	0.13	0.18	0.39	0.02	0.02
其他的内分泌腺	C75	0	0.00	0.00	0.00	0.00	0.00	1	0.13	0.18	0.12	0.01	0.01
霍奇金病	C81	4	0.35	0.70	0.77	0.00	0.12	1	0.13	0.18	0.12	0.01	0.01
非霍奇金淋巴瘤	C82–C85;C96	11	0.96	1.92	2.20	0.07	0.14	6	0.80	1.10	0.94	0.02	0.09
免疫增生性疾病	C88	0	0.00	0.00	0.00	0.00	0.00	0	0.00	0.00	0.00	0.00	0.00
多发性骨髓瘤	C90	3	0.26	0.52	0.94	0.03	0.03	2	0.27	0.37	0.40	0.03	0.06
淋巴样白血病	C91	5	0.44	0.87	0.90	0.02	0.13	2	0.27	0.37	0.27	0.01	0.01
髓样白血病	C92–C94	4	0.35	0.70	0.65	0.01	0.15	4	0.54	0.73	0.56	0.03	0.03
白血病，未特指	C95	20	1.75	3.49	3.75	0.19	0.32	17	2.28	3.12	3.40	0.15	0.30
其他的或未指明部位的	O&U	19	1.67	3.31	4.40	0.07	0.15	17	2.28	3.12	3.01	0.10	0.31
骨髓增殖性疾病	MPD	0	0.00	0.00	0.00	0.00	0.00	1	0.13	0.18	0.17	0.00	0.04
骨髓增生异常综合征	MDS	2	0.18	0.35	0.36	0.00	0.00	3	0.40	0.55	0.73	0.00	0.00
合计	ALL	1 140	100.00	198.73	239.87	6.47	17.32	747	100.00	136.94	135.65	4.61	11.64
所有部位除外 C44	ALL but C44	1 134	99.47	197.69	238.95	6.45	17.25	740	99.06	135.66	133.80	4.57	11.60

表 6-2-10b 2014 年河南省孟津县恶性肿瘤死亡主要指标

部位		男性						女性					
		病例数	构成 (%)	粗率 (1/10^5)	世标率 (1/10^5)	累积率 (%) 0~64	累积率 (%) 0~74	病例数	构成 (%)	粗率 (1/10^5)	世标率 (1/10^5)	累积率 (%) 0~64	累积率 (%) 0~74
唇	C00	0	0.00	0.00	0.00	0.00	0.00	0	0.00	0.00	0.00	0.00	0.00
舌	C01–C02	0	0.00	0.00	0.00	0.00	0.00	1	0.38	0.44	0.36	0.00	0.09
口	C03–C06	0	0.00	0.00	0.00	0.00	0.00	1	0.38	0.44	0.35	0.04	0.04
唾液腺	C07–C08	0	0.00	0.00	0.00	0.00	0.00	0	0.00	0.00	0.00	0.00	0.00
扁桃体	C09	1	0.25	0.43	0.39	0.00	0.06	0	0.00	0.00	0.00	0.00	0.00
其他的口咽	C10	0	0.00	0.00	0.00	0.00	0.00	0	0.00	0.00	0.00	0.00	0.00
鼻咽	C11	1	0.25	0.43	0.39	0.00	0.06	0	0.00	0.00	0.00	0.00	0.00
喉咽	C12–C13	0	0.00	0.00	0.00	0.00	0.00	0	0.00	0.00	0.00	0.00	0.00
咽，部位不明	C14	1	0.25	0.43	0.25	0.03	0.03	0	0.00	0.00	0.00	0.00	0.00
食管	C15	51	12.72	22.06	18.88	0.35	2.07	49	18.77	21.45	12.88	0.13	1.38
胃	C16	99	24.69	42.82	35.53	1.11	4.51	34	13.03	14.89	10.11	0.32	1.48
小肠	C17	1	0.25	0.43	0.39	0.00	0.10	5	1.92	2.19	1.25	0.00	0.06
结肠	C18	7	1.75	3.03	2.72	0.02	0.35	2	0.77	0.88	0.71	0.04	0.13
直肠	C19–C20	14	3.49	6.06	4.86	0.14	0.73	6	2.30	2.63	1.33	0.00	0.09
肛门	C21	0	0.00	0.00	0.00	0.00	0.00	2	0.77	0.88	0.60	0.00	0.06
肝脏	C22	51	12.72	22.06	17.63	1.04	1.88	30	11.49	13.13	9.58	0.29	1.37
胆囊及其他	C23–C24	12	2.99	5.19	4.95	0.14	0.40	14	5.36	6.13	4.23	0.15	0.55
胰腺	C25	7	1.75	3.03	2.43	0.06	0.45	8	3.07	3.50	2.35	0.12	0.28
鼻、鼻窦及其他	C30–C31	0	0.00	0.00	0.00	0.00	0.00	0	0.00	0.00	0.00	0.00	0.00
喉	C32	1	0.25	0.43	0.25	0.03	0.03	1	0.38	0.44	0.16	0.00	0.00
气管、支气管、肺	C33–C34	90	22.44	38.93	31.63	1.04	2.76	46	17.62	20.14	12.62	0.60	1.36
其他的胸腔器官	C37–C38	1	0.25	0.43	0.34	0.03	0.03	0	0.00	0.00	0.00	0.00	0.00
骨	C40–C41	5	1.25	2.16	1.44	0.11	0.11	1	0.38	0.44	0.39	0.00	0.06
皮肤的黑色素瘤	C43	1	0.25	0.43	0.34	0.03	0.03	0	0.00	0.00	0.00	0.00	0.00
其他的皮肤	C44	1	0.25	0.43	0.25	0.03	0.03	2	0.77	0.88	0.51	0.03	0.03
间皮瘤	C45	0	0.00	0.00	0.00	0.00	0.00	0	0.00	0.00	0.00	0.00	0.00
卡波西肉瘤	C46	0	0.00	0.00	0.00	0.00	0.00	0	0.00	0.00	0.00	0.00	0.00
周围神经、其他结缔组织、软组织	C47;C49	1	0.25	0.43	0.25	0.03	0.03	0	0.00	0.00	0.00	0.00	0.00
乳房	C50	—	—	—	—	—	—	16	6.13	7.01	5.20	0.41	0.65
外阴	C51	—	—	—	—	—	—	0	0.00	0.00	0.00	0.00	0.00
阴道	C52	—	—	—	—	—	—	0	0.00	0.00	0.00	0.00	0.00
子宫颈	C53	—	—	—	—	—	—	7	2.68	3.06	2.39	0.07	0.41
子宫体	C54	—	—	—	—	—	—	4	1.53	1.75	1.36	0.09	0.15
子宫，部位不明	C55	—	—	—	—	—	—	2	0.77	0.88	0.51	0.03	0.03
卵巢	C56	—	—	—	—	—	—	3	1.15	1.31	0.90	0.04	0.11
其他的女性生殖器	C57	—	—	—	—	—	—	0	0.00	0.00	0.00	0.00	0.00
胎盘	C58	—	—	—	—	—	—	0	0.00	0.00	0.00	0.00	0.00
阴茎	C60	0	0.00	0.00	0.00	0.00	0.00	—	—	—	—	—	—
前列腺	C61	2	0.50	0.87	0.88	0.00	0.00	—	—	—	—	—	—
睾丸	C62	0	0.00	0.00	0.00	0.00	0.00	—	—	—	—	—	—
其他的男性生殖器	C63	0	0.00	0.00	0.00	0.00	0.00	—	—	—	—	—	—
肾	C64	4	1.00	1.73	1.42	0.03	0.29	2	0.77	0.88	0.51	0.04	0.04
肾盂	C65	0	0.00	0.00	0.00	0.00	0.00	0	0.00	0.00	0.00	0.00	0.00
输尿管	C66	0	0.00	0.00	0.00	0.00	0.00	0	0.00	0.00	0.00	0.00	0.00
膀胱	C67	5	1.25	2.16	1.71	0.03	0.26	0	0.00	0.00	0.00	0.00	0.00
其他的泌尿器官	C68	0	0.00	0.00	0.00	0.00	0.00	0	0.00	0.00	0.00	0.00	0.00
眼	C69	0	0.00	0.00	0.00	0.00	0.00	0	0.00	0.00	0.00	0.00	0.00
脑、神经系统	C70–C72	13	3.24	5.62	4.81	0.16	0.42	9	3.45	3.94	3.65	0.17	0.37
甲状腺	C73	2	0.50	0.87	0.63	0.03	0.03	2	0.77	0.88	0.37	0.00	0.00
肾上腺	C74	1	0.25	0.43	0.25	0.03	0.03	0	0.00	0.00	0.00	0.00	0.00
其他的内分泌腺	C75	1	0.25	0.43	0.34	0.03	0.03	0	0.00	0.00	0.00	0.00	0.00
霍奇金病	C81	0	0.00	0.00	0.00	0.00	0.00	0	0.00	0.00	0.00	0.00	0.00
非霍奇金淋巴瘤	C82–C85;C96	6	1.50	2.60	2.28	0.08	0.15	4	1.53	1.75	1.08	0.03	0.12
免疫增生性疾病	C88	0	0.00	0.00	0.00	0.00	0.00	0	0.00	0.00	0.00	0.00	0.00
多发性骨髓瘤	C90	1	0.25	0.43	0.39	0.00	0.06	0	0.00	0.00	0.00	0.00	0.00
淋巴样白血病	C91	2	0.50	0.87	0.82	0.07	0.07	0	0.00	0.00	0.00	0.00	0.00
髓样白血病	C92–C94	1	0.25	0.43	0.34	0.04	0.04	0	0.00	0.00	0.00	0.00	0.00
白血病，未特指	C95	9	2.24	3.89	3.48	0.19	0.26	5	1.92	2.19	1.33	0.10	0.10
其他的或未指明部位的	O&U	9	2.24	3.89	3.22	0.20	0.33	5	1.92	2.19	1.28	0.10	0.10
骨髓增殖性疾病	MPD	0	0.00	0.00	0.00	0.00	0.00	0	0.00	0.00	0.00	0.00	0.00
骨髓增生异常综合征	MDS	0	0.00	0.00	0.00	0.00	0.00	0	0.00	0.00	0.00	0.00	0.00
合计	ALL	401	100.00	173.44	143.51	5.11	15.62	261	100.00	114.27	76.01	2.80	9.08
所有部位除外 C44	ALL but C44	400	99.75	173.01	143.26	5.08	15.59	259	99.23	113.40	75.50	2.77	9.05

表 6-2-11b　2014 年河南省南阳市恶性肿瘤死亡主要指标

部位		男性						女性					
		病例数	构成 (%)	粗率 (1/10^5)	世标率 (1/10^5)	累积率 (%) 0~64	累积率 (%) 0~74	病例数	构成 (%)	粗率 (1/10^5)	世标率 (1/10^5)	累积率 (%) 0~64	累积率 (%) 0~74
唇	C00	0	0.00	0.00	0.00	0.00	0.00	0	0.00	0.00	0.00	0.00	0.00
舌	C01–C02	2	0.20	0.43	0.32	0.03	0.03	4	0.79	0.90	0.73	0.07	0.07
口	C03–C06	3	0.31	0.64	0.60	0.00	0.07	4	0.79	0.90	0.70	0.00	0.05
唾液腺	C07–C08	1	0.10	0.21	0.26	0.02	0.02	1	0.20	0.23	0.14	0.01	0.01
扁桃体	C09	0	0.00	0.00	0.00	0.00	0.00	0	0.00	0.00	0.00	0.00	0.00
其他的口咽	C10	1	0.10	0.21	0.13	0.00	0.00	0	0.00	0.00	0.00	0.00	0.00
鼻咽	C11	3	0.31	0.64	0.65	0.04	0.08	4	0.79	0.90	0.74	0.01	0.09
喉咽	C12–C13	0	0.00	0.00	0.00	0.00	0.00	0	0.00	0.00	0.00	0.00	0.00
咽，部位不明	C14	1	0.10	0.21	0.18	0.00	0.00	1	0.20	0.23	0.13	0.02	0.02
食管	C15	175	17.91	37.40	33.07	0.99	3.27	59	11.61	13.28	10.96	0.30	1.13
胃	C16	211	21.60	45.10	40.56	1.61	4.38	74	14.57	16.66	14.07	0.46	1.24
小肠	C17	5	0.51	1.07	0.88	0.03	0.16	5	0.98	1.13	0.77	0.02	0.07
结肠	C18	26	2.66	5.56	5.00	0.06	0.43	10	1.97	2.25	1.83	0.05	0.23
直肠	C19–C20	30	3.07	6.41	6.12	0.29	0.71	19	3.74	4.28	3.41	0.25	0.39
肛门	C21	1	0.10	0.21	0.19	0.00	0.05	0	0.00	0.00	0.00	0.00	0.00
肝脏	C22	141	14.43	30.14	26.96	1.39	3.22	49	9.65	11.03	8.96	0.50	1.17
胆囊及其他	C23–C24	4	0.41	0.85	0.79	0.07	0.07	1	0.20	0.23	0.16	0.01	0.01
胰腺	C25	3	0.31	0.64	0.51	0.00	0.09	8	1.57	1.80	1.39	0.10	0.15
鼻、鼻窦及其他	C30–C31	0	0.00	0.00	0.00	0.00	0.00	1	0.20	0.23	0.13	0.00	0.00
喉	C32	4	0.41	0.85	0.73	0.04	0.08	0	0.00	0.00	0.00	0.00	0.00
气管、支气管、肺	C33–C34	254	26.00	54.29	47.70	1.82	5.02	72	14.17	16.21	13.05	0.55	1.45
其他的胸腔器官	C37–C38	4	0.41	0.85	0.62	0.03	0.08	4	0.79	0.90	0.68	0.02	0.07
骨	C40–C41	11	1.13	2.35	2.01	0.10	0.28	9	1.77	2.03	1.48	0.10	0.15
皮肤的黑色素瘤	C43	1	0.10	0.21	0.21	0.00	0.04	1	0.20	0.23	0.18	0.01	0.01
其他的皮肤	C44	2	0.20	0.43	0.43	0.02	0.07	1	0.20	0.23	0.18	0.01	0.01
间皮瘤	C45	1	0.10	0.21	0.14	0.01	0.01	0	0.00	0.00	0.00	0.00	0.00
卡波西肉瘤	C46	0	0.00	0.00	0.00	0.00	0.00	0	0.00	0.00	0.00	0.00	0.00
周围神经、其他结缔组织、软组织	C47;C49	2	0.20	0.43	0.33	0.02	0.02	0	0.00	0.00	0.00	0.00	0.00
乳房	C50	—	—	—	—	—	—	58	11.42	13.06	11.07	0.90	1.16
外阴	C51	—	—	—	—	—	—	0	0.00	0.00	0.00	0.00	0.00
阴道	C52	—	—	—	—	—	—	0	0.00	0.00	0.00	0.00	0.00
子宫颈	C53	—	—	—	—	—	—	39	7.68	8.78	7.51	0.54	0.85
子宫体	C54	—	—	—	—	—	—	8	1.57	1.80	1.61	0.13	0.18
子宫，部位不明	C55	—	—	—	—	—	—	5	0.98	1.13	1.12	0.06	0.14
卵巢	C56	—	—	—	—	—	—	15	2.95	3.38	2.69	0.20	0.29
其他的女性生殖器	C57	—	—	—	—	—	—	1	0.20	0.23	0.18	0.01	0.01
胎盘	C58	—	—	—	—	—	—	0	0.00	0.00	0.00	0.00	0.00
阴茎	C60	2	0.20	0.43	0.25	0.00	0.00	—	—	—	—	—	—
前列腺	C61	6	0.61	1.28	1.04	0.00	0.04	—	—	—	—	—	—
睾丸	C62	2	0.20	0.43	0.30	0.00	0.00	—	—	—	—	—	—
其他的男性生殖器	C63	0	0.00	0.00	0.00	0.00	0.00	—	—	—	—	—	—
肾	C64	2	0.20	0.43	0.36	0.02	0.05	2	0.39	0.45	0.31	0.00	0.00
肾盂	C65	1	0.10	0.21	0.15	0.01	0.01	0	0.00	0.00	0.00	0.00	0.00
输尿管	C66	2	0.20	0.43	0.38	0.04	0.04	0	0.00	0.00	0.00	0.00	0.00
膀胱	C67	10	1.02	2.14	2.08	0.05	0.26	1	0.20	0.23	0.21	0.00	0.05
其他的泌尿器官	C68	2	0.20	0.43	0.34	0.04	0.04	2	0.39	0.45	0.38	0.03	0.03
眼	C69	0	0.00	0.00	0.00	0.00	0.00	0	0.00	0.00	0.00	0.00	0.00
脑、神经系统	C70–C72	19	1.94	4.06	3.75	0.16	0.27	9	1.77	2.03	1.88	0.08	0.19
甲状腺	C73	3	0.31	0.64	0.54	0.05	0.05	13	2.56	2.93	2.12	0.23	0.23
肾上腺	C74	0	0.00	0.00	0.00	0.00	0.00	0	0.00	0.00	0.00	0.00	0.00
其他的内分泌腺	C75	1	0.10	0.21	0.21	0.00	0.04	0	0.00	0.00	0.00	0.00	0.00
霍奇金病	C81	3	0.31	0.64	0.75	0.04	0.04	3	0.59	0.68	0.59	0.01	0.10
非霍奇金淋巴瘤	C82–C85;C96	10	1.02	2.14	1.77	0.05	0.18	6	1.18	1.35	1.42	0.11	0.17
免疫增生性疾病	C88	0	0.00	0.00	0.00	0.00	0.00	0	0.00	0.00	0.00	0.00	0.00
多发性骨髓瘤	C90	0	0.00	0.00	0.00	0.00	0.00	0	0.00	0.00	0.00	0.00	0.00
淋巴样白血病	C91	2	0.20	0.43	0.36	0.02	0.05	1	0.20	0.23	0.18	0.01	0.01
髓样白血病	C92–C94	1	0.10	0.21	0.26	0.02	0.02	1	0.20	0.23	0.30	0.01	0.01
白血病，未特指	C95	9	0.92	1.92	1.43	0.10	0.10	7	1.38	1.58	1.48	0.06	0.15
其他的或未指明部位的	O&U	15	1.54	3.21	3.02	0.16	0.38	10	1.97	2.25	1.98	0.13	0.22
骨髓增殖性疾病	MPD	0	0.00	0.00	0.00	0.00	0.00	0	0.00	0.00	0.00	0.00	0.00
骨髓增生异常综合征	MDS	0	0.00	0.00	0.00	0.00	0.00	0	0.00	0.00	0.00	0.00	0.00
合计	ALL	977	100.00	208.83	185.51	7.36	19.75	508	100.00	114.37	94.70	5.01	10.14
所有部位除外 C44	ALL but C44	975	99.80	208.40	185.08	7.33	19.68	507	99.80	114.14	94.53	5.00	10.12

表 6-2-12b 2014 年河南省内乡县恶性肿瘤死亡主要指标

部位		男性						女性					
		病例数	构成 (%)	粗率 (1/10^5)	世标率 (1/10^5)	累积率 (%) 0~64	累积率 (%) 0~74	病例数	构成 (%)	粗率 (1/10^5)	世标率 (1/10^5)	累积率 (%) 0~64	累积率 (%) 0~74
唇	C00	2	0.27	0.54	0.42	0.00	0.04	0	0.00	0.00	0.00	0.00	0.00
舌	C01–C02	0	0.00	0.00	0.00	0.00	0.00	0	0.00	0.00	0.00	0.00	0.00
口	C03–C06	1	0.13	0.27	0.27	0.00	0.04	0	0.00	0.00	0.00	0.00	0.00
唾液腺	C07–C08	0	0.00	0.00	0.00	0.00	0.00	0	0.00	0.00	0.00	0.00	0.00
扁桃体	C09	1	0.13	0.27	0.25	0.03	0.03	0	0.00	0.00	0.00	0.00	0.00
其他的口咽	C10	1	0.13	0.27	0.27	0.00	0.04	1	0.26	0.29	0.15	0.00	0.00
鼻咽	C11	1	0.13	0.27	0.27	0.00	0.04	1	0.26	0.29	0.24	0.02	0.02
喉咽	C12–C13	2	0.27	0.54	0.39	0.04	0.04	0	0.00	0.00	0.00	0.00	0.00
咽，部位不明	C14	0	0.00	0.00	0.00	0.00	0.00	0	0.00	0.00	0.00	0.00	0.00
食管	C15	227	30.47	61.67	50.98	2.69	6.53	107	27.79	30.51	22.67	0.78	3.08
胃	C16	239	32.08	64.93	52.49	2.94	6.93	70	18.18	19.96	14.38	0.65	1.87
小肠	C17	0	0.00	0.00	0.00	0.00	0.00	0	0.00	0.00	0.00	0.00	0.00
结肠	C18	6	0.81	1.63	1.46	0.12	0.20	7	1.82	2.00	1.56	0.11	0.21
直肠	C19–C20	26	3.49	7.06	5.79	0.31	0.82	17	4.42	4.85	3.66	0.20	0.44
肛门	C21	0	0.00	0.00	0.00	0.00	0.00	0	0.00	0.00	0.00	0.00	0.00
肝脏	C22	57	7.65	15.48	12.74	0.90	1.66	27	7.01	7.70	6.19	0.31	0.84
胆囊及其他	C23–C24	4	0.54	1.09	0.99	0.05	0.10	2	0.52	0.57	0.42	0.00	0.05
胰腺	C25	8	1.07	2.17	1.80	0.12	0.28	7	1.82	2.00	1.57	0.10	0.20
鼻、鼻窦及其他	C30–C31	0	0.00	0.00	0.00	0.00	0.00	0	0.00	0.00	0.00	0.00	0.00
喉	C32	3	0.40	0.81	0.76	0.06	0.11	1	0.26	0.29	0.22	0.00	0.06
气管、支气管、肺	C33–C34	119	15.97	32.33	26.78	1.53	3.79	43	11.17	12.26	9.03	0.55	0.95
其他的胸腔器官	C37–C38	1	0.13	0.27	0.16	0.00	0.00	0	0.00	0.00	0.00	0.00	0.00
骨	C40–C41	4	0.54	1.09	1.00	0.09	0.09	3	0.78	0.86	0.55	0.04	0.04
皮肤的黑色素瘤	C43	0	0.00	0.00	0.00	0.00	0.00	0	0.00	0.00	0.00	0.00	0.00
其他的皮肤	C44	2	0.27	0.54	0.45	0.02	0.08	1	0.26	0.29	0.12	0.00	0.00
间皮瘤	C45	2	0.27	0.54	0.50	0.02	0.07	0	0.00	0.00	0.00	0.00	0.00
卡波西肉瘤	C46	0	0.00	0.00	0.00	0.00	0.00	0	0.00	0.00	0.00	0.00	0.00
周围神经、其他结缔组织、软组织	C47;C49	0	0.00	0.00	0.00	0.00	0.00	1	0.26	0.29	0.26	0.03	0.03
乳房	C50	—	—	—	—	—	—	34	8.83	9.69	7.07	0.62	0.76
外阴	C51	—	—	—	—	—	—	0	0.00	0.00	0.00	0.00	0.00
阴道	C52	—	—	—	—	—	—	2	0.52	0.57	0.38	0.03	0.03
子宫颈	C53	—	—	—	—	—	—	13	3.38	3.71	2.90	0.21	0.43
子宫体	C54	—	—	—	—	—	—	16	4.16	4.56	3.42	0.19	0.51
子宫，部位不明	C55	—	—	—	—	—	—	0	0.00	0.00	0.00	0.00	0.00
卵巢	C56	—	—	—	—	—	—	8	2.08	2.28	1.81	0.15	0.19
其他的女性生殖器	C57	—	—	—	—	—	—	0	0.00	0.00	0.00	0.00	0.00
胎盘	C58	—	—	—	—	—	—	0	0.00	0.00	0.00	0.00	0.00
阴茎	C60	0	0.00	0.00	0.00	0.00	0.00	—	—	—	—	—	—
前列腺	C61	5	0.67	1.36	1.23	0.00	0.18	—	—	—	—	—	—
睾丸	C62	0	0.00	0.00	0.00	0.00	0.00	—	—	—	—	—	—
其他的男性生殖器	C63	1	0.13	0.27	0.31	0.00	0.00	—	—	—	—	—	—
肾	C64	1	0.13	0.27	0.27	0.00	0.04	1	0.26	0.29	0.26	0.03	0.03
肾盂	C65	1	0.13	0.27	0.25	0.03	0.03	0	0.00	0.00	0.00	0.00	0.00
输尿管	C66	0	0.00	0.00	0.00	0.00	0.00	0	0.00	0.00	0.00	0.00	0.00
膀胱	C67	2	0.27	0.54	0.41	0.03	0.03	2	0.52	0.57	0.49	0.02	0.06
其他的泌尿器官	C68	0	0.00	0.00	0.00	0.00	0.00	0	0.00	0.00	0.00	0.00	0.00
眼	C69	0	0.00	0.00	0.00	0.00	0.00	0	0.00	0.00	0.00	0.00	0.00
脑、神经系统	C70–C72	7	0.94	1.90	1.88	0.13	0.13	8	2.08	2.28	2.01	0.14	0.24
甲状腺	C73	1	0.13	0.27	0.27	0.00	0.04	2	0.52	0.57	0.81	0.05	0.05
肾上腺	C74	0	0.00	0.00	0.00	0.00	0.00	0	0.00	0.00	0.00	0.00	0.00
其他的内分泌腺	C75	1	0.13	0.27	0.18	0.02	0.02	0	0.00	0.00	0.00	0.00	0.00
霍奇金病	C81	2	0.27	0.54	0.41	0.05	0.05	1	0.26	0.29	0.21	0.02	0.02
非霍奇金淋巴瘤	C82–C85;C96	11	1.48	2.99	2.25	0.18	0.22	1	0.26	0.29	0.24	0.02	0.02
免疫增生性疾病	C88	0	0.00	0.00	0.00	0.00	0.00	1	0.26	0.29	0.19	0.00	0.00
多发性骨髓瘤	C90	0	0.00	0.00	0.00	0.00	0.00	0	0.00	0.00	0.00	0.00	0.00
淋巴样白血病	C91	0	0.00	0.00	0.00	0.00	0.00	0	0.00	0.00	0.00	0.00	0.00
髓样白血病	C92–C94	2	0.27	0.54	0.50	0.04	0.04	2	0.52	0.57	0.40	0.03	0.03
白血病，未特指	C95	1	0.13	0.27	0.27	0.00	0.04	3	0.78	0.86	1.08	0.06	0.06
其他的或未指明部位的	O&U	4	0.54	1.09	0.84	0.05	0.10	3	0.78	0.86	0.66	0.07	0.07
骨髓增殖性疾病	MPD	0	0.00	0.00	0.00	0.00	0.00	0	0.00	0.00	0.00	0.00	0.00
骨髓增生异常综合征	MDS	0	0.00	0.00	0.00	0.00	0.00	0	0.00	0.00	0.00	0.00	0.00
合计	ALL	745	100.00	202.38	166.82	9.45	21.85	385	100.00	109.77	82.95	4.43	10.31
所有部位除外 C44	ALL but C44	743	99.73	201.84	166.36	9.43	21.77	384	99.74	109.48	82.83	4.43	10.31

表 6-2-13b　2014 年河南省汝阳县恶性肿瘤死亡主要指标

部位		男性						女性					
		病例数	构成 (%)	粗率 ($1/10^5$)	世标率 ($1/10^5$)	累积率 (%) 0~64	累积率 (%) 0~74	病例数	构成 (%)	粗率 ($1/10^5$)	世标率 ($1/10^5$)	累积率 (%) 0~64	累积率 (%) 0~74
唇	C00	0	0.00	0.00	0.00	0.00	0.00	0	0.00	0.00	0.00	0.00	0.00
舌	C01–C02	0	0.00	0.00	0.00	0.00	0.00	0	0.00	0.00	0.00	0.00	0.00
口	C03–C06	0	0.00	0.00	0.00	0.00	0.00	2	0.78	0.81	0.60	0.00	0.11
唾液腺	C07–C08	2	0.42	0.76	0.61	0.05	0.05	0	0.00	0.00	0.00	0.00	0.00
扁桃体	C09	0	0.00	0.00	0.00	0.00	0.00	1	0.39	0.41	0.17	0.00	0.00
其他的口咽	C10	1	0.21	0.38	0.23	0.00	0.00	1	0.39	0.41	0.17	0.00	0.00
鼻咽	C11	2	0.42	0.76	0.61	0.06	0.06	1	0.39	0.41	0.43	0.00	0.11
喉咽	C12–C13	1	0.21	0.38	0.28	0.03	0.03	1	0.39	0.41	0.51	0.00	0.08
咽，部位不明	C14	0	0.00	0.00	0.00	0.00	0.00	0	0.00	0.00	0.00	0.00	0.00
食管	C15	89	18.74	33.67	29.88	1.15	4.00	45	17.44	18.32	12.50	0.25	1.25
胃	C16	122	25.68	46.16	41.76	1.39	4.75	46	17.83	18.73	13.95	0.32	1.71
小肠	C17	0	0.00	0.00	0.00	0.00	0.00	0	0.00	0.00	0.00	0.00	0.00
结肠	C18	1	0.21	0.38	0.29	0.02	0.02	3	1.16	1.22	1.04	0.05	0.16
直肠	C19–C20	7	1.47	2.65	2.29	0.08	0.08	7	2.71	2.85	1.73	0.03	0.14
肛门	C21	0	0.00	0.00	0.00	0.00	0.00	0	0.00	0.00	0.00	0.00	0.00
肝脏	C22	40	8.42	15.13	13.05	0.88	1.41	19	7.36	7.74	5.38	0.28	0.47
胆囊及其他	C23–C24	5	1.05	1.89	1.50	0.06	0.14	9	3.49	3.66	2.92	0.09	0.39
胰腺	C25	5	1.05	1.89	1.70	0.14	0.24	8	3.10	3.26	2.56	0.08	0.24
鼻、鼻窦及其他	C30–C31	0	0.00	0.00	0.00	0.00	0.00	0	0.00	0.00	0.00	0.00	0.00
喉	C32	2	0.42	0.76	0.63	0.00	0.10	0	0.00	0.00	0.00	0.00	0.00
气管、支气管、肺	C33–C34	143	30.11	54.10	48.87	1.47	5.61	46	17.83	18.73	14.38	0.81	1.58
其他的胸腔器官	C37–C38	0	0.00	0.00	0.00	0.00	0.00	1	0.39	0.41	0.31	0.04	0.04
骨	C40–C41	4	0.84	1.51	1.38	0.09	0.09	0	0.00	0.00	0.00	0.00	0.00
皮肤的黑色素瘤	C43	0	0.00	0.00	0.00	0.00	0.00	0	0.00	0.00	0.00	0.00	0.00
其他的皮肤	C44	2	0.42	0.76	0.82	0.00	0.00	4	1.55	1.63	1.28	0.04	0.04
间皮瘤	C45	0	0.00	0.00	0.00	0.00	0.00	0	0.00	0.00	0.00	0.00	0.00
卡波西肉瘤	C46	0	0.00	0.00	0.00	0.00	0.00	0	0.00	0.00	0.00	0.00	0.00
周围神经、其他结缔组织、软组织	C47;C49	0	0.00	0.00	0.00	0.00	0.00	0	0.00	0.00	0.00	0.00	0.00
乳房	C50	—	—	—	—	—	—	15	5.81	6.11	5.49	0.42	0.69
外阴	C51	—	—	—	—	—	—	0	0.00	0.00	0.00	0.00	0.00
阴道	C52	—	—	—	—	—	—	0	0.00	0.00	0.00	0.00	0.00
子宫颈	C53	—	—	—	—	—	—	11	4.26	4.48	3.70	0.24	0.43
子宫体	C54	—	—	—	—	—	—	2	0.78	0.81	0.66	0.06	0.06
子宫，部位不明	C55	—	—	—	—	—	—	0	0.00	0.00	0.00	0.00	0.00
卵巢	C56	—	—	—	—	—	—	2	0.78	0.81	0.71	0.08	0.08
其他的女性生殖器	C57	—	—	—	—	—	—	0	0.00	0.00	0.00	0.00	0.00
胎盘	C58	—	—	—	—	—	—	0	0.00	0.00	0.00	0.00	0.00
阴茎	C60	0	0.00	0.00	0.00	0.00	0.00	—	—	—	—	—	—
前列腺	C61	6	1.26	2.27	1.75	0.00	0.00	—	—	—	—	—	—
睾丸	C62	1	0.21	0.38	0.31	0.03	0.03	—	—	—	—	—	—
其他的男性生殖器	C63	0	0.00	0.00	0.00	0.00	0.00	—	—	—	—	—	—
肾	C64	0	0.00	0.00	0.00	0.00	0.00	2	0.78	0.81	0.35	0.00	0.00
肾盂	C65	0	0.00	0.00	0.00	0.00	0.00	0	0.00	0.00	0.00	0.00	0.00
输尿管	C66	2	0.42	0.76	0.63	0.00	0.10	0	0.00	0.00	0.00	0.00	0.00
膀胱	C67	5	1.05	1.89	1.88	0.05	0.22	2	0.78	0.81	0.72	0.00	0.08
其他的泌尿器官	C68	0	0.00	0.00	0.00	0.00	0.00	0	0.00	0.00	0.00	0.00	0.00
眼	C69	0	0.00	0.00	0.00	0.00	0.00	0	0.00	0.00	0.00	0.00	0.00
脑、神经系统	C70–C72	9	1.89	3.41	3.17	0.11	0.28	10	3.88	4.07	3.62	0.22	0.30
甲状腺	C73	1	0.21	0.38	0.40	0.00	0.10	3	1.16	1.22	0.96	0.08	0.08
肾上腺	C74	0	0.00	0.00	0.00	0.00	0.00	0	0.00	0.00	0.00	0.00	0.00
其他的内分泌腺	C75	2	0.42	0.76	0.71	0.03	0.13	0	0.00	0.00	0.00	0.00	0.00
霍奇金病	C81	0	0.00	0.00	0.00	0.00	0.00	0	0.00	0.00	0.00	0.00	0.00
非霍奇金淋巴瘤	C82–C85;C96	2	0.42	0.76	0.61	0.06	0.06	2	0.78	0.81	1.01	0.00	0.17
免疫增生性疾病	C88	0	0.00	0.00	0.00	0.00	0.00	0	0.00	0.00	0.00	0.00	0.00
多发性骨髓瘤	C90	1	0.21	0.38	0.23	0.00	0.00	0	0.00	0.00	0.00	0.00	0.00
淋巴样白血病	C91	1	0.21	0.38	0.32	0.02	0.02	1	0.39	0.41	0.37	0.02	0.02
髓样白血病	C92–C94	2	0.42	0.76	0.63	0.05	0.05	1	0.39	0.41	0.21	0.00	0.00
白血病，未特指	C95	9	1.89	3.41	3.03	0.19	0.26	8	3.10	3.26	2.43	0.13	0.21
其他的或未指明部位的	O&U	5	1.05	1.89	1.81	0.03	0.31	5	1.94	2.04	1.37	0.13	0.13
骨髓增殖性疾病	MPD	1	0.21	0.38	0.31	0.03	0.03	0	0.00	0.00	0.00	0.00	0.00
骨髓增生异常综合征	MDS	2	0.42	0.76	0.65	0.08	0.08	0	0.00	0.00	0.00	0.00	0.00
合计	ALL	475	100.00	179.71	160.36	6.10	18.27	258	100.00	105.05	79.53	3.36	8.58
所有部位除外 C44	ALL but C44	473	99.58	178.96	159.53	6.10	18.27	254	98.45	103.42	78.25	3.33	8.54

表 6-2-14b 2014 年河南省三门峡市恶性肿瘤死亡主要指标

部位		男性						女性					
		病例数	构成 (%)	粗率 ($1/10^5$)	世标率 ($1/10^5$)	累积率 (%) 0~64	累积率 (%) 0~74	病例数	构成 (%)	粗率 ($1/10^5$)	世标率 ($1/10^5$)	累积率 (%) 0~64	累积率 (%) 0~74
唇	C00	0	0.00	0.00	0.00	0.00	0.00	0	0.00	0.00	0.00	0.00	0.00
舌	C01–C02	0	0.00	0.00	0.00	0.00	0.00	0	0.00	0.00	0.00	0.00	0.00
口	C03–C06	1	0.36	0.68	0.40	0.04	0.04	0	0.00	0.00	0.00	0.00	0.00
唾液腺	C07–C08	0	0.00	0.00	0.00	0.00	0.00	0	0.00	0.00	0.00	0.00	0.00
扁桃体	C09	0	0.00	0.00	0.00	0.00	0.00	0	0.00	0.00	0.00	0.00	0.00
其他的口咽	C10	2	0.71	1.37	0.91	0.00	0.00	0	0.00	0.00	0.00	0.00	0.00
鼻咽	C11	2	0.71	1.37	0.81	0.00	0.09	0	0.00	0.00	0.00	0.00	0.00
喉咽	C12–C13	0	0.00	0.00	0.00	0.00	0.00	0	0.00	0.00	0.00	0.00	0.00
咽，部位不明	C14	1	0.36	0.68	0.41	0.05	0.05	0	0.00	0.00	0.00	0.00	0.00
食管	C15	17	6.05	11.63	8.04	0.31	1.27	8	5.00	5.46	3.47	0.05	0.48
胃	C16	36	12.81	24.62	16.69	0.87	1.94	15	9.38	10.24	5.52	0.25	0.43
小肠	C17	1	0.36	0.68	0.57	0.00	0.09	0	0.00	0.00	0.00	0.00	0.00
结肠	C18	7	2.49	4.79	2.94	0.07	0.34	5	3.13	3.41	1.78	0.11	0.11
直肠	C19–C20	25	8.90	17.10	10.09	0.33	0.83	20	12.50	13.65	8.62	0.19	0.98
肛门	C21	0	0.00	0.00	0.00	0.00	0.00	1	0.63	0.68	0.25	0.00	0.00
肝脏	C22	44	15.66	30.10	19.00	0.85	2.18	14	8.75	9.56	5.00	0.18	0.53
胆囊及其他	C23–C24	2	0.71	1.37	0.79	0.00	0.14	5	3.13	3.41	2.09	0.00	0.19
胰腺	C25	8	2.85	5.47	3.30	0.14	0.41	9	5.63	6.14	3.88	0.08	0.44
鼻、鼻窦及其他	C30–C31	0	0.00	0.00	0.00	0.00	0.00	0	0.00	0.00	0.00	0.00	0.00
喉	C32	2	0.71	1.37	0.88	0.00	0.14	0	0.00	0.00	0.00	0.00	0.00
气管、支气管、肺	C33–C34	91	32.38	62.24	37.60	1.25	3.56	33	20.63	22.53	13.01	0.78	1.32
其他的胸腔器官	C37–C38	2	0.71	1.37	0.91	0.00	0.00	1	0.63	0.68	0.56	0.07	0.07
骨	C40–C41	6	2.14	4.10	2.76	0.03	0.26	1	0.63	0.68	0.56	0.07	0.07
皮肤的黑色素瘤	C43	0	0.00	0.00	0.00	0.00	0.00	0	0.00	0.00	0.00	0.00	0.00
其他的皮肤	C44	1	0.36	0.68	0.58	0.00	0.00	2	1.25	1.37	1.12	0.07	0.16
间皮瘤	C45	0	0.00	0.00	0.00	0.00	0.00	0	0.00	0.00	0.00	0.00	0.00
卡波西肉瘤	C46	0	0.00	0.00	0.00	0.00	0.00	0	0.00	0.00	0.00	0.00	0.00
周围神经、其他结缔组织、软组织	C47;C49	0	0.00	0.00	0.00	0.00	0.00	0	0.00	0.00	0.00	0.00	0.00
乳房	C50	—	—	—	—	—	—	16	10.00	10.92	7.07	0.44	0.75
外阴	C51	—	—	—	—	—	—	0	0.00	0.00	0.00	0.00	0.00
阴道	C52	—	—	—	—	—	—	0	0.00	0.00	0.00	0.00	0.00
子宫颈	C53	—	—	—	—	—	—	7	4.38	4.78	2.73	0.24	0.24
子宫体	C54	—	—	—	—	—	—	4	2.50	2.73	1.88	0.08	0.30
子宫，部位不明	C55	—	—	—	—	—	—	1	0.63	0.68	0.56	0.07	0.07
卵巢	C56	—	—	—	—	—	—	2	1.25	1.37	0.97	0.10	0.10
其他的女性生殖器	C57	—	—	—	—	—	—	0	0.00	0.00	0.00	0.00	0.00
胎盘	C58	—	—	—	—	—	—	0	0.00	0.00	0.00	0.00	0.00
阴茎	C60	0	0.00	0.00	0.00	0.00	0.00	—	—	—	—	—	—
前列腺	C61	6	2.14	4.10	2.85	0.07	0.07	—	—	—	—	—	—
睾丸	C62	1	0.36	0.68	0.62	0.04	0.04	—	—	—	—	—	—
其他的男性生殖器	C63	0	0.00	0.00	0.00	0.00	0.00	—	—	—	—	—	—
肾	C64	6	2.14	4.10	3.63	0.19	0.32	1	0.63	0.68	0.25	0.00	0.00
肾盂	C65	0	0.00	0.00	0.00	0.00	0.00	0	0.00	0.00	0.00	0.00	0.00
输尿管	C66	3	1.07	2.05	1.15	0.00	0.00	0	0.00	0.00	0.00	0.00	0.00
膀胱	C67	3	1.07	2.05	0.91	0.00	0.00	1	0.63	0.68	0.47	0.00	0.00
其他的泌尿器官	C68	0	0.00	0.00	0.00	0.00	0.00	0	0.00	0.00	0.00	0.00	0.00
眼	C69	0	0.00	0.00	0.00	0.00	0.00	0	0.00	0.00	0.00	0.00	0.00
脑、神经系统	C70–C72	1	0.36	0.68	0.40	0.04	0.04	5	3.13	3.41	2.29	0.07	0.28
甲状腺	C73	1	0.36	0.68	0.41	0.03	0.03	2	1.25	1.37	1.07	0.05	0.17
肾上腺	C74	0	0.00	0.00	0.00	0.00	0.00	0	0.00	0.00	0.00	0.00	0.00
其他的内分泌腺	C75	0	0.00	0.00	0.00	0.00	0.00	0	0.00	0.00	0.00	0.00	0.00
霍奇金病	C81	0	0.00	0.00	0.00	0.00	0.00	0	0.00	0.00	0.00	0.00	0.00
非霍奇金淋巴瘤	C82–C85;C96	4	1.42	2.74	1.52	0.03	0.13	2	1.25	1.37	0.73	0.00	0.12
免疫增生性疾病	C88	0	0.00	0.00	0.00	0.00	0.00	0	0.00	0.00	0.00	0.00	0.00
多发性骨髓瘤	C90	1	0.36	0.68	0.55	0.00	0.14	0	0.00	0.00	0.00	0.00	0.00
淋巴样白血病	C91	1	0.36	0.68	0.57	0.00	0.09	0	0.00	0.00	0.00	0.00	0.00
髓样白血病	C92–C94	4	1.42	2.74	1.76	0.11	0.20	1	0.63	0.68	0.60	0.04	0.04
白血病，未特指	C95	0	0.00	0.00	0.00	0.00	0.00	0	0.00	0.00	0.00	0.00	0.00
其他的或未指明部位的	O&U	2	0.71	1.37	0.95	0.05	0.19	4	2.50	2.73	1.71	0.11	0.23
骨髓增殖性疾病	MPD	0	0.00	0.00	0.00	0.00	0.00	0	0.00	0.00	0.00	0.00	0.00
骨髓增生异常综合征	MDS	0	0.00	0.00	0.00	0.00	0.00	0	0.00	0.00	0.00	0.00	0.00
合计	ALL	281	100.00	192.20	121.99	4.49	12.61	160	100.00	109.22	66.18	3.06	7.08
所有部位除外 C44	ALL but C44	280	99.64	191.52	121.42	4.49	12.61	158	98.75	107.86	65.07	2.99	6.92

表 6-2-15b 2014 年河南省沈丘县恶性肿瘤死亡主要指标

部位		男性						女性					
		病例数	构成 (%)	粗率 ($1/10^5$)	世标率 ($1/10^5$)	累积率 (%) 0~64	累积率 (%) 0~74	病例数	构成 (%)	粗率 ($1/10^5$)	世标率 ($1/10^5$)	累积率 (%) 0~64	累积率 (%) 0~74
唇	C00	0	0.00	0.00	0.00	0.00	0.00	0	0.00	0.00	0.00	0.00	0.00
舌	C01–C02	2	0.14	0.34	0.20	0.00	0.03	3	0.33	0.52	0.30	0.02	0.02
口	C03–C06	3	0.21	0.50	0.42	0.02	0.05	2	0.22	0.34	0.16	0.00	0.00
唾液腺	C07–C08	0	0.00	0.00	0.00	0.00	0.00	0	0.00	0.00	0.00	0.00	0.00
扁桃体	C09	1	0.07	0.17	0.20	0.02	0.02	0	0.00	0.00	0.00	0.00	0.00
其他的口咽	C10	3	0.21	0.50	0.58	0.05	0.05	0	0.00	0.00	0.00	0.00	0.00
鼻咽	C11	5	0.34	0.84	0.68	0.05	0.08	7	0.77	1.20	1.25	0.13	0.13
喉咽	C12–C13	1	0.07	0.17	0.15	0.02	0.02	0	0.00	0.00	0.00	0.00	0.00
咽，部位不明	C14	1	0.07	0.17	0.12	0.00	0.03	0	0.00	0.00	0.00	0.00	0.00
食管	C15	177	12.16	29.66	24.60	1.20	2.87	123	13.52	21.17	14.84	0.53	1.75
胃	C16	204	14.01	34.18	28.64	1.36	3.53	116	12.75	19.97	13.51	0.55	1.47
小肠	C17	7	0.48	1.17	0.88	0.03	0.08	1	0.11	0.17	0.07	0.00	0.00
结肠	C18	23	1.58	3.85	3.37	0.21	0.47	22	2.42	3.79	3.09	0.22	0.39
直肠	C19–C20	45	3.09	7.54	6.75	0.44	0.99	40	4.40	6.89	4.77	0.28	0.48
肛门	C21	0	0.00	0.00	0.00	0.00	0.00	0	0.00	0.00	0.00	0.00	0.00
肝脏	C22	341	23.42	57.14	50.36	3.60	5.89	133	14.62	22.89	18.57	1.25	2.22
胆囊及其他	C23–C24	9	0.62	1.51	1.48	0.10	0.18	19	2.09	3.27	2.35	0.08	0.32
胰腺	C25	18	1.24	3.02	2.63	0.18	0.35	12	1.32	2.07	1.24	0.02	0.14
鼻、鼻窦及其他	C30–C31	0	0.00	0.00	0.00	0.00	0.00	1	0.11	0.17	0.15	0.00	0.02
喉	C32	11	0.76	1.84	1.46	0.09	0.17	1	0.11	0.17	0.15	0.00	0.02
气管、支气管、肺	C33–C34	435	29.88	72.89	60.74	3.39	7.29	211	23.19	36.32	26.91	1.41	3.19
其他的胸腔器官	C37–C38	1	0.07	0.17	0.15	0.02	0.02	1	0.11	0.17	0.16	0.02	0.02
骨	C40–C41	19	1.30	3.18	3.08	0.25	0.39	6	0.66	1.03	0.91	0.07	0.07
皮肤的黑色素瘤	C43	0	0.00	0.00	0.00	0.00	0.00	0	0.00	0.00	0.00	0.00	0.00
其他的皮肤	C44	6	0.41	1.01	0.95	0.09	0.12	6	0.66	1.03	0.70	0.03	0.05
间皮瘤	C45	0	0.00	0.00	0.00	0.00	0.00	0	0.00	0.00	0.00	0.00	0.00
卡波西肉瘤	C46	0	0.00	0.00	0.00	0.00	0.00	0	0.00	0.00	0.00	0.00	0.00
周围神经、其他结缔组织、软组织	C47;C49	1	0.07	0.17	0.12	0.00	0.03	0	0.00	0.00	0.00	0.00	0.00
乳房	C50	—	—	—	—	—	—	64	7.03	11.02	9.54	0.81	1.00
外阴	C51	—	—	—	—	—	—	0	0.00	0.00	0.00	0.00	0.00
阴道	C52	—	—	—	—	—	—	0	0.00	0.00	0.00	0.00	0.00
子宫颈	C53	—	—	—	—	—	—	41	4.51	7.06	5.46	0.29	0.75
子宫体	C54	—	—	—	—	—	—	5	0.55	0.86	0.84	0.08	0.10
子宫，部位不明	C55	—	—	—	—	—	—	0	0.00	0.00	0.00	0.00	0.00
卵巢	C56	—	—	—	—	—	—	15	1.65	2.58	2.15	0.15	0.26
其他的女性生殖器	C57	—	—	—	—	—	—	0	0.00	0.00	0.00	0.00	0.00
胎盘	C58	—	—	—	—	—	—	1	0.11	0.17	0.10	0.01	0.01
阴茎	C60	0	0.00	0.00	0.00	0.00	0.00	—	—	—	—	—	—
前列腺	C61	10	0.69	1.68	1.32	0.05	0.13	—	—	—	—	—	—
睾丸	C62	1	0.07	0.17	0.12	0.00	0.03	—	—	—	—	—	—
其他的男性生殖器	C63	1	0.07	0.17	0.08	0.00	0.00	—	—	—	—	—	—
肾	C64	10	0.69	1.68	1.37	0.08	0.20	5	0.55	0.86	0.69	0.04	0.09
肾盂	C65	2	0.14	0.34	0.27	0.00	0.05	0	0.00	0.00	0.00	0.00	0.00
输尿管	C66	1	0.07	0.17	0.19	0.02	0.02	0	0.00	0.00	0.00	0.00	0.00
膀胱	C67	29	1.99	4.86	3.80	0.09	0.50	8	0.88	1.38	0.91	0.01	0.15
其他的泌尿器官	C68	0	0.00	0.00	0.00	0.00	0.00	0	0.00	0.00	0.00	0.00	0.00
眼	C69	0	0.00	0.00	0.00	0.00	0.00	0	0.00	0.00	0.00	0.00	0.00
脑、神经系统	C70–C72	36	2.47	6.03	4.99	0.31	0.53	28	3.08	4.82	3.91	0.23	0.48
甲状腺	C73	2	0.14	0.34	0.28	0.02	0.02	4	0.44	0.69	0.57	0.03	0.08
肾上腺	C74	1	0.07	0.17	0.19	0.02	0.02	1	0.11	0.17	0.12	0.00	0.03
其他的内分泌腺	C75	0	0.00	0.00	0.00	0.00	0.00	0	0.00	0.00	0.00	0.00	0.00
霍奇金病	C81	7	0.48	1.17	0.92	0.03	0.12	2	0.22	0.34	0.36	0.04	0.04
非霍奇金淋巴瘤	C82–C85;C96	15	1.03	2.51	2.25	0.17	0.31	7	0.77	1.20	1.01	0.08	0.14
免疫增生性疾病	C88	0	0.00	0.00	0.00	0.00	0.00	1	0.11	0.17	0.15	0.00	0.02
多发性骨髓瘤	C90	2	0.14	0.34	0.31	0.02	0.05	1	0.11	0.17	0.07	0.00	0.00
淋巴样白血病	C91	4	0.27	0.67	0.70	0.03	0.06	2	0.22	0.34	0.38	0.02	0.02
髓样白血病	C92–C94	0	0.00	0.00	0.00	0.00	0.00	0	0.00	0.00	0.00	0.00	0.00
白血病，未特指	C95	19	1.30	3.18	2.84	0.18	0.28	21	2.31	3.61	3.35	0.23	0.39
其他的或未指明部位的	O&U	3	0.21	0.50	0.42	0.02	0.05	0	0.00	0.00	0.00	0.00	0.00
骨髓增殖性疾病	MPD	0	0.00	0.00	0.00	0.00	0.00	0	0.00	0.00	0.00	0.00	0.00
骨髓增生异常综合征	MDS	0	0.00	0.00	0.00	0.00	0.00	0	0.00	0.00	0.00	0.00	0.00
合计	ALL	1 456	100.00	243.97	207.61	12.18	25.06	910	100.00	156.65	118.72	6.60	13.85
所有部位除外 C44	ALL but C44	1 450	99.59	242.97	206.66	12.09	24.94	904	99.34	155.62	118.02	6.57	13.80

表 6-2-16b 2014 年河南省西平县恶性肿瘤死亡主要指标

部位		男性						女性					
		病例数	构成(%)	粗率($1/10^5$)	世标率($1/10^5$)	累积率(%) 0~64	累积率(%) 0~74	病例数	构成(%)	粗率($1/10^5$)	世标率($1/10^5$)	累积率(%) 0~64	累积率(%) 0~74
唇	C00	0	0.00	0.00	0.00	0.00	0.00	0	0.00	0.00	0.00	0.00	0.00
舌	C01–C02	1	0.12	0.22	0.13	0.00	0.00	0	0.00	0.00	0.00	0.00	0.00
口	C03–C06	2	0.24	0.44	0.29	0.01	0.01	0	0.00	0.00	0.00	0.00	0.00
唾液腺	C07–C08	1	0.12	0.22	0.16	0.02	0.02	1	0.18	0.24	0.17	0.02	0.02
扁桃体	C09	1	0.12	0.22	0.13	0.00	0.00	0	0.00	0.00	0.00	0.00	0.00
其他的口咽	C10	0	0.00	0.00	0.00	0.00	0.00	1	0.18	0.24	0.18	0.01	0.01
鼻咽	C11	3	0.36	0.67	0.53	0.04	0.09	3	0.53	0.71	0.46	0.04	0.04
喉咽	C12–C13	2	0.24	0.44	0.33	0.03	0.03	0	0.00	0.00	0.00	0.00	0.00
咽，部位不明	C14	0	0.00	0.00	0.00	0.00	0.00	0	0.00	0.00	0.00	0.00	0.00
食管	C15	118	14.05	26.23	21.52	0.58	1.88	74	13.17	17.42	9.67	0.12	0.91
胃	C16	98	11.67	21.78	17.68	0.52	1.49	45	8.01	10.59	6.36	0.24	0.59
小肠	C17	3	0.36	0.67	0.57	0.03	0.10	3	0.53	0.71	0.45	0.03	0.03
结肠	C18	16	1.90	3.56	3.03	0.11	0.26	12	2.14	2.82	1.84	0.06	0.21
直肠	C19–C20	15	1.79	3.33	2.58	0.14	0.37	21	3.74	4.94	3.42	0.21	0.31
肛门	C21	0	0.00	0.00	0.00	0.00	0.00	0	0.00	0.00	0.00	0.00	0.00
肝脏	C22	155	18.45	34.45	26.76	1.77	2.59	70	12.46	16.48	10.61	0.51	1.06
胆囊及其他	C23–C24	12	1.43	2.67	2.33	0.08	0.16	26	4.63	6.12	3.83	0.21	0.29
胰腺	C25	18	2.14	4.00	3.19	0.09	0.38	13	2.31	3.06	2.27	0.11	0.28
鼻、鼻窦及其他	C30–C31	1	0.12	0.22	0.16	0.02	0.02	1	0.18	0.24	0.17	0.01	0.01
喉	C32	6	0.71	1.33	1.29	0.04	0.15	1	0.18	0.24	0.16	0.02	0.02
气管、支气管、肺	C33–C34	264	31.43	58.67	46.55	1.68	4.68	119	21.17	28.01	16.95	0.65	1.52
其他的胸腔器官	C37–C38	2	0.24	0.44	0.33	0.03	0.03	2	0.36	0.47	0.34	0.00	0.03
骨	C40–C41	6	0.71	1.33	1.28	0.03	0.13	9	1.60	2.12	1.35	0.07	0.14
皮肤的黑色素瘤	C43	0	0.00	0.00	0.00	0.00	0.00	2	0.36	0.47	0.35	0.00	0.07
其他的皮肤	C44	4	0.48	0.89	0.83	0.00	0.08	2	0.36	0.47	0.18	0.00	0.00
间皮瘤	C45	0	0.00	0.00	0.00	0.00	0.00	1	0.18	0.24	0.21	0.03	0.03
卡波西肉瘤	C46	0	0.00	0.00	0.00	0.00	0.00	0	0.00	0.00	0.00	0.00	0.00
周围神经、其他结缔组织、软组织	C47;C49	4	0.48	0.89	0.65	0.05	0.05	1	0.18	0.24	0.15	0.00	0.00
乳房	C50	—	—	—	—	—	—	50	8.90	11.77	8.52	0.70	0.87
外阴	C51	—	—	—	—	—	—	0	0.00	0.00	0.00	0.00	0.00
阴道	C52	—	—	—	—	—	—	1	0.18	0.24	0.17	0.02	0.02
子宫颈	C53	—	—	—	—	—	—	19	3.38	4.47	3.25	0.26	0.37
子宫体	C54	—	—	—	—	—	—	10	1.78	2.35	1.69	0.09	0.23
子宫，部位不明	C55	—	—	—	—	—	—	5	0.89	1.18	0.86	0.07	0.10
卵巢	C56	—	—	—	—	—	—	12	2.14	2.82	2.11	0.09	0.27
其他的女性生殖器	C57	—	—	—	—	—	—	0	0.00	0.00	0.00	0.00	0.00
胎盘	C58	—	—	—	—	—	—	0	0.00	0.00	0.00	0.00	0.00
阴茎	C60	0	0.00	0.00	0.00	0.00	0.00	—	—	—	—	—	—
前列腺	C61	12	1.43	2.67	2.40	0.03	0.11	—	—	—	—	—	—
睾丸	C62	1	0.12	0.22	0.17	0.02	0.02	—	—	—	—	—	—
其他的男性生殖器	C63	0	0.00	0.00	0.00	0.00	0.00	—	—	—	—	—	—
肾	C64	3	0.36	0.67	0.75	0.04	0.07	0	0.00	0.00	0.00	0.00	0.00
肾盂	C65	1	0.12	0.22	0.17	0.02	0.02	1	0.18	0.24	0.16	0.02	0.02
输尿管	C66	1	0.12	0.22	0.17	0.00	0.04	1	0.18	0.24	0.16	0.00	0.04
膀胱	C67	8	0.95	1.78	1.35	0.07	0.13	2	0.36	0.47	0.26	0.02	0.02
其他的泌尿器官	C68	0	0.00	0.00	0.00	0.00	0.00	0	0.00	0.00	0.00	0.00	0.00
眼	C69	0	0.00	0.00	0.00	0.00	0.00	1	0.18	0.24	0.21	0.03	0.03
脑、神经系统	C70–C72	24	2.86	5.33	5.17	0.26	0.44	15	2.67	3.53	2.34	0.12	0.25
甲状腺	C73	2	0.24	0.44	0.32	0.04	0.04	1	0.18	0.24	0.10	0.00	0.00
肾上腺	C74	0	0.00	0.00	0.00	0.00	0.00	0	0.00	0.00	0.00	0.00	0.00
其他的内分泌腺	C75	1	0.12	0.22	0.13	0.00	0.00	0	0.00	0.00	0.00	0.00	0.00
霍奇金病	C81	0	0.00	0.00	0.00	0.00	0.00	1	0.18	0.24	0.15	0.00	0.00
非霍奇金淋巴瘤	C82–C85;C96	16	1.90	3.56	2.85	0.25	0.25	10	1.78	2.35	1.65	0.11	0.21
免疫增生性疾病	C88	0	0.00	0.00	0.00	0.00	0.00	0	0.00	0.00	0.00	0.00	0.00
多发性骨髓瘤	C90	5	0.60	1.11	0.78	0.02	0.09	1	0.18	0.24	0.16	0.02	0.02
淋巴样白血病	C91	5	0.60	1.11	0.93	0.08	0.08	4	0.71	0.94	0.87	0.07	0.07
髓样白血病	C92–C94	8	0.95	1.78	1.45	0.12	0.12	7	1.25	1.65	0.94	0.06	0.06
白血病，未特指	C95	5	0.60	1.11	1.12	0.05	0.09	6	1.07	1.41	0.95	0.07	0.10
其他的或未指明部位的	O&U	10	1.19	2.22	1.93	0.11	0.15	6	1.07	1.41	1.30	0.04	0.08
骨髓增殖性疾病	MPD	0	0.00	0.00	0.00	0.00	0.00	1	0.18	0.24	0.10	0.00	0.00
骨髓增生异常综合征	MDS	5	0.60	1.11	1.13	0.07	0.10	1	0.18	0.24	0.19	0.00	0.03
合计	ALL	840	100.00	186.69	151.29	6.45	14.27	562	100.00	132.27	85.25	4.12	8.35
所有部位除外 C44	ALL but C44	836	99.52	185.80	150.46	6.45	14.18	560	99.64	131.80	85.07	4.12	8.35

表 6-2-17b　2014 年河南省开封市祥符区恶性肿瘤死亡主要指标

部位		男性						女性					
		病例数	构成 (%)	粗率 (1/10^5)	世标率 (1/10^5)	累积率 (%) 0~64	累积率 (%) 0~74	病例数	构成 (%)	粗率 (1/10^5)	世标率 (1/10^5)	累积率 (%) 0~64	累积率 (%) 0~74
唇	C00	0	0.00	0.00	0.00	0.00	0.00	0	0.00	0.00	0.00	0.00	0.00
舌	C01–C02	2	0.38	0.56	0.49	0.00	0.05	0	0.00	0.00	0.00	0.00	0.00
口	C03–C06	0	0.00	0.00	0.00	0.00	0.00	1	0.37	0.29	0.15	0.00	0.00
唾液腺	C07–C08	0	0.00	0.00	0.00	0.00	0.00	1	0.37	0.29	0.28	0.00	0.07
扁桃体	C09	0	0.00	0.00	0.00	0.00	0.00	0	0.00	0.00	0.00	0.00	0.00
其他的口咽	C10	1	0.19	0.28	0.17	0.02	0.02	0	0.00	0.00	0.00	0.00	0.00
鼻咽	C11	2	0.38	0.56	0.42	0.05	0.05	1	0.37	0.29	0.33	0.03	0.03
喉咽	C12–C13	0	0.00	0.00	0.00	0.00	0.00	0	0.00	0.00	0.00	0.00	0.00
咽，部位不明	C14	0	0.00	0.00	0.00	0.00	0.00	0	0.00	0.00	0.00	0.00	0.00
食管	C15	62	11.81	17.34	14.98	0.52	1.61	20	7.49	5.77	3.84	0.06	0.44
胃	C16	79	15.05	22.10	19.92	1.07	2.50	38	14.23	10.97	7.76	0.27	1.05
小肠	C17	8	1.52	2.24	1.80	0.17	0.22	3	1.12	0.87	0.49	0.00	0.07
结肠	C18	18	3.43	5.04	4.60	0.27	0.54	3	1.12	0.87	0.50	0.03	0.03
直肠	C19–C20	17	3.24	4.76	4.13	0.12	0.40	9	3.37	2.60	1.74	0.02	0.23
肛门	C21	4	0.76	1.12	1.14	0.08	0.13	2	0.75	0.58	0.42	0.05	0.05
肝脏	C22	67	12.76	18.74	17.31	1.38	1.99	19	7.12	5.48	4.62	0.26	0.65
胆囊及其他	C23–C24	10	1.90	2.80	2.30	0.10	0.23	13	4.87	3.75	2.49	0.10	0.27
胰腺	C25	15	2.86	4.20	3.81	0.17	0.55	7	2.62	2.02	1.33	0.12	0.12
鼻、鼻窦及其他	C30–C31	0	0.00	0.00	0.00	0.00	0.00	3	1.12	0.87	0.52	0.00	0.07
喉	C32	4	0.76	1.12	0.83	0.08	0.08	1	0.37	0.29	0.17	0.02	0.02
气管、支气管、肺	C33–C34	170	32.38	47.56	43.68	1.36	5.50	74	27.72	21.36	15.98	0.63	2.10
其他的胸腔器官	C37–C38	3	0.57	0.84	0.88	0.06	0.06	0	0.00	0.00	0.00	0.00	0.00
骨	C40–C41	4	0.76	1.12	1.02	0.11	0.11	3	1.12	0.87	0.56	0.04	0.04
皮肤的黑色素瘤	C43	3	0.57	0.84	0.85	0.06	0.13	2	0.75	0.58	0.24	0.00	0.00
其他的皮肤	C44	2	0.38	0.56	0.56	0.03	0.08	2	0.75	0.58	0.60	0.00	0.10
间皮瘤	C45	0	0.00	0.00	0.00	0.00	0.00	0	0.00	0.00	0.00	0.00	0.00
卡波西肉瘤	C46	0	0.00	0.00	0.00	0.00	0.00	0	0.00	0.00	0.00	0.00	0.00
周围神经、其他结缔组织、软组织	C47;C49	2	0.38	0.56	0.55	0.05	0.05	1	0.37	0.29	0.28	0.00	0.07
乳房	C50	—	—	—	—	—	—	11	4.12	3.18	2.46	0.23	0.23
外阴	C51	—	—	—	—	—	—	0	0.00	0.00	0.00	0.00	0.00
阴道	C52	—	—	—	—	—	—	0	0.00	0.00	0.00	0.00	0.00
子宫颈	C53	—	—	—	—	—	—	13	4.87	3.75	2.85	0.20	0.32
子宫体	C54	—	—	—	—	—	—	6	2.25	1.73	1.30	0.09	0.16
子宫，部位不明	C55	—	—	—	—	—	—	0	0.00	0.00	0.00	0.00	0.00
卵巢	C56	—	—	—	—	—	—	6	2.25	1.73	1.48	0.08	0.20
其他的女性生殖器	C57	—	—	—	—	—	—	0	0.00	0.00	0.00	0.00	0.00
胎盘	C58	—	—	—	—	—	—	0	0.00	0.00	0.00	0.00	0.00
阴茎	C60	0	0.00	0.00	0.00	0.00	0.00	—	—	—	—	—	—
前列腺	C61	2	0.38	0.56	0.48	0.00	0.00	—	—	—	—	—	—
睾丸	C62	0	0.00	0.00	0.00	0.00	0.00	—	—	—	—	—	—
其他的男性生殖器	C63	0	0.00	0.00	0.00	0.00	0.00	—	—	—	—	—	—
肾	C64	2	0.38	0.56	0.51	0.06	0.06	0	0.00	0.00	0.00	0.00	0.00
肾盂	C65	2	0.38	0.56	0.55	0.03	0.03	2	0.75	0.58	0.40	0.00	0.05
输尿管	C66	0	0.00	0.00	0.00	0.00	0.00	0	0.00	0.00	0.00	0.00	0.00
膀胱	C67	11	2.10	3.08	2.70	0.03	0.18	2	0.75	0.58	0.29	0.00	0.00
其他的泌尿器官	C68	0	0.00	0.00	0.00	0.00	0.00	0	0.00	0.00	0.00	0.00	0.00
眼	C69	0	0.00	0.00	0.00	0.00	0.00	0	0.00	0.00	0.00	0.00	0.00
脑、神经系统	C70–C72	10	1.90	2.80	2.50	0.08	0.21	7	2.62	2.02	1.96	0.14	0.21
甲状腺	C73	1	0.19	0.28	0.15	0.00	0.00	3	1.12	0.87	0.66	0.05	0.05
肾上腺	C74	1	0.19	0.28	0.26	0.03	0.03	0	0.00	0.00	0.00	0.00	0.00
其他的内分泌腺	C75	1	0.19	0.28	0.15	0.00	0.00	0	0.00	0.00	0.00	0.00	0.00
霍奇金病	C81	0	0.00	0.00	0.00	0.00	0.00	0	0.00	0.00	0.00	0.00	0.00
非霍奇金淋巴瘤	C82–C85;C96	7	1.33	1.96	1.51	0.06	0.06	0	0.00	0.00	0.00	0.00	0.00
免疫增生性疾病	C88	0	0.00	0.00	0.00	0.00	0.00	0	0.00	0.00	0.00	0.00	0.00
多发性骨髓瘤	C90	1	0.19	0.28	0.31	0.00	0.08	2	0.75	0.58	0.50	0.06	0.06
淋巴样白血病	C91	5	0.95	1.40	1.51	0.08	0.08	5	1.87	1.44	1.09	0.05	0.12
髓样白血病	C92–C94	2	0.38	0.56	0.47	0.03	0.03	4	1.50	1.15	0.97	0.07	0.07
白血病，未特指	C95	6	1.14	1.68	1.66	0.06	0.21	2	0.75	0.58	0.58	0.00	0.12
其他的或未指明部位的	O&U	1	0.19	0.28	0.31	0.00	0.08	1	0.37	0.29	0.15	0.00	0.00
骨髓增殖性疾病	MPD	0	0.00	0.00	0.00	0.00	0.00	0	0.00	0.00	0.00	0.00	0.00
骨髓增生异常综合征	MDS	0	0.00	0.00	0.00	0.00	0.00	0	0.00	0.00	0.00	0.00	0.00
合计	ALL	525	100.00	146.87	132.52	6.16	15.35	267	100.00	77.07	56.97	2.60	6.99
所有部位除外 C44	ALL but C44	523	99.62	146.31	131.96	6.12	15.27	265	99.25	76.49	56.37	2.60	6.89

表 6-2-18b 2014 年河南省新安县恶性肿瘤死亡主要指标

部位		男性						女性					
		病例数	构成 (%)	粗率 ($1/10^5$)	世标率 ($1/10^5$)	累积率 (%) 0~4	累积率 (%) 0~74	病例数	构成 (%)	粗率 ($1/10^5$)	世标率 ($1/10^5$)	累积率 (%) 0~64	累积率 (%) 0~74
唇	C00	0	0.00	0.00	0.00	0.00	0.00	0	0.00	0.00	0.00	0.00	0.00
舌	C01–C02	0	0.00	0.00	0.00	0.00	0.00	1	0.27	0.39	0.17	0.00	0.00
口	C03–C06	0	0.00	0.00	0.00	0.00	0.00	0	0.00	0.00	0.00	0.00	0.00
唾液腺	C07–C08	0	0.00	0.00	0.00	0.00	0.00	0	0.00	0.00	0.00	0.00	0.00
扁桃体	C09	0	0.00	0.00	0.00	0.00	0.00	0	0.00	0.00	0.00	0.00	0.00
其他的口咽	C10	1	0.18	0.36	0.27	0.00	0.07	0	0.00	0.00	0.00	0.00	0.00
鼻咽	C11	3	0.54	1.09	0.78	0.05	0.05	3	0.82	1.16	0.54	0.03	0.03
喉咽	C12–C13	0	0.00	0.00	0.00	0.00	0.00	0	0.00	0.00	0.00	0.00	0.00
咽，部位不明	C14	0	0.00	0.00	0.00	0.00	0.00	0	0.00	0.00	0.00	0.00	0.00
食管	C15	75	13.49	27.22	20.69	0.84	2.62	46	12.60	17.78	12.39	0.54	1.68
胃	C16	126	22.66	45.73	33.01	0.99	3.99	69	18.90	26.66	17.80	0.67	2.04
小肠	C17	0	0.00	0.00	0.00	0.00	0.00	0	0.00	0.00	0.00	0.00	0.00
结肠	C18	11	1.98	3.99	2.90	0.21	0.27	3	0.82	1.16	1.03	0.03	0.17
直肠	C19–C20	21	3.78	7.62	5.41	0.07	0.89	11	3.01	4.25	3.03	0.21	0.35
肛门	C21	1	0.18	0.36	0.33	0.00	0.05	0	0.00	0.00	0.00	0.00	0.00
肝脏	C22	92	16.55	33.39	25.06	1.13	2.97	64	17.53	24.73	17.06	0.60	2.19
胆囊及其他	C23–C24	3	0.54	1.09	0.89	0.03	0.10	15	4.11	5.80	3.36	0.08	0.39
胰腺	C25	11	1.98	3.99	3.03	0.15	0.38	10	2.74	3.86	2.47	0.19	0.19
鼻、鼻窦及其他	C30–C31	0	0.00	0.00	0.00	0.00	0.00	0	0.00	0.00	0.00	0.00	0.00
喉	C32	3	0.54	1.09	0.79	0.07	0.07	1	0.27	0.39	0.31	0.00	0.08
气管、支气管、肺	C33–C34	145	26.08	52.63	39.00	1.85	4.54	66	18.08	25.50	16.50	0.60	1.88
其他的胸腔器官	C37–C38	0	0.00	0.00	0.00	0.00	0.00	0	0.00	0.00	0.00	0.00	0.00
骨	C40–C41	4	0.72	1.45	1.19	0.10	0.17	3	0.82	1.16	1.02	0.13	0.13
皮肤的黑色素瘤	C43	0	0.00	0.00	0.00	0.00	0.00	0	0.00	0.00	0.00	0.00	0.00
其他的皮肤	C44	1	0.18	0.36	0.30	0.00	0.00	0	0.00	0.00	0.00	0.00	0.00
间皮瘤	C45	0	0.00	0.00	0.00	0.00	0.00	0	0.00	0.00	0.00	0.00	0.00
卡波西肉瘤	C46	0	0.00	0.00	0.00	0.00	0.00	0	0.00	0.00	0.00	0.00	0.00
周围神经、其他结缔组织、软组织	C47;C49	0	0.00	0.00	0.00	0.00	0.00	0	0.00	0.00	0.00	0.00	0.00
乳房	C50	—	—	—	—	—	—	18	4.93	6.96	5.23	0.36	0.57
外阴	C51	—	—	—	—	—	—	0	0.00	0.00	0.00	0.00	0.00
阴道	C52	—	—	—	—	—	—	0	0.00	0.00	0.00	0.00	0.00
子宫颈	C53	—	—	—	—	—	—	21	5.75	8.11	6.73	0.45	0.92
子宫体	C54	—	—	—	—	—	—	1	0.27	0.39	0.28	0.02	0.02
子宫，部位不明	C55	—	—	—	—	—	—	9	2.47	3.48	1.96	0.06	0.12
卵巢	C56	—	—	—	—	—	—	1	0.27	0.39	0.28	0.02	0.02
其他的女性生殖器	C57	—	—	—	—	—	—	0	0.00	0.00	0.00	0.00	0.00
胎盘	C58	—	—	—	—	—	—	0	0.00	0.00	0.00	0.00	0.00
阴茎	C60	0	0.00	0.00	0.00	0.00	0.00	—	—	—	—	—	—
前列腺	C61	13	2.34	4.72	3.22	0.06	0.17	—	—	—	—	—	—
睾丸	C62	1	0.18	0.36	0.27	0.00	0.07	—	—	—	—	—	—
其他的男性生殖器	C63	1	0.18	0.36	0.33	0.00	0.05	—	—	—	—	—	—
肾	C64	7	1.26	2.54	1.88	0.05	0.18	4	1.10	1.55	0.96	0.06	0.06
肾盂	C65	0	0.00	0.00	0.00	0.00	0.00	0	0.00	0.00	0.00	0.00	0.00
输尿管	C66	1	0.18	0.36	0.27	0.00	0.07	0	0.00	0.00	0.00	0.00	0.00
膀胱	C67	3	0.54	1.09	0.87	0.00	0.19	0	0.00	0.00	0.00	0.00	0.00
其他的泌尿器官	C68	0	0.00	0.00	0.00	0.00	0.00	0	0.00	0.00	0.00	0.00	0.00
眼	C69	0	0.00	0.00	0.00	0.00	0.00	0	0.00	0.00	0.00	0.00	0.00
脑、神经系统	C70–C72	12	2.16	4.36	3.10	0.18	0.24	11	3.01	4.25	3.27	0.26	0.34
甲状腺	C73	3	0.54	1.09	0.86	0.07	0.07	0	0.00	0.00	0.00	0.00	0.00
肾上腺	C74	0	0.00	0.00	0.00	0.00	0.00	0	0.00	0.00	0.00	0.00	0.00
其他的内分泌腺	C75	0	0.00	0.00	0.00	0.00	0.00	0	0.00	0.00	0.00	0.00	0.00
霍奇金病	C81	1	0.18	0.36	0.30	0.00	0.00	0	0.00	0.00	0.00	0.00	0.00
非霍奇金淋巴瘤	C82–C85;C96	2	0.36	0.73	0.57	0.00	0.07	1	0.27	0.39	0.31	0.00	0.08
免疫增生性疾病	C88	0	0.00	0.00	0.00	0.00	0.00	0	0.00	0.00	0.00	0.00	0.00
多发性骨髓瘤	C90	0	0.00	0.00	0.00	0.00	0.00	0	0.00	0.00	0.00	0.00	0.00
淋巴样白血病	C91	2	0.36	0.73	0.74	0.04	0.04	0	0.00	0.00	0.00	0.00	0.00
髓样白血病	C92–C94	0	0.00	0.00	0.00	0.00	0.00	2	0.55	0.77	0.65	0.03	0.10
白血病，未特指	C95	5	0.90	1.81	1.38	0.04	0.10	0	0.00	0.00	0.00	0.00	0.00
其他的或未指明部位的	O&U	6	1.08	2.18	1.60	0.07	0.20	5	1.37	1.93	1.45	0.07	0.22
骨髓增殖性疾病	MPD	1	0.18	0.36	0.27	0.00	0.07	0	0.00	0.00	0.00	0.00	0.00
骨髓增生异常综合征	MDS	1	0.18	0.36	0.14	0.00	0.00	0	0.00	0.00	0.00	0.00	0.00
合计	ALL	556	100.00	201.81	149.46	6.03	17.68	365	100.00	141.04	96.80	4.41	11.58
所有部位除外 C44	ALL but C44	555	99.82	201.45	149.16	6.03	17.68	365	100.00	141.04	96.80	4.41	11.58

表 6-2-19b 2014 年河南省宜阳县恶性肿瘤死亡主要指标

部位		男性						女性					
		病例数	构成(%)	粗率($1/10^5$)	世标率($1/10^5$)	累积率(%) 0~64	累积率(%) 0~74	病例数	构成(%)	粗率($1/10^5$)	世标率($1/10^5$)	累积率(%) 0~64	累积率(%) 0~74
唇	C00	0	0.00	0.00	0.00	0.00	0.00	0	0.00	0.00	0.00	0.00	0.00
舌	C01–C02	0	0.00	0.00	0.00	0.00	0.00	0	0.00	0.00	0.00	0.00	0.00
口	C03–C06	0	0.00	0.00	0.00	0.00	0.00	0	0.00	0.00	0.00	0.00	0.00
唾液腺	C07–C08	0	0.00	0.00	0.00	0.00	0.00	0	0.00	0.00	0.00	0.00	0.00
扁桃体	C09	0	0.00	0.00	0.00	0.00	0.00	0	0.00	0.00	0.00	0.00	0.00
其他的口咽	C10	0	0.00	0.00	0.00	0.00	0.00	0	0.00	0.00	0.00	0.00	0.00
鼻咽	C11	1	0.14	0.28	0.23	0.03	0.03	1	0.23	0.30	0.31	0.00	0.05
喉咽	C12–C13	1	0.14	0.28	0.26	0.00	0.07	0	0.00	0.00	0.00	0.00	0.00
咽，部位不明	C14	0	0.00	0.00	0.00	0.00	0.00	0	0.00	0.00	0.00	0.00	0.00
食管	C15	246	33.38	68.76	60.62	1.90	6.59	128	29.16	37.90	27.43	0.84	3.31
胃	C16	194	26.32	54.22	49.45	1.67	5.52	98	22.32	29.02	21.93	0.85	2.39
小肠	C17	2	0.27	0.56	0.48	0.02	0.08	0	0.00	0.00	0.00	0.00	0.00
结肠	C18	6	0.81	1.68	1.45	0.08	0.14	5	1.14	1.48	0.98	0.04	0.11
直肠	C19–C20	7	0.95	1.96	2.15	0.15	0.20	9	2.05	2.66	2.15	0.09	0.25
肛门	C21	0	0.00	0.00	0.00	0.00	0.00	0	0.00	0.00	0.00	0.00	0.00
肝脏	C22	69	9.36	19.29	18.13	0.88	2.11	41	9.34	12.14	8.24	0.26	0.78
胆囊及其他	C23–C24	8	1.09	2.24	1.98	0.03	0.16	5	1.14	1.48	1.15	0.00	0.17
胰腺	C25	4	0.54	1.12	0.86	0.10	0.10	5	1.14	1.48	1.34	0.08	0.13
鼻、鼻窦及其他	C30–C31	1	0.14	0.28	0.25	0.02	0.02	0	0.00	0.00	0.00	0.00	0.00
喉	C32	1	0.14	0.28	0.23	0.03	0.03	2	0.46	0.59	0.47	0.00	0.06
气管、支气管、肺	C33–C34	149	20.22	41.65	38.01	1.19	4.04	75	17.08	22.21	16.39	0.83	1.66
其他的胸腔器官	C37–C38	0	0.00	0.00	0.00	0.00	0.00	2	0.46	0.59	0.37	0.02	0.02
骨	C40–C41	2	0.27	0.56	0.45	0.05	0.05	2	0.46	0.59	0.55	0.03	0.03
皮肤的黑色素瘤	C43	0	0.00	0.00	0.00	0.00	0.00	0	0.00	0.00	0.00	0.00	0.00
其他的皮肤	C44	2	0.27	0.56	0.76	0.00	0.05	1	0.23	0.30	0.20	0.02	0.02
间皮瘤	C45	0	0.00	0.00	0.00	0.00	0.00	0	0.00	0.00	0.00	0.00	0.00
卡波西肉瘤	C46	0	0.00	0.00	0.00	0.00	0.00	0	0.00	0.00	0.00	0.00	0.00
周围神经、其他结缔组织、软组织	C47;C49	0	0.00	0.00	0.00	0.00	0.00	0	0.00	0.00	0.00	0.00	0.00
乳房	C50	—	—	—	—	—	—	19	4.33	5.63	4.39	0.29	0.53
外阴	C51	—	—	—	—	—	—	0	0.00	0.00	0.00	0.00	0.00
阴道	C52	—	—	—	—	—	—	0	0.00	0.00	0.00	0.00	0.00
子宫颈	C53	—	—	—	—	—	—	14	3.19	4.15	3.29	0.20	0.52
子宫体	C54	—	—	—	—	—	—	1	0.23	0.30	0.20	0.02	0.02
子宫，部位不明	C55	—	—	—	—	—	—	1	0.23	0.30	0.20	0.03	0.03
卵巢	C56	—	—	—	—	—	—	10	2.28	2.96	2.66	0.11	0.39
其他的女性生殖器	C57	—	—	—	—	—	—	0	0.00	0.00	0.00	0.00	0.00
胎盘	C58	—	—	—	—	—	—	0	0.00	0.00	0.00	0.00	0.00
阴茎	C60	0	0.00	0.00	0.00	0.00	0.00	—	—	—	—	—	—
前列腺	C61	2	0.27	0.56	0.50	0.03	0.09	—	—	—	—	—	—
睾丸	C62	1	0.14	0.28	0.23	0.03	0.03	—	—	—	—	—	—
其他的男性生殖器	C63	0	0.00	0.00	0.00	0.00	0.00	—	—	—	—	—	—
肾	C64	4	0.54	1.12	0.88	0.07	0.12	0	0.00	0.00	0.00	0.00	0.00
肾盂	C65	0	0.00	0.00	0.00	0.00	0.00	0	0.00	0.00	0.00	0.00	0.00
输尿管	C66	0	0.00	0.00	0.00	0.00	0.00	0	0.00	0.00	0.00	0.00	0.00
膀胱	C67	5	0.68	1.40	1.19	0.06	0.11	1	0.23	0.30	0.14	0.00	0.00
其他的泌尿器官	C68	0	0.00	0.00	0.00	0.00	0.00	0	0.00	0.00	0.00	0.00	0.00
眼	C69	0	0.00	0.00	0.00	0.00	0.00	0	0.00	0.00	0.00	0.00	0.00
脑、神经系统	C70–C72	9	1.22	2.52	2.29	0.11	0.22	5	1.14	1.48	1.50	0.04	0.22
甲状腺	C73	2	0.27	0.56	0.45	0.03	0.03	0	0.00	0.00	0.00	0.00	0.00
肾上腺	C74	1	0.14	0.28	0.30	0.00	0.05	0	0.00	0.00	0.00	0.00	0.00
其他的内分泌腺	C75	0	0.00	0.00	0.00	0.00	0.00	0	0.00	0.00	0.00	0.00	0.00
霍奇金病	C81	0	0.00	0.00	0.00	0.00	0.00	0	0.00	0.00	0.00	0.00	0.00
非霍奇金淋巴瘤	C82–C85;C96	2	0.27	0.56	0.47	0.06	0.06	1	0.23	0.30	0.21	0.01	0.01
免疫增生性疾病	C88	0	0.00	0.00	0.00	0.00	0.00	0	0.00	0.00	0.00	0.00	0.00
多发性骨髓瘤	C90	0	0.00	0.00	0.00	0.00	0.00	0	0.00	0.00	0.00	0.00	0.00
淋巴样白血病	C91	1	0.14	0.28	0.40	0.02	0.02	1	0.23	0.30	0.21	0.01	0.01
髓样白血病	C92–C94	1	0.14	0.28	0.19	0.02	0.02	0	0.00	0.00	0.00	0.00	0.00
白血病，未特指	C95	6	0.81	1.68	1.33	0.04	0.15	4	0.91	1.18	1.27	0.10	0.10
其他的或未指明部位的	O&U	9	1.22	2.52	2.38	0.08	0.20	8	1.82	2.37	1.91	0.15	0.20
骨髓增殖性疾病	MPD	0	0.00	0.00	0.00	0.00	0.00	0	0.00	0.00	0.00	0.00	0.00
骨髓增生异常综合征	MDS	0	0.00	0.00	0.00	0.00	0.00	0	0.00	0.00	0.00	0.00	0.00
合计	ALL	737	100.00	205.99	186.19	6.70	20.36	439	100.00	129.99	97.49	4.03	11.00
所有部位除外 C44	ALL but C44	735	99.73	205.43	185.43	6.70	20.31	438	99.77	129.69	97.29	4.01	10.99

表 6-2-20b 2014 年河南省虞城县恶性肿瘤死亡主要指标

部位		男性						女性					
		病例数	构成(%)	粗率($1/10^5$)	世标率($1/10^5$)	累积率(%)		病例数	构成(%)	粗率($1/10^5$)	世标率($1/10^5$)	累积率(%)	
						0~64	0~74					0~64	0~74
唇	C00	0	0.00	0.00	0.00	0.00	0.00	0	0.00	0.00	0.00	0.00	0.00
舌	C01–C02	0	0.00	0.00	0.00	0.00	0.00	2	0.26	0.38	0.34	0.02	0.05
口	C03–C06	0	0.00	0.00	0.00	0.00	0.00	0	0.00	0.00	0.00	0.00	0.00
唾液腺	C07–C08	2	0.23	0.35	0.33	0.02	0.05	2	0.26	0.38	0.31	0.03	0.03
扁桃体	C09	1	0.11	0.17	0.18	0.00	0.03	1	0.13	0.19	0.12	0.00	0.00
其他的口咽	C10	0	0.00	0.00	0.00	0.00	0.00	0	0.00	0.00	0.00	0.00	0.00
鼻咽	C11	2	0.23	0.35	0.30	0.03	0.03	9	1.16	1.69	1.46	0.08	0.22
喉咽	C12–C13	1	0.11	0.17	0.15	0.02	0.02	0	0.00	0.00	0.00	0.00	0.00
咽，部位不明	C14	5	0.57	0.87	0.81	0.06	0.09	2	0.26	0.38	0.31	0.02	0.06
食管	C15	106	12.03	18.50	16.80	0.77	2.54	131	16.82	24.59	21.50	1.69	2.85
胃	C16	229	25.99	39.97	34.43	1.19	4.26	80	10.27	15.02	12.21	0.68	1.67
小肠	C17	17	1.93	2.97	2.50	0.11	0.25	9	1.16	1.69	1.28	0.09	0.12
结肠	C18	22	2.50	3.84	3.33	0.14	0.52	14	1.80	2.63	2.08	0.10	0.29
直肠	C19–C20	41	4.65	7.16	6.48	0.22	0.88	21	2.70	3.94	3.24	0.13	0.45
肛门	C21	1	0.11	0.17	0.09	0.00	0.00	2	0.26	0.38	0.20	0.01	0.01
肝脏	C22	125	14.19	21.82	19.33	0.73	2.49	100	12.84	18.77	15.67	1.10	2.22
胆囊及其他	C23–C24	12	1.36	2.09	1.76	0.06	0.27	4	0.51	0.75	0.64	0.02	0.08
胰腺	C25	6	0.68	1.05	0.90	0.07	0.14	7	0.90	1.31	1.11	0.07	0.18
鼻、鼻窦及其他	C30–C31	0	0.00	0.00	0.00	0.00	0.00	1	0.13	0.19	0.19	0.00	0.03
喉	C32	12	1.36	2.09	1.87	0.09	0.27	11	1.41	2.06	1.74	0.10	0.24
气管、支气管、肺	C33–C34	197	22.36	34.38	30.40	1.26	4.16	99	12.71	18.58	14.78	0.92	1.91
其他的胸腔器官	C37–C38	1	0.11	0.17	0.18	0.00	0.03	0	0.00	0.00	0.00	0.00	0.00
骨	C40–C41	4	0.45	0.70	0.57	0.03	0.06	6	0.77	1.13	1.08	0.08	0.14
皮肤的黑色素瘤	C43	1	0.11	0.17	0.29	0.01	0.01	1	0.13	0.19	0.15	0.00	0.04
其他的皮肤	C44	3	0.34	0.52	0.53	0.04	0.04	1	0.13	0.19	0.15	0.02	0.02
间皮瘤	C45	0	0.00	0.00	0.00	0.00	0.00	0	0.00	0.00	0.00	0.00	0.00
卡波西肉瘤	C46	0	0.00	0.00	0.00	0.00	0.00	0	0.00	0.00	0.00	0.00	0.00
周围神经、其他结缔组织、软组织	C47;C49	0	0.00	0.00	0.00	0.00	0.00	0	0.00	0.00	0.00	0.00	0.00
乳房	C50	—	—	—	—	—	—	94	12.07	17.64	14.52	0.98	1.86
外阴	C51	—	—	—	—	—	—	1	0.13	0.19	0.14	0.01	0.01
阴道	C52	—	—	—	—	—	—	4	0.51	0.75	0.64	0.00	0.14
子宫颈	C53	—	—	—	—	—	—	37	4.75	6.95	5.48	0.28	0.74
子宫体	C54	—	—	—	—	—	—	19	2.44	3.57	2.60	0.20	0.27
子宫，部位不明	C55	—	—	—	—	—	—	3	0.39	0.56	0.46	0.04	0.08
卵巢	C56	—	—	—	—	—	—	47	6.03	8.82	6.33	0.31	0.73
其他的女性生殖器	C57	—	—	—	—	—	—	0	0.00	0.00	0.00	0.00	0.00
胎盘	C58	—	—	—	—	—	—	0	0.00	0.00	0.00	0.00	0.00
阴茎	C60	2	0.23	0.35	0.29	0.00	0.00	—	—	—	—	—	—
前列腺	C61	15	1.70	2.62	2.00	0.00	0.24	—	—	—	—	—	—
睾丸	C62	2	0.23	0.35	0.24	0.00	0.04	—	—	—	—	—	—
其他的男性生殖器	C63	0	0.00	0.00	0.00	0.00	0.00	—	—	—	—	—	—
肾	C64	5	0.57	0.87	0.72	0.00	0.04	2	0.26	0.38	0.27	0.00	0.04
肾盂	C65	3	0.34	0.52	0.46	0.04	0.04	1	0.13	0.19	0.12	0.00	0.00
输尿管	C66	2	0.23	0.35	0.40	0.00	0.00	0	0.00	0.00	0.00	0.00	0.00
膀胱	C67	7	0.79	1.22	0.95	0.02	0.08	7	0.90	1.31	1.18	0.07	0.17
其他的泌尿器官	C68	0	0.00	0.00	0.00	0.00	0.00	0	0.00	0.00	0.00	0.00	0.00
眼	C69	0	0.00	0.00	0.00	0.00	0.00	0	0.00	0.00	0.00	0.00	0.00
脑、神经系统	C70–C72	11	1.25	1.92	1.77	0.10	0.23	10	1.28	1.88	1.36	0.10	0.13
甲状腺	C73	9	1.02	1.57	1.21	0.04	0.11	10	1.28	1.88	1.51	0.10	0.17
肾上腺	C74	1	0.11	0.17	0.18	0.02	0.02	0	0.00	0.00	0.00	0.00	0.00
其他的内分泌腺	C75	1	0.11	0.17	0.15	0.00	0.04	2	0.26	0.38	0.27	0.02	0.02
霍奇金病	C81	0	0.00	0.00	0.00	0.00	0.00	0	0.00	0.00	0.00	0.00	0.00
非霍奇金淋巴瘤	C82–C85;C96	6	0.68	1.05	0.95	0.09	0.09	7	0.90	1.31	0.80	0.03	0.11
免疫增生性疾病	C88	0	0.00	0.00	0.00	0.00	0.00	0	0.00	0.00	0.00	0.00	0.00
多发性骨髓瘤	C90	0	0.00	0.00	0.00	0.00	0.00	0	0.00	0.00	0.00	0.00	0.00
淋巴样白血病	C91	0	0.00	0.00	0.00	0.00	0.00	4	0.51	0.75	0.60	0.00	0.11
髓样白血病	C92–C94	2	0.23	0.35	0.32	0.01	0.04	1	0.13	0.19	0.17	0.02	0.02
白血病，未特指	C95	13	1.48	2.27	2.04	0.12	0.19	15	1.93	2.82	2.49	0.14	0.34
其他的或未指明部位的	O&U	12	1.36	2.09	1.94	0.14	0.17	12	1.54	2.25	1.92	0.09	0.22
骨髓增殖性疾病	MPD	0	0.00	0.00	0.00	0.00	0.00	0	0.00	0.00	0.00	0.00	0.00
骨髓增生异常综合征	MDS	0	0.00	0.00	0.00	0.00	0.00	0	0.00	0.00	0.00	0.00	0.00
合计	ALL	881	100.00	153.77	135.13	5.46	17.47	779	100.00	146.23	119.43	7.53	15.74
所有部位除外 C44	ALL but C44	878	99.66	153.25	134.60	5.42	17.43	778	99.87	146.04	119.27	7.51	15.72

表 6-2-21b　2014 年河南省禹州市恶性肿瘤死亡主要指标

部位		男性						女性					
		病例数	构成 (%)	粗率 (1/10^5)	世标率 (1/10^5)	累积率 (%) 0~64	累积率 (%) 0~74	病例数	构成 (%)	粗率 (1/10^5)	世标率 (1/10^5)	累积率 (%) 0~64	累积率 (%) 0~74
唇	C00	0	0.00	0.00	0.00	0.00	0.00	0	0.00	0.00	0.00	0.00	0.00
舌	C01–C02	0	0.00	0.00	0.00	0.00	0.00	0	0.00	0.00	0.00	0.00	0.00
口	C03–C06	0	0.00	0.00	0.00	0.00	0.00	0	0.00	0.00	0.00	0.00	0.00
唾液腺	C07–C08	0	0.00	0.00	0.00	0.00	0.00	0	0.00	0.00	0.00	0.00	0.00
扁桃体	C09	0	0.00	0.00	0.00	0.00	0.00	0	0.00	0.00	0.00	0.00	0.00
其他的口咽	C10	1	0.09	0.17	0.09	0.00	0.00	0	0.00	0.00	0.00	0.00	0.00
鼻咽	C11	2	0.18	0.33	0.32	0.00	0.05	5	0.84	0.93	0.93	0.07	0.07
喉咽	C12–C13	0	0.00	0.00	0.00	0.00	0.00	0	0.00	0.00	0.00	0.00	0.00
咽，部位不明	C14	1	0.09	0.17	0.16	0.00	0.03	0	0.00	0.00	0.00	0.00	0.00
食管	C15	114	10.14	19.05	14.76	0.36	2.08	49	8.21	9.14	5.23	0.17	0.53
胃	C16	107	9.52	17.88	12.66	0.35	1.39	35	5.86	6.53	3.68	0.08	0.34
小肠	C17	5	0.44	0.84	0.71	0.03	0.11	3	0.50	0.56	0.34	0.00	0.04
结肠	C18	16	1.42	2.67	2.03	0.06	0.31	8	1.34	1.49	0.93	0.01	0.11
直肠	C19–C20	22	1.96	3.68	2.33	0.10	0.16	23	3.85	4.29	2.60	0.05	0.31
肛门	C21	0	0.00	0.00	0.00	0.00	0.00	0	0.00	0.00	0.00	0.00	0.00
肝脏	C22	237	21.09	39.61	30.73	1.72	3.74	89	14.91	16.61	11.42	0.61	1.47
胆囊及其他	C23–C24	2	0.18	0.33	0.24	0.00	0.04	5	0.84	0.93	0.47	0.00	0.04
胰腺	C25	8	0.71	1.34	1.15	0.04	0.11	7	1.17	1.31	0.96	0.04	0.11
鼻、鼻窦及其他	C30–C31	0	0.00	0.00	0.00	0.00	0.00	0	0.00	0.00	0.00	0.00	0.00
喉	C32	4	0.36	0.67	0.49	0.01	0.09	3	0.50	0.56	0.37	0.03	0.03
气管、支气管、肺	C33–C34	540	48.04	90.25	69.15	1.99	8.33	178	29.82	33.21	21.18	0.53	2.54
其他的胸腔器官	C37–C38	0	0.00	0.00	0.00	0.00	0.00	0	0.00	0.00	0.00	0.00	0.00
骨	C40–C41	7	0.62	1.17	0.82	0.02	0.07	4	0.67	0.75	0.71	0.04	0.11
皮肤的黑色素瘤	C43	0	0.00	0.00	0.00	0.00	0.00	0	0.00	0.00	0.00	0.00	0.00
其他的皮肤	C44	5	0.44	0.84	0.49	0.00	0.04	1	0.17	0.19	0.07	0.00	0.00
间皮瘤	C45	0	0.00	0.00	0.00	0.00	0.00	0	0.00	0.00	0.00	0.00	0.00
卡波西肉瘤	C46	0	0.00	0.00	0.00	0.00	0.00	0	0.00	0.00	0.00	0.00	0.00
周围神经、其他结缔组织、软组织	C47;C49	0	0.00	0.00	0.00	0.00	0.00	0	0.00	0.00	0.00	0.00	0.00
乳房	C50	—	—	—	—	—	—	88	14.74	16.42	12.42	0.81	1.50
外阴	C51	—	—	—	—	—	—	0	0.00	0.00	0.00	0.00	0.00
阴道	C52	—	—	—	—	—	—	0	0.00	0.00	0.00	0.00	0.00
子宫颈	C53	—	—	—	—	—	—	65	10.89	12.13	8.15	0.49	1.08
子宫体	C54	—	—	—	—	—	—	1	0.17	0.19	0.10	0.00	0.00
子宫，部位不明	C55	—	—	—	—	—	—	0	0.00	0.00	0.00	0.00	0.00
卵巢	C56	—	—	—	—	—	—	5	0.84	0.93	0.63	0.05	0.08
其他的女性生殖器	C57	—	—	—	—	—	—	0	0.00	0.00	0.00	0.00	0.00
胎盘	C58	—	—	—	—	—	—	0	0.00	0.00	0.00	0.00	0.00
阴茎	C60	0	0.00	0.00	0.00	0.00	0.00	—	—	—	—	—	—
前列腺	C61	5	0.44	0.84	0.62	0.01	0.05	—	—	—	—	—	—
睾丸	C62	0	0.00	0.00	0.00	0.00	0.00	—	—	—	—	—	—
其他的男性生殖器	C63	0	0.00	0.00	0.00	0.00	0.00	—	—	—	—	—	—
肾	C64	4	0.36	0.67	0.56	0.00	0.10	2	0.34	0.37	0.31	0.01	0.04
肾盂	C65	0	0.00	0.00	0.00	0.00	0.00	0	0.00	0.00	0.00	0.00	0.00
输尿管	C66	0	0.00	0.00	0.00	0.00	0.00	0	0.00	0.00	0.00	0.00	0.00
膀胱	C67	10	0.89	1.67	1.16	0.04	0.12	1	0.17	0.19	0.07	0.00	0.00
其他的泌尿器官	C68	0	0.00	0.00	0.00	0.00	0.00	0	0.00	0.00	0.00	0.00	0.00
眼	C69	0	0.00	0.00	0.00	0.00	0.00	0	0.00	0.00	0.00	0.00	0.00
脑、神经系统	C70–C72	18	1.60	3.01	2.77	0.19	0.25	17	2.85	3.17	2.46	0.07	0.28
甲状腺	C73	0	0.00	0.00	0.00	0.00	0.00	0	0.00	0.00	0.00	0.00	0.00
肾上腺	C74	0	0.00	0.00	0.00	0.00	0.00	0	0.00	0.00	0.00	0.00	0.00
其他的内分泌腺	C75	0	0.00	0.00	0.00	0.00	0.00	0	0.00	0.00	0.00	0.00	0.00
霍奇金病	C81	0	0.00	0.00	0.00	0.00	0.00	0	0.00	0.00	0.00	0.00	0.00
非霍奇金淋巴瘤	C82–C85;C96	0	0.00	0.00	0.00	0.00	0.00	0	0.00	0.00	0.00	0.00	0.00
免疫增生性疾病	C88	0	0.00	0.00	0.00	0.00	0.00	0	0.00	0.00	0.00	0.00	0.00
多发性骨髓瘤	C90	0	0.00	0.00	0.00	0.00	0.00	0	0.00	0.00	0.00	0.00	0.00
淋巴样白血病	C91	0	0.00	0.00	0.00	0.00	0.00	0	0.00	0.00	0.00	0.00	0.00
髓样白血病	C92–C94	0	0.00	0.00	0.00	0.00	0.00	0	0.00	0.00	0.00	0.00	0.00
白血病，未特指	C95	0	0.00	0.00	0.00	0.00	0.00	0	0.00	0.00	0.00	0.00	0.00
其他的或未指明部位的	O&U	16	1.42	2.67	2.08	0.11	0.18	8	1.34	1.49	1.04	0.02	0.15
骨髓增殖性疾病	MPD	0	0.00	0.00	0.00	0.00	0.00	0	0.00	0.00	0.00	0.00	0.00
骨髓增生异常综合征	MDS	0	0.00	0.00	0.00	0.00	0.00	0	0.00	0.00	0.00	0.00	0.00
合计	ALL	1 124	100.00	187.86	143.34	5.03	17.26	597	100.00	111.38	74.09	3.06	8.83
所有部位除外 C44	ALL but C44	1 119	99.56	187.03	142.84	5.03	17.22	596	99.83	111.20	74.01	3.06	8.83

表 6-2-22b 2014 年河南省漯河市召陵区恶性肿瘤死亡主要指标

部位		男性						女性					
		病例数	构成(%)	粗率($1/10^5$)	世标率($1/10^5$)	累积率(%) 0~64	累积率(%) 0~74	病例数	构成(%)	粗率($1/10^5$)	世标率($1/10^5$)	累积率(%) 0~64	累积率(%) 0~74
唇	C00	0	0.00	0.00	0.00	0.00	0.00	0	0.00	0.00	0.00	0.00	0.00
舌	C01–C02	0	0.00	0.00	0.00	0.00	0.00	4	1.94	1.73	1.25	0.07	0.07
口	C03–C06	0	0.00	0.00	0.00	0.00	0.00	1	0.49	0.43	0.17	0.00	0.00
唾液腺	C07–C08	0	0.00	0.00	0.00	0.00	0.00	0	0.00	0.00	0.00	0.00	0.00
扁桃体	C09	0	0.00	0.00	0.00	0.00	0.00	0	0.00	0.00	0.00	0.00	0.00
其他的口咽	C10	0	0.00	0.00	0.00	0.00	0.00	0	0.00	0.00	0.00	0.00	0.00
鼻咽	C11	0	0.00	0.00	0.00	0.00	0.00	1	0.49	0.43	0.30	0.02	0.02
喉咽	C12–C13	0	0.00	0.00	0.00	0.00	0.00	0	0.00	0.00	0.00	0.00	0.00
咽，部位不明	C14	0	0.00	0.00	0.00	0.00	0.00	0	0.00	0.00	0.00	0.00	0.00
食管	C15	42	10.74	17.13	16.02	0.43	2.05	20	9.71	8.64	6.41	0.08	0.55
胃	C16	28	7.16	11.42	10.96	0.30	0.89	12	5.83	5.18	3.52	0.11	0.45
小肠	C17	1	0.26	0.41	0.24	0.00	0.00	0	0.00	0.00	0.00	0.00	0.00
结肠	C18	9	2.30	3.67	3.23	0.13	0.35	5	2.43	2.16	1.71	0.03	0.30
直肠	C19–C20	16	4.09	6.53	5.94	0.06	0.63	10	4.85	4.32	3.02	0.13	0.22
肛门	C21	0	0.00	0.00	0.00	0.00	0.00	0	0.00	0.00	0.00	0.00	0.00
肝脏	C22	86	21.99	35.08	31.97	1.55	3.83	20	9.71	8.64	6.39	0.51	0.66
胆囊及其他	C23–C24	2	0.51	0.82	0.84	0.05	0.12	0	0.00	0.00	0.00	0.00	0.00
胰腺	C25	13	3.32	5.30	4.87	0.24	0.73	3	1.46	1.30	1.34	0.00	0.22
鼻、鼻窦及其他	C30–C31	0	0.00	0.00	0.00	0.00	0.00	0	0.00	0.00	0.00	0.00	0.00
喉	C32	0	0.00	0.00	0.00	0.00	0.00	0	0.00	0.00	0.00	0.00	0.00
气管、支气管、肺	C33–C34	156	39.90	63.64	57.73	2.31	7.20	58	28.16	25.06	18.69	0.64	2.03
其他的胸腔器官	C37–C38	0	0.00	0.00	0.00	0.00	0.00	0	0.00	0.00	0.00	0.00	0.00
骨	C40–C41	4	1.02	1.63	1.42	0.07	0.14	1	0.49	0.43	0.38	0.05	0.05
皮肤的黑色素瘤	C43	0	0.00	0.00	0.00	0.00	0.00	0	0.00	0.00	0.00	0.00	0.00
其他的皮肤	C44	0	0.00	0.00	0.00	0.00	0.00	1	0.49	0.43	0.37	0.04	0.04
间皮瘤	C45	0	0.00	0.00	0.00	0.00	0.00	0	0.00	0.00	0.00	0.00	0.00
卡波西肉瘤	C46	0	0.00	0.00	0.00	0.00	0.00	0	0.00	0.00	0.00	0.00	0.00
周围神经、其他结缔组织、软组织	C47;C49	0	0.00	0.00	0.00	0.00	0.00	0	0.00	0.00	0.00	0.00	0.00
乳房	C50	—	—	—	—	—	—	47	22.82	20.31	15.84	1.02	1.72
外阴	C51	—	—	—	—	—	—	0	0.00	0.00	0.00	0.00	0.00
阴道	C52	—	—	—	—	—	—	0	0.00	0.00	0.00	0.00	0.00
子宫颈	C53	—	—	—	—	—	—	3	1.46	1.30	1.34	0.00	0.22
子宫体	C54	—	—	—	—	—	—	5	2.43	2.16	1.69	0.10	0.28
子宫，部位不明	C55	—	—	—	—	—	—	3	1.46	1.30	1.30	0.07	0.14
卵巢	C56	—	—	—	—	—	—	2	0.97	0.86	0.63	0.05	0.05
其他的女性生殖器	C57	—	—	—	—	—	—	0	0.00	0.00	0.00	0.00	0.00
胎盘	C58	—	—	—	—	—	—	0	0.00	0.00	0.00	0.00	0.00
阴茎	C60	0	0.00	0.00	0.00	0.00	0.00	—	—	—	—	—	—
前列腺	C61	2	0.51	0.82	0.61	0.04	0.04	—	—	—	—	—	—
睾丸	C62	0	0.00	0.00	0.00	0.00	0.00	—	—	—	—	—	—
其他的男性生殖器	C63	0	0.00	0.00	0.00	0.00	0.00	—	—	—	—	—	—
肾	C64	5	1.28	2.04	2.04	0.13	0.28	0	0.00	0.00	0.00	0.00	0.00
肾盂	C65	0	0.00	0.00	0.00	0.00	0.00	0	0.00	0.00	0.00	0.00	0.00
输尿管	C66	0	0.00	0.00	0.00	0.00	0.00	0	0.00	0.00	0.00	0.00	0.00
膀胱	C67	5	1.28	2.04	2.90	0.00	0.17	0	0.00	0.00	0.00	0.00	0.00
其他的泌尿器官	C68	0	0.00	0.00	0.00	0.00	0.00	0	0.00	0.00	0.00	0.00	0.00
眼	C69	0	0.00	0.00	0.00	0.00	0.00	0	0.00	0.00	0.00	0.00	0.00
脑、神经系统	C70–C72	9	2.30	3.67	3.18	0.33	0.33	3	1.46	1.30	1.00	0.09	0.09
甲状腺	C73	1	0.26	0.41	0.39	0.05	0.05	0	0.00	0.00	0.00	0.00	0.00
肾上腺	C74	0	0.00	0.00	0.00	0.00	0.00	0	0.00	0.00	0.00	0.00	0.00
其他的内分泌腺	C75	0	0.00	0.00	0.00	0.00	0.00	0	0.00	0.00	0.00	0.00	0.00
霍奇金病	C81	4	1.02	1.63	1.31	0.03	0.20	0	0.00	0.00	0.00	0.00	0.00
非霍奇金淋巴瘤	C82–C85;C96	0	0.00	0.00	0.00	0.00	0.00	0	0.00	0.00	0.00	0.00	0.00
免疫增生性疾病	C88	0	0.00	0.00	0.00	0.00	0.00	0	0.00	0.00	0.00	0.00	0.00
多发性骨髓瘤	C90	0	0.00	0.00	0.00	0.00	0.00	0	0.00	0.00	0.00	0.00	0.00
淋巴样白血病	C91	5	1.28	2.04	1.92	0.16	0.25	4	1.94	1.73	1.36	0.03	0.10
髓样白血病	C92–C94	1	0.26	0.41	0.23	0.00	0.00	1	0.49	0.43	0.15	0.00	0.00
白血病，未特指	C95	0	0.00	0.00	0.00	0.00	0.00	0	0.00	0.00	0.00	0.00	0.00
其他的或未指明部位的	O&U	2	0.51	0.82	0.48	0.03	0.03	2	0.97	0.86	0.67	0.06	0.06
骨髓增殖性疾病	MPD	0	0.00	0.00	0.00	0.00	0.00	0	0.00	0.00	0.00	0.00	0.00
骨髓增生异常综合征	MDS	0	0.00	0.00	0.00	0.00	0.00	0	0.00	0.00	0.00	0.00	0.00
合计	ALL	391	100.00	159.51	146.27	5.90	17.28	206	100.00	89.00	67.51	3.10	7.28
所有部位除外 C44	ALL but C44	391	100.00	159.51	146.27	5.90	17.28	205	99.51	88.57	67.14	3.06	7.25

表 6-2-23b　2014 年河南省偃师市恶性肿瘤死亡主要指标

部位		男性						女性					
		病例数	构成 (%)	粗率 ($1/10^5$)	世标率 ($1/10^5$)	累积率 (%) 0~64	累积率 (%) 0~74	病例数	构成 (%)	粗率 ($1/10^5$)	世标率 ($1/10^5$)	累积率 (%) 0~64	累积率 (%) 0~74
唇	C00	0	0.00	0.00	0.00	0.00	0.00	0	0.00	0.00	0.00	0.00	0.00
舌	C01–C02	0	0.00	0.00	0.00	0.00	0.00	0	0.00	0.00	0.00	0.00	0.00
口	C03–C06	0	0.00	0.00	0.00	0.00	0.00	1	0.27	0.33	0.11	0.00	0.00
唾液腺	C07–C08	0	0.00	0.00	0.00	0.00	0.00	1	0.27	0.33	0.26	0.02	0.02
扁桃体	C09	0	0.00	0.00	0.00	0.00	0.00	0	0.00	0.00	0.00	0.00	0.00
其他的口咽	C10	0	0.00	0.00	0.00	0.00	0.00	1	0.27	0.33	0.26	0.00	0.06
鼻咽	C11	0	0.00	0.00	0.00	0.00	0.00	1	0.27	0.33	0.11	0.00	0.00
喉咽	C12–C13	1	0.19	0.32	0.30	0.00	0.05	0	0.00	0.00	0.00	0.00	0.00
咽，部位不明	C14	2	0.37	0.64	0.40	0.02	0.02	0	0.00	0.00	0.00	0.00	0.00
食管	C15	114	21.11	36.39	28.79	0.81	2.88	69	18.75	22.46	13.87	0.25	1.85
胃	C16	113	20.93	36.07	28.20	0.88	2.92	45	12.23	14.65	9.19	0.24	0.99
小肠	C17	2	0.37	0.64	0.54	0.03	0.10	2	0.54	0.65	0.39	0.02	0.02
结肠	C18	10	1.85	3.19	2.66	0.20	0.20	8	2.17	2.60	1.44	0.03	0.08
直肠	C19–C20	19	3.52	6.07	4.78	0.20	0.44	4	1.09	1.30	0.80	0.08	0.08
肛门	C21	0	0.00	0.00	0.00	0.00	0.00	0	0.00	0.00	0.00	0.00	0.00
肝脏	C22	83	15.37	26.50	20.86	1.21	2.38	36	9.78	11.72	7.61	0.46	0.86
胆囊及其他	C23–C24	8	1.48	2.55	2.02	0.02	0.21	9	2.45	2.93	1.76	0.08	0.21
胰腺	C25	8	1.48	2.55	2.37	0.02	0.38	3	0.82	0.98	0.52	0.00	0.06
鼻、鼻窦及其他	C30–C31	0	0.00	0.00	0.00	0.00	0.00	0	0.00	0.00	0.00	0.00	0.00
喉	C32	1	0.19	0.32	0.30	0.00	0.05	1	0.27	0.33	0.26	0.00	0.06
气管、支气管、肺	C33–C34	103	19.07	32.88	25.26	0.96	2.53	69	18.75	22.46	14.46	0.53	1.72
其他的胸腔器官	C37–C38	3	0.56	0.96	0.70	0.09	0.09	0	0.00	0.00	0.00	0.00	0.00
骨	C40–C41	2	0.37	0.64	0.70	0.03	0.03	3	0.82	0.98	0.64	0.06	0.06
皮肤的黑色素瘤	C43	0	0.00	0.00	0.00	0.00	0.00	2	0.54	0.65	0.57	0.02	0.07
其他的皮肤	C44	3	0.56	0.96	0.77	0.00	0.00	3	0.82	0.98	0.46	0.00	0.00
间皮瘤	C45	0	0.00	0.00	0.00	0.00	0.00	0	0.00	0.00	0.00	0.00	0.00
卡波西肉瘤	C46	0	0.00	0.00	0.00	0.00	0.00	0	0.00	0.00	0.00	0.00	0.00
周围神经、其他结缔组织、软组织	C47;C49	2	0.37	0.64	0.40	0.02	0.02	1	0.27	0.33	0.22	0.02	0.02
乳房	C50	—	—	—	—	—	—	31	8.42	10.09	7.21	0.50	0.90
外阴	C51	—	—	—	—	—	—	0	0.00	0.00	0.00	0.00	0.00
阴道	C52	—	—	—	—	—	—	2	0.54	0.65	0.37	0.00	0.06
子宫颈	C53	—	—	—	—	—	—	8	2.17	2.60	1.70	0.09	0.22
子宫体	C54	—	—	—	—	—	—	6	1.63	1.95	1.01	0.05	0.05
子宫，部位不明	C55	—	—	—	—	—	—	1	0.27	0.33	0.24	0.02	0.02
卵巢	C56	—	—	—	—	—	—	11	2.99	3.58	2.34	0.06	0.28
其他的女性生殖器	C57	—	—	—	—	—	—	1	0.27	0.33	0.16	0.00	0.00
胎盘	C58	—	—	—	—	—	—	0	0.00	0.00	0.00	0.00	0.00
阴茎	C60	0	0.00	0.00	0.00	0.00	0.00	—	—	—	—	—	—
前列腺	C61	8	1.48	2.55	2.18	0.00	0.19	—	—	—	—	—	—
睾丸	C62	0	0.00	0.00	0.00	0.00	0.00	—	—	—	—	—	—
其他的男性生殖器	C63	0	0.00	0.00	0.00	0.00	0.00	—	—	—	—	—	—
肾	C64	4	0.74	1.28	0.89	0.02	0.09	3	0.82	0.98	0.72	0.00	0.10
肾盂	C65	0	0.00	0.00	0.00	0.00	0.00	0	0.00	0.00	0.00	0.00	0.00
输尿管	C66	1	0.19	0.32	0.19	0.02	0.02	0	0.00	0.00	0.00	0.00	0.00
膀胱	C67	3	0.56	0.96	0.70	0.00	0.07	4	1.09	1.30	0.92	0.03	0.15
其他的泌尿器官	C68	0	0.00	0.00	0.00	0.00	0.00	1	0.27	0.33	0.15	0.00	0.00
眼	C69	0	0.00	0.00	0.00	0.00	0.00	0	0.00	0.00	0.00	0.00	0.00
脑、神经系统	C70–C72	17	3.15	5.43	4.42	0.28	0.47	18	4.89	5.86	4.69	0.31	0.54
甲状腺	C73	1	0.19	0.32	0.30	0.00	0.05	3	0.82	0.98	0.73	0.02	0.15
肾上腺	C74	0	0.00	0.00	0.00	0.00	0.00	0	0.00	0.00	0.00	0.00	0.00
其他的内分泌腺	C75	0	0.00	0.00	0.00	0.00	0.00	0	0.00	0.00	0.00	0.00	0.00
霍奇金病	C81	0	0.00	0.00	0.00	0.00	0.00	0	0.00	0.00	0.00	0.00	0.00
非霍奇金淋巴瘤	C82–C85;C96	11	2.04	3.51	3.15	0.09	0.40	7	1.90	2.28	1.52	0.14	0.14
免疫增生性疾病	C88	0	0.00	0.00	0.00	0.00	0.00	0	0.00	0.00	0.00	0.00	0.00
多发性骨髓瘤	C90	2	0.37	0.64	0.42	0.00	0.00	0	0.00	0.00	0.00	0.00	0.00
淋巴样白血病	C91	0	0.00	0.00	0.00	0.00	0.00	1	0.27	0.33	0.76	0.03	0.03
髓样白血病	C92–C94	0	0.00	0.00	0.00	0.00	0.00	1	0.27	0.33	0.33	0.03	0.03
白血病，未特指	C95	11	2.04	3.51	3.31	0.15	0.30	10	2.72	3.26	2.72	0.24	0.24
其他的或未指明部位的	O&U	7	1.30	2.23	1.60	0.05	0.10	1	0.27	0.33	0.11	0.00	0.00
骨髓增殖性疾病	MPD	0	0.00	0.00	0.00	0.00	0.00	0	0.00	0.00	0.00	0.00	0.00
骨髓增生异常综合征	MDS	0	0.00	0.00	0.00	0.00	0.00	0	0.00	0.00	0.00	0.00	0.00
合计	ALL	540	100.00	172.38	136.39	5.12	14.01	368	100.00	119.80	78.63	3.32	9.07
所有部位除外 C44	ALL but C44	537	99.44	171.42	135.62	5.12	14.01	365	99.18	118.82	78.16	3.32	9.07

表 6-2-24b 2014 年河南省嵩县恶性肿瘤死亡主要指标

部位		男性						女性					
		病例数	构成 (%)	粗率 ($1/10^5$)	世标率 ($1/10^5$)	累积率 (%) 0~64	累积率 (%) 0~74	病例数	构成 (%)	粗率 ($1/10^5$)	世标率 ($1/10^5$)	累积率 (%) 0~64	累积率 (%) 0~74
唇	C00	0	0.00	0.00	0.00	0.00	0.00	0	0.00	0.00	0.00	0.00	0.00
舌	C01–C02	1	0.16	0.32	0.22	0.03	0.03	0	0.00	0.00	0.00	0.00	0.00
口	C03–C06	1	0.16	0.32	0.36	0.00	0.09	2	0.54	0.70	0.53	0.07	0.07
唾液腺	C07–C08	1	0.16	0.32	0.24	0.02	0.02	0	0.00	0.00	0.00	0.00	0.00
扁桃体	C09	0	0.00	0.00	0.00	0.00	0.00	0	0.00	0.00	0.00	0.00	0.00
其他的口咽	C10	0	0.00	0.00	0.00	0.00	0.00	0	0.00	0.00	0.00	0.00	0.00
鼻咽	C11	1	0.16	0.32	0.25	0.03	0.03	2	0.54	0.70	0.53	0.05	0.05
喉咽	C12–C13	0	0.00	0.00	0.00	0.00	0.00	0	0.00	0.00	0.00	0.00	0.00
咽，部位不明	C14	1	0.16	0.32	0.23	0.02	0.02	1	0.27	0.35	0.18	0.00	0.00
食管	C15	155	24.49	49.40	39.55	1.89	4.87	100	27.03	35.06	26.40	1.06	3.44
胃	C16	216	34.12	68.85	54.91	2.68	6.41	78	21.08	27.35	19.51	0.98	2.10
小肠	C17	1	0.16	0.32	0.31	0.00	0.00	1	0.27	0.35	0.28	0.03	0.03
结肠	C18	6	0.95	1.91	1.51	0.05	0.16	6	1.62	2.10	1.34	0.07	0.16
直肠	C19–C20	16	2.53	5.10	4.02	0.21	0.36	5	1.35	1.75	1.18	0.00	0.12
肛门	C21	0	0.00	0.00	0.00	0.00	0.00	0	0.00	0.00	0.00	0.00	0.00
肝脏	C22	64	10.11	20.40	16.54	0.93	2.09	36	9.73	12.62	8.90	0.50	1.10
胆囊及其他	C23–C24	4	0.63	1.27	0.92	0.09	0.09	3	0.81	1.05	0.66	0.03	0.03
胰腺	C25	13	2.05	4.14	3.44	0.24	0.42	7	1.89	2.45	2.25	0.03	0.37
鼻、鼻窦及其他	C30–C31	1	0.16	0.32	0.31	0.00	0.00	2	0.54	0.70	0.51	0.06	0.06
喉	C32	2	0.32	0.64	0.49	0.00	0.06	1	0.27	0.35	0.25	0.03	0.03
气管、支气管、肺	C33–C34	95	15.01	30.28	24.71	1.20	2.85	46	12.43	16.13	10.74	0.51	1.11
其他的胸腔器官	C37–C38	2	0.32	0.64	0.57	0.03	0.12	1	0.27	0.35	0.25	0.03	0.03
骨	C40–C41	3	0.47	0.96	0.97	0.03	0.21	3	0.81	1.05	0.83	0.02	0.12
皮肤的黑色素瘤	C43	0	0.00	0.00	0.00	0.00	0.00	0	0.00	0.00	0.00	0.00	0.00
其他的皮肤	C44	4	0.63	1.27	0.97	0.06	0.06	2	0.54	0.70	0.65	0.03	0.10
间皮瘤	C45	0	0.00	0.00	0.00	0.00	0.00	0	0.00	0.00	0.00	0.00	0.00
卡波西肉瘤	C46	0	0.00	0.00	0.00	0.00	0.00	0	0.00	0.00	0.00	0.00	0.00
周围神经、其他结缔组织、软组织	C47;C49	0	0.00	0.00	0.00	0.00	0.00	0	0.00	0.00	0.00	0.00	0.00
乳房	C50	—	—	—	—	—	—	20	5.41	7.01	5.42	0.48	0.67
外阴	C51	—	—	—	—	—	—	0	0.00	0.00	0.00	0.00	0.00
阴道	C52	—	—	—	—	—	—	1	0.27	0.35	0.25	0.03	0.03
子宫颈	C53	—	—	—	—	—	—	14	3.78	4.91	3.71	0.32	0.38
子宫体	C54	—	—	—	—	—	—	6	1.62	2.10	1.37	0.06	0.15
子宫，部位不明	C55	—	—	—	—	—	—	2	0.54	0.70	0.25	0.00	0.00
卵巢	C56	—	—	—	—	—	—	4	1.08	1.40	1.10	0.05	0.15
其他的女性生殖器	C57	—	—	—	—	—	—	0	0.00	0.00	0.00	0.00	0.00
胎盘	C58	—	—	—	—	—	—	0	0.00	0.00	0.00	0.00	0.00
阴茎	C60	0	0.00	0.00	0.00	0.00	0.00	—	—	—	—	—	—
前列腺	C61	6	0.95	1.91	1.77	0.00	0.15	—	—	—	—	—	—
睾丸	C62	0	0.00	0.00	0.00	0.00	0.00	—	—	—	—	—	—
其他的男性生殖器	C63	0	0.00	0.00	0.00	0.00	0.00	—	—	—	—	—	—
肾	C64	1	0.16	0.32	0.22	0.03	0.03	2	0.54	0.70	0.56	0.00	0.06
肾盂	C65	1	0.16	0.32	0.16	0.00	0.00	0	0.00	0.00	0.00	0.00	0.00
输尿管	C66	0	0.00	0.00	0.00	0.00	0.00	0	0.00	0.00	0.00	0.00	0.00
膀胱	C67	2	0.32	0.64	0.55	0.03	0.08	0	0.00	0.00	0.00	0.00	0.00
其他的泌尿器官	C68	0	0.00	0.00	0.00	0.00	0.00	0	0.00	0.00	0.00	0.00	0.00
眼	C69	0	0.00	0.00	0.00	0.00	0.00	0	0.00	0.00	0.00	0.00	0.00
脑、神经系统	C70–C72	16	2.53	5.10	4.74	0.24	0.65	5	1.35	1.75	1.32	0.14	0.14
甲状腺	C73	2	0.32	0.64	0.60	0.02	0.11	3	0.81	1.05	0.72	0.06	0.06
肾上腺	C74	1	0.16	0.32	0.36	0.03	0.03	1	0.27	0.35	0.18	0.00	0.00
其他的内分泌腺	C75	0	0.00	0.00	0.00	0.00	0.00	1	0.27	0.35	0.19	0.00	0.00
霍奇金病	C81	0	0.00	0.00	0.00	0.00	0.00	0	0.00	0.00	0.00	0.00	0.00
非霍奇金淋巴瘤	C82–C85;C96	1	0.16	0.32	0.22	0.03	0.03	1	0.27	0.35	0.42	0.02	0.02
免疫增生性疾病	C88	0	0.00	0.00	0.00	0.00	0.00	0	0.00	0.00	0.00	0.00	0.00
多发性骨髓瘤	C90	1	0.16	0.32	0.25	0.03	0.03	0	0.00	0.00	0.00	0.00	0.00
淋巴样白血病	C91	2	0.32	0.64	0.47	0.04	0.04	1	0.27	0.35	0.28	0.03	0.03
髓样白血病	C92–C94	0	0.00	0.00	0.00	0.00	0.00	0	0.00	0.00	0.00	0.00	0.00
白血病，未特指	C95	4	0.63	1.27	1.27	0.10	0.10	6	1.62	2.10	2.40	0.09	0.24
其他的或未指明部位的	O&U	9	1.42	2.87	2.29	0.12	0.23	7	1.89	2.45	1.93	0.13	0.13
骨髓增殖性疾病	MPD	0	0.00	0.00	0.00	0.00	0.00	0	0.00	0.00	0.00	0.00	0.00
骨髓增生异常综合征	MDS	0	0.00	0.00	0.00	0.00	0.00	0	0.00	0.00	0.00	0.00	0.00
合计	ALL	633	100.00	201.76	163.38	8.17	19.37	370	100.00	129.72	95.10	4.92	11.00
所有部位除外 C44	ALL but C44	629	99.37	200.48	162.41	8.12	19.31	368	99.46	129.02	94.46	4.88	10.91

表 6-2-25b　2014 年河南省漯河市恶性肿瘤死亡主要指标

部位		男性						女性					
		病例数	构成 (%)	粗率 (1/10^5)	世标率 (1/10^5)	累积率 (%) 0~64	累积率 (%) 0~74	病例数	构成 (%)	粗率 (1/10^5)	世标率 (1/10^5)	累积率 (%) 0~64	累积率 (%) 0~74
唇	C00	0	0.00	0.00	0.00	0.00	0.00	0	0.00	0.00	0.00	0.00	0.00
舌	C01–C02	0	0.00	0.00	0.00	0.00	0.00	4	1.94	1.73	1.25	0.07	0.07
口	C03–C06	0	0.00	0.00	0.00	0.00	0.00	1	0.49	0.43	0.17	0.00	0.00
唾液腺	C07–C08	0	0.00	0.00	0.00	0.00	0.00	0	0.00	0.00	0.00	0.00	0.00
扁桃体	C09	0	0.00	0.00	0.00	0.00	0.00	0	0.00	0.00	0.00	0.00	0.00
其他的口咽	C10	0	0.00	0.00	0.00	0.00	0.00	0	0.00	0.00	0.00	0.00	0.00
鼻咽	C11	0	0.00	0.00	0.00	0.00	0.00	1	0.49	0.43	0.30	0.02	0.02
喉咽	C12–C13	0	0.00	0.00	0.00	0.00	0.00	0	0.00	0.00	0.00	0.00	0.00
咽，部位不明	C14	0	0.00	0.00	0.00	0.00	0.00	0	0.00	0.00	0.00	0.00	0.00
食管	C15	42	10.74	17.13	16.02	0.43	2.05	20	9.71	8.64	6.41	0.08	0.55
胃	C16	28	7.16	11.42	10.96	0.30	0.89	12	5.83	5.18	3.52	0.11	0.45
小肠	C17	1	0.26	0.41	0.24	0.00	0.00	0	0.00	0.00	0.00	0.00	0.00
结肠	C18	9	2.30	3.67	3.23	0.13	0.35	5	2.43	2.16	1.71	0.03	0.30
直肠	C19–C20	16	4.09	6.53	5.94	0.06	0.63	10	4.85	4.32	3.02	0.13	0.22
肛门	C21	0	0.00	0.00	0.00	0.00	0.00	0	0.00	0.00	0.00	0.00	0.00
肝脏	C22	86	21.99	35.08	31.97	1.55	3.83	20	9.71	8.64	6.39	0.51	0.66
胆囊及其他	C23–C24	2	0.51	0.82	0.84	0.05	0.12	0	0.00	0.00	0.00	0.00	0.00
胰腺	C25	13	3.32	5.30	4.87	0.24	0.73	3	1.46	1.30	1.34	0.00	0.22
鼻、鼻窦及其他	C30–C31	0	0.00	0.00	0.00	0.00	0.00	0	0.00	0.00	0.00	0.00	0.00
喉	C32	0	0.00	0.00	0.00	0.00	0.00	0	0.00	0.00	0.00	0.00	0.00
气管、支气管、肺	C33–C34	156	39.90	63.64	57.73	2.31	7.20	58	28.16	25.06	18.69	0.64	2.03
其他的胸腔器官	C37–C38	0	0.00	0.00	0.00	0.00	0.00	0	0.00	0.00	0.00	0.00	0.00
骨	C40–C41	4	1.02	1.63	1.42	0.07	0.14	1	0.49	0.43	0.38	0.05	0.05
皮肤的黑色素瘤	C43	0	0.00	0.00	0.00	0.00	0.00	0	0.00	0.00	0.00	0.00	0.00
其他的皮肤	C44	0	0.00	0.00	0.00	0.00	0.00	1	0.49	0.43	0.37	0.04	0.04
间皮瘤	C45	0	0.00	0.00	0.00	0.00	0.00	0	0.00	0.00	0.00	0.00	0.00
卡波西肉瘤	C46	0	0.00	0.00	0.00	0.00	0.00	0	0.00	0.00	0.00	0.00	0.00
周围神经、其他结缔组织、软组织	C47;C49	0	0.00	0.00	0.00	0.00	0.00	0	0.00	0.00	0.00	0.00	0.00
乳房	C50	—	—	—	—	—	—	47	22.82	20.31	15.84	1.02	1.72
外阴	C51	—	—	—	—	—	—	0	0.00	0.00	0.00	0.00	0.00
阴道	C52	—	—	—	—	—	—	0	0.00	0.00	0.00	0.00	0.00
子宫颈	C53	—	—	—	—	—	—	3	1.46	1.30	1.34	0.00	0.22
子宫体	C54	—	—	—	—	—	—	5	2.43	2.16	1.69	0.10	0.28
子宫，部位不明	C55	—	—	—	—	—	—	3	1.46	1.30	1.30	0.07	0.14
卵巢	C56	—	—	—	—	—	—	2	0.97	0.86	0.63	0.05	0.05
其他的女性生殖器	C57	—	—	—	—	—	—	0	0.00	0.00	0.00	0.00	0.00
胎盘	C58	—	—	—	—	—	—	0	0.00	0.00	0.00	0.00	0.00
阴茎	C60	0	0.00	0.00	0.00	0.00	0.00	—	—	—	—	—	—
前列腺	C61	2	0.51	0.82	0.61	0.04	0.04	—	—	—	—	—	—
睾丸	C62	0	0.00	0.00	0.00	0.00	0.00	—	—	—	—	—	—
其他的男性生殖器	C63	0	0.00	0.00	0.00	0.00	0.00	—	—	—	—	—	—
肾	C64	5	1.28	2.04	2.04	0.13	0.28	0	0.00	0.00	0.00	0.00	0.00
肾盂	C65	0	0.00	0.00	0.00	0.00	0.00	0	0.00	0.00	0.00	0.00	0.00
输尿管	C66	0	0.00	0.00	0.00	0.00	0.00	0	0.00	0.00	0.00	0.00	0.00
膀胱	C67	5	1.28	2.04	2.90	0.00	0.17	0	0.00	0.00	0.00	0.00	0.00
其他的泌尿器官	C68	0	0.00	0.00	0.00	0.00	0.00	0	0.00	0.00	0.00	0.00	0.00
眼	C69	0	0.00	0.00	0.00	0.00	0.00	0	0.00	0.00	0.00	0.00	0.00
脑、神经系统	C70–C72	9	2.30	3.67	3.18	0.33	0.33	3	1.46	1.30	1.00	0.09	0.09
甲状腺	C73	1	0.26	0.41	0.39	0.05	0.05	0	0.00	0.00	0.00	0.00	0.00
肾上腺	C74	0	0.00	0.00	0.00	0.00	0.00	0	0.00	0.00	0.00	0.00	0.00
其他的内分泌腺	C75	0	0.00	0.00	0.00	0.00	0.00	0	0.00	0.00	0.00	0.00	0.00
霍奇金病	C81	4	1.02	1.63	1.31	0.03	0.20	0	0.00	0.00	0.00	0.00	0.00
非霍奇金淋巴瘤	C82–C85;C96	0	0.00	0.00	0.00	0.00	0.00	0	0.00	0.00	0.00	0.00	0.00
免疫增生性疾病	C88	0	0.00	0.00	0.00	0.00	0.00	0	0.00	0.00	0.00	0.00	0.00
多发性骨髓瘤	C90	0	0.00	0.00	0.00	0.00	0.00	0	0.00	0.00	0.00	0.00	0.00
淋巴样白血病	C91	5	1.28	2.04	1.92	0.16	0.25	4	1.94	1.73	1.36	0.03	0.10
髓样白血病	C92–C94	1	0.26	0.41	0.23	0.00	0.00	1	0.49	0.43	0.15	0.00	0.00
白血病，未特指	C95	0	0.00	0.00	0.00	0.00	0.00	0	0.00	0.00	0.00	0.00	0.00
其他的或未指明部位的	O&U	2	0.51	0.82	0.48	0.03	0.03	2	0.97	0.86	0.67	0.06	0.06
骨髓增殖性疾病	MPD	0	0.00	0.00	0.00	0.00	0.00	0	0.00	0.00	0.00	0.00	0.00
骨髓增生异常综合征	MDS	0	0.00	0.00	0.00	0.00	0.00	0	0.00	0.00	0.00	0.00	0.00
合计	ALL	391	100.00	159.51	146.27	5.90	17.28	206	100.00	89.00	67.51	3.10	7.28
所有部位除外 C44	ALL but C44	391	100.00	159.51	146.27	5.90	17.28	205	99.51	88.57	67.14	3.06	7.25

表 6-2-26b 2014 年河南省栾川县恶性肿瘤死亡主要指标

部位		男性						女性					
		病例数	构成 (%)	粗率 (1/10^5)	世标率 (1/10^5)	累积率 (%) 0~64	累积率 (%) 0~74	病例数	构成 (%)	粗率 (1/10^5)	世标率 (1/10^5)	累积率 (%) 0~64	累积率 (%) 0~74
唇	C00	0	0.00	0.00	0.00	0.00	0.00	0	0.00	0.00	0.00	0.00	0.00
舌	C01–C02	0	0.00	0.00	0.00	0.00	0.00	0	0.00	0.00	0.00	0.00	0.00
口	C03–C06	0	0.00	0.00	0.00	0.00	0.00	0	0.00	0.00	0.00	0.00	0.00
唾液腺	C07–C08	1	0.38	0.54	0.43	0.00	0.07	0	0.00	0.00	0.00	0.00	0.00
扁桃体	C09	0	0.00	0.00	0.00	0.00	0.00	0	0.00	0.00	0.00	0.00	0.00
其他的口咽	C10	0	0.00	0.00	0.00	0.00	0.00	0	0.00	0.00	0.00	0.00	0.00
鼻咽	C11	2	0.76	1.08	0.60	0.05	0.05	1	0.70	0.62	0.34	0.00	0.00
喉咽	C12–C13	0	0.00	0.00	0.00	0.00	0.00	0	0.00	0.00	0.00	0.00	0.00
咽，部位不明	C14	0	0.00	0.00	0.00	0.00	0.00	0	0.00	0.00	0.00	0.00	0.00
食管	C15	42	16.03	22.58	15.22	0.60	1.90	30	21.13	18.64	11.38	0.23	0.89
胃	C16	83	31.68	44.62	29.47	1.74	3.17	18	12.68	11.18	7.51	0.46	0.70
小肠	C17	0	0.00	0.00	0.00	0.00	0.00	0	0.00	0.00	0.00	0.00	0.00
结肠	C18	3	1.15	1.61	1.11	0.03	0.10	1	0.70	0.62	0.44	0.06	0.06
直肠	C19–C20	6	2.29	3.23	2.39	0.08	0.37	8	5.63	4.97	3.58	0.21	0.56
肛门	C21	0	0.00	0.00	0.00	0.00	0.00	0	0.00	0.00	0.00	0.00	0.00
肝脏	C22	42	16.03	22.58	15.94	0.96	1.88	14	9.86	8.70	6.36	0.41	0.80
胆囊及其他	C23–C24	0	0.00	0.00	0.00	0.00	0.00	2	1.41	1.24	1.03	0.00	0.22
胰腺	C25	3	1.15	1.61	1.15	0.09	0.16	3	2.11	1.86	1.18	0.00	0.08
鼻、鼻窦及其他	C30–C31	0	0.00	0.00	0.00	0.00	0.00	0	0.00	0.00	0.00	0.00	0.00
喉	C32	3	1.15	1.61	1.22	0.03	0.26	0	0.00	0.00	0.00	0.00	0.00
气管、支气管、肺	C33–C34	46	17.56	24.73	17.52	0.84	2.21	23	16.20	14.29	9.29	0.33	1.16
其他的胸腔器官	C37–C38	0	0.00	0.00	0.00	0.00	0.00	0	0.00	0.00	0.00	0.00	0.00
骨	C40–C41	4	1.53	2.15	1.65	0.04	0.30	1	0.70	0.62	0.62	0.04	0.04
皮肤的黑色素瘤	C43	0	0.00	0.00	0.00	0.00	0.00	0	0.00	0.00	0.00	0.00	0.00
其他的皮肤	C44	1	0.38	0.54	0.22	0.00	0.00	1	0.70	0.62	0.44	0.00	0.00
间皮瘤	C45	0	0.00	0.00	0.00	0.00	0.00	0	0.00	0.00	0.00	0.00	0.00
卡波西肉瘤	C46	0	0.00	0.00	0.00	0.00	0.00	0	0.00	0.00	0.00	0.00	0.00
周围神经、其他结缔组织、软组织	C47;C49	0	0.00	0.00	0.00	0.00	0.00	0	0.00	0.00	0.00	0.00	0.00
乳房	C50	—	—	—	—	—	—	6	4.23	3.73	3.07	0.25	0.38
外阴	C51	—	—	—	—	—	—	1	0.70	0.62	0.44	0.06	0.06
阴道	C52	—	—	—	—	—	—	0	0.00	0.00	0.00	0.00	0.00
子宫颈	C53	—	—	—	—	—	—	12	8.45	7.45	4.97	0.33	0.49
子宫体	C54	—	—	—	—	—	—	0	0.00	0.00	0.00	0.00	0.00
子宫，部位不明	C55	—	—	—	—	—	—	2	1.41	1.24	1.00	0.00	0.17
卵巢	C56	—	—	—	—	—	—	3	2.11	1.86	1.37	0.13	0.13
其他的女性生殖器	C57	—	—	—	—	—	—	0	0.00	0.00	0.00	0.00	0.00
胎盘	C58	—	—	—	—	—	—	0	0.00	0.00	0.00	0.00	0.00
阴茎	C60	0	0.00	0.00	0.00	0.00	0.00	—	—	—	—	—	—
前列腺	C61	0	0.00	0.00	0.00	0.00	0.00	—	—	—	—	—	—
睾丸	C62	0	0.00	0.00	0.00	0.00	0.00	—	—	—	—	—	—
其他的男性生殖器	C63	0	0.00	0.00	0.00	0.00	0.00	—	—	—	—	—	—
肾	C64	2	0.76	1.08	0.65	0.00	0.07	0	0.00	0.00	0.00	0.00	0.00
肾盂	C65	0	0.00	0.00	0.00	0.00	0.00	0	0.00	0.00	0.00	0.00	0.00
输尿管	C66	1	0.38	0.54	0.32	0.00	0.00	0	0.00	0.00	0.00	0.00	0.00
膀胱	C67	2	0.76	1.08	0.61	0.00	0.00	0	0.00	0.00	0.00	0.00	0.00
其他的泌尿器官	C68	0	0.00	0.00	0.00	0.00	0.00	0	0.00	0.00	0.00	0.00	0.00
眼	C69	0	0.00	0.00	0.00	0.00	0.00	0	0.00	0.00	0.00	0.00	0.00
脑、神经系统	C70–C72	4	1.53	2.15	1.82	0.18	0.18	7	4.93	4.35	3.35	0.36	0.36
甲状腺	C73	1	0.38	0.54	0.45	0.00	0.11	0	0.00	0.00	0.00	0.00	0.00
肾上腺	C74	1	0.38	0.54	0.22	0.00	0.00	0	0.00	0.00	0.00	0.00	0.00
其他的内分泌腺	C75	0	0.00	0.00	0.00	0.00	0.00	0	0.00	0.00	0.00	0.00	0.00
霍奇金病	C81	1	0.38	0.54	0.47	0.04	0.04	0	0.00	0.00	0.00	0.00	0.00
非霍奇金淋巴瘤	C82–C85;C96	0	0.00	0.00	0.00	0.00	0.00	0	0.00	0.00	0.00	0.00	0.00
免疫增生性疾病	C88	0	0.00	0.00	0.00	0.00	0.00	0	0.00	0.00	0.00	0.00	0.00
多发性骨髓瘤	C90	0	0.00	0.00	0.00	0.00	0.00	0	0.00	0.00	0.00	0.00	0.00
淋巴样白血病	C91	0	0.00	0.00	0.00	0.00	0.00	0	0.00	0.00	0.00	0.00	0.00
髓样白血病	C92–C94	0	0.00	0.00	0.00	0.00	0.00	0	0.00	0.00	0.00	0.00	0.00
白血病，未特指	C95	0	0.00	0.00	0.00	0.00	0.00	0	0.00	0.00	0.00	0.00	0.00
其他的或未指明部位的	O&U	14	5.34	7.53	5.69	0.40	0.77	9	6.34	5.59	5.04	0.33	0.41
骨髓增殖性疾病	MPD	0	0.00	0.00	0.00	0.00	0.00	0	0.00	0.00	0.00	0.00	0.00
骨髓增生异常综合征	MDS	0	0.00	0.00	0.00	0.00	0.00	0	0.00	0.00	0.00	0.00	0.00
合计	ALL	262	100.00	140.85	97.15	5.09	11.63	142	100.00	88.21	61.42	3.18	6.49
所有部位除外 C44	ALL but C44	261	99.62	140.31	96.93	5.09	11.63	141	99.30	87.59	60.98	3.18	6.49

表 6-2-27b 2014 年河南省睢县恶性肿瘤死亡主要指标

部位		男性						女性					
		病例数	构成(%)	粗率(1/10^5)	世标率(1/10^5)	累积率(%)		病例数	构成(%)	粗率(1/10^5)	世标率(1/10^5)	累积率(%)	
						0~64	0~74					0~64	0~74
唇	C00	0	0.00	0.00	0.00	0.00	0.00	0	0.00	0.00	0.00	0.00	0.00
舌	C01–C02	0	0.00	0.00	0.00	0.00	0.00	0	0.00	0.00	0.00	0.00	0.00
口	C03–C06	1	0.14	0.23	0.28	0.00	0.05	2	0.48	0.49	0.35	0.00	0.04
唾液腺	C07–C08	0	0.00	0.00	0.00	0.00	0.00	0	0.00	0.00	0.00	0.00	0.00
扁桃体	C09	1	0.14	0.23	0.29	0.00	0.00	0	0.00	0.00	0.00	0.00	0.00
其他的口咽	C10	2	0.27	0.45	0.43	0.05	0.05	0	0.00	0.00	0.00	0.00	0.00
鼻咽	C11	3	0.41	0.68	0.63	0.02	0.06	3	0.71	0.73	0.62	0.06	0.06
喉咽	C12–C13	1	0.14	0.23	0.13	0.00	0.00	0	0.00	0.00	0.00	0.00	0.00
咽，部位不明	C14	0	0.00	0.00	0.00	0.00	0.00	0	0.00	0.00	0.00	0.00	0.00
食管	C15	34	4.63	7.70	7.33	0.14	0.93	23	5.46	5.63	3.82	0.13	0.44
胃	C16	80	10.90	18.12	16.90	0.60	1.94	36	8.55	8.81	5.74	0.24	0.50
小肠	C17	1	0.14	0.23	0.19	0.02	0.02	3	0.71	0.73	0.46	0.03	0.03
结肠	C18	11	1.50	2.49	2.56	0.06	0.36	4	0.95	0.98	0.69	0.06	0.06
直肠	C19–C20	21	2.86	4.76	4.68	0.19	0.54	16	3.80	3.92	2.58	0.17	0.26
肛门	C21	0	0.00	0.00	0.00	0.00	0.00	0	0.00	0.00	0.00	0.00	0.00
肝脏	C22	241	32.83	54.59	48.84	3.04	5.95	88	20.90	21.54	14.80	0.63	1.65
胆囊及其他	C23–C24	12	1.63	2.72	3.03	0.05	0.37	27	6.41	6.61	4.66	0.21	0.55
胰腺	C25	20	2.72	4.53	3.72	0.24	0.40	11	2.61	2.69	1.60	0.02	0.22
鼻、鼻窦及其他	C30–C31	1	0.14	0.23	0.23	0.01	0.01	1	0.24	0.24	0.23	0.03	0.03
喉	C32	1	0.14	0.23	0.13	0.00	0.00	0	0.00	0.00	0.00	0.00	0.00
气管、支气管、肺	C33–C34	210	28.61	47.57	43.16	1.61	5.76	83	19.71	20.32	13.51	0.63	1.29
其他的胸腔器官	C37–C38	0	0.00	0.00	0.00	0.00	0.00	0	0.00	0.00	0.00	0.00	0.00
骨	C40–C41	8	1.09	1.81	1.48	0.05	0.16	6	1.43	1.47	1.04	0.07	0.10
皮肤的黑色素瘤	C43	0	0.00	0.00	0.00	0.00	0.00	0	0.00	0.00	0.00	0.00	0.00
其他的皮肤	C44	2	0.27	0.45	0.45	0.02	0.02	0	0.00	0.00	0.00	0.00	0.00
间皮瘤	C45	0	0.00	0.00	0.00	0.00	0.00	0	0.00	0.00	0.00	0.00	0.00
卡波西肉瘤	C46	0	0.00	0.00	0.00	0.00	0.00	0	0.00	0.00	0.00	0.00	0.00
周围神经、其他结缔组织、软组织	C47;C49	0	0.00	0.00	0.00	0.00	0.00	0	0.00	0.00	0.00	0.00	0.00
乳房	C50	—	—	—	—	—	—	27	6.41	6.61	4.95	0.39	0.51
外阴	C51	—	—	—	—	—	—	0	0.00	0.00	0.00	0.00	0.00
阴道	C52	—	—	—	—	—	—	0	0.00	0.00	0.00	0.00	0.00
子宫颈	C53	—	—	—	—	—	—	9	2.14	2.20	1.77	0.08	0.23
子宫体	C54	—	—	—	—	—	—	3	0.71	0.73	0.51	0.03	0.03
子宫，部位不明	C55	—	—	—	—	—	—	1	0.24	0.24	0.23	0.03	0.03
卵巢	C56	—	—	—	—	—	—	4	0.95	0.98	0.64	0.04	0.08
其他的女性生殖器	C57	—	—	—	—	—	—	0	0.00	0.00	0.00	0.00	0.00
胎盘	C58	—	—	—	—	—	—	0	0.00	0.00	0.00	0.00	0.00
阴茎	C60	0	0.00	0.00	0.00	0.00	0.00	—	—	—	—	—	—
前列腺	C61	2	0.27	0.45	0.41	0.00	0.05	—	—	—	—	—	—
睾丸	C62	0	0.00	0.00	0.00	0.00	0.00	—	—	—	—	—	—
其他的男性生殖器	C63	0	0.00	0.00	0.00	0.00	0.00	—	—	—	—	—	—
肾	C64	2	0.27	0.45	0.43	0.05	0.05	1	0.24	0.24	0.09	0.00	0.00
肾盂	C65	0	0.00	0.00	0.00	0.00	0.00	0	0.00	0.00	0.00	0.00	0.00
输尿管	C66	0	0.00	0.00	0.00	0.00	0.00	0	0.00	0.00	0.00	0.00	0.00
膀胱	C67	5	0.68	1.13	1.01	0.00	0.16	2	0.48	0.49	0.37	0.03	0.03
其他的泌尿器官	C68	0	0.00	0.00	0.00	0.00	0.00	0	0.00	0.00	0.00	0.00	0.00
眼	C69	1	0.14	0.23	0.22	0.03	0.03	0	0.00	0.00	0.00	0.00	0.00
脑、神经系统	C70–C72	44	5.99	9.97	9.65	0.54	0.90	49	11.64	11.99	8.91	0.60	1.00
甲状腺	C73	2	0.27	0.45	0.44	0.00	0.11	0	0.00	0.00	0.00	0.00	0.00
肾上腺	C74	1	0.14	0.23	0.29	0.00	0.00	1	0.24	0.24	0.52	0.03	0.03
其他的内分泌腺	C75	0	0.00	0.00	0.00	0.00	0.00	0	0.00	0.00	0.00	0.00	0.00
霍奇金病	C81	3	0.41	0.68	0.59	0.05	0.10	2	0.48	0.49	0.26	0.00	0.04
非霍奇金淋巴瘤	C82–C85;C96	2	0.27	0.45	0.43	0.03	0.08	1	0.24	0.24	0.17	0.02	0.02
免疫增生性疾病	C88	0	0.00	0.00	0.00	0.00	0.00	0	0.00	0.00	0.00	0.00	0.00
多发性骨髓瘤	C90	0	0.00	0.00	0.00	0.00	0.00	0	0.00	0.00	0.00	0.00	0.00
淋巴样白血病	C91	4	0.54	0.91	1.04	0.06	0.06	4	0.95	0.98	0.57	0.03	0.03
髓样白血病	C92–C94	7	0.95	1.59	1.68	0.05	0.21	4	0.95	0.98	0.58	0.04	0.04
白血病，未特指	C95	8	1.09	1.81	2.02	0.11	0.26	8	1.90	1.96	1.66	0.13	0.17
其他的或未指明部位的	O&U	3	0.41	0.68	0.64	0.02	0.13	2	0.48	0.49	0.37	0.01	0.05
骨髓增殖性疾病	MPD	0	0.00	0.00	0.00	0.00	0.00	0	0.00	0.00	0.00	0.00	0.00
骨髓增生异常综合征	MDS	0	0.00	0.00	0.00	0.00	0.00	0	0.00	0.00	0.00	0.00	0.00
合计	ALL	734	100.00	166.26	153.32	7.06	18.75	421	100.00	103.05	71.71	3.77	7.50
所有部位除外 C44	ALL but C44	732	99.73	165.81	152.87	7.04	18.73	421	100.00	103.05	71.71	3.77	7.50